NEUROTOXICOLOGY

Volume 1

Neurotoxicology

Volume 1

Edited by

Leon Roizin, M.D.
Department of Neuropathology and
Neurotoxicology
New York State Psychiatric Institute
New York, New York

Hirotsugu Shiraki, M.D.
Institute of Brain Research
Tokyo University Medical School
Tokyo, Japan

Nenad Grčević, M.D.
Department of Neuropathology
University of Zagreb
Clinical Medical Center Rebro
Zagreb, Yugoslavia

Raven Press ▪ New York

Raven Press, 1140 Avenue of the Americas, New York, New York 10036

Made in the United States of America

Library of Congress Cataloging in Publication Data

Main entry under title:

Neurotoxicology.

     Includes bibliographical references and index.
     1. Nervous system – Diseases. 2. Toxicology.
I. Roizin, Leon. II. Shiraki, Hirotsugu, 1917–
III. Grčević, Nenad. [DNLM: 1. Pharmacology.
2. Nervous system – drug effects. 3. Drug
therapy – Adverse effects. 4. Poisoning. QV76.5
N496]
RC346.N46   615.9   77–4632
ISBN 0–89004–148–2

Preface

The principal concern of this volume is the problem of adverse and toxic reactions of the nervous system to a variety of drugs and environmental toxic agents, including their clinical, biochemical, pharmacological, toxicological, genetic, teratogenic and pathological aspects. Pathogenic mechanisms encompass alcohol-drug and food-drug interactions, the effects of alcoholism on the nervous system and its relationship to B-vitamin malnutrition, the blood-brain barrier, and the multifactor concept of the chemogenic lesion.

Multidisciplinary methodologies provide a more comprehensive insight into the understanding of the biological complexities of the nervous system, and the interpretation of some pathologic processes in terms of underlying biochemical changes. They also have shown repeatedly the significant interrelation between altered function and structure (in morphologic terms).

Review papers provided a fundamental framework of existing knowledge, while original contributions delineated new achievements, and pointed out the possible future trends of advancement.

It is clear from the papers in this volume that: a) the clinical side effects may "merely be the floating tip of an iceberg, with much of the difficulty hidden beneath the surface of our awareness"[2]; b) selective toxicity is often a temporary rather than permanent condition; c) many drugs show multiple "targets" of interaction and produce a multiplicity of side effects; d) "complexity is inherent in all biological processes"[1]; and e) the toxic or adverse reactions (chemogenic lesions) are generally the compounded effects of multiple chemo- and biopathological cofactors (neural and extraneural). In final analysis, there is general agreement that the knowledge of the mode of action of chemical agents enables the physician to use more efficiently the required medication both alone and in various combinations, and that the awareness of their potential pathogenic mechanisms may suggest safeguards or development of prophylactic measures for the prevention of unwarranted reactions.

The Editors would like to express their gratitude to the chairmen of the scientific sessions at the conference on which this volume is based: Dr. J. B. Cavanagh, Dr. J. Levine, Dr. H. Brill, Dr. H. F. Butts, Dr. S. Malitz, Dr. H. Shiraki, Dr. O. Steinwall, Dr. M. R. Krigman, Dr. A. Bischoff, Dr. D. W. King, Dr. N. Grčević, and Dr. G. C. Salmoiraghi.

Our sincere thanks are due to the Editorial staff of Raven Press, and particularly to Dr. Diana Schneider and Mrs. Berta Steiner Rosenberg for their kind cooperation, helpful suggestions, and assistance to expedite the publication of this book.

Leon Roizin

---

[1] Albert, A. (1960): Preface. In: *Selective Toxicity*. J. Wiley & Sons, Inc., New York, p. V.
[2] Lasagna, L. (1964): The diseases drugs cause. *Perspect. Biol. Med.,* 7:457–470.

Contents

xx   *Foreword*
xxi   *Introduction*

Tranquilizers

1   Neurotoxicology of Major Tranquilizers
G. M. Simpson

9   Pharmacokinetics of Therapeutic and Toxic Reactions: I. Phenothiazines
J. M. Perel and A. A. Manian

15   Selective Neurotoxicity of 6-Hydroxydopamine
S. Garattini and R. Samanin

25   Neuropathologic Findings After Neuroleptic Long-Term Therapy
K. Jellinger

43   Neuropathology of "Grumus Degeneration" of the Cerebellar Dentate Nucleus with Special Reference to Certain Neurotoxic Disorders and other Pathological Processes
H. Shiraki, A. Okumura, and Sh. Oyahagi

57   Alternative Diagnosis to Tardive Dyskinesia: Neuropathologic Findings in Three Suspected Cases
M. A. Kaufman

Narcotics and Anesthetics

63   Biochemical Effects of the Use of Narcotic Analgesic Drugs
D. H. Clouet

71   Methadone Maintenance in the Treatment of Heroin Addicts in New York City: A Ten-Year Overview
F. R. Gearing

81   Drugs-of-Abuse Detection in Biological Specimens
R. L. Stiller and D. Pierson

93   Drug Detection and Identification: Direct Immunoassay of Urinary Specimens Adsorbed on Papers Loaded with Ion Exchange Resins
G. J. Alexander, S. M. Machiz, and S. Marynowski

103   Certification of Deaths from Drug Addiction
M. Helpern

111   Ultrastructural Investigation of the Hypothalamus in Chronically Heroin Addicted Monkeys
L. Roizin and J. C. Liu

137   Review of Effects of Chronic Exposure to Low Levels of Halothane
A. W. Dudley, Jr., L. W. Chang, M. A. Dudley, R. E. Bowman, and J. Katz

Stimulants, Antidepressants, and Hallucinogens

147   Drug Interactions: Methylphenidate
L. C. Mark, J. Perel, and L. Brand

149   Cortical Atrophy Caused by Long-Term Therapy with Antidepressive and Neuroleptic Drugs: A Clinical and Experimental Study
N. Sabuncu, S. Salaçin, R. Saygill, K. Kumral, and T. Örnek

157   Pharmacokinetics of Therapeutic and Toxic Reactions: II. Tricyclic Antidepressants
J. Perel

163   Effects of Nortriptyline and Other Psychotropic Drugs on Neurons and Glia *In Vitro:* An Ultrastructural Study
M. L. Grunnet

171   Lithium Toxicity: A Review
G. M. Dempsey and H. L. Meltzer

185   Ultrastructural Findings of the Central Nervous System in Lithium Neurotoxicology
K. Akai, L. Roizin, and J. C. Liu

205   Clinical Aspects of Psychotomimetic Drugs
H. C. B. Denber

215   Hallucinogen Compounds: Biochemical Aspects
D. N. Teller

227   Effects of LSD on Membranous Organelles in Cultured Neurons
N. J. Willson, L. Roizin, J. F. Schneider, and J. C. Liu

Heavy and Trace Metals

235   Neuropathology of Minamata Disease in Kumamoto: Especially at the
      Chronic Stage
      T. Takeuchi

247   Essential Neuropathology of Alkylmercury Intoxication in Humans
      from the Acute to the Chronic Stage with Special Reference to Experi-
      mental Whole Body Autoradiographic Study Using Labeled Mercury
      Compounds
      H. Shiraki and K. Nagashima

261   Neuropathology of Methylmercury Intoxication in Niigata and Chronic
      Effect in Monkeys
      T. Sato and F. Ikuta

271   Chemotoxic Blood-Brain Barrier Damage with Special Regard to
      Some Mercurial Effects
      O. Steinwall

275   Modification of the Neurotoxic Effects of Methyl Mercury by Selenium
      *L. W. Chang, A. W. Dudley, Jr., M. A. Dudley, H. E. Ganther, and M. L.
      Sunde*

283   Metabolic Mechanisms of Neurotoxicity Caused by Mercury
      J. B. Cavanagh

289   Subcellular Mechanisms in Lead Toxicity: Significance in Childhood
      Encephalopathy, Neurological Sequelae, and Late Dementias
      W. J. Niklowitz

299   An Appraisal of Rodent Models of Lead Encephalopathy
      M. R. Krigman, P. Mushak, and T. W. Bouldin

303   Relationship of Blood and Brain Lead Levels to Morphologic Changes
      in Lead-Induced Chick Embryo Encephalopathy. I. Morphologic
      Studies
      A. Hirano and J. A. Kochen

309   Relationship of Blood and Brain Lead Levels to Morphologic Changes
      in Lead-Induced Chick Embryo Encephalopathy. II. Biochemical
      Studies
      J. A. Kochen, Y. Greener, and A. Hirano

313   Neurotoxicity of Aluminum
      *H. M. Wisniewski, J. K. Korthals, L. M. Kopeloff, R. Ferszt, J. G.
      Chusid, and R. D. Terry*

317   Effect of Triethyltin on the Developing Brain of the Mouse
      I. Watanabe

Antimicrobials

327 Neuropathology of Subacute Myeloopticoneuropathy in Humans with Special Reference to Experimental Whole Body Autoradiographic Studies Using Labeled Quinoform Compounds
H. Shiraki

345 Experimental and Subacute Myeloopticoneuropathy
J. Tateishi, S. Kuroda, H. Ikeda, and S. Otsuki

353 Neuropathology of Subacute Myeloopticoneuropathy (Clioquinol Intoxication) in Humans and Experimental Animals
F. Ikuta, T. Atsumi, T. Makifuchi, T. Sato, and T. Tsubaki

361 Neurotoxic Effects of Chinoform Studied on Nervous Tissue Maintained *In Vitro*
T. Yonezawa, T. Saida, A. Nakano, and M. Hasegawa

371 Neuronal Storage Dystrophy in Chronic Chloroquine Intoxication
G. W. Klinghardt

381 Hexachlorophene Neurotoxicity
H. C. Powell and P. W. Lampert

391 Neurotoxicity of Actinomycin D and Related Inhibitors of RNA Synthesis: The Role of Nuclear Heterochromatinization
H. Koenig, R. Nayyar, P. Sanghavi, C. Y. Lu, and C. Hughes

403 Examination of the Developing Nervous System of *Xenopus* Tadpoles with Differential Interference Microscopy: A New Assay Procedure for Neurotoxicologists
H. deF. Webster, T. Tabira, and P. J. Reier

413 Fine Structure of Sciatic Nerves in Nitrofurantoin Neuropathy Induced in Rats
A. J. Behar, N. Livni, and D. Soffer

419 Degeneration of Choroid Plexus Epithelium Induced by Some Tertiary Amines
S. Levine

Industrial Chemicals

427 Industrial Neuropathies
P. S. Spencer and H. H. Schaumburg

431 Tri-Ortho-Cresyl Phosphate Neurotoxicology
A. Bischoff

443   Kepone Poisoning: Cliniconeuropathological Study
       A. J. Martinez, J. R. Taylor, S. A. Houff, and E. R. Isaacs

Pesticides

457   Parathion-Induced Alterations in Acetylcholinesterase of the Rat
       Nervous System: A Histochemical, Biochemical, and Isoenzyme
       Study
       R. H. Brownson, H. D. McDouglas, D. B. Suter, and V. K. Vijayan

469   Cerebral Changes in Paraquat Poisoning
       N. Grčević, D. Jadro-Šantel, and S. Jukić

Anorexic Agents

485   Ultrastructural Observations on the Cytoplasmic Inclusion of Nervous
       Tissue and the Peripheral Neuropathy Induced in Suckling Mice by
       Chlorphentermine Administration
       A. P. Anzil, H. Herrlinger, and K. Blinzinger

497   Neurotoxic Effects of Chlorphentermine on Rats
       M. Adachi, L. Schenck, and B. W. Volk

Pathogenic Considerations in Neurotoxicology

503   Alcohol-Drug Interactions
       C. M. Smith

511   Food and Drug Interactions
       C. J. Carr

517   Some Observations on the Neurological Effects of Alcohol Intoxication
       and Withdrawal
       M. Victor

529   Malnutrition-Alcoholism: Histopathology of Peripheral Nerves and
       B-Vitamins in Nerves, Blood, and CSF
       *D. K. Dastur, A. Dewan, N. Santhadevi, D. K. Manghani, and Z. A.
       Razzak*

549   Hepatotropic Effects of Phenothiazines and Narcotics: Histopathologic
       and Electron Microscope Observations
       A. Goldfield, L. Roizin, S. Hashimoto, and J. C. Liu

577   Pathologic Aspects of the Blood-Brain Barrier
       I. Klatzo

585   Effects of Central Nervous System Active and Nonactive Drugs on
       the Fetal Nervous System
       W. F. Geber

595   Effects of Prolonged Administration of "Street Heroin" on the Chromosomes of *Macaca mulatta* (Rhesus) Monkeys
H. K. Fischman, L. Roizin, E. Moralishvili, C. Joy, and J. D. Rainer

603   Primary and Secondary Alterations in Cerebellar Morphology in Carnivore (Ferret) and Rodent (Rat) After Exposure to Methylazoxymethanol Acetate
R. Haddad, A. Rabe, J. Shek, S. Donahue, and R. Dumas

613   Chemogenic Lesion: A Multifactor Pathogenic Concept
L. Roizin

649   *Subject Index*

Contributors

Masa Adachi, M.D.
*Isaac Albert Research Institute of Kingsbrook
   Jewish Medical Center
Rutland Road and East 49th Street
Brooklyn, New York 11203*

Keiichiro Akai, M.D.
*Department of Pathology
Kyorin University School of Medicine
6-20-2, Shinkawa
Mitakashi, Tokyo-181, Japan*

George Alexander, Ph.D.
*Department of Neurotoxicology
New York State Psychiatric Institute
722 West 168th Street
New York, New York 10032*

Archinto P. Anzil, M.D.
*Max-Planck-Institute of Psychiatry
8 München 40
Kraepelinstrasse 2
Postfach 401240, West Germany*

T. Atsumi, M.D.
*Department of Neuropathology
Brain Research Institute
Niigata University
1 Asahimachi
Niigata City, Japan 951*

Albert Behar, M.D.
*Department of Pathology
The Hebrew University
Hadassah Medical School
Jerusalem, Israel*

Albert Bischoff, M.D.
*Department of Neurology
University of Berne Medical School
Inselpital
3010 Berne, Switzerland*

K. Blinzinger, M.D.
*Max-Planck-Institute of Psychiatry
8 München 40
Kraepelinstrasse 2
Postfach 401240, West Germany*

T. W. Bouldin, M.D.
*Department of Pathology
School of Medicine
University of North Carolina
Chapel Hill, North Carolina 27514*

Robert E. Bowman, Ph.D.
*Department of Psychology
The University of Wisconsin Medical School
Madison, Wisconsin 53706*

Leonard Brand, M.D.
*Department of Anesthesiology
Columbia University
630 West 168th Street
New York, New York 10032*

Robert H. Brownson, Ph.D.
*Department of Human Anatomy
School of Medicine
University of California
Davis, California 95616*

C. Jelleff Carr, Ph.D.
*Federation of American Societies for Experimental
   Biology
9650 Rockville Pike
Bethesda, Maryland 20014*

John B. Cavanagh, M.D.
*Institute of Neurology
8-11 Queen Square
London WC1N 3AR, England*

Louis W. Chang, Ph.D.
*Department of Pathology
University of Arkansas for Medical Sciences
Little Rock, Arkansas 72201
and
National Center for Toxicological Research
Jefferson, Arkansas 72709*

J. G. Chusid, M.D.
*St. Vincent's Hospital and Medical Center
New York, New York 10011*

Doris H. Clouet, Ph.D.
New York State Office of Drug Abuse Services
Testing and Research Laboratories
80 Hanson Place
Brooklyn, New York 11217

Darab K. Dastur, M.D.
Neuropathology Unit
Grant Medical College and J. J. Group of Hospitals
Bombay 400–008, India

G. Michael Dempsey, M.D.
Veterans Administration Hospital
Lexington, Kentucky 40201

Herman C. B. Denber, M.D.
University of Louisville
School of Medicine
Health Sciences Center
Louisville, Kentucky 40201

Anita Dewan, M.S.
Neuropathology Unit
Grant Medical College and J. J. Group of Hospitals
Bombay 400–008, India

Sheila Donahue, M.D.
New York State Institute for Research in Mental
  Retardation
1050 Forest Hill Road
Staten Island, New York 10314

Alden W. Dudley, M.D.
Department of Pathology
University of South Alabama Medical School
Mobile, Alabama 36688

Mary A. Dudley, Ph.D.
Department of Pathology
University of South Alabama Medical School
Mobile, Alabama 36688

Ruth Dumas, M.A.
New York State Institute for Research in Mental
  Retardation
1050 Forest Hill Road
Staten Island, New York 10314

R. Ferszt, M.D.
Albert Einstein College of Medicine
Bronx, New York 10461

Harlow K. Fischman, Ph.D.
Cytogenetics Laboratory
New York State Psychiatric Institute
722 West 168th Street
New York, New York 10032

Howard E. Ganther, Ph.D.
Department of Nutritional Sciences
University of Wisconsin
470 North Charter Street
Madison, Wisconsin 53706

Silvio Garattini, M.D.
Istituto di Ricerche Farmacologiche "Mario Negri"
Via Eritrea, 62
20157 Milano, Italy

Frances Rowe Gearing, M.D.
Columbia University
School of Public Health
60 Haven Avenue
New York, New York 10032

William F. Geber, Ph.D.
Medical College of Georgia
Pharmacology Department
Augusta, Georgia 30902

Albert Goldfield, M.D.
Buffalo Psychiatric Center
400 Forest Avenue
Buffalo, New York 14213

Nenad Grčević, M.D.
Department of Neuropathology
University of Zagreb
Clinical Medical Center Rebro
41000 Zagreb, Yugoslavia

Yigal Greener, M.D.
Pediatric Hematology Service
Albert Einstein College of Medicine
Montefiore Hospital and Medical Center
111 East 210 Street
New York, New York 10467

Margaret L. Grunnet, M.D.
Department of Neurology
University of Utah
50 North Medical Center Drive
Salt Lake City, Utah 84117

Raef Haddad, Ph.D.
New York State Institute for Research in Mental
  Retardation
1050 Forest Hill Road
Staten Island, New York 10314

Michinori Hasegawa, M.D.
Kyoto Prefectural University of Medicine
Kawaramachi-Hirokoji
Kyoto, Japan

Shigeo Hashimoto, M.D.
Buffalo Psychiatric Center
400 Forest Avenue
Buffalo, New York 14213

Milton Helpern, M.D.[1]
Retired Chief Medical Examiner
City of New York;
Department of Forensic Medicine
New York University
School of Medicine
New York, New York 10022

H. Herrlinger, M.D.
Max-Planck-Institute of Psychiatry
8 München 40
Kraepelinstrasse 2
Postfach 401240, West Germany

Asao Hirano, M.D.
Division of Neuropathology
Montefiore Hospital and Medical Center
111 East 210th Street
Bronx, New York 10467

Sidney A. Houff, M.D.
Medical College of Virginia
Virginia Commonwealth University
1100 Marshall Street, Box 17
Richmond, Virginia 23298

Charles Hughes, M.D.
Neurology Service
Veterans Administration Lakeside Hospital;
Neurology Department
Northwestern University Medical School
Chicago, Illinois 60611

H. Ikeda, M.D.
Department of Neuropsychiatry
Okayama University Medical School
700 Okayama, Japan

Fusahiro Ikuta, M.D.
Department of Neuropathology
Brain Research Institute
Niigata University
l Asahimachi
Niigata City, Japan 951

Edward R. Isaacs, M.D.
Medical College of Virginia
Virginia Commonwealth University
1100 Marshall Street, Box 17
Richmond, Virginia 23298

Dubrauka Jadro-Šantel, M.D.
Department of Neuropathology
University of Zagreb
Clinical Medical Center Rebro
41000 Zagreb, Yugoslavia

Kurt Jellinger, M.D.
Neurological Institute
University of Vienna Medical School;
L. Boltzmann-Institute of Neurobiology
Lainz Hospital
A 1130 Vienna, Austria

Catherine Joy, B.A.
Department of Medical Genetics
New York State Psychiatric Institute
722 West 168th Street
New York, New York 10032

Stanko Jukić, M.D.
General Hospital
Vinkovci, Yugoslavia

Jordan Katz, M.D.
Department of Anesthesiology
The University of Wisconsin
Medical School
Madison, Wisconsin 53706

Mavis A. Kaufman, M.D.
Department of Neuropathology
New York State Psychiatric Institute
722 West 168th Street
New York, New York 10032

Igor Klatzo, M.D.
Laboratory of Neuropathology and
Neuroanatomical Sciences
National Institutes of Health
Bethesda, Maryland 20014

Georg Klinghardt, M.D.
Max-Planck Institute for Brain Research
6 Frankfurt a.M.-Niederrad
Deutschordenstr. 46, West Germany

Joseph A. Kochen, M.D.
Pediatric Hematology Service
Albert Einstein College of Medicine
Montefiore Hospital and Medical Center
111 East 210 Street
New York, New York 10467

Harold Koenig, M.D.
Neurology Service
Veterans Administration Lakeside Hospital;
Neurology Department
Northwestern University Medical School
Chicago, Illinois 60611

[1] Deceased.

L. M. Kopeloff, Ph.D.
New York State Psychiatric Institute
722 West 168th Street
New York, New York 10032

J. K. Korthals, M.D.
Albert Einstein College of Medicine
Montefiore Hospital and Medical Center
111 East 210 Street
New York, New York 10461

Martin R. Krigman, M.D.
Department of Pathology
School of Medicine
University of North Carolina
Chapel Hill, North Carolina 27514

K. Kumral, M.D.
Department of Pathology
Ege University Medical School
Bornova–Izmir, Turkey

S. Kuroda, M.D.
Department of Neuropsychiatry
Okayama University Medical School
700 Okayama, Japan

P. W. Lampert, M.D.
Department of Pathology
University of California at San Diego
La Jolla, California 92037

Seymour Levine, M.D.
New York Medical College
Bird S. Coler Hospital
Roosevelt Island, New York 10017

Jevons C. Liu, M.S.
Department of Neuropathology
New York State Psychiatric Institute
722 West 168th Street
New York, New York 10032

Nelly Livni, M.D.
Department of Pathology
The Hebrew University
Hadassah Medical School
Jerusalem, Israel

Chung Y. Lu, M.D.
Neurology Service
Veterans Administration Lakeside Hospital
Chicago, Illinois 60611

Sandra Machiz, B.A.
Department of Neurotoxicology
New York State Psychiatric Institute
722 West 168th Street
New York, New York 10032

Albert A. Manian, Ph.D.
Psychopharmacology Research Branch
National Institute of Mental Health
Rockville, Maryland 20852

T. Makifuchi, M.D.
Department of Neuropathology
Brain Research Institute
Niigata University
1 Asahimachi
Niigata City, Japan 951

Daya K. Manghani, Ph.D.
Nerve-Muscle Research Division
Bombay Hospital
Bombay 20 India

Lester C. Mark, Ph.D.
Department of Anesthesiology
Columbia University
630 West 168th Street
New York, New York 10032

A. Julio Martinez, M.D.
Presbyterian–University Hospital
Neuropathology Division
230 Lothrop Street
Pittsburgh, Pennsylvania 15213

Stanley Marynowski, B.S.
Department of Neurotoxicology
New York State Psychiatric Institute
722 West 168th Street
New York, New York 10032

H. D. McDouglas, M.D.
Department of Human Anatomy
School of Medicine
University of California
Davis, California 95616

Herbert L. Meltzer, Ph.D.
Department of Internal Medicine
New York State Psychiatric Institute
722 West 168th Street
New York, New York 10032

Emilia Moralishvili, M.S.
Department of Medical Genetics
New York State Psychiatric Institute
722 West 168th Street
New York, New York 10032

Paul Mushak, M.D.
Department of Pathology
School of Medicine
University of North Carolina
Chapel Hill, North Carolina 27514

K. Nagashima, M.D.
Department of Pathology
Tokyo University Medical School
Tokyo, Japan

Rajinder Nayyar, M.D.
Neurology Service
Veterans Administration Lakeside Hospital
Chicago, Illinois 60611

Werner J. Niklowitz, Ph.D.
Indiana University Medical Center
Division of Neuropathology
1100 West Michigan Street
Indianapolis, Indiana 46202

Akira Nakano, M.D.
Kyoto Prefectural University of Medicine
Kawaramachi–Hirokoji
Kyoto, Japan

A. Okumura, M.D.
Institute of Brain Research
Tokyo University Medical School
7–3–1 Hongo, Bunkyo-ku
Tokyo, Japan

T. Örnek, M.D.
Department of Pathology
Ege University Medical School
Bornova–Izmir, Turkey

S. Otsuki, M.D.
Department of Neuropsychiatry
Okayama University Medical School
700 Okayama, Japan

Sh. Oyahagi, M.D.
Institute of Brain Research
Tokyo University Medical School
7–3–1 Hongo, Bunkyo-ku
Tokyo, Japan

James M. Perel, Ph.D.
Department of Biological Psychiatry
New York State Psychiatric Institute
722 West 168th Street
New York, New York 10032

D. Pierson, M.S.
Department of Neurotoxicology
New York State Psychiatric Institute
722 West 168th Street
New York, New York 10032

Henry C. Powell, M.B.
Department of Pathology
University of California at San Diego
La Jolla, California 92037

Ausma Rabe, Ph.D.
New York State Institute for Research in
* Mental Retardation*
1050 Forest Hill Road
Staten Island, New York 10314

John D. Rainer, M.D.
Department of Medical Genetics
New York State Psychiatric Institute
722 West 168th Street
New York, New York 10032

Zohra A. Razzak, Ph.D.[2]
Neuropathology Unit
Grant Medical College and
* Sir J. J. Group of Hospitals*
Bombay 400–008 India

Paul J. Reier, M.D.
Laboratory of Neuropathology and
* Neuroanatomical Sciences*
National Institute of Neurological
* and Communicative Disorders and Stroke*
Bethesda, Maryland 20014

Leon Roizin, M.D.
Department of Neuropathology and
* Neurotoxicology*
New York State Psychiatric Institute
722 West 168th Street
New York, New York 10032

Nejat Sabuncu, M.D.
Department of Pathology
Ege University Medical School
Bornova–Izmir, Turkey

T. Saida, M.D.
Department of Pathology
Kyoto Prefectural University of Medicine
Kyoto, Japan

S. Salaçin, M.D.
Department of Pathology
Ege University Medical School
Bornova–Izmir, Turkey

[2] Deceased.

R. Samanin, M.D.
Istituto di Richerce Farmacologiche
"Mario Negri"
Via Eritrea 62
20157 Milan, Italy

Panna Sanghavi, M.D.
Neurology Service
Veterans Administration Hospital
Lakeside Hospital
Chicago, Illinois 60611

N. Santhadevi, Ph.D.
Neuropathology Unit
Grant Medical College and
* Sir J. J. Group of Hospitals*
Bombay 400–008 India

Takeshi Sato, M.D.
Department of Neuropathology
Brain Research Institute
Niigata University
1 Asahimachi
Niigata City, Japan 951

R. Saygill, M.D.
Department of Pathology
Ege University Medical School
Bornova-Izmir, Turkey

Herbert H. Schaumburg, M.D.
Neurotoxicology Unit
Albert Einstein College of Medicine
1300 Morris Park Avenue
Bronx, New York 10461

L. Schenck, M.D.
Isaac Albert Research Institute of
* Kingsbrook Jewish Medical Center*
Rutland Road and East 49th Street
Brooklyn, New York 11203

Joseph Schneider, M.D.
New York State Institute for Research
* in Mental Retardation*
1050 Forest Hill Road
Staten Island, New York 10032

Judy Shek, M.D.
New York State Institute for Research
* in Mental Retardation*
1050 Forest Hill Road
Staten Island, New York 10314

Hirotsugu Shiraki, M.D.
Institute of Brain Research
Tokyo University Medical School
7–3–1, Hongo, Bunkyo-ku
Tokyo, Japan

George Simpson, M.B., Ch.B.
Rockland Psychiatric Center
Orangeburg, New York 10962

Cedric M. Smith, M.D.
Research Institute on Alcoholism
1021 Main Street
Buffalo, New York 14203

Dov Soffer, M.D.
Department of Pathology
The Hebrew University
Hadassah Medical School
Jerusalem, Israel

Peter S. Spencer, M.D.
Neurotoxicology Unit
Albert Einstein College of Medicine
1300 Morris Park Avenue
Bronx, New York 10461

Oskar Steinwall, M.D.
Department of Neurology
Sahlgrenska sjukhuset
S-41345 Goteborg, Sweden

Richard Stiller, M.D.
Department of Neurotoxicology
New York State Psychiatric Institute
722 West 168th Street
New York, New York 10032

Milton L. Sunde, Ph.D.
Department of Pathology
The University of Wisconsin Medical School
Madison, Wisconsin 53706

D. B. Suter, M.D.
Department of Biology
Eastern Mennonite College
Harrisonburg, Virginia 22801

Takeshi Tabira, M.D.
Laboratory of Neuropathology and
* Neuroanatomical Sciences*
National Institute of Neurological and
* Communicative Disorders and Stroke*
Bethesda, Maryland 20014

Tadao Takeuchi, M.D.
Department of Pathology
Kumamoto University School of Medicine
2–2–1, Honjyo-machi
Kumamoto City, Japan

J. Tateishi, M.D.
Department of Neuropathology
Brain Research Institute
Niigata University
1 Asahimachi
Niigata City, Japan 951

John R. Taylor, M.D.
Medical College of Virginia
Virginia Commonwealth University
1100 Marshall Street, Box 17
Richmond, Virginia 23298

David N. Teller, Ph.D.
Department of Psychiatry and
Behavioral Sciences
P.O. Box 1055-MDR 517
Louisville, Kentucky 40201

R. D. Terry, M.D.
Albert Einstein College of Medicine
1300 Morris Park Avenue
Bronx, New York 10461

T. Tsubaki, M.D.
Department of Neuropathology
Brain Research Institute
Niigata University
1 Asahimachi
Niigata City, Japan 951

Maurice Victor, M.D.
Case Western Reserve University
School of Medicine
Cleveland, Ohio 44106

V. K. Vijayan, M.D.
Department of Human Anatomy
School of Medicine
University of California
Davis, California 95616

B. W. Volk, M.D.
Isaac Albert Research Institute of
Kingsbrook Jewish Medical Center
Rutland Road and East 49th Street
Brooklyn, New York 11203

Itaru Watanabe, M.D.
Veterans Administration Hospital
4801 Linwood Boulevard
Kansas City, Missouri 64128

Henry deF. Webster, M.D.
Laboratory of Neuropathology and
Neuroanatomical Sciences
National Institute of Neurological and
Communicative Disorders and Stroke
Bethesda, Maryland 20014

Nicholas Willson, M.D.
Department of Neuropathology
New York State Psychiatric Institute
722 West 168th Street
New York, New York 10032

H. M. Wisniewski, M.D.
New York State Institute for
Basic Research in Mental Retardation
Staten Island, New York 10314

Takeshi Yonezawa, M.D.
Kyoto Prefectural University of Medicine
Kawaramachi-Hirokoji
Kyoto, Japan

Foreword

As one who is responsible for the care service for the mentally ill, the retarded and the drug abusers in the State of New York, I am constantly touched and confronted by the tragic consequences of the neurotoxic effects of both our powerful therapeutic psychopharmaceuticals as well as by the serious behavioral and brain malfunctions produced by drugs used for hedonistic purposes or to escape pain and anxiety.

While the scientific and professional communities have known for decades of the effects of certain chemical agents upon the brain, it is only recently we have developed an awareness of the long term toxic effects of both older and newer agents, sometimes involving the succeeding generations. The newer agents, developed as a consequence of the rapidly expanding researches in chemistry and biochemistry which have moved forward rapidly through researches in both the academic and industrial circles have changed the world in which we live. We now enjoy worldwide many useful material substances as well as chemotherapeutic agents as the result of this work.

What societies worldwide failed to realize, astounded as they have been by these important advantages to mankind, were the equally significant disadvantages of certain of the related technological and industrial movements.

Perhaps no other series of events so emphatically enlightened the general public of the need to understand and establish preventive measures and public controls than the embryogenetic defects produced by the phenothiazine Thalidomide in Germany or the tragedy of extensive methyl mercurial poisoning which occurred in Japan. As for the phenothiazines, they were available early, but overlooked, indications of the embryogenetic effects of phenothiazines. Here I refer particularly to the early work of Dr. Leon Roizin. Today, in New York, we face the serious consequences of unlimited discharge of the chemical PCB into one of our most important and most beautiful water resources, the Hudson River. Perhaps the tragedies to people and their environment so dramatically exposed by the neurotoxic consequences of these scientifically ill-thought through industrial adventures have fortunately now forced upon people worldwide a sensitivity to the necessity for careful study, establishment of appropriate public health controls and environmental protection and the need for exploration of means for development of blocking antidotes. You undoubtedly join me in these hopes.

Lawrence C. Kolb, M.D.

Commissioner
Department of Mental Hygiene;
Professor of Psychiatry
College of Physicians and Surgeons
Columbia University
New York, New York

Introduction

Leon Roizin

The recognition of the authority of the fact, the justification of the particular and the rule of the law. (73,102)

In the course of progress, from time to time, it seems appropriate to pause in order to reexamine and reevaluate some older definitions, theories, or concepts in the light of current observations and newly acquired knowledge (76).

Harvey (37), in discussing the manner of acquiring knowledge, elaborates on Seneca's distinction, "As art is a habit with reference to things to be done, so is science a habit of things to be known. . . ." And, when on "the road of knowledge," it is necessary to proceed from the particulars to the universals. Bacon (3) insisted that it is the method of investigation that is essential, whereas Bernard (5) thought that "scientists not only correct their ideas on the basis of experience but bring them in harmony with the facts and nearer to the truth." However, when Virchow (103) tried to correlate clinical "facts" with Morgani's "anatomical idea" (60) and Bichat's (8) "tissue concept," he realized that, at times, a point is reached when the previous methods and tools of observation no longer suffice for the investigation of processes taking place in a disease (103). Thus, the idea of the macroscopic "localization" had to be extended to the invisible world, the living cell, and its physicochemical environment. Fortunately, this was accomplished with the discovery of the microscope and the subsequent extraordinary development of various optical, biophysical, and biochemical technologies that are also the testimony of the scientific triumph of the 20th century. In addition, Virchow (102)

emphasized that hypotheses, when based on analogies with scientific laws, are indispensable in research, because they lead science beyond the hitherto established facts and thus permit it to progress. In light of these considerations, "each worker is dependent on the thoughts of his time, utilizes formulations suggested by others, and is inspired or influenced by particular circumstances of his own ear" (14).

Among several medicobiological developments, our current era is characterized by chemical welfare, the drug explosion, polypharmacy, or drug culture, with its by-product, the myth of the pill.

During recent decades, psychotropic agents have become the most widely used chemotherapy for behavioral and mental disorders (20,57). For instance, prochlorperazine (Compazine®, SKF) alone, one of the common tranquilizers, has been used for the treatment of millions of cases. Although there is undeniable evidence of beneficial effects for this drug as well as for many other phenothiazines, intolerance and side effects occasionally occur, even with therapeutic doses. These reactions involve the central nervous system (CNS), liver, kidney, cardiovascular, gastrointestinal, secretory, endocrine, and reproductive functions, thermoregulating, immunochemical hemopoetic mechanisms, etc. (2,23,83,93). Generally, most of these disorders are reversible when promptly taken care of. However, irreversible alterations also develop that, in some instances, may even have a fatal outcome (1,19,25,40,45,50,66,71,83,87).

The problem of adverse and toxic effects of neuropsychotropic drugs becomes even more significant when the following facts are taken into consideration: (a) the dosage of most tranquilizers, in order to exercise beneficial psychiatric effects, must frequently be increased until the patient shows adverse reactions, such as extrapyramidal symptoms; (b) patients must often be treated for long periods of time, thus increasing the toxic hazard; (c) psychotropic agents show potentiating interaction with sedatives, anesthetics, analgesics, antihistamines, and alcohol; and (d) growing drug abuse and narcotic addiction have become major health problems (4,27,38,56,69,78,81).

Concerning drug abuse, in 1972 (38) drug addiction was "the greatest single cause of death among adolescents and young adults from 15–35 — exceeding deaths from any other single cause: accidents, suicide, homocide, or natural diseases."[1] What is so alarming is that this condition affects all socioeconomical levels irrespective of age, sex, race, or culture. It is almost incomprehensible to see our supersophisticated society and responsible governments engaging in prolific debates while drug-abused or addicted mothers continue to conceive in unhealthy conditions, thereby risking the delivery of an unpredictable number of genetically or prenatally affected babies (24,59,90). This deplorable situation should cause even more concern in the light of inadequate knowledge about the "psychochemosomatic"[2] future development of these newly born innocent victims (89,91,92,98,

111,112), as can be surmised also from experimental investigations (28,30,35,36,41, 43,54,58,106). Various embryopathies, teratogenesis, and mutagenicity have been described following prenatal administration of phenothiazines (9,13,15,46,61,67, 68,82,83,84,100,104,107), rauwolfia derivatives (32,96), sedatives and hypnotics (7,63,97), stimulants (48,64,65), antidepressants (17,18,36,54,74), monoamine oxidase inhibitors (72,108,109), diphenylmetane derivatives (51,100), hallucinogens (2,21,28,49,79), marihuana (extract, refs. 2,29), miscellaneous drugs (24,33,47,105, 108,110), and heavy and trace metals (39,86,95).

After World War II and in the 1950s drug abuse and drug dependence dominated the drug scene, especially in the United States. More recently, a drug wave has rapidly expanded in Europe (22,34,53,75), and amphetamine abuse has become a major concern in Japan (11). In the same country Minamata disease, attributed to the toxicity of mercurial compounds, severely affected significant proportions of the population, particularly in the regions of Minamata, Miigata, and Cumamoto (52,86,95). Toxic effects of industrial chemicals and heavy and trace metals on the central and peripheral nervous system, as well as other body systems or tissues, have been recorded in many countries, including the USSR (26).

In addition, indiscriminant technological advances, burgeoning industrialization, modernization of agriculture, and multiplication of commercial enterprises have contaminated the atmosphere with threatening pollutants, fed the waters with poisonous chemicals, insecticides, pesticides, detergents, radioisotope discards, etc., despoiled the earth with a variety of minerals and fertilizers, weed controls, etc., and artificially enriched canned foods with various synthetic preservatives and additives, the consumption of which has continued to increase. Moreover, qualitative

---

[1] The National Institute of Drug Abuse has recently released the results of four new national surveys on legal and illegal drug use. They show that consumption of these drugs is continuing at high levels in various regions of the United States (ref. 113).

[2] Biochemical changes of the CNS (62,99), as well as CNS and liver (62), were also detected following prenatal administration of neuropsychotropic agents.

and quantitative malnutrition depletes the individual's essential metabolic storage. As a consequence, the whole terrestrial ecology is becoming insidiously permeated and progressively affected by organic and inorganic chemical agents or their by-products. And, as if this caleidoscopic pathobiological situation were not convincing enough, the chemoprone or chemoreceptive *Homo sapien* continues to indulge in unwholesome social drinking, which hastens with extra deleterious fuel (81,88,101) the decay of the struggling chemopathic[3] organism (25,27,81).

Furthermore, the medicoscientific scene is handicapped by inadequacies in the study of pathogenic mechanisms. Although several validation criteria have been devised for drug reaction in human cases (42), some difficulties are still encountered in evaluating retrospective drug reactions in patients (80). These are some of the problems: (a) incomplete information about how the dosage relates to the patient's drug profile and drug history, (b) different medicobiological conditions of patients, (c) multiple drug or chemical intakes, (d) methodological uncertainties regarding chemical identification of drugs or their metabolites, particularly in polypharmacy, (e) uncertainties about the temporal relationship between the intake of the drug or chemical agents and the appearance and duration of the adverse reaction, (f) existence of inborn or acquired predisposing or facilitating factors to certain drug or chemical reactions (idiosyncrasies, incompatibilities), (g) inadequate surveillance or follow-up of cases from outpatient clinics, and (h) insufficient knowledge of the body's limited means of tolerance.

To facilitate or at least lay the groundwork for some fundamental drug reaction profiles, animal experiments may help to establish: (a) the pharmacodynamics of drug administration, (b) the sites of drug

---

[3] Denotes chemically abnormal or pathological.

distribution (body fluids and anatomical allocation), (c) the sequence of physiological and toxicological reactions, (d) the short and prolonged (chronic) effect of medications, (e) the temporal relationship between drug administration and chemical, histometabolic, and structural examinations, (f) a monitoring system, marked by close surveillance and direct observation of reaction patterns of the organism, (g) the role of age, sex, and race or strain variables, and (h) the correlation of *in vivo* and *in vitro* experiments with control studies, etc.

Although animal model experiments may be informative, delayed effects are little known, and causal associations with various environmental conditions, actually an integral part of human life, are artificially excluded. Furthermore, no single animal may be adequate for all studies at all times with regard to disease processes in man (80). A few human cases may, at times, be more crucial than hundreds of animal experiments (55). It is well established that the experimental animal or the laboratory *in vitro* procedures are not satisfactory substitutes for humans, although they serve as very useful and even essential preclinical research models.

To circumvent some of these problems, we organized a multidisciplinary volume on neurotoxicology. The organization of this first volume aims to focus attention principally on some of the most current neurotoxicologic topics of common interest and includes presentations and discussions on the toxic effects of phenothiazines and tranquilizers, narcotics and anesthetics, stimulants, antidepressants, hallucinogens, heavy and trace metals, antiinflammatory and immunosuppressor agents, antiinfectives, industrial chemicals, insecticides, herbicides, and anorexic chemical agents. The chapters consider clinical, pharmacological, biochemical, and toxicological (including research and diagnostic methodologies) aspects of these topics with special emphasis on neuropathology, teratogenesis, and pathogenic mechanisms. The volume shows that a direct exchange of ideas among many professional disciplines with converging interests and the integration of a multilateral knowledge into a coherent sum can provide better understanding of the modern toxicogenic dilemma under discussion. It is hoped that this comprehensive information will stimulate further research toward the following: (a) serial measurements of drug profiles to evaluate individual drug response, incompatibility, or intolerance, (b) the establishment of pharmacokinetics to control long-term therapies, (c) the identification of biological variables to prevent adverse or toxic reactions, and (d) the development of inhibitors or blocking agents and antidotes, etc.

Even in some unpredictable or uncontrollable instances, hope should not be lost, since "en etudiant attentivement le mechanisme de la mort dans les divers empoisonments, il s'instruit par voie indirect sur le mechanisme physiologique de la vie" (6)—in the careful study of the mechanism of death in various poisonings, one is taught indirectly the physiological mechanism of life.

As a matter of fact, this optimism is already justified by some current clinical observations, biochemical examinations, and ultracellular investigations demonstrating that some toxicological effects and histochemical reaction patterns caused by certain neuropsychotropic agents, particularly morphine and opiates, can be blocked or inhibited for a certain period of time by antagonists such as nalorphine (16,94), lavellorphan (85), naloxone (70), cyclazocine (12,31), etc. (10,44).

Stimulated by these recent achievements, motivated clinicians and scientists will continue to heed the advice, "Lege, lege, relege, ora, labora et invenis"—read, read, reread, pray, toil and thou shall find (77).

The neurotoxicological multidisciplinary research and diagnostic methodologies will, in the final analysis, benefit the patient and safeguard society.

REFERENCES

1. Arseni, C., Nerentiu, P., Nicolescu, P., and Horvath, L. (1976): Encephalopathy subsequent to accidental poisoning with chlorpromazine. *Eur. Neurol.,* 14:29–38.
2. Auerbach, R., and Rugowski, J. A. (1967): Lysergic acid diethylamide: Effect on embryos. *Science,* 157:1325–1326.
3. Bacon, F. (1962): Standpoints in scientific medicine (1847). In: *Disease, Life, and Man, Selected Essays by Rudolf Virchow,* translated and with introduction by L. J. Rather, pp. 40–42. Collier Books, New York.
4. Baden, M. M. (1971): Methadone related deaths in New York City. In: *Methadone Maintenance,* edited by S. Einstein, pp. 143–152. Dekker, New York.
5. Bernard, C. (1962): Introduction a l'étude de la médicine expérimentale (1865). In: *Disease, Life, and Man, Selected Essays by Rudolf Virchow,* translated and with introduction by L. J. Rather, pp. 19–25. Collier Books, New York.
6. Bernard, C. (1957): La science expérimentale, Baillière, Paris (1878), p. 237. H. B. Stoner and P. N. Magee. *P. N. Br. Med. Bull.,* 13:102–106.
7. Bertrand, M. (1960): Effets du méprobamate sur l'évolution de la gestation chez la ratte. *CR Soc. Biol.,* 154:2309–2312.
8. Bichat, M. F. X. (1962): Anatomie générale appliquée a la physiologie et la médicine (1801). In: *Disease, Life, and Man, Selected Essays by Rudolf Virchow,* translated and with introduction by L. J. Rather, p. 33. Collier Books, New York.
9. Bovet-Nitti, F., and Bovet, D. (1959): Action of some sympatholytic agents on pregnancy in the rat. *Proc. Soc. Exp. Biol. Med.,* 100:555–557.
10. Bramwell, G. J., and Bradley, P. B. (1974): Actions and interactions of narcotic agonists and antagonists on brain stem neurons. *Brain Res.,* 73:167–170.
11. Brill, H., and Hirose, T. (1969): Rise and fall of a methamphetamine epidemic. *Semin. Psychiatry,* 1:179–194.
12. Brill, L., and Laskowitz, D. (1972): Cyclazocine in the treatment of narcotic addiction. Another look. In: *Drug Abuse: Current Concepts and Research,* edited by W. Keup, pp. 407–417. Charles C Thomas, Springfield, Ill.
13. Brock, N., and von Kreybig, T. (1964): Experimenteller Beitrag zur Prufung teratogener Wirkungen von Arzneimitteln an der Laboratoriumstratte. *Naunyn Schmiedebergs Arch. Exp. Pathol.,* 249:117–145.

14. Campbell, C. M. (1937): Perspectives in psychiatry. *Am. J. Psychiatry,* 94:1–14.
15. Chambon, Y. (1955): Action de la chlorpromazine sur l'évolution et l'avenir de la gestation chez la rate. *Ann. Endocrinol (Paris),* 16:912–922.
16. Cox, B. M., and Weinstock, M. (1964): Quantitative studies of the antagonism by nalorphine of some of the actions of morphine-like analgesic drugs. *Br. J. Pharmacol.,* 22:289–300.
17. Coyle, I. R., and Singer, G. (1975): The interactive effects of prenatal imipramine exposure and postnatal rearing conditions on behaviour and histology. *Psychopharmacologia,* 44:253–256.
18. Coyle, I. R. (1975): Changes in developing behavior following prenatal administration of imipramine. *Pharmacol. Biochem. Behav.,* 3:799–807.
19. Cristensen, E., Möller, J. E., and Faurbye, A. (1970): Neuropathological investigations of 28 brains from patients with dyskinesia. *Acta Psychiatr. Scand.,* 46:14–23.
20. Delay, J., and Deniker, P. (1968): Drug-induced extrapyramidal syndrome. In: *Handbook of Clinical Neurology,* Vol. 6, edited by P. J. Vinken and G. W. Bruyn, pp. 248–267. North-Holland Publ., Amsterdam.
21. DiPaolo, J. A., Givelber, H. M., and Erwin, H. (1968): Evaluation of teratogenicity of lysergic acid diethylamide. *Nature,* 220:490–491.
22. Ehrhardt, H. E. (1972): Drug abuse in Europe: Medical and legal aspects. In: *Drug Abuse: Current Concepts and Research,* edited by W. Keup, pp. 27–35. Charles C Thomas, Springfield, Ill.
23. Fann, W. E., Sullivan, J. L., and Richman, B. W. (1976): Dyskinesias associated with tricyclic antidepressants. *Br. J. Psychiatry,* 128:490–493.
24. Forfar, J. O. (1976): What drugs are unsafe in pregnancy? *Rassegna Med.,* 53:14–28 (English ed.)
25. Forrest, F. M., Forrest, D. S., and Roizin, L. (1963): Clinical, biochemical and postmortem studies on a patient treated with chlorpromazine. *Agressologie,* 4:259–265.
26. Friberg, L. T., and Vostal, J. J. (1972): *Mercury in the Environment: A Toxicological and Epidemiological Appraisal.* CRC Press, Cleveland.
27. Gearing, F. (1971): The evoluation of methadone maintenance treatment program. In: *Methadone Maintenance,* edited by S. Einstein. Dekker, New York.
28. Geber, W. F. (1967): Congenital malformations induced by mescaline, lysergic acid diethylamide, and bromolysergic acid in the hamster. *Science,* 158:265–267.
29. Geber, W. F., and Schramm, L. C. (1969): Effect of marihuana extract on fetal hamsters and rabbits. *Toxicol. Appl. Pharmacol.,* 14:276–282.
30. Geber, W. F. (1970): Blockade of teratogenic effect of morphine and dihydromorphinone by nalorphine and cyclazocine. *Pharmacologist,* 12:296.
31. Geber, W. F. (1972): Blockade of teratogenic effect of morphine, dihydromorphine and methadone by nalorphine, cyclazocine, and naloxone in the fetal hamster. In: *Drug Abuse: Current Concepts and Research,* edited by W. Keup, pp. 117–122. Charles C Thomas, Springfield, Ill.
32. Goldman, A. S., and Yakovac, W. C. (1965): Teratogenic action in rats of reserpine alone and in combination with salicylate and immobilization. *Proc. Soc. Exp. Biol. Med.,* 118:857–862.
33. Haddad, R., Rabe, A., Shek, J., Donahue, S., and Dumas, R. (1977): Primary and secondary alterations in cerebellar morphology in carnivore (Ferret) and rodent (Rat) after exposure to methylazoxymethanol acetate. (*This volume.*)
34. Haenel, T. A. (1970): Kulturgeschichte und heutige Problematik des Haschisch. *Pharmakopsychiatr. Neuropsychopharmakol.,* 3:89–115.
35. Harpel, H. S., Jr., and Gautieri, R. F. (1968): Morphine-induced fetal malformations. I. Enecephalopathy and axial skeletal fusions. *J. Pharm. Sci.,* 57:1590–1597.
36. Harper, K. H., Palmer, A. K., and Davies, R. E. (1965): Effect of imipramine upon the pregnancy of laboratory animals. *Arzneim. Forsch.,* 15:1218–1221.
37. Harvey, W. (1962): *The Works of William Harvey (1847),* translated from the Latin with *A Life of the Author,* by R. Willis. Quoted by L. R. Rather, pp. 13–18. Collier Books, New York.
38. Helpern, M. (1972): Deaths resulting from narcotic addiction. A major health problem. In: *Drug Abuse: Current Concepts and Research,* edited by W. Keup, pp. 51–63. Charles C Thomas, Springfield, Ill.
39. Hirano, A., and Kochen, J. A. (1977): Relationship of blood and brain lead levels to morphologic changes in lead-induced chick embryo encephalopathy. I. Morphologic studies. (*This volume.*)
40. Hollister, L. E., and Kosek, J. C. (1965): Sudden death during treatment with phenothiazine derivatives. *JAMA,* 192:1035–1038.
41. Hutchings, D. E., Hunt, H. F., Towey, J. P., Rosen, T. S., and Gorinson, H. S. (1976): Methadone during pregnancy in the rat: Dose level effects on maternal and perinatal mortality and growth in the offspring. *J. Pharmacol. Exp. Ther.,* 197(1):171–179.
42. Irey, N. S. (1970): Registry of tissue reactions to drugs. AFIP. *Presented at Int. Conf. Adverse Reaction Reporting Systems, Washington, D.C., Oct. 22–23.*
43. Iuliucci, J. D., and Gautieri, R. F. (1971): Morphine-induced fetal malformations. II. Influence of histamine and diphenhydramine. *J. Pharm. Sci.,* 60:420.
44. Jasinsi, D. R. (1972): Studies on the subjective effects of narcotic antagonists. In: *Drug Abuse: Current Concepts and Research,* edited by

W. Keup, pp. 270–276. Charles C Thomas, Springfield, Ill.

45. Jellinger, K. (1977): Neuropathological findings after neuroleptic long-term therapy. (*This volume.*)

46. Jewett, R. E., and Norton, S. (1966): Effects of tranquilizing drugs on postnatal behavior. *Exp. Neurol.*, 14:33–43.

47. Kalter, H. (1972): Teratogenicity, embryolethality and mutagenicity of drugs of dependence. In: *Chemical and Biological Aspects of Drug Dependence,* edited by S. J. Mulé, and H. Brill, pp. 413–445. CRC Press, Cleveland.

48. Kasirsky, G., and Tansy, M. F. (1971): Teratogenic effects of methamphetamine in mice and rabbits. *Teratology,* 4:131–134.

49. Kato, T., Jarvik, L. F., Roizin, L., and Moralishvili, E. (1970): Chromosome studies in pregnant rhesus macaque given LSD-25. *Dis. Nerv. Syst.,* 31:245–250.

50. Kaufman, M. A. (1977): Alternate diagnoses of tardive dyskinesia: Neuropathological findings in three suspected cases. (*This volume.*)

51. King, C. T. G., and Howell, J. (1966): Teratogenic effect of buclizine and hydroxyzine in the rat and chlorcyclizine in the mouse. *Am. J. Obstet. Gynecol.,* 95:109–111.

52. Kitamura, S. (1968): Determination on mercury content in bodies in inhabitants, cats, fishes and shells in Minamata district and in the mud of Minamata bay. In: *Minamata Disease: Study Group of Minamata Disease,* edited by M. Kutsuna, pp. 257–266. Kumamoto University, Japan.

53. Ladewig, D. (1969): Neuere Suchttrends bei Jugendlichen. *Schweiz. Med. Wochenschr.,* 99:781–783.

54. Larsen, V. (1963): The teratogenic effects of thalidomide, imipramine HCl and imipramine-N-oxide HCl on white Danish rabbits. *Acta Pharmacol.,* 20:186–200.

55. Long, J. W. (1970): Problems related to the dissemination of drug adverse reaction information. *Presented at Int. Conf. Adverse Reaction Reporting Systems, Washington, D.C., Oct. 22–23.*

56. Louria, D. B., Hensle, T., and Rose, J. (1967): The major medical complications of heroin addiction. *Ann. Intern. Med.,* 67:1–22.

57. Malitz, S., and Hoch, P. H. (1959): Drug therapy: Neuroleptics and tranquilizers. In: *American Handbook of Psychiatry,* Vol. 3, edited by S. Arieti, pp. 458–476. Basic Books, New York.

58. Markham, J. K., Emmerson, J. L., and Owen, N. V. (1971): Teratogenicity studies of methadone HCl in rats and rabbits. *Nature,* 233:342–343.

59. Ministry of Health (1964): *Deformities Caused by Thalidomide,* p. 70. Report #112, London.

60. Morgagni, G. B. (1962): De Sedibus et Causis Morborum per Anatomen Indagatis (1761). In: *Selected Essays by Rudolf Virchow: Disease, Life, and Man,* translated and with introduction by L. J. Rather, p. 33. Collier Books, New York.

61. Murphree, O. D., Monroe, B. L., and Seager, L. D. (1962): Survival of offspring of rats administered phenothiazines during pregnancy. *J. Neuropsychiatry,* 3:295–297.

62. Nair, V., Bau, D., and Siegel, S. (1970): Effect of LSD in pregnancy on the biochemical development of brain and liver in the offspring. *Pharmacologist,* 12:296.

63. Nishikawa, M. (1963): Effect of the administration of meprobamate to pregnant mice on the development of the fetus. *Acta Anat. Nippon.,* 38:258–263 (In Japanese with English summary.)

64. Nora, J. J., Trasler, D. G., and Fraser, F. C. (1965): Malformations in mice induced by dextroamphetamine sulphate. *Lancet,* 2:1021–1022.

65. Nora, J. J., Sommerville, R. J., and Fraser, F. C. (1968): Homologies for congenital heart diseases: Murine models, influenced by dextroamphetamine. *Teratology,* 1:413–416.

66. Olchanskii, Y. O., and Morozov, V. V. (1962): Death due to necrotizing nephrosis following aminozine. *Zh. Nevropatol. Psikhiatr.,* 62:762–764.

67. Ordy, J. M., Latanick, A., Johnson, R., and Massopust, L. C. (1963): Chlorpromazine effects on pregnancy and offspring in mice. *Proc. Soc. Exp. Biol. Med.,* 113:833–836.

68. Ordy, J. M., Samorajski, T., Collins, R. L., and Rolsten, C. (1966): Prenatal chlorpromazine effects on liver, survival and behavior of mice offspring. *J. Pharmacol. Exp. Ther.,* 151:110–125.

69. Pearson, J., Challenor, Y., Baden, M., and Richter, R. (1972): The neuropathology of heroin addiction. *J. Neuropathol. Exp. Neurol.,* 31:165–166.

70. Pert, C. B., and Synder, S. H. (1973): Opiate receptor: Demonstration in nervous tissue. *Science,* 174:1011–1014.

71. Popova, E. N., and Krivitskaya, G. N. (1975): The influence of some psychotropic drugs on brain structures. *Zh. Nevropatol. Psikhiatr.,* 75:1064–1069.

72. Poulson, E., and Robson, J. M. (1964): Effect of phenelzine and some related compounds on pregnancy and on sexual development. *J. Endocrinol.,* 30:205–215.

73. Rather, L. J. (translator with an introduction) (1962): *Selected Essays by Rudolf Virchow: Disease, Life, and Man,* pp. 13–183. Collier Books, New York.

74. Robson, J. M., and Sullivan, F. M. (1963): The production of foetal abnormalities in rabbits by imipramine. *Lancet,* 1:638–639.

75. Remschmidt, H., and Dauner, I. (1970): Klinische und soziale Aspekte der Drogenabhdngigkeit bei Jugenlichen. *Med. Klinik,* 65:1993–1997.

76. Roizin, L. (1963): Presidential address: Some basic principles of "molecular pathology:" 3. Ultracellular organelles as structural-metabolic and pathogenic gradients. *J. Neuropathol. Exp. Neurol.,* 23:209–252.

77. Roizin, L. (1970): Van Gieson, a visionary of psychiatric research. *Am. J. Psychiatry,* 127:98–103.
78. Roizin, L., Baden, M., Kaufman, M. A., Willson, N., Alexander, G., Hashimoto, S., Liu, J. C., and Eisenberg-Gelber, B. (1975): Neuropathology of drug narcotism syndrome (pathogenic considerations). In: *VIIth Int. Congr. Neuropathology,* edited by St. Környey, St. Tariska, and G. Gosztonyi, pp. 343–348. Excerpta Medica, Amsterdam.
79. Roizin, L., Gold, G., Alexander, G., Miles, B., Kaufman, M. A., Lawler, C., and Akai, K. (1972): Prenatal effects of hallucinogens. In: *Drug Abuse: Current Concepts and Research,* edited by W. Keup, pp. 123–127. Charles C Thomas, Springfield, Ill.
80. Roizin, L., Helpern, M., Baden, M., Kaufman, M. A., and Akai, K. (1972): Toxosynpathies (A multifactor concept). In: *Drug Abuse: Current Concepts and Research,* edited by W. Keup, pp. 97–116. Charles C Thomas, Springfield, Ill.
81. Roizin, L., Helpern, M., Baden, M., Kaufman, M. A., Hashimoto, S., Liu, J. C., and Eisenberg-Gelber, B. (1972); Methadone fatalities in heroin addicts. *Psychiatr. Q.,* 46:393–410.
82. Roizin, L., Lazar, M., and Gold, G. (1966): Prenatal effects of phenothiazines. *Fed. Proc.,* 25:353.
83. Roizin, L., True, C., and Knight, M. (1959): Structural effects of tranquilizers. The effect of pharmacologic agents. *Proc. Assoc. Res. Nerv. Ment. Dis.,* 37:285–324.
84. Roux, C. (1959): Action tératogène de la prochlorpémazine. *Arch. Fr. Pediatr.,* 16:968–971.
85. Seevers, M. H., and Deneau, G. A. (1962): A critique of the "dual action" hypothesis of morphine physical dependence. *Arch. Int. Pharmacodyn. Ther.,* 140:514–520.
86. Shiraki, H. (1977): The neuropathology of alkylmercury intoxications at different stages in humans — with special reference to. the time-dependent autoradiograms in monkeys using labeled inorganic and organic mercury compounds. (*This volume.*)
87. Shiraki, H. (1977): Morphological background; Grumous degeneration of cerebellar nucleus for tardive dyskinesia induced by antipsychotic drugs in schizophrenia. (*This volume.*)
88. Smith, C. M. (1977): Alcohol-drug interactions. (*This volume.*)
89. Smithells, R. W. (1966): Drugs and human malformations. *Adv. Teratol.,* 1:251–278.
90. Somers, G. F. (1962): Thalidomide and congenital abnormalities. *Lancet,* 1:912–913.
91. Stern, R. (1966): The pregnant addict. A study of 66 case histories. *Obstet. Gynecol.,* 94:253.
92. Strauss, M. E. (1975): Behavior of narcotics-addicted newborns. *Child Dev.,* 46:887–893.
93. Simpson, G. (1977): Neurotoxicology of major tranquilizers. (*This volume.*)
94. Takemori, A. E. (1962): Studies on cellular adaptation to morphine and its reversal by nalor-phine in cerebral cortical slices of rats. *J. Pharmacol. Exp. Ther.,* 135:89–93.
95. Takeuchi, T. (1977): Neuropathology of Minamata disease in Kumamoto, especially at chronic stage. (*This volume.*)
96. Tuchmann-Duplessis, H., and Mercier-Parot, L. (1961): Malformations foetales chez le rat traité par de fortes doses de desérpidine. *CR Soc. Biol.,* 155:2291.
97. Tuchmann-Duplessis, H., and Mercier-Parot, L. (1963): Répercussion d'un somnifére, le gluté-thimide, sur la gestation et le développement foetal du rat, de la souris et du lapin. *CR Acad. Sci.,* 256:1841–1843.
98. Van Leeuwen, G., Guthrice, R., and Stange, F. (1965): Narcotic withdrawal reaction in a newborn infant due to codeine. *Pediatrics,* 36:635–636.
99. Vernadakis, A., and Clark, C. V. H. (1970): Effects of prenatal administration of psychotropic drugs to rats on butylcholinesterase activity at birth. *Brain Res.,* 21:460–463.
100. Vichi, F. (1969): Neuroleptic drugs in experimental teratogenesis. In: *Teratology,* edited by A. Bertilli, and L. Donati, pp. 87–101. Excerpta Medica, Amsterdam.
101. Victor, M. (1977): The effect of alcohol on the nervous system. (*This volume.*)
102. Virchow, R. (1962): Cellular pathology (1855). In: *Disease, Life, and Man, Selected Essays by Rudolph Virchow,* translated and with introduction by L. J. Rather, p. 87. Collier Books, New York.
103. Virchow, R. (1962): Cellular pathology (1855). In: *Disease, Life, and Man, Selected Essays by Rudolph Virchow,* translated and with an introduction by L. J. Rather, pp. 86–115. Collier Books, New York.
104. Webster, R. L., and McNew, J. (1967): Adverse effects on offspring of tranquilizing drugs during pregnancy. *Nature,* 215:182–183.
105. Wechsler, W. (1976): Acute and late effects of prenatal and transplacental exposure to rats, hamsters, and mice to ethylnitrosourea. First International Symposium of Neurotoxicology, New York.
106. Werboff, J., and Kesner, R. (1963): Learning deficits of offspring after administration of tranquilizing drugs to the mothers. *Nature,* 197:106–107.
107. Werboff, J., and Dembicki, E. L. (1962): Toxic effects of tranquilizers administered to gravid rats. *J. Neuropsychiatry,* 4:87–91.
108. Werboff, J., Gottlieb, J. S., Dembicki, E. L., and Havlena, J. (1961): Postnatal effect of antidepressant drugs administered during gestation. *Exp. Neurol.,* 3:542–555.
109. Werboff, J., Gottlieb, J. S., Havlena, J., and Wood, T. J. (1961): Behavioral effects of prenatal drug administration in the white rat. *Pediatrics,* 27:318–324.
110. Wilson, J. G. (1964): Teratogenic interaction of chemical agents in the rat. *J. Pharmacol. Exp. Ther.,* 144:429–436.

111. Yakovleva, A. I., and Sorokina, M. N. (1966): Effect of indopan on albino rats and their progeny. *Farmakol. Toksikol.,* 29:224–229. (In Russian with English summary.)

112. Zelson, C., Sook, J. L., and Casalino, M. (1973): Neonatal narcotic addiction. Comparative effects of maternal intake of heroin and methadone. *N. Engl. J. Med.,* 289:1216–1220.

113. National Institute of Drug Abuse (1976): *Psychiatric News,* 11:23.

Neurotoxicology, edited by L. Roizin, H. Shiraki, and N. Grčević. Raven Press, New York © 1977.

Neurotoxicity of Major Tranquilizers

George M. Simpson

Rockland Research Institute, Orangeburg, New York 10962

Following the introduction of chlorpromazine and other phenothiazines in the 1950s, it was almost immediately apparent that this group of drugs and the ones that were to follow affected many areas of the central nervous system. The early phenothiazines were found to affect temperature regulation, have antiemetic properties, produce sedation, and have effects on the autonomic nervous system as well as on the extrapyramidal system. These effects were all in addition to and perhaps even related to their main therapeutic use as antipsychotic agents. Because of this multiplicity of action, it is not surprising that the neurotoxicity of these drugs is wide ranging and complex. However, at the onset it should be stated that serious complications with these agents are uncommon and that in relation to their therapeutic efficacy they are indeed valuable and worthwhile drugs.

SEDATIVE AND AUTONOMIC EFFECTS

Sedation is a common side effect but is more a characteristic of the less potent drugs than the more potent piperazines or drugs such as haloperidol. When these agents are given in very high dosages, the sedation can become quite profound, although it differs significantly from the sedation produced by previous drugs in that it does not depress the respiratory center to the same extent. It is for this reason that these drugs are relatively safe to use, if required, in large dosages. With extreme overdosage, coma and death can result, but it should be noted that these effects only occur when many times the therapeutic dosage has been taken. Less common but more dramatic side effects, such as toxic confusional states, can take place early in treatment particularly in the elderly; these are likely to be related to the atropine-like side effects of the drugs, and, therefore, would be more common with the more sedative drugs or if (as is all too frequently done) the drugs are combined with antiparkinson agents. This confusional state is an easily recognized, disturbing phenomenon that disappears with discontinuation of the medication.

These agents generally lower temperature, but on rare occasions they produce an elevation in temperature that can exceed 104°F and result in coma and death. This has been called a malignant hyperthermia and, although rare, its existence has to be borne in mind. It is probably an idiosyncratic sensitivity reaction as are the behavioral effects described below.

The problem of sudden death in patients on neuroleptics is a complicated one. It is rare, and indeed there is dispute whether it occurs or not because there are studies to show that the death rate at each age in mental hospitals has not changed since the introduction of these drugs (3). The fact that these drugs resulted in a tremendous diminution in the hospital population and in an improvement in patient care confounds the issue. Even if we accept that neuroleptic-related sudden deaths do occur, it is unclear whether they result from an effect on the central nervous system or from a direct effect on the heart.

All major tranquilizers lower the seizure threshold, and, therefore, patients receiving neuroleptics may have grand mal seizures. This is an uncommon phenomenon but more common than sudden deaths and hyperthermia. In general, the more sedative drugs have a greater effect on the seizure threshold than the more potent ones; thus, with a patient who has had a convulsion while receiving a neuroleptic, rather than giving continuous anticonvulsants, it might be better to change him to a more potent neuroleptic and observe him. The addition of anticonvulsants confuses the treatment, as they are likely to have an effect on the metabolism of the neuroleptic and are not without side effects themselves.

NEUROLOGICAL EFFECTS

The neurological effects (together with the autonomic and sedative effects) are the most commonly occurring side effects of these drugs. They can be seen in almost every case where therapeutic dosages are employed, suggesting these are implicit actions of the drugs as opposed to idiosyncratic reactions of patients. The extrapyramidal disturbances may conveniently be described under four headings: the acute dystonic reaction, akathisia, pseudoparkinsonism, and tardive dyskinesia.

Acute Dystonic Reaction

Acute dystonic reactions are of sudden onset and consist of bizarre muscular spasms that have been misdiagnosed as tetany or hysteria (particularly because emotional reactions can contribute to their precipitation and because patients can occasionally be talked out of them). The muscles of the head and neck are predominantly affected, and the most commonly noted feature is macroglossia, with or without tongue protrusion, leading to difficulties in speaking and swallowing. The patient may be able to tell you that he is unable to speak or to swallow and then proceed to demonstrate this, again contributing to the feeling that this is an hysterical type of reaction. The masseter muscles may be tightly contracted so that the mouth cannot be opened and, on rare occasions, this can lead to damage to the teeth, tongue, or even the mandible. The possibility that such reactions can be fatal does exist, particularly if they occur during eating. The neck muscles are also frequently affected; thus, opisthotonus, torticollis, etc. can occur and may be associated with oculogyric crises. The back, arm, and leg muscles are less frequently affected, but when they are, the most bizarre gaits are noted, on occasion reminiscent of a "Frankenstein monster" walk.

Acute dystonic reactions usually take place within 24 to 48 hr of starting medication, although occasionally they take place when there is an increase in dosage. They are easily treated by injection of a wide variety of agents, e.g., antihistamines, barbiturates, phenothiazines, antiparkinson agents, caffeine, and sodium benzoate. Continued medication, however, is not required. Rare individuals (men more than women) continue to have these reactions from time to time and probably represent a separate or distinct group of people. The young and the brain-damaged seem predisposed to these recurring reactions.

Akathisia

Essentially akathisia is a restlessness that may be intense and is associated with an inability to sit still. Conventionally, it is associated with a subjective feeling of anxiety. The patient needs to walk up and down, and the restlessness can even interfere with his sleeping. In lesser varieties of akathisia, which are common in the early part of treatment, the subjective feelings of tension and anxiety are frequent and difficult for the patient to describe. Here, misdiagnoses can result in increasing medication, thus worsening the condition. In the more chronic conditions the subjective aspects are more difficult to elicit.

Akathisia usually occurs within a few days of starting medication. The administration of parenteral antiparkinson medication is indicated and can remove the symptoms almost immediately. It is as dramatic here as in the treatment of the acute dystonias. Continued antiparkinson medication is frequently not required (as in the dystonic reactions); this is true particularly for early akathisias. It should be noted, however, that the presence of akathisia, especially in outpatients, makes one much more inclined to continue antiparkinson medication, than does the isolated occurrence of a dystonic phenomenon. Late onset akathisia, which may begin weeks, months, or years after the onset of treatment, is much more difficult to treat; in fact, it is virtually untreatable. It may occur on its own, but the very late onset variety is frequently associated with tardive dyskinesia.

Pseudoparkinsonism

This condition, indistinguishable from postencephalitic parkinsonism, occurs at varying time intervals after commencing treatment. Like the dystonias, it can be patient- or drug-related. Thus, extremely high doses of medication can literally produce a parkinsonian picture within 24 hr. With the usual mode of prescribing medication, however, pseudoparkinsonism normally develops at the end of 2 to 3 weeks. The first signs are usually the loss of arm movements. Thus, although the patient may walk normally, he loses the swing of his arms. Perhaps associated with this is diminished facial movements and the appearance of a positive glabella tap response.

As the severity of the condition increases, complete loss of arm movements can develop, with flexion of the arms culminating in the classic stoop, shuffling gait with pill-rolling movements of the hands, and excessive salivation. The motor abnormalities are similar in every way to those associated with the postencephalitic or classic parkinsonism.

This particular extrapyramidal effect leads to difficulties in performing motor tasks and to typical cramping changes in handwriting. A full-blown picture is rarely seen because, unless one initiates treatment with high dosages of parenteral medication, such unwanted effects develop gradually, can be detected early, and antiparkinson medication can be added or the dosage reduced or both. Minor handwriting changes probably antedate all of these signs in the vast majority of patients.

Akinesia, a loss of all mobility, which occurs very early in treatment, is a side effect that is not always recognized (13). It is probably an early parkinsonian symptom, and the treatment is the same, i.e., reduction of dosage or even the addition of an antiparkinson agent as a treatment or diagnostic test.

Individual susceptibility to extrapyramidal side effects varies widely, but it is consistent within the patient. Thus, in one study (19), we found that the neuroleptic threshold (the dosage required to produce minimal effects) varied 200-fold across patients, but when the same drug was administered on a second occasion, in addition to finding a similar dosage range, it was clear that each patient's neuroleptic threshold was the same on the two occasions. This also holds true across the different neuroleptics and different chemical groups. In other words, the patient who develops extrapyramidal side effects on a low dosage of a phenothiazine will develop the same effects on low dosages of a butyrophenone or thioxanthene. There is also an age factor in terms of susceptibility: generally, the older the patient, the lower the dosage required to produce extrapyramidal side effects. This is distinct from idiosyncratic reactions.

When neuroleptics are discontinued, it has been shown that extrapyramidal side effects can be present for up to 3 months following the discontinuation (18). If an antiparkinson agent has been administered in conjunction with a neuroleptic and both are discontinued, there is frequently an upsurge in extrapyramidal side effects for several weeks following. Abrupt discontinuation of combinations of antiparkinson agents and neuroleptics can produce withdrawal effects (nausea, vomiting, rigidity, and tremor) that have occasionally been attributed to the neuroleptic. However, in several studies examining this issue, it was demonstrated that the offending agent was the antiparkinson medication (17,19).

The use of very high doses of neuroleptics (up to ten times the recommended dosage) was of considerable interest in the late 1960s, particularly in France. I personally examined patients of Lambert in Chambrey receiving from 400 to 800 mg of trifluoperazine/day. All of them had visible tremor, but none had any other signs of extrapyramidal disorders. Specifically, rigidity and akathisia were absent. I could not help but feel that our routine "small" amounts of neuroleptics "stimulate" the extrapyramidal system and that these large dosages, if anything, anesthetize it. The beneficial effects of high dosages have been confirmed recently by studies in the United States. Prien et al. (9,10) showed that patients receiving high dosages of chlorpromazine or of trifluoperazine did better than patients receiving lower doses. Both dosages were, however, fixed. Rifkin et al. (12), in addition to reviewing the literature, reported on a study employing high dosage neuroleptic treatment in a small series of patients. Their findings were similar to those of the French workers (5,6)—high dosages of fluphenazine caused no more side effects than low

dosages and did result in behavioral improvement in patients who had failed to respond to orthodox dosages. In a later controlled study (11), they were unable to confirm this. In another study, we were able to show that high dosages of fluphenazine (up to 800 mg/day) produced improvement in patients who had failed to respond to regular or routine, recommended dosages, but found that extrapyramidal effects were more frequent at high dosages (14). In any event, as long-term side effects of neuroleptics are now more widely recognized, very high dosages are not to be recommended. On the other hand, patients who do not respond at the neuroleptic threshold, that is, patients who are treatment failures, do warrant a trial on a high dosage regimen if treatment with orthodox dosages of the structurally different neuroleptics has failed.

Tardive Dyskinesia

Tardive dyskinesia, a "late onset" side effect, can develop some months after the institution of treatment but is more likely to occur following years of neuroleptic therapy. It is very difficult to obtain precise epidemiological data on the disorder, and estimates of its prevalence range up to 40% (4). However, the majority of studies have been carried out in hospitals where chronic patients (those with the highest risk) are the only ones left. Unfortunately, data are not so readily available on outpatients. Unquestionably in an elderly population who are at risk, a figure of 40% would not seem an exaggeration, whereas in a younger group who are still chronically institutionalized and receiving neuroleptics more or less continuously figures of under 20% are likely.

The disorder is characterized by a variety of involuntary movements involving the face, mouth, and tongue—the so-called buccolingual masticatory syndrome—which are frequently associated with choreoathetoid movements of the fingers and occasionally the arms and feet. Akathisia may also be present.

Tongue movements are usually the first sign of the disorder, although occasionally the condition begins with blinking, tics, and grimacing, which can be confused with schizophrenic illness. Exaggerated chewing movements or licking of the lips may be the next sign that progresses further to constant mouthing, chewing, pouting, and licking of lips as well as protrusion of the tongue. In some cases, the tongue movements can be very dramatic, e.g., the so-called fly catcher's tongue, where the tongue protrudes to a great extent and appears to curl up. Usually associated with this is the "bon-bon" sign, a protrusion of the cheek so named because it gives the impression that the patient is eating a candy or chewing a large wad of gum. Actually, it is the highly mobile tongue pushing against the cheek. This can be clearly seen if the patient is told to open his mouth; the tongue will continue to move and indeed will turn on its axis in a manner that could not be achieved voluntarily.

The oral movements may comprise the total picture, although they are often associated with mild movements of the fingers which at first may seem to be mannerisms or stereotyped behavior. These finger movements may progress to waving movements of the fingers and the toes (the toes may contract and relax continuously); in severe cases, the wrists and arms may be involved, culminating in movements similar to those seen in Huntington's chorea. Thus, the patient may have abrupt gross movements that end up in purposeful-like movements, e.g., patting down the hair, rubbing the face or legs. Other features may involve full-blown ballistic movements and rocking movements of the pelvis (axial hyperkinesis) which can produce various bizarre gyrations or copulatory types of movements. In some cases, the diaphragm may be involved, and breathing becomes complicated, often associated with grunting sounds. The akathisia frequently present may consist merely of constant swinging of the legs when crossed, but there may also be a rocking movement when the patient stands up or a continuous pacing up and down. This is often not associated with any feeling of discomfort (particularly in schizophrenics); indeed, many of the patients with tardive dyskinesia have no complaints whatsoever.

Long-term neuroleptic treatment is believed to be the primary causal factor, although individual susceptibility appears to play a role. Thus, elderly women are the most frequently affected, and there is some evidence organicity may be implicated (16). However, the condition can occur in younger people even on quite low dosages of neuroleptics, hence, in nonschizophrenic disorders, neuroleptics should be avoided. There is also evidence to suggest that the concomitant use of antiparkinson agents can exacerbate or precipitate this condition (7).

Treatment of the disorder presents many problems, and at the moment the only solution, albeit partial, is the judicious use of these agents. The most dramatic remissions occur following an increase in the dosage of neuroleptics, but ultimately symptom break-through occurs. In addition, this approach to treatment, in effect, contributes to the disorder while producing only a temporary remission at best. The use of lithium, deanol, clozapine, and other agents is still in an experimental stage. At the moment such treatments arise either from serendipitous findings (e.g., when a misdiagnosed manic, who has been treated as schizophrenic, develops a dyskinetic disorder, is evaluated and given lithium, and the disorder disappears), or from theories concerning the action of neuroleptics on dopamine or cholinergic fibers. The similarity, clinically, of the disorder to L-DOPA-induced dyskinesias and to Huntington's chorea has also stimulated interest and theories concerning etiology and treatment, but these are still in the very early stages. The best treatment, at the moment, is the gradual withdrawal of neuroleptics with the substitution of minor tranquilizers to relieve anxiety. The potential of neuroleptics to produce dyskinesia, a serious complication, in a considerable number of patients would indicate that an attempt should be made to withdraw neuroleptics in every patient. Many patients who have required medication in the past may have stabilized at a lower level of functioning and can manage without drugs. In others, it may at least be possible to decrease the dosage to a minimum.

The fact that tardive dyskinesia generally develops after many years of neuroleptic therapy following a trial on almost every drug and drug combination available makes it almost impossible to determine the potential of the individual neuroleptic for inducing dyskinetic syndromes.

All neuroleptics currently on the market produce extrapyramidal side effects, and it is hypothesized that the development of dyskinesias may be related to the extrapyramidal side effect potential. Clozapine, a new antipsychotic agent which is available in Europe, has been shown to be therapeutically active but is without extrapyramidal side effects (16). This compound has also been shown to suppress dyskinetic symptoms and may well be the treatment of choice for schizophrenics with tardive dyskinesia (20). It is possible it may not produce dyskinesias during long-term therapy. Certainly one direction psychopharmacology should take is the development of drugs free of these disabling and unpleasant side effects.

Finally, neuroleptics can produce behavioral toxicity. These effects fortunately are not too frequent but are quite important. Perhaps the most common is a toxic confusional state, which is more likely to appear in the elderly or at the beginning of treatment. Typically, the patient is excited and hallucinated with confusion and dis-

orientation; reduction in the dosage of the medication or the antiparkinson agent (if it is being administered concomitantly) may be all that is required. Alternately, a more potent and therefore less anticholinergic drug may be added. Occasionally, an exacerbation of psychotic symptoms is seen at the beginning of treatment that really represents an exaggeration of the underlying illness and can easily be dealt with by rapidly increasing the dosage. A more difficult-to-diagnose syndrome is that where too much of a neuroleptic is being administered. The patient in this case may *seem* to have an exaggeration of his illness, although in this case there is a clouding component, with confusional, infantile, demanding, histrionic behavior frequently compounding the already existing psychotic behavior. The treatment consists in the withdrawal of medication, and improvement usually takes place in a few days. Catatonic type behavior has been described (8), as have other types of mute behavior (2) [including akinetic mutism (1)] and psychotic exacerbations associated with extrapyramidal symptoms (21). These usually respond to antiparkinson medication. A comprehensive description of behavioral abnormalities can be found in an earlier study of mine (15).

SUMMARY

The neurotoxicity of major tranquilizers embraces a variety of symptoms and syndromes, the most ubiquitous being the extrapyramidal effects. These manifestations, including tardive dyskinesia, are described in detail. Other more idiosyncratic effects of the drugs are discussed together with several types of behavioral toxicities. The treatment of these effects are included.

REFERENCES

1. Angus, J. W. S., and Simpson, G. M. (1970): Hysteria and drug induced dystonia. *Acta Psychiatr. Scand. [Suppl.]*, 212:25–58.

2. Behrman, S. (1972): Mutism induced by phenothiazines. *Br. J. Psychiatry*, 121:599–604.
3. Brill, H., and Patton, R. E. (1962): Clinical statistical analysis of population changes in New York State mental hospitals since the introduction of psychotropic drugs. *Am. J. Psychiatry*, 119:20–35.
4. Crane, G. D. (1973): Persistent dyskinesia. *Br. J. Psychiatry*, 122:395–406.
5. Fouks, L. (1967): Originalite et specificite de la fluphenazine. In: *Proc. Vth Congr. Neuropsychopharmacol., Washington, D.C., 1966*, pp. 1128–1134. Int. Congr. Ser., No. 192. Excerpta Medica, Amsterdam.
6. Gayral, L., and Lambert, P. (1967): La dichorhyrate de fluphenazine: Etude des doses eleves et des traitments de longue duree. In: *Proc. Vth Int. Congr. Neuropsychopharmacol., Washington, D.C., 1966*, pp. 1128–1134. Int. Congr. Ser., No. 129. Excerpta Medica, Amsterdam.
7. Kiloh, L. G., Smith, J. S., and Williams, S. E. (1973): Antiparkinson drugs as causal agents in tardive dyskinesia. *Med. J. Aust.*, 2:591–593.
8. May, P. H. (1959): Catatonic-like states following phenothiazine therapy. *Am. J. Psychiatry*, 115(12):1119–1120.
9. Prien, R. F., and Cole, J. O. (1968): High dose chlorpromazine therapy in chronic schizophrenia. *Arch. Gen. Psychiatry*, 18:482–495.
10. Prien, R. F., Levine, J., and Cole, J. O. (1969): High dose trifluoperazine therapy in chronic schizophrenia. *Am. J. Psychiatry*, 126:305–313.
11. Quitkin, F., Rifkin, A., and Klein, D. F. (1975): A double-blind study of very high dosage vs. standard dosage fluphenazine in non-chronic treatment-refractory schizophrenics. *Arch. Gen. Psychiatry*, 32(10):1276–1281.
12. Rifkin, A., Quitkin, F., Carrillo, C., and Klein, D. F. (1971): Very high dosage fluphenazine for non-chronic treatment-refractory patients. *Arch. Gen. Psychiatry*, 25:5,398–403.
13. Rifkin, A., Quitkin, F., and Klein, D. F. (1975): Akinesia: a poorly recognized drug induced extrapyramidal behavioral disorder. *Arch. Gen. Psychiatry*, 32:672–674.
14. Sanseigne, A., and Simpson, G. M.: A comparison of high and low dosage fluphenazine. (*Unpublished manuscript.*)
15. Simpson, G. M. (1975): CNS effects of neuroleptics. *Psychiatr. Ann.*, 5:53.
16. Simpson, G. M. (1974): Prognosis and diagnosis of tardive dyskinesia. Presented at: *Collegium Int. Neuropsychopharmacol. Congr., Paris*.
17. Simpson, G. M., Amin, M., and Kunz, E. (1965): Withdrawal effects of phenothiazines. *Compr. Psychiatry*, 6:347–351.
18. Simpson, G. M., Amuso, D., Blair, J. H., and Farkas, T. (1964): Pheothiazine-produced extrapyramidal system disturbance. *Arch. Gen. Psychiatry*, 10:199–208.
19. Simpson, G. M., and Kunz-Bartholini, E. (1970): The relationship of individual tolerance, behavior, and phenothiazine-produced extrapyramidal system disturbance. *Acta Psychiat. Scand.*, 212:52–55.
20. Simpson, G. M., and Varga E. (1974): Clozapine —A new antipsychotic agent. *Curr. Ther. Res.*, 16(7):679–686.
21. Van Putten, T., Mutalipassi, L. R., and Malkin, M. D. (1974): Phenothiazine-induced decompensation. *Arch. Gen. Psychiatry*, 30:102–105.

Neurotoxicology, edited by L. Roizin, H. Shiraki, and N. Grčević. Raven Press, New York © 1977.

Pharmacokinetics of Therapeutic and Toxic Reactions: I. Phenothiazines

James M. Perel and Albert A. Manian

Department of Psychiatry, Columbia University, College of Physicians and Surgeons, and the New York State Psychiatric Institute, New York, New York 10032; Psychopharmacology Research Branch, National Institute of Mental Health, Rockville, Maryland 20852

The therapeutic effectiveness of a psychoactive agent depends on its interaction with tissue sites. Therefore, factors that influence the concentration at the "receptor" site, such as rates and sites of absorption, plasma and tissue levels, plasma and tissue protein bindings, rates and routes of metabolism (biotransformation), and excretion, play an integral part in determining the quality and duration of drug action (Fig. 1).

In common with other drugs, phenothiazines such as chlorpromazine, undergo extensive metabolism mainly via hepatic and intestinal microsomal mixed function oxygenases through the participation of cytochrome P-450 and its variant hemoprotein, cytochrome P-448, electron transport systems (19,24). Forrest et al. (11) were among the first to demonstrate that oxidative biotransformation leads to a large number of different sulfoxides, aromatic hydroxy, N-desmethyl, and N-oxide (partially microsomal) metabolites. With the exception of the inactive sulfoxides, the metabolites show varying degrees of potential antipsychotic effects so that the total therapeutic action of a phenothiazine is a composite of the activities from the parent compound and products, as indicated by the work of Mackay et al. (16) and Axelsson et al. (1).

Due to the wide individual variation of response to each unit of oral dose, the more recent therapeutic studies of chlorpromazine have sought a correlation between response and blood levels of parent compound and selected metabolites. A wide range of concentrations have been found in patients given similar doses of chlorpromazine. This variation appears to be primarily related to individual differences in drug oxidation and secondarily to differences in rates of absorption. At present, as shown in Table 1, two main conclusions appear to be emerging: (a) patients producing mainly active metabolites respond better than the ones producing inactive metabolites although the plasma levels of chlorpromazine itself might be similar (16,21), and (b) optimal therapeutic ranges have been found for plasma chlorpromazine and presumably tissue concentrations *below* and *above* which treatment fails, i.e., a curvilinear relationship with a defined "therapeutic window" (8,20). Those patients who manifested toxicity in the form

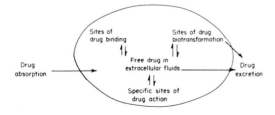

FIG. 1. Schematic representation of drug kinetics with possible sites of interaction in the body.

TABLE 1. *Average plasma concentrations (ng/ml) of chlorpromazine (CPZ) and its metabolites — their relationship to therapeutic control*

Global control	CPZ	CPZ	7-OH-CPZ	7-OH-CPZ / CPZ	7-OH-CPZ / CPZ-SO
Poor	59 ± 20 (10)	61 ± 21 (10)	26 ± 11 (4)	0.75 ± 0.02 (4)	0.4 ± 0.1 (4)
Moderate	46 ± 9 (26)	41 ± 9 (26)	34 ± 4 (11)	1.0 ± 0.2 (11)	0.8 ± 0.1 (11)
Good	30 ± 6 (36)	19 ± 4 (36)	42 ± 7 (8)	1.2 ± 0.3 (8)	2.2 ± 0.3 (8)
			Range plasma CPZ (ng/ml)		
Response			50–300; 30–400		
Poor or no response		< 30–50		500; 700–1,000*	

Based on Curry (8), Rivera-Calimlin et al. (20), and MacKay et al. (16). Values inside parentheses are number of patients.
* Toxicity manifested by tremors and convulsions.

of tremors and convulsions were shown to have very high plasma levels (750 to 1,000 ng/ml). All these findings should still be viewed as tentative, because other reports such as Kolakowska et al. (14) have not found a relationship between therapeutic effects and plasma chlorpromazine levels; furthermore, there is a disagreement on whether 7-hydroxychlorpromazine is present in more than small quantities in the plasma of responding patients (9).

Although chlorpromazine is extensively bound to human serum proteins (mostly albumin), Bickel (2) has determined that the values of binding affinity and capacity to microsomes are much higher than those of serum proteins, so that intracellular localization would be strongly favored. The high lipid solubility would further enhance the passive transport of the "free" or unbound form of the drug into tissues (7,10). During chronic treatment (steady-state), binding to tissue constituents is important in determining the overall pharmacokinetics because the calculated apparent volume of distribution (V_{dss}), obtained by using a two-compartment model, is a measure of tissue localization; the larger volumes of distributions (average 11.2 liters/kg) are obtained with patients having lower bindings to plasma proteins. One of the consequences is that, in these patients, there is greater

concentration of chlorpromazine and less polar metabolites in the brain as measured in cerebrospinal fluid samples. Also, fluctuations in chlorpromazine concentrations are probably caused by small changes in protein binding that lead to redistribution of the drug into tissues. The significance of those changes has been treated theoretically by Curry (6).

Information has been recently obtained indicating that red blood cell (RBC) binding of chlorpromazine might be a better indicator of therapeutic effectiveness and toxic reactions (12,15). Manian et al. (15) speculated that stronger chlorpromazine binding by RBC could explain a lack of response on the part of a patient because transfer of the drug molecule to the receptor site of the brain would be thermodynamically unfavorable. This explanation received support from Garver and associates (12) when they found that RBC butaperazine levels differentiated better in those subjects in whom dystonias would develop than in those in whom they did not. Dystonic reactions occurred in patients with slower rates of butaperazine disappearance from RBC.

The pharmacokinetics of tissue localization are also important in elucidating the mechanisms of toxic reactions. The recent finding of 7,8-dihydroxychlorpromazine as an urinary metabolite in schizophrenic patients on long-term therapy (22) provides an opportunity for postulating the formation of a reactive intermediate in the hydroxylation. As shown in Fig. 2, a reactive arene oxide, the 7,8-epoxide, would be initially formed by microsomal oxidation. This intermediate rearranges non- enzymatically to the 7-hydroxy and/or 8-hydroxy metabolite; and/or would react with glutathione for the eventual formation of nontoxic premercapturic acids; and/or be attacked by epoxidehydrase (microsomal) to form diols that, in turn, become the observed 7,8-dihydroxy-chlorpromazine; and/or covalently bind

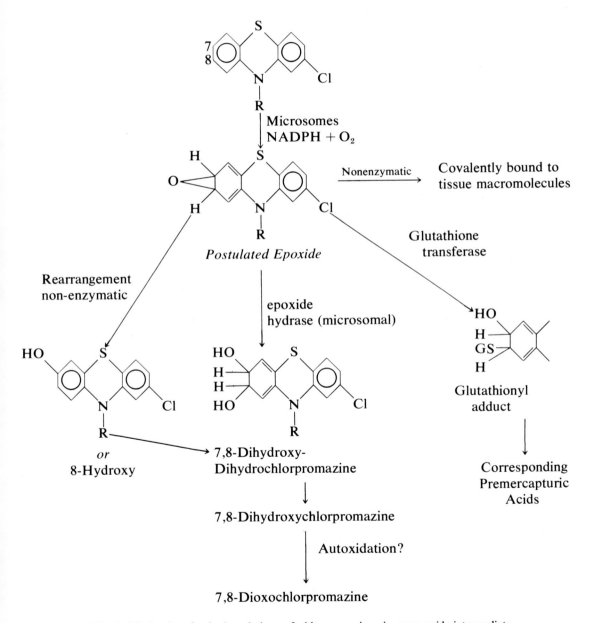

FIG. 2. Mechanism for hydroxylations of chlorpromazine via arene oxide intermediate.

with the sulfhydryl groups in tissue macro-molecules (13). The formation of potentially toxic metabolites such as the 7,8-dihydroxy and the production of covalently-bonded adducts to tissue components (3,23) would provide an explanation and perhaps a treatment for some of the observed toxicity of phenothiazines. The use of glutathione as described by Mitchell et al. (18) would channel the overall metabolic pathway into the formation of relatively nontoxic premercapturic acids.

In view of the toxic effects of phenothiazines during therapy, it is of importance that soluble proteins, particularly serum proteins and cytoplasmic proteins of the liver, have been shown to irreversibly bind phenothiazines and/or its metabolites. It can be assumed that the irreversibly protein-bound molecule, when present in the blood stream, has a haptenic property and that antibodies are formed against this drug in the body during therapy.

There is evidence that toxic neurologic effects, such as dystonic reactions and tardive dyskinesias, are more directly related to the accumulation of the parent phenothiazine at critical functional central nervous sites (5). In general, it appears that the incidence of tardive dyskinesia increases directly with the total amount of phenothiazine received, regardless of the mode of administration. Thus, McAndrew et al. (17) showed that the median drug intake, expressed as chlorpromazine equivalents, was 403 g over a median of 32.5 months for dyskinetic children versus 8.7 g over 3.9 months in the nondyskinetic group. There is also evidence for central nervous system tissue damage in adults. Christensen et al. (4) studied 28 brains from neuroleptically treated schizophrenic patients who, at the time of death, were manifesting oral dyskinesia. They found cell degeneration in the substantia nigra of 27 of the 28 and gliosis in the midbrain and brainstem of 25 of 28. Untreated controls had degeneration in seven of 28 and abnormalities in the mid-

brain and brainstem of four of the 28 controls.

On the 25th anniversary of the introduction of chlorpromazine as an antipsychotic agent, we find that its mechanisms of therapeutic and toxic effects are far from established. Nevertheless, by striving to learn about the bases of its clinical effects we are hopefully setting the necessary scientific foundations for the more accurate evaluations and studies of other future neuroleptics.

ACKNOWLEDGMENT

The work reported here has been supported in part by USPHS grant no. MH-17044.

REFERENCES

1. Axelsson, S., Jönsson, S., and Nordgreen, L. (1975): Cerebrospinal fluid levels of chlorpromazine and its metabolites in schizophrenia. *Arch. Psychiatr. Nervenkr.*, 221:167–170.
2. Bickel, M. H. (1974): Binding of phenothiazines and related compounds to tissues and cell constituents. *Adv. Biochem. Psychopharmacol.*, 9:163–166.
3. Bolt, A. G., and Forrest, I. S. (1968): Metabolic studies of chlorpromazine induced hyperpigmentation of the skin in psychiatric patients. *Agressologie*, 9:201–207.
4. Christensen, E., Møeller, J. E. and Faurbye, A. (1970): Neuropathological investigation of 28 brains from patients with dyskinesia. *Acta Psychiatr. Scand.*, 46:14–23.
5. Crane, G. E. (1973): Persistent dyskinesia. *Br. J. Psychiatry*, 122:395–495.
6. Curry, S. H. (1970): Theoretical changes in drug distribution resulting from changes in binding to plasma proteins and to tissues. *J. Pharm. Pharmacol.*, 22:753–757.
7. Curry, S. H. (1972): Relation between binding to plasma protein, apparent volume of distribution, and rate constants of disposition and elimination for chlorpromazine in three species. *J. Pharm. Pharmacol.*, 24:818–819.
8. Curry, S. H. (1976): Gas chromatographic methods for the study of chlorpromazine and some of its metabolites in human plasma. *Psychopharmacol. Commun.*, 2:1–15.
9. Curry, S. H., and Evans, S. (1975): Assay of 7-hydroxychlorpromazine, and failure to detect more than small quantities, in plasma of responding schizophrenics. *Psychopharmacol. Commun.*, 1:481–490.

10. Dayton, P. G., and Perel, J. M. (1973): Influence of binding on drug metabolism and distribution. *Ann. NY. Acad. Sci.,* 226:172–194.

11. Forrest, I. S., Bolt, A. G., and Aber, R. C. (1968): Metabolic pathways for the detoxication of chlorpromazine in various mammalian species. *Agressologie,* 9:259–263.

12. Garver, D. L., Davis, J. M., DeKirmenjian, H., Jones, F. D., Casper, R., and Haraszti, J. (1976): Pharmacokinetics of red blood cell phenothiazine and clinical effects. *Arch. Gen. Psychiatry,* 33:862–866.

13. Gillette, J. R. (1975): Formation of reactive drug metabolites as a basis of drug action and toxicity. *Isr. J. Chem.,* 14:193–204.

14. Kolakowska, T., Wiles, D. H., Gelder, M. G., and McNeilly, A. S. (1976): Clinical significance of plasma chlorpromazine levels. *Psychopharmacol.,* 49:101–107.

15. Manian, A. A., Piette, L. H., Holland, D., Grover, T., and Leterrier, F. (1974): Red blood cell drug binding as a possible mechanism for tranquilization. *Adv. Biochem. Psychopharmacol.,* 9:149–161.

16. MacKay, H. V. P., Healey, H. F., and Baker, J. (1974): The relationship of plasma chlorpromazine to its 7-hydroxy and sulphoxy metabolites in a large population of chronic schizophrenics. *Br. J. Clin. Pharmacol.,* 1:425–430.

17. McAndrew, J. B., Case, Q., and Treffert, D. A. (1972): Effects of prolonged phenothiazine intake on psychotic and other hospitalized children. *J. Autism Child. Schizo.,* 2:75–91.

18. Mitchell, J. R., Jollow, D. J., Potter, W. Z., Gillette, J. R., and Brodie, B. B. (1973): Acetoaminophen-induced hepatic necrosis. IV. Protective role of glutathione. *J. Pharmacol. Exp. Therap.,* 187:211–217.

19. Perel, J. M., O'Brien, L., Black, N. B., Bellward, G., and Dayton, P. G. (1974): Imipramine and chlorpromazine in hepatic microsomal systems. *Adv. Biochem. Psychopharmacol.,* 9:201–212.

20. Rivera-Calimlin, L., Nasrallah, H., Strauss, J., and Lasagna, L. (1976): Clinical response and plasma levels: Effect of dose, dosage schedules, and drug interactions on plasma chlorpromazine levels. *Am. J. Psychiatry,* 133:646–652.

21. Sakalis, G., Curry, S. H., Mould, G. P., and Lader, M. H. (1972): Physiologic and clinical effects of chlorpromazine and their relationship to plasma level. *Clin. Pharmacol. Ther.,* 13: 931–946.

22. Turano, P., Turner, W. J., and Manian, A. (1973): Thin-layer chromatography of chloropromazine metabolites. Attempt to identify each of the metabolites appearing in blood, urine and feces of chronically medicated schizophrenics. *J. Chromagr.,* 75:277–293.

23. Van Woert, M. H. (1968): Isolation of chlorpromazine pigments in man. *Nature,* 219:1054–1056.

24. Wattenberg, L. W., and Leong, J. L. (1965): Effects of phenothiazines on protective systems against polycyclic hydrocarbons. *Cancer Res.,* 25:365–370.

Neurotoxicology, edited by L. Roizin, H. Shiraki, and N. Grčević. Raven Press, New York © 1977.

Selective Neurotoxicity of 6-Hydroxydopamine

S. Garattini and R. Samanin

Istituto di Ricerche Farmacologiche 'Mario Negri,' Via Eritrea, 62, 20157 Milan, Italy

EFFECTS OF 6-HYDROXYDOPAMINE ON CATECHOLAMINES — MECHANISM OF ACTION

When injected into the cerebral ventricles, 6-hydroxydopamine (6-OHDA) produces a long-lasting depletion of norepinephrine and dopamine in various parts of the central nervous system (CNS) (62). Tyrosine hydroxylase (7,62) and dopamine β-hydroxylase (44) as well as the uptake of catecholamines into the nerve terminals are found to be similarly reduced by 6-OHDA (7,34).

In analogy with observations made in the periphery (57,58), these effects have been attributed to a degeneration of catecholamine-containing neurons, as suggested by the fact that electron microscopic signs of neuronal degeneration and disappearance of specific fluorescence in brain areas rich in catecholaminergic terminals have been observed in animals injected intracerebrally with 6-OHDA (6,36,60).

The intimate mechanism by which 6-OHDA produces this effect is not yet completely understood. The formation of oxidative products of 6-OHDA that can undergo covalent binding with nucleophilic groups of some important constituents of the neuronal membrane is considered the most likely mechanism of its neurotoxic action (9,51,52).

The formation of hydrogen peroxide can also contribute to the degeneration of neuronal elements (20,21). In order to exert its destructive effects on catecholamine-containing neurons, it appears necessary that 6-OHDA be accumulated into the neurons, as indicated by the fact that drugs interfering with the membrane transport mechanism for norepinephrine and other phenylethylamines completely prevent the effect of 6-OHDA on noradrenergic neurons (8,27).

Moreover the cytoplasmic concentrations of 6-OHDA appear to be of greater importance than the binding of 6-OHDA into the granules in determining its destructive effects, since reserpine, which prevents the binding of 6-OHDA to the storage granules, does not significantly modify the effect of 6-OHDA (29,35,36).

SPECIFICITY OF 6-OHDA

With the exception of a reported decrease of serotonin (5-HT) in cats (42), the action of 6-OHDA on catecholamine is rather selective since no changes in brain levels of acetylcholine (ACh), γ-aminobutyric acid (GABA), and other central putative transmitters have been reported following the intracerebral administration of 6-OHDA (26). Table 1 reports the selective effect of 6-OHDA on catecholamine with respect to 5-HT and ACh in the rat brain. On the other hand, it should be considered that 6-OHDA can produce a general toxic effect of neuronal elements, and

TABLE 1. *The effect of an intraventricular injection of 6-OHDA on brain levels of norepinephrine, dopamine, 5-HT, and ACh in the rat*

Treatment	Brain levels (μg/g $\pm$ SE)			
	NE	DA	5-HT	ACh
Vehicle	0.44 ± 0.02	1.11 ± 0.06	0.43 ± 0.02	2.18 ± 0.05
6-OHDA (2×200 μg)	0.06 ± 0.02^a	0.52 ± 0.05^a	0.45 ± 0.02	2.13 ± 0.04

Each value is the mean $\pm$ SE of six animals. NE, norepinephrine; DA, dopamine.

The two doses of 6-OHDA were administered at an interval of 24 hr. Biochemical determinations were performed 10 days after the last injection. 6-OHDA was dissolved in 20 μl of saline containing ascorbic acid (0.1 mg/ml).

Norepinephrine and dopamine were determined according to the method of Chang (9) and Laverty and Taylor (33). 5-HT was assayed according to the method of Giacalone and Valzelli (18). ACh was measured radiochemically according to the method of Saelens et al. (46).

[a] $p < 0.01$ when compared with vehicle (Student's t-test).

its specificity of action is the result of its specific accumulation into catecholamine-containing nerve terminals. Therefore, particularly when it is applied directly into cerebral tissue, 6-OHDA can produce unspecific damage if precautions such as appropriate dose/volume ratio, composition of the vehicle, and others are not considered carefully. Accurate studies have been performed in order to establish the best conditions to minimize the risk of unspecific damage to neuronal tissue (1,22).

Despite this selective effect of 6-OHDA on catecholamine neurons, biochemical changes, particularly in the serotonergic system, have been reported in animals treated with 6-OHDA. Thus an increase of brain 5-HT synthesis and 5-hydroxy-indolacetic acid (5-HIAA) levels have been found after an intracerebral injection of 6-OHDA in rats (5).

However, in agreement with the hypothesis of a relationship between noradrenergic and serotonergic neurons in the brain (49), these changes have been considered a consequence of the action on noradrenergic neurons rather than a direct effect on 5-HT. Therefore in experiments using 6-OHDA the possibility of secondary changes in the serotonergic system should be considered in interpreting the various results.

MODULATION OF THE EFFECTS OF 6-OHDA ON CATECHOLAMINE

When injected intraventricularly or intracisternally, 6-OHDA is much more effective in reducing brain norepinephrine than brain dopamine. The reasons for this difference are not clear. A higher affinity of 6-OHDA for the membrane transport in the noradrenergic than in dopaminergic neurons (23), a different anatomical distribution of catecholamine neurons, different intraneuronal concentrations or distribution of catecholamines in their respective nerve terminals, or both, have been considered possible factors (45).

It has been found that pretreatment with a monoamine oxidase inhibitor markedly potentiates that effect of 6-OHDA on dopamine, probably because 6-OHDA is also metabolized by this enzyme (8,28). Because of the higher sensitivity of norepinephrine neurons to the action of 6-OHDA, small (25 to 50 μg), repeated doses of this compound, applied intraventricularly, produce a marked reduction of brain norepinephrine levels with little or no effect on brain dopamine (24).

On the other hand, it is possible to obtain a selective decrease of brain dopamine by injecting 6-OHDA into animals pretreated with desipramine which, as men-

TABLE 2. *The effect of various intraventricular 6-OHDA treatments on the levels of norepinephrine and dopamine in the rat brain*

Treatment	Brain levels ($\mu g/g \pm SE$)	
	NE	DA
Vehicle	0.40 ± 0.04	1.12 ± 0.15
6-OHDA		
3 × 25 μg[a]	0.12 ± 0.02[e]	0.98 ± 0.06
2 × 250 μg[b]	0.06 ± 0.01[e]	0.46 ± 0.06[e]
Pargyline + 250 μg[c]	0.06 ± 0.01[e]	0.26 ± 0.05[e]
DMI + 250 μg[d]	0.38 ± 0.02	0.46 ± 0.04[e]

Each value is the mean ± SE of six animals. Biochemical determinations were performed 10 days after the last injection. NE, norepinephrine; DA, dopamine; DMI, desipramine.

6-OHDA was dissolved in 20 μl of saline containing ascorbic acid (0.1 mg/ml) and administered intraventricularly according to the method of Noble et al. (41).

[a] The doses of 6-OHDA were administered at intervals of 2 days.

[b] An interval of 24 hr between the two doses was used.

[c] Pargyline was administered intraperitoneally at a dose of 50 mg/kg 30 min before 6-OHDA.

[d] DMI (30 mg/kg) was injected intraperitoneally 1 hr before the 6-OHDA administration.

[e] $p < 0.01$ when compared with vehicle (Duncan's Test).

tioned before, completely prevents the decrease of brain norepinephrine induced by 6-OHDA (8,27).

These possibilities for modulating the effect of 6-OHDA on catecholamine neurons constitute a useful tool for producing a selective degeneration of norepinephrine or dopamine neurons in the brain and for contributing to the clarification of the differential role of catecholamine in various situations (32).

Table 2 summarizes some intraventricular 6-OHDA treatments and their effect on brain catecholamine.

In order to obtain a selective effect on either norepinephrine or dopamine, 6-OHDA has been applied directly in areas particularly rich in noradrenergic or dopaminergic neurons.

Thus the injection of small quantities of 6-OHDA at the level of the ventral or dorsal noradrenergic bundles, or both, in the mesencephalon produces a marked selective decrease of norepinephrine in various brain areas (16). On the other hand, the application of 6-OHDA at the level of the nigrostriatal dopaminergic bundle or in areas rich in dopaminergic terminals such as the corpus striatum and the nucleus accumbens produces a marked decrease of dopamine in these areas with little or no effects on the levels of brain norepinephrine, particularly if the animals were pretreated with desipramine (1,22,25).

In Table 3 are shown the effects on catecholamine of various intracerebral injections of 6-OHDA.

As mentioned before, when 6-OHDA is applied directly to cerebral tissue, particular care should be taken to minimize the unspecific tissue damage produced by this drug.

BEHAVIORAL EFFECTS OF 6-OHDA

Various effects produced by an intraventricular injection of 6-OHDA have been described. These include a reserpine-like syndrome, hypothermia, food and water intake reduction, increased irritability, decrease of locomotion and exploratory activity, and others (28). Although no complete homogeneity exists among the various authors in describing the presence and the characteristics of these signs, there is general agreement that, with the possible exception of the increased irritability and the decrease of exploratory activity (32,40) most signs disappear within a period of a few hours or days, so that 7 to 10 days after the 6-OHDA administration the gross behavior of animals appears largely normal in spite of the low levels of brain catecholamine. The reasons for the recovery of normal behavior in a relatively short period of time are not known. Among the various explanations, the development of a state of

TABLE 3. *The effect of an injection of 6-OHDA at the level of the dorsal–ventral norepinephrine bundles or into the striatum on brain catecholamines in the rat*

Site of injection	6-OHDA (one side)	Amine levels (μg/g + SE)			
		Striatum	n. Accumbens	Hypothalamus	Telencephalon
		DA		NE	
Controls	–	9.26 ± 0.42	6.50 ± 0.32	1.25 ± 0.08	0.42 ± 0.02
Dorsal-ventral norepinephrine bundles	$2 \times 4\ \mu$g	9.84 ± 0.75	6.12 ± 0.40	0.18 ± 0.02^b	0.08 ± 0.01
Striatum[a]	$2 \times 20\ \mu$g	0.45 ± 0.02^b	4.20 ± 0.37^b	1.30 ± 0.09	0.40 ± 0.01

Each value is the mean ± SE of six animals. 6-OHDA was administered in a constant ratio of 2 μg/1 μl and was delivered at the rate of 1 μl/min. The following stereotaxic coordinates (from König and Klippel, ref. 31) were used for the 6-OHDA injections:
Dorsal NE bundle   A + 2.2   L 0.8   H −0.6;   Ventral NE bundle   A + 1   L 1.3   H −1.9;
Striatum   A + 7.9   L 2.6   H +0.5 and   A +7.9   L 2.6   H +0.5
Biochemical determinations were performed 15 days after the 6-OHDA administration. NE, norepinephrine; DA, dopamine; DMI, desipramine.
[a] These animals received DMI (30 mg/kg i.p.) 1 hr before the 6-OHDA administration.
[b] $p < 0.01$ when compared with vehicle (Duncan's test).

supersensitivity of postsynaptic receptors in the dopaminergic or noradrenergic system, or both, has been postulated as the most likely mechanism of the functional compensation. Although this phenomenon has been directly observed in the periphery (11,19), some indirect evidence suggests that it can be present also in the CNS. A situation in which this phenomenon has been postulated as operative in the CNS is the rotational model, first described by Ungerstedt and Arbuthnott (61).

Rats, injected unilaterally with 6-OHDA into the substantia nigra or at the level of the ascending dopaminergic nigrostriatal bundle show a strong rotational behavior following the administration of various stimulant drugs. In particular it has been observed that amphetamine and apomorphine make the animals turn, respectively, toward the ipsilateral- and controlateral-lesioned side (59). The explanation offered for these different effects is the following: amphetamine, which acts mainly by releasing dopamine from the presynaptic terminals, stimulates the side with intact dopamine neurons, making the animals turn toward the opposite side (i.e., the lesioned one). On the contrary, apomorphine, which acts mainly by stimulating directly the dopamine receptors, stimulates preferentially the lesioned side, revealing the developed supersensitivity in the degenerated dopaminergic system. An increase of stereotyped behavior induced by apomorphine (38) as well as an increase of dopamine-stimulated adenylate cyclase in the striatum of rats treated intracerebrally with 6-OHDA (37) have also been considered evidence of denervation supersensitivity.

Much more dramatic behavioral changes are observed in animals receiving a bilateral injection of 6-OHDA in the substantia nigra or at various levels of the dopamine nigrostriatal system. Soon after the 6-OHDA administration these animals develop such severe aphagia, adipsia, and hypokinesia that most of them would normally die if not fed intragastrically. These findings have led to the suggestion that the dopamine nigrostriatal system can be involved in the regulation of eating and drinking, although the extent by which the consumatory behavior is influenced by the impairment of motor behavior observed in these animals is not yet clear.

6-OHDA AS A TOOL TO STUDY THE INTERACTION OF PSYCHOTROPIC DRUGS WITH BRAIN CATECHOLAMINES

Despite the above discussed limitations, an appropriate use of 6-OHDA makes it a very useful tool to investigate the interaction between various drugs and brain catecholamines. Particularly interesting are some recent findings on the differential role of brain norepinephrine and dopamine in the pharmacological actions of amphetamine.

On the basis of comparisons between the potencies of (+) and (−)amphetamine in producing biochemical and behavioral effects, it has been suggested that norepinephrine is selectively involved in the increase of locomotor activity induced by amphetamine (54). However, further studies did not confirm this hypothesis (53,55). Recent experiments in which 6-OHDA was injected intracerebrally in either noradrenergic or dopaminergic brain areas clearly suggest a preferential role of brain dopamine in the stereotypy and increase of locomotion induced by amphetamine (3,30,43, 56).

In particular we have found that an intrastriatal injection of 6-OHDA in rats pre-treated with desipramine, which protects the noradrenergic neurons from the action of 6-OHDA, reduces both these effects of amphetamine without affecting significantly the anoretic effect (Table 4).

It has been found recently that an intraventricular injection of 6-OHDA in rats pretreated with pargyline markedly antagonizes the anoretic effect of amphetamine (14,48). These findings, together with the fact that the anoretic effect of amphetamine is found to be reduced in rats with selective lesions of noradrenergic neurons in the brain (2), appear to suggest a preferential role for brain norepinephrine in amphetamine anorexia. However, various authors have found antagonism towards amphetamine anorexia with some neuroleptics believed to exert a specific effect in blocking dopamine receptors in the brain (10,15). Therefore the exact role of brain norepinephrine and dopamine in the anoretic action needs to be further explored.

6-OHDA has been also used to investigate the possible interaction of morphine with brain catecholamine, but the results have been less consistent. Thus potentiation or antagonism of morphine analgesia has been found in animals injected intraventricularly with 6-OHDA (4,47). This difference appears to be due mainly to the

TABLE 4. *The effect of an intrastriatal injection of 6-OHDA on various pharmacological effects of (+) amphetamine*

Experimental group	Food intake (g/rat/2 hr ± SE)	Stereotypy[a] (proportion of positive animals)	Locomotor activity[b] (counts/10 min ± SE)
Vehicle			
Saline	8.0 ± 0.4	0/6	−
(+)Amphetamine	2.4 ± 0.3[c]	10/10	203 ± 26
6-OHDA			
Saline	8.8 ± 0.7	0/6	−
(+)Amphetamine	3.9 ± 0.4	0/10[d]	110 ± 20[d]

6-OHDA (20 μg × 2) was administered bilaterally in the striatum, and the experiments were performed 10 days after. (+)Amphetamine sulphate was administered intraperitoneally at doses of 1.5, 2.5, and 10 mg/kg, respectively, for locomotor activity, food intake, and stereotypy.

[a] Animals showing continuous licking, biting, or gnawing 120 min after amphetamine were considered positive.
[b] Recorded by an actometer (Basile, Italy) 30 min after the injection of (+)amphetamine sulphate.
[c] $p < 0.01$ when compared with saline.
[d] $p < 0.01$ when compared with the vehicle group receiving (+)amphetamine.

TABLE 5. *The effect of various 6-OHDA treatments on morphine analgesia in the rat*

Treatment	Analgesic index $\pm$ SE
Vehicle	0.62 ± 0.08
Intraventricular 6-OHDA	
2 $\times$ 250 μg	0.90 ± 0.05^a
Pargyline + 250 μg	0.35 ± 0.02^a
DMI + 250 μg	0.32 ± 0.04^a
Intrastriatal 6-OHDA	
2 $\times$ 20 μg	0.40 ± 0.02^a

Each value is the mean $\pm$ SE of eight animals. See Tables 2 and 3 for details of the 6-OHDA treatments. DMI, desipramine.

A dose of 5 mg/kg s.c. of morphine hydrochloride was used. The analgesic effect was evaluated according to the tail compression. Test previously described (From Samanin et al., ref. 50). The analgesic index was calculated according to the method described by Cox et al. (12).

[a] $p < 0.01$ when compared with vehicle (Duncan's test).

extent of either norepinephrine or dopamine depletion. In fact, by using more selective procedures to affect either dopamine or norepinephrine, it seems that a selective decrease of brain dopamine constantly reduces the effect of morphine, whereas a selective decrease of norepinephrine tends to potentiate it (13,39). Table 5 summarizes some of these findings.

An interesting application of 6-OHDA has been the study of the possible localization of psychoactive drugs in catecholamine-containing neurons in the brain (Table 6).

Thus, decreased levels of reserpine in various brain structures, particularly in the corpus striatum, have been found in rats injected intraventricularly with 6-OHDA (17). The changes of reserpine levels appear to be related to the extent of catecholamine depletion in the various areas (*unpublished results*), suggesting that the integrity of catecholaminergic neurons is an important condition to maintain normal levels of brain reserpine.

Also the striatal levels of amphetamine have been found to be reduced in animals pretreated with 6-OHDA but not in animals treated with 5,6-dihydroxytryptamine, which is known to produce a selective decrease of brain 5-HT (17). These findings clearly indicate that amphetamine is mainly concentrated in catecholamine-containing neurons.

In conclusion, when used appropriately, 6-OHDA is a very useful tool for investigating the functional role of catecholamine in the CNS as well as the interaction of

TABLE 6. *Reserpine levels in encephalic areas from controls and 6-OHDA pretreated female rats*

	15 Min			6 Hr		
	A: Control	B: 6-OHDA	B/A $\times$ 100	A: Control	B: 6-OHDA	B/A $\times$ 100
Hemispheres	39.0 ± 4.3	33.2 ± 3.5	85	6.5 ± 0.1	3.7 ± 0.5^b	57
Striata	71.4 ± 21.7	44.0 ± 8.4	62	83.0 ± 9.1	14.1 ± 6.3^b	17
Diencephalon	43.2 ± 5.8	36.2 ± 8.2	84	13.6 ± 1.0	9.3 ± 0.5^b	68
Mesencephalon pons and medulla oblongata	35.2 ± 7.0	30.7 ± 6.5	87	10.0 ± 0.5	5.8 ± 0.3^b	58
Cerebellum	38.2 ± 4.0	28.9 ± 5.8^a	76	2.3 ± 0.3	0.7 ± 0.2^b	30
Plasma	63.4 ± 8.5	70.3 ± 14.7	111	2.5 ± 0.4	2.5 ± 0.3	100

Figures are ng reserpine/g tissue (averages of 4 determinations + SD) at stated intervals after intravenous administration of 0.5 mg/kg of tritium-labeled reserpine. At 15 min individual specimens and at 6 hr pools of two each were processed. 6-OHDA 250 μg/20 μl/rat was administered intraventricularly 10 days before reserpine and all of the animals (including controls) received pargyline 50 mg/kg i.p. 30 min prior to 6-OHDA. (From Garattini et al., ref. 17.)

[a] $p < 0.05$
[b] $p < 0.01$ Student's *t*-test.

various psychotropic drugs with these brain substances.

REFERENCES

1. Agid, Y., Javoy, F., Glowinski, J., Bouvet, D., and Sotelo, C. (1973): Injection of 6-hydroxy-dopamine into the substantia nigra of the rat. II. Diffusion and specificity. *Brain Res.,* 58:291–301.
2. Ahlskog, J. E. (1974): Food intake and ampheta-mine anorexia after selective forebrain norepi-nephrine loss. *Brain Res.,* 82:211–240.
3. Asher, I. M., and Aghajanian, G. K. (1974): 6-Hydroxydopamine lesions of olfactory tubercles and caudate nuclei: Effect on amphetamine-induced stereotyped behavior in rats. *Brain Res.,* 82:1–12.
4. Ayhan, I. H. (1972): Effect of 6-hydroxydopa-mine on morphine analgesia. *Psychopharma-cologia,* 25:183–188.
5. Blondaux, C., Juge, A., Sordet, F., Chouvet, G., Jouvet, M., and Pujol, J. F. (1973): Modification du métabolisme de la sérotonine (5-HT) cérébrale induite chez le rat par administration de 6-hy-droxydopamine. *Brain Res.,* 50:101–114.
6. Bloom, F. E. (1971): Fine structural changes in rat brain after intracisternal injection of 6-hy-droxydopamine. In: *6-Hydroxydopamine and Catecholamine Neurons,* edited by T. Malmfors and H. Thoenen, pp. 135–150. North-Holland, Amsterdam.
7. Breese, G. R., and Traylor, T. D. (1970): Effect of 6-hydroxydopamine on brain norepinephrine and dopamine: Evidence for selective degeneration of catecholamine neurons. *J. Pharmacol. Exp. Ther.,* 174:413–420.
8. Breese, G. R., and Traylor, T. D. (1971): Deple-tion of brain noradrenaline and dopamine by 6-hy-droxydopamine. *Br. J. Pharmacol.,* 42:88–99.
9. Chang, C. C. (1964): A sensitive method for spec-trophotofluorimetric assay of catecholamines. *Int. J. Neuropharmacol.,* 3:643–649.
10. Clineschmidt, B. V., McGuffin, J. C., and Werner, A. B. (1974): Role of monoamines in the anorexi-genic actions of fenfluramine, amphetamine, and *p*-chloromethamphetamine. *Eur. J. Pharmacol.,* 27:313–323.
11. Coleman, R. A., and Levy, G. P. (1972): Mecha-nisms of 6-hydroxydopamine-induced supersensi-tivity in guinea-pig isolated intact trachea. *Br. J. Pharmacol.,* 46:528P–529P.
12. Cox, B. M., Ginsburg, M., and Osman, O. H. (1968): Acute tolerance to narcotic analgesic drugs in rats. *Br. J. Pharmacol.,* 33:245–256.
13. Elchisak, M. A., and Rosecrans, J. A. (1973): Effect of central catecholamine depletions by 6-hydroxydopamine on morphine antinociception in rats. *Res. Commun. Chem. Pathol. Pharmacol.,* 6:349–352.
14. Fibiger, H. C., Zis, A. P., and McGeer, E. G. (1973): Feeding and drinking deficits after 6-hy-droxydopamine administration in the rat: Simi-larities to the lateral hypothalamic syndrome. *Brain Res.,* 55:135–148.
15. Frey, H.-H., and Schulz, R. (1973): On the cen-tral mediation of anorexigenic drug effects. *Bio-chem. Pharmacol.,* 22:3041–3049.
16. Fuxe, K., Eneroth, P., Gustavsson, J. Å., Hökfelt, T., Jonsson, G., Löfström, A., and Skett, P. (1975): Effects of 6-OH-DA induced lesions of the ascending noradrenaline and adrenaline path-ways to the tel- and diencephalon on FSH, LH and prolactin secretion in the ovariectomized female rat. In: *Chemical Tools in Catechol-amine Research,* Vol. I, edited by G. Jonsson, T. Malmfors, and Ch. Sachs, pp. 273–283. North-Holland, Amsterdam.
17. Garattini, S., Jori, A., Manara, L., and Samanin, R. (1975): 6-Hydroxydopamine, a tool to study distribution of drugs in the catecholaminergic system. In: *Chemical Tools in Catecholamine Re-search,* Vol. I, edited by G. Jonsson, T. Malmfors, and Ch. Sachs, pp. 303–309. North-Holland, Amsterdam.
18. Giacalone, E., and Valzelli, L. (1969): A spectro-fluorometric method for the simultaneous determination of 2-(5-hydroxyindol-3-yl) ethylamine (Serotonin) and 5-hydroxyindol-3-yl-acetic acid in the brain. *Pharmacology,* 2:171–175.
19. Haeusler, G., Haefely, W., and Huerlimann, A. (1969): Zum mechanismus der adrenerg blockie-renden Wirkung von Bretylium und Guanethidin. *Naunyn-Schmiedebergs Arch. Pharmakol. Exp. Pathol.,* 264:241–243.
20. Heikkila, R., and Cohen, G. (1971): Inhibition of biogenic amine uptake by hydrogen peroxide: A mechanism for toxic effects of 6-hydroxydopa-mine. *Science,* 172:1257–1258.
21. Heikkila, R., and Cohen, G. (1972): Further studies on the generation of hydrogen peroxide by 6-hydroxydopamine. *Mol. Pharmacol.,* 8:241–248.
22. Hökfelt, T., and Ungerstedt, U. (1973): Spec-ificity of 6-hydroxydopamine induced degenera-tion of central monoamine neurones: An electron and fluorescence microscopic study with special reference to intracerebral injection on the nigro-striatal dopamine system. *Brain Res.,* 60:269–297.
23. Iversen, L. L. (1970): Inhibition of catechol-amine uptake by 6-hydroxydopamine in rat brain. *Eur. J. Pharmacol.,* 10:408–410.
24. Iversen, L. L., and Uretsky, N. J. (1971): Bio-chemical effects of 6-hydroxydopamine on cate-cholamine-containing neurones in the rat central nervous system. In: *6-Hydroxydopamine and Catecholamine Neurons,* edited by T. Malmfors and H. Thoenen, pp. 171–186. North-Holland, Amsterdam.
25. Iversen, S. D., and Kelly, P. H. (1975): The use of 6-hydroxydopamine (6-OHDA) techniques for studying the pathways involved in drug-induced motor behaviours. In: *Chemical Tools in Cate-cholamine Research,* Vol. I, edited by G. Jonsson, T. Malmfors, and Ch. Sachs, pp. 327–333. North-Holland, Amsterdam.

26. Jacks, B. R., De Champlain, J., and Cordeau, J.-P. (1972): Effects of 6-hydroxydopamine on putative transmitter substances in the central nervous system. *Eur. J. Pharmacol.,* 18:353–360.

27. Jonsson, G. (1971): Effects of 6-hydroxydopamine on the uptake, storage and subcellular distribution of noradrenaline. In: *6-Hydroxydopamine and Catecholamine Neurons,* edited by T. Malmfors and H. Thoenen, pp. 87–99. North-Holland, Amsterdam.

28. Jonsson, G., Malmfors, T., and Sachs, Ch. (1972): Effects of drugs on the 6-hydroxydopamine induced degeneration of adrenergic nerves. *Res. Commun. Chem. Pathol. Pharmacol.,* 3:543–556.

29. Jonsson, G., and Sachs, Ch. (1970): Effects of 6-hydroxydopamine on the uptake and storage of noradrenaline in sympathetic adrenergic neurons. *Eur. J. Pharmacol.,* 9:141–155.

30. Kelly, P. H., Seviour, P. W., and Iversen, S. D. (1975): Amphetamine and apomorphine responses in the rat following 6-OHDA lesions of the nucleus accumbens septi and corpus striatum. *Brain Res.,* 94:507–522.

31. König, J. F. R., and Klippel, R. A. (1963): *The Rat Brain. A Stereotaxic Atlas of the Forebrain and Lower Parts of the Brain Stem.* Williams & Wilkins, Baltimore.

32. Kostrzewa, R. M., and Jacobowitz, D. M. (1974): Pharmacological actions of 6-hydroxydopamine. *Pharmacol. Rev.,* 26:199–288.

33. Laverty, R., and Taylor, K. M. (1968): The fluorometric assay of catecholamines and related compounds: Improvements and extensions to the hydroxyindole technique. *Anal. Biochem.,* 22:269–279.

34. Laverty, R., and Taylor, K. M. (1970): Effects of intraventricular 2,4,5-trihydroxyphenylethylamine (6-hydroxydopamine) on rat behavior and brain catecholamine metabolism. *Br. J. Pharmacol.,* 40:836–846.

35. Malmfors, T. (1971): The influence of drugs on the effect of 6-hydroxydopamine. In: *6-Hydroxydopamine and Catecholamine Neurons,* edited by T. Malmfors and H. Thoenen, pp. 239–242. North-Holland, Amsterdam.

36. Malmfors, T., and Sachs, Ch. (1968): Degeneration of adrenergic nerves produced by 6-hydroxydopamine. *Eur. J. Pharmacol.,* 3:89–92.

37. Mishra, R. K., Gardner, E. L., Katzman, R., and Makman, M. H. (1974): Enhancement of dopamine-stimulated adenylate cyclase activity in rat caudate after lesions in substantia nigra: Evidence for denervation supersensitivity. *Proc. Natl. Acad. Sci. USA,* 71:3883–3887.

38. Nahorski, S. R. (1975): Behavioural supersensitivity to apomorphine following cerebral dopaminergic denervation by 6-hydroxydopamine. *Psychopharmacologia,* 42:159–162.

39. Nakamura, K., Kuntzman, R., Maggio, A. C., Augulis, V., and Conney, A. H. (1973): Influence of 6-hydroxydopamine on the effect of morphine on the tail-flick latency. *Psychopharmacologia,* 31:177–189.

40. Nakamura, K., and Thoenen, H. (1972): Increased irritability: A permanent behavior change induced in the rat by intraventricular administration of 6-hydroxydopamine. *Psychopharmacologia,* 24:359–372.

41. Noble, E. P., Wurtman, R. J., and Axelrod, J. (1967): A simple and rapid method for injecting H^3-norepinephrine into the lateral ventricle of the rat brain. *Life Sci.,* 6:281–291.

42. Petitjean, F., Laguzzi, R., Sordet, F., Jouvet, F., and Pujol, J. F. (1972): Effets de l'injection intraventriculaire de 6-hydroxydopamine. I. Sur les monoamines cérébrales du chat. *Brain Res.,* 48:281–293.

43. Pijnenburg, A. J. J., and Van Rossum, J. M. (1973): Stimulation of locomotor activity following injection of dopamine into the nucleus accumbens. *J. Pharm. Pharmacol.,* 25:1003–1005.

44. Reis, D. J., and Molinoff, P. B. (1972): Brain dopamine-β-hydroxylase: Regional distribution and effects of lesions 6-hydroxy-dopamine on activity. *J. Neurochem.,* 19:195–204.

45. Sachs, Ch., and Jonsson, G. (1975): Mechanisms of action of 6-hydroxydopamine. *Biochem. Pharmacol.,* 24:1–8.

46. Saelens, J. K., Allen, M. P., and Simke, J. P. (1970): Determination of acetylcholine and choline by an enzymatic assay. *Arch. Int. Pharmacodyn. Ther.,* 186:279–286.

47. Samanin, R., and Bernasconi, S. (1972): Effects of intraventricular injected 6-OH dopamine or midbrain raphe lesion on morphine analgesia in rats. *Psychopharmacologia,* 25:175–182.

48. Samanin, R., Bernasconi, S., and Garattini, S. (1975): The effect of selective lesioning of brain catecholamine-containing neurons on the activity of various anorectics in the rat. *Eur. J. Pharmacol.,* 34:373–375.

49. Samanin, R., and Garattini, S. (1975): The serotonergic system in the brain and its possible functional connections with other aminergic systems. *Life Sci.,* 17:1201–1210.

50. Samanin, R., Gumulka, W., and Valzelli, L. (1970): Reduced effect of morphine in midbrain raphe lesioned rats. *Eur. J. Pharmacol.,* 10:339–343.

51. Saner, A., and Thoenen, H. (1971): Contributions to the molecular mechanism of action of 6-hydroxydopamine. In: *6-Hydroxydopamine and Catecholamine Neurons,* edited by T. Malmfors and H. Thoenen, pp. 265–275. North-Holland, Amsterdam.

52. Saner, A., and Thoenen, H. (1971): Model experiments on the molecular mechanism of action of 6-hydroxydopamine. *Mol. Pharmacol.,* 7:147–154.

53. Scheel-Krüger, J. (1972): Behavioural and biochemical comparison of amphetamine derivatives, cocaine, benztropine and tricyclic anti-depressant drugs. *Eur. J. Pharmacol.,* 18:63–73.

54. Taylor, K. M., and Snyder, S. H. (1971): Differential effects of d- and l-amphetamine on behaviour and on catecholamine disposition in

dopamine and norepinephrine containing neurones of rat brain. *Brain Res.,* 28:295–309.
55. Thornburg, J. E., and Moore, K. E. (1973):
Dopamine and norepinephrine uptake by rat brain
synaptosomes: Relative inhibitory potencies of
l- and d-amphetamine and amantadine. *Res.
Commun. Chem. Pathol. Pharmacol.,* 5:81–89.
56. Thornburg, J. E., and Moore, K. E. (1973): The
relative importance of dopaminergic and noradrenergic neuronal systems for the stimulation of
locomotor activity induced by amphetamine and
other drugs. *Neuropharmacology,* 12:853–866.
57. Tranzer, J. P., and Thoenen, H. (1967): Ultra-
morphologische Veränderungen der sympathi-
schen Nervenendigungen der Katze nach Vorbe-
handlung mit 5- und 6-Hydroxy-Dopamin.
*Naunyn-Schmiedebergs Arch. Pharmakol. Exp.
Pathol.,* 257:343–344.
58. Tranzer, J. P., and Thoenen, H. (1968): An electron microscopic study of selective, acute de-

generation of sympathetic nerve terminals after
administration of 6-hydroxydopamine. *Experientia,* 24:155–156.
59. Ungerstedt, U. (1971): Postsynaptic supersensitivity after 6-hydroxy-dopamine induced degeneration of the nigrostriatal dopamine system.
Acta Physiol. Scand. (Suppl.), 367:69–93.
60. Ungerstedt, U. (1971): Adipsia and aphagia after
6-hydroxydopamine induced degeneration of the
nigro-striatal dopamine system. *Acta Physiol.
Scand. (Suppl.),* 367:95–122.
61. Ungerstedt, U., and Arbuthnott, G. W. (1970):
Quantitative recording of rotational behavior in
rats after 6-hydroxydopamine lesions of the nigrostriatal dopamine system. *Brain Res.,* 24:485–
493.
62. Uretsky, N. J., and Iversen, L. L. (1970): Effects
of 6-hydroxydopamine on catecholamine containing neurons in the rat brain. *J. Neurochem.,* 17:
269–278.

Neurotoxicology, edited by L. Roizin, H. Shiraki, and N. Grčević. Raven Press, New York © 1977.

Neuropathologic Findings after Neuroleptic Long-Term Therapy

Kurt Jellinger

Division of Neuropathology, Neurological Institute of the University of Vienna Medical School, and L. Boltzmann-Institute of Neurobiology, Lainz Hospital, A 1130 Vienna, Austria

There are several theories explaining the main tranquilizing action and side effects of neuroleptic (NL) and related antipsychotic drugs that are thought to act on dopamine (DA) receptor sites in brain (12,14,29,56, 93).

1. The receptor–blockage hypothesis states that the NL drugs specifically attach to striatal DA receptors (90,93), thus inhibiting DA-sensitive adenyl cyclase (44), increasing the firing rate of DAergic nigral neurons, and accelerating DA turnover and synthesis (2,28,68). There is no simple and direct quantitative relationship, however, between any of these NL actions and their antipsychotic potencies (79).

2. As the strionigral GABA-ergic system is suggested to influence the nigrostriatal DA-ergic systems (7), NL-induced decrease of γ-aminobutyric acid in strionigral neurons may result in decreased inhibition of DA-ergic nigrostriatal neurons and thus activate the turnover of DA in the striatum (47).

3. The coupling–blocking hypothesis of NL action recognizes that the NLs are fat-soluble and surface-active drugs that accumulate in cell membranes (78) blocking nerve membrane impulses, enhancing the spontaneous release of the transmitter, or modulating the coupling between impulses and neurosecretion (23). There is recent evidence of a direct correlation between the antipsychotic activity of NL drugs and their ability to block the presynaptic impulse-coupled release of DA (79). Whatever the mechanism of NL inhibition of DA release, a presynaptic site of NL action in the small striatal DA neuron terminals might explain many of the chronic NL effects in brain (79), which also have been related to a state of denervation hypersensitivity of postsynaptic DA receptors with a resulting increase in DA-ergic activity (12,40,48,87,93).

Although clinical and experimental data on both acute intoxication and chronic treatment with NL drugs suggest some morphologic changes in the central nervous system (CNS), the problems of chronic brain damage due to long-term NL therapy and of the kind of lesion accounting for the clinical syndromes [e.g., parkinsonism and tardive and persistent dyskinesias (6,19,22, 48,71)] are poorly understood.

The results of neuropathologic studies after both acute intoxication and prolonged treatment with NL drugs are controversial, and surprisingly little is known of the anatomic substrate of drug-induced encephalopathies (31,43,72).

ACUTE INTOXICATION

After acute intoxication with NL drugs, CNS changes in both man and experimental animals

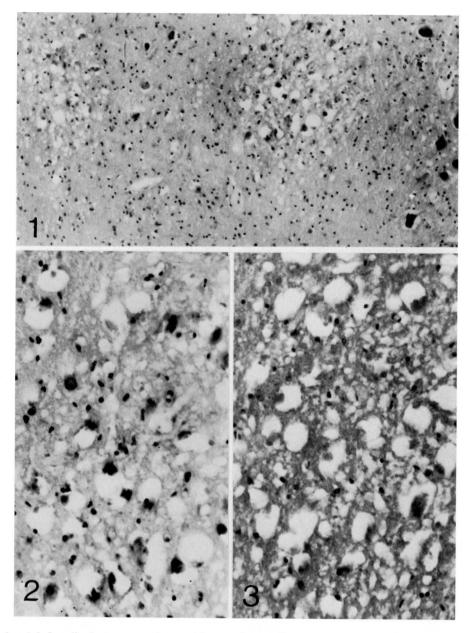

FIGS. 1 and 2. Localized status spongiosus with astroglial swelling and mild neuronal damage in Westphal–Edinger nuclei after fatal overdosage of nialamide. H. & E. Fig. 1, ×90. Fig. 2, ×250.
FIG. 3. Severe spongy changes with neuronal and axonal changes in inferior olive after acute fatal intoxication with thioridazine. C. V. ×250.

include cerebral edema and nonspecific neuronal changes, including reversible neuronal swelling and vacuolation, often superimposed on by secondary anoxic and vasocirculatory lesions (for review, see 13,25,43,58). Necroses of the cerebral gray matter with gliovascular re-action found in a cerebral biopsy of an infant 9 months after accidental poisoning with chlorpromazine (CPZ) were attributed to chronic hypoxia (5). In one case of acute fatal intoxication with thioridazine (Melleril®, 6,000 mg), and in two cases of acute death following overdoses of nialamide, a monoamine oxidase (MAO) inhibitor, given in doses of 1,500 mg/day, we observed localized spongy changes of the neuropil with astroglial swelling and neuronal damage in both the Westphal–Edinger nuclei (Figs. 1 and 2) and inferior olives (Fig. 3). Similar changes experimentally induced in dogs by heavy dosing and chronic application of MAO inhibitors were attributed to a vasoconstrictor action of serotonine in the brain, with associated edema (70,91).

Nonspecific neuronal changes in the striatum, substantia nigra, hypothalamus, and cerebral cortex of experimental animals after application of high doses of NL drugs are often unrelated to clinical signs (73), and their separation from artifacts may be difficult. Ultrastructural demonstration of increased glycogen in astroglia and dendrites of hypothalamus and globus pallidus after therapeutic doses of CPZ and trifluoperazine (haloperidol) (50–52) are suggested to result from blockage of glycolysis and oxidative processes (24). Neuronal swelling with dilated endoplasmic reticulum (ER), increase in the number of mitochondria and profiles of granular ER (4) and of microvesicles in dendrites and presynaptic terminals are related to a partial—probably reversible—blockage of rapid axonal transport induced by CPZ and other tranquilizers (23). Increased pinocytosis of capillary endothelial cells after intracisternal application of CPZ indicates disorders of the blood-brain barrier (24).

In vitro application of CPZ and antidepressant drugs induces neuronal swelling with dilatation of the ER and mitochondria, and accumulation of concentric multilamellated dense bodies (MLB), often related to rough ER or resulting from stimulation of the lysosomal system with accumulation of phospholipids (10,35,36). Although similar MLBs were observed after chronic phenothiazine treatment in rats and in a human biopsy case after acute CPZ intoxication (5), these changes were not seen in human brains after chronic CPZ treatment (36). Similar changes induced by a variety of drugs [e.g., LSD, chloroquine, and antidepressant and anorexic drugs (3,49,60,61,76,85)] are thought to result from impairment of phospholipid turnover, thus representing some kind of experimental lipidosis.

CHRONIC EXPERIMENTS

Neuropathologic studies after long-term administration of phenothiazines and related drugs, summarized in Table 1, revealed nonspecific neuronal changes, neuronal loss, and gliosis in cerebral cortex, limbic system, brain stem, and cerebellar nuclei, with changes in the glioneuronal ratio in dentate nuclei and superior olives (38). Neuronal hyperchromia in cerebral cortex is associated with increase in the RNS content, accumulation of glycogen, and decreased activities of oxidative enzymes (77), some of these changes being dose dependent (81). Neuronal changes and gliosis in the limbic system (20,81) could be related to a blockage of DA receptors in the (meso)limbic system that project to the hypothalamus and nucleus accumbens septi (67,86).

Electron microscopic studies in rabbits with extrapyramidal syndromes after prolonged application of CPZ and haloperidole showed synaptic changes in the pallidum and hypothalamus (53–55,88) that were considered the results of partial blockage of glycolysis and/or axonal transport. Increased cytoplasmic membranes in the presynaptic axons of the globus pallidus (54) are probably related either to the interaction of phenothiazines with synaptosomal membranes (18) or to hyperplasia of the smooth ER resulting from disorders in the physiologic remodeling of synapses seen in a large variety of conditions (83). Changes of the postsynaptic dendrites with deposition of granular and fibrillar material, shrunken boutons embraced by astroglia, and vacuolation of presynaptic axon terminals in the hypothalamus (55) are similar to antegrade axonal degeneration following neuritic transection (1,82) and to degeneration of striatal boutons after experimental damage to the substantia nigra with degeneration of the DA-ergic nigroneostriatal pathway (39,46). Changes in the glioneuronal ratio (38) and synaptic changes in the brainstem, therefore, are tentatively related to chronic "biochemical denervation" of striatal DA- or GABA-ergic neuronal systems.

HUMAN NL ENCEPHALOPATHY

Neuropathologic experience in man after long-term NL treatment is still limited, and its results are controversial (see Table 2). A suggested increase of mortality in schizophrenic patients after prolonged NL treatment (64) needs further statistical confirmation. The majority of the morphologic CNS changes reported in the literature are nonspecific or related to normal aging, extraneural disease, or agonal and postmortem phenomena.

Chronic liver damage may induce hepatic encephalopathy with occurrence of Alzheimer type II astroglia. Drug-induced agranulocytosis and coagulation disorders may induce cerebral

TABLE 1. *CNS morphology in animals following long-term administration of NLs*

Author (ref. no.)	Animal	Drugs	Dosage/day (mg/kg)	Duration	CNS changes	Location
Kemali et al. (45)	Rabbit	CPZ, reserp.	7.5	12 d	Neuronal lesion, gliosis	Basal ganglia, hypothalamus
Roizin et al. (75a)	Rat, monkey	CPZ	12.5	8 mo	Chromatolysis, neuronophagia, gliosis	Diffuse
Guyeniseman (37)	Rat	CPZ	5.0	30 d	Neuronal lesion	Diffuse
Palmer & Noel (70)	Dog	MAO-inhibitors	5–35	3 mo	Focal neuronal loss, spongy necrosis, gliosis, myelin damage	Inf. olives, cerebellar nucl., caud. nucl.
Mackiewicz & Gershon (63)	Guinea pig	CPZ	10	4–13 wk	Neuronal lesion, gliosis, capill. hyperplasia	Reticular formation
Cazzullo et al. (15)	Rabbit	CPZ	Clin. dose	12 mo	Neuronal swelling	Brainstem
Dom (20)	Rat	Haloper.	Ther. dose	4 mo	Gliosis	Limbic system
Worden et al. (91)	Dog	MAO-inhibitors	?	wk	Stat. spong., neuron. loss, myelin lesion	Inf. olives, Cerebell.; nuclei
Romasenko & Jacobson (77)	Rat	Trifluoper.	20	4 wk	Neuron. hyperchromasia, RNS, AcPase, SDH[a]	Cerebral cortex
Sommer & Quandt (81)	Rabbit	CPZ Prothioop.	3–16.7	6 mo	Neuron. loss, gliosis, glycogen increase	Cortex, Ammon's horn
Koizumi & Shiraishi (54,55)	Rabbit	CPZ Haloper.	2.0 15	2–5 mo	Presyn. axon degen. Postsyn. dendrite	Glob. pallidus Hypothalam.
Hackenberg & Lange (38)	Rat	CPZ	10–15	6–8 wk	Neuron. degeneration, neuron. loss, gliosis (diffuse)	Dent. nucl., sup. olive

[a] RNS, ribonucleic acid; AcPase, acid phosphatase; SDH, succinic dehydrogenase.

TABLE 2. *Morphology of human brains following long-term NL therapy*

Author (ref. no.)	No. cases	Drug	Dosage (mg/d)	Duration	Dyskinesia	Autopsy	Neuropathology
Ayd (6)	1	CPZ	400	4 yr	–	Ac. death	Neuron. swelling bas. ggl.
Bom (9)	1	Megaph.	400	17 d	–	Ac. death	Neuron. swelling striatum
Grünthal & Bühl (34)	1	Perph.	550	13 d	Perioral	Pneum.	Edema, chromatolysis inf. olivary neurons
Roizin et al. (75)	17	CPZ	50–1200 mg	3–6 mo	Parkinson	?	Lipofuscinosis (general), cortical neuronophagia (4 cases)
Forrest et al. (27)	1	CPZ Trifluoper.	?	? yr	–	?	Neuronophag. putamen depigmentation nigra
Greiner & Nicolson (30)	12	CPZ	225	0.4–9 yr	–	Increas. melanine	Generalized lipofuscinosis
Hunter et al. (41)	1	CPZ	1–200	2.5 yr	Perioral	Pneum.	Gliosis striatum, thal., mild nigral lesion
Same	1	CPZ Trifluoper.	Same	6 yr	Perioral	Pneum.	Moderate nigral lesion
Same		Same	10	6 mo	Perioral	Liver dm.	Nigrostrial myelin damage
Christensen et al. (17)	28 (21)	CPZ Thior. Reserp.	Same	6 yr	Perioral	Myoc. inf.	27/28 nigral lesion; 25/28 brainstem gliosis
Same	28	Same	75–600 mg	1–40 mo	–	?	7/28 nigral lesion; 4/28 brainstem gliosis
Eijk-Bots (25)	1	Thiop.	Similar	1–43 mo	Perioral	Shock	Edema, lipofuscinosis
Personal series (31,33,43)	14	CPZ	20	? mo	Hyperkin. (9)	Pneum.	8/14 caudate lesions
Same		Var. NL	Ther. dose	3–11 yr (int)[a]	Akinetic (5)	Bolus	2/13 pallid. lesion
Same	14	Similar	Similar	2–11 yr	None	Similar	5/14 caudate lesion

[a] Int = intermittent.

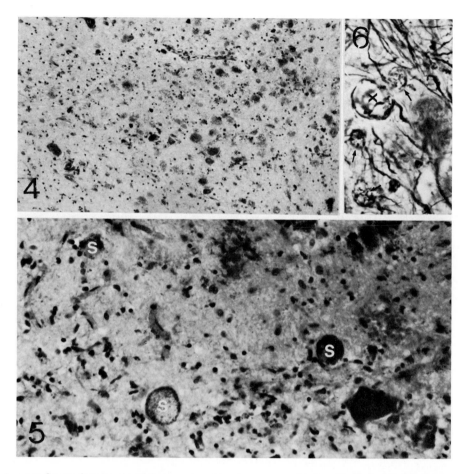

FIGS. 4 and 5. Severe increase in glial pigment and numerous axonal spheroids (S) in the reticular zone of substantia nigra of schizophrenic man aged 65 without dyskinesia. C. V. Fig. 4, ×90. Fig. 2,×280.
FIG. 6. Terminal axonal swellings (x, *arrows*) in globus pallidus of schizophrenic woman on long-term NL treatment. Bodian's silver impregnation. ×560.

edema, microhemorrhages, capillary thromboses with microcirculation disorders, and ischemic lesions. Frequent cerebral edema in psychiatric autopsy material can only rarely be related to chronic psychopharmacotherapy (26). Frequent but nonspecific phenomena are chromatolysis and increased lipid in neurons and other visceral organs (13,26,30,75).

Lesions of substantia nigra with depigmentation and neuronal loss occasionally seen in drug-induced dyskinesia (17,27,41) are *not* considered significant in view of the advanced age of most of these patients, the average age in the dyskinesia material of Christensen et al. (17) being 74 years. Reduction in the number of melanin-containing neurons in elderly subjects has been shown by semiquantitative and automatic counting procedures (16,69) but was not ob-

served in a personal series I conducted of 28 autopsy cases after prolonged NL treatment where the average age at death was 56 years (see discussion below).

Axonal swellings ("spheroids") in the reticular zone of substantia nigra (Figs. 4 and 5) and globus pallidus (Fig. 6), described in some cases of drug-induced dyskinesia (32,33), are also considered age-dependent changes *unrelated* to NL treatment. "Dystrophic" axonal changes represent a nonspecific and experimentally reproducible degenerating phenomenon of the neuron, the intensity of which in some constantly affected sites of the human CNS is clearly related to age without relation to any basic disease (42). However, the occurrence of dystrophic axons in the reticulata nigrae has been shown to be significantly elevated in Parkinson's disease and chronic alcoholism (42). This latter condition and advanced age are suggested to be responsible for the presence of these axonal changes in some elderly patients with drug-induced dyskinesia.

Diffuse gliosis in the striatum and thalamus, and mild chronic degeneration of myelin of questionable significance in the pallidonigral system were observed in phenothiazine-induced dyskinesia (41). Christensen et al. (17) reported gliosis in the brainstem in 25 of 28 brains with drug-induced dyskinesia, a condition rarely seen in age-matched controls. However, these changes, which in combination with damage to substantia nigra were considered to account for the clinical syndromes, were not confirmed by other investigators (31–34).

Damage to large neurons in the *caudate nucleus* with increased glial satellitosis, occasional neuronophagia, and mild gliomesenchymal reaction in the brains of patients with dyskinesia was reported by Gross et al. (31–34). These changes, observed in the striatum of other patients who died after prolonged treatment with CPZ and triflupromazine (27,74) but not seen in normal controls, were taken to be related to the drug-induced clinical syndrome.

PERSONAL INVESTIGATIONS

In order to further elucidate this problem, a histologic study of 28 brains following long-term NL treatment with persistent extrapyramidal symptoms in 14, was performed. The series included 16 men and 12 women, ranging in age from 21 to 74 years (average 56.1 years). There were 24 schizophrenics, four depressives, and two organic psychoses to whom NL and tranquilizers had been administered for, on the average, 5 years (range from 2 months to 11 years), although in most of the patients intermittent treatment was given. The drugs administered were CPZ, trifluoroperazine, chlorprothixen, reserpine, thioridazine, tricyclic antidepressants, and tranquilizers, alone or in combination. Fourteen patients developed extrapyramidal disorders with rigid akinetic parkinsonism in five and choreiform or perioral hyperkinesias in nine (Table 3). The duration of dyskinesia ranged from 4 months to

7 years. The average age at death was 54.3 years; the average duration of drug treatment was 5 years. The control group included 14 patients with an average age at death of 57.8 years who never developed extrapyramidal symptoms in the course of NL medication with an average duration of 4.4 years (Table 4).

The *pathologic changes* in brains of both groups consisted of:

1. nonspecific lesions related to age or lethal basic disease, e.g., cerebral edema, atrophy, atherosclerosis, lipid deposition in the neurons, and dystrophic axons in substantia nigra (Figs. 4 and 5), globus pallidus, and Goll's nucleus;
2. incidental findings unrelated to NL treatment, e.g., two cases of abortive Fahr's syndrome (mineralization of the basal ganglia), and lipoma of the hypothalamus;
3. no observed damage to substantia nigra and gliosis in the brainstem although this had been previously reported;
4. changes in the *caudate nucleus* in 13 cases, i.e., 46% of the total series, with swelling of large neurons, increased glial satellitosis, and occasional neuronophagia, associated with slight proliferation of astroglia and preservation of small neurons (Figs. 7–11). These changes were usually conspicuous in the rostral two-thirds of the caudate nucleus with almost bilaterally symmetrical intensity, but were rarely seen in the caudal part of the nucleus. Similar, much less pronounced, changes in the putamen and globus pallidus were seen in five of the affected cases, but were never observed in other subcortical nuclei or in the cerebral cortex. In some cases, multiple terminal axonal swellings in the globus pallidus next to swollen neurons with central chromatolysis or ballooned cytoplasm (Fig. 6) were noted. All these changes were unrelated to general autopsy findings and to the cause of death, basic lethal disorder, or duration of agonia (Tables 3 and 4).

TABLE 3. CNS changes following long-term NL therapy with extrapyramidal disorders

Case no.	Age, sex	Clinical diagnosis	Duration NL Th. (yr/int)[a]	Extrapyr. symptoms		Autopsy	Neuropathology findings		
				Parkinson.[b]	Hyperkinesia		Caud.	Pallid.	Others
11/66	55, M	Schizo.	3	+	Perioral	Bolus death	++	−	Edema
18/67	50, M	MDP[c] alc. chron.	4	+	Perioral	Myoc. Inf.	++	−	Edema
23/67	40, F	Schizo.	3	+	Choreif.	Pneumonia	+	−	Cer. atrophy
17/68	48, F	Schizo.	5	+	Perioral	Pneumonia	−	−	Abort. Fahr's dis.
26/68	51, M	Schizo.	4	+	Dyskinet.	Nephritis	++	+	Cer. atrophy
5/69	55, M	Invol. psych.	8	+	Perioral	Card. decomp.	−	−	Vasc. encephalop.
20-69	55, F	Schizo.	11	+	Perioral	Pneumonia	++	−	Bil. lobotomy
348-70	56, M	Schizo.	11	−	Choreoathet.	Pneumonia	−	−	Hydroceph. int.
388-70	70, M	Schizo.	9	−	Choreif. + tremor	Pneumonia	++	−	−
18/63	38, M	Hebephr.	2 yr	++	−	Pneumonia	−	−	Edema
56/65	66, M	Vasc. dementia	4	++	−	Pneumonia	−	−	Pontine dystrophy
16 67	44, M	Hebephr.	9	++	−	Pulm. edema	+	−	Edema
16/68	56, M	Schizo.	5	+	−	Bolus death	+	+	−
182-72	66, F	Schizo.	11	++	−	Pneumonia	−	−	Abort. Fahr's dis.

[a]Yr/int = years/intermittent application.
[b]+ = slight; ++ = moderate.
[c]MDP = manic–depressive psychosis.

TABLE 4. *CNS changes following long-term NL therapy without extrapyramidal symptoms*

Case no.	Age, sex	Clinical diagnosis	Duration NL Th.	Autopsy	Neuropathology findings		
					Caud.[b]	Pall.	Others
22/63	65, M	Schizo., alc.	3 yr	Tuberc., myoc. inf.	++	−	−
17/65	70, M	Schizo.	7 yr/int[a]	Pneumonia	+	−	Diff. cer. atroph.
42/65	29, M	Schizo. suic.	6 yr/int	Shock, aort. stab.	+	−	Cerebr. edema
3–68	65, M	Schizo. suic.	5 yr/int	Pneum. shock	+	−	Atherosclerosis II
49–69	60, M	Depression	2 mo	Tuberculosis	+	−	Diff. gliosis
22/67	40, F	Schizo.	3 yr	Bronchopneum.	−	−	Neuron. lipidosis
275–69	56, F	Schizo.	6 yr/int	Hem. cystitis	−	−	Cerebr. edema
434–70	21, F	Schizo.	1 yr	Pneumonia	−	−	Cerebr. edema
14–71	69, F	Depression	2 yr	Pneumonia	−	−	
66–71	72, F	Mixed psych.	2 mo	Enteritis, pneum.	−	−	Cerebr. edema (mild)
389–71	74, F	Schizo. defect.	6 yr/int	Hypertension	−	−	Lipoma hypothalamus
14–72	66, F	Schizo.	6 yr/int	Tuberculosis	−	−	Cerebr. edema
78–72	68, F	Schizo.	8 yr/int	GI carcinoma	−	−	Cerebr. edema
177–72	60, F	Schizo. defect.	7 yr/int	Pulm. embolism	−	−	Edema (mild)

[a] Yr/int = years/intermittent application
[b] + = slight; ++ = moderate.

As these lesions in the caudate nuclei were only observed in 4% of an age-matched control group of psychotics without long-term NL treatment and in less than 2% of a large neuropathologic routine group of patients, they were tentatively considered significant. Caudal lesions of this type were seen in nine of 14 cases, i.e., 57% of the dyskinesia group, and in only five of 35 cases, 7% of the cases without extrapyramidal disorders (Table 2). Although these changes were more pronounced in cases with choreiform and perioral hyperkinesias than in akinetic parkinsonism and controls, there was no definite correlation between the intensity of the morphologic changes and the clinical syndrome.

Electron microscopic studies performed on formalin-fixed and osmium-postfixed autopsy material of the caudate nucleus and globus pallidus of two patients with late dyskinesias following prolonged treatment with CPZ and other NL drugs (cases 348–70 and 388–70, Table 3) gave the following preliminary results: in addition to considerable postmortem changes and nonspecific neuronal and astroglial changes including lipofuscin accumulation, there were neuronal processes and mildly enlarged axons with a variety of altered organelles including mitochondrial, multigranular bodies (MB) with accumulation of glycogen, and concentric multilamellar bodies and loose membranous whorls (Fig. 12). These "myelin bodies" resembled those observed in degenerating and dystrophic axoplasm (42,57) and in neurons of aging brain (74) rather than the drug-induced MLBs (10,49,60,61,76).

The pathogenesis of the changes in the caudate nuclei following prolonged NL treatment and their relation to the biochemical effects of NL drugs are obscure. The possible mechanisms underlying the caudate lesions, which are believed to represent the only constant light microscopic findings in drug-induced dyskinesia, could be the following.

1. Nonspecific damage to the large caudate neurons associated with increased glial satellitosis, and occasional neuronophagia are consistent with some chronic sublethal neuronal lesions, e.g., as seen in chronic denervation.

2. Although ultrastructural data indicate nonspecific neuronal changes and axonal

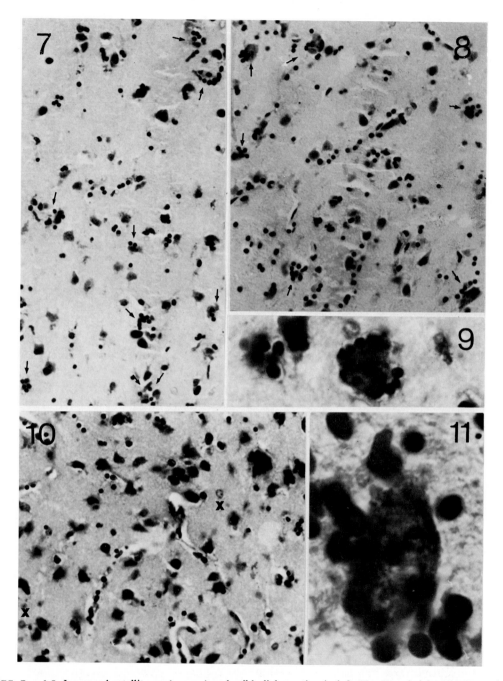

FIGS. 7 and 8. Increased satellitoses (*arrows*) and mild glial reaction in left (**Fig. 7**) and right (**Fig. 8**) caudate nuclei of schizophrenic man aged 55 with persistent dyskinesia. C. V. Both figures, ×90.
FIG. 9. Satellitosis around large neuron and small glial nodule in caudate nucleus of same patient. C. V. ×540.
FIG. 10. Occasional glial satellitosis and mild glial reaction (x) in caudate nucleus of schizophrenic man aged 65 on long-term NL therapy without dyskinesia. C. V. ×240.
FIG. 11. Glial satellitosis around large caudate neuron in same patient. C. V. ×1,500.

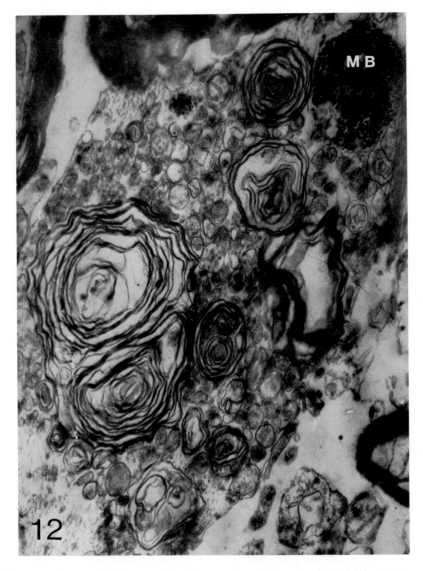

FIG. 12. Enlarged axon in caudate nucleus of schizophrenic patient on prolonged NL treatment, showing increased number of mitochondria, some MB and many concentric MLB and loose-lamellated whorls. ×10,000.

degeneration, some similarities with experimental striatal changes following prolonged NL administration (53–55) and lesion of the nigrostriatal pathway (7,39) indicate that these changes may be the results of chronic biochemical denervation in some striatal neuronal systems.

3. The phenothiazines and related NL drugs are thought to act by blocking DA receptor sites, thus chemically denervating DA receptors of the striatal afferents, which are most probably the small and medium spiny neurons (7,46), whereas dendrites originating from the sparse population of larger caudate neurons are believed to send their axons to the substantia nigra (84), thus forming a strioneostriatal loop system. The prominent changes in the large caudate neurons after prolonged NL treatment, therefore, might result from *in-*

direct damage, although the selective vulnerability of the large striatal neurons to different noxae is well established (65).

Although biochemical and experimental data are in favor of some relationship between hyperkinesia and lesions in the caudate nuclei (59), the clinical significance of the caudate changes after long-term NL treatment remains to be elucidated. The similarities between NL-induced dyskinesias and those following levodopa therapy of parkinsonism have been emphasized (12,48), both disorders probably being related to excessive inhibition of the striatal DA neurons. So far, however, no anatomic substrate of the levodopa-induced syndrome has been found (21,92). The question remains, therefore, why some patients on chronic NL treatment develop parkinsonism or tardive dyskinesia with or without caudate lesions, whereas others on equal or even higher doses do not show any extrapyramidal disorders even in the presence of some anatomic changes in the caudate nuclei.

Alternative Diagnoses to NL Encephalopathy

Clinical problems may arise from the "masking" of extrapyramidal degenerative disorders, e.g., Huntington's chorea, by NL treatment, and from difficulties in the clinical distinction between drug-induced encephalopathies and organic brain disease, including Creutzfeldt–Jakob disease and Huntington's chorea.

Long-term NL treatment may inhibit the clinical manifestation of Huntington's chorea, as observed in a demented woman aged 63, presenting with schizophrenia, who received intermittent NL treatment for 11 years without developing hyperkinesia. At autopsy, the brain showed the characteristic features of Huntington's chorea, without pallidal lesions often associated with rigid akinetic forms of this disease (11). This is in keeping with clinical experience indicating favorable influence

of NL drugs on Huntington's chorea (40,80), which is morphologically characterized by loss of small striatal neurons (11) with preserved striatal DA receptors, and no or very little decrease in striatal DA content (8).

Although NL-induced dyskinesia usually differs from Huntington's chorea, NL-induced encephalopathy may be occasionally mimicked by the latter disease showing initial psychotic features with delayed development of extrapyramidal symptoms (33,89). We observed three cases of Huntington's chorea, confirmed at autopsy, that had been clinically interpreted as chronic schizophrenia with NL-induced dyskinesia. Later, positive family histories of Huntington's chorea were found in two of these patients. Any causal relationship to or triggering of Huntington's chorea, a hereditary degenerative disease, by NL treatment, however, can be strictly denied.

Cerebral Phlebitis

A rare type of *cerebrovascular lesion* should be mentioned that may or may not be related to prolonged NL treatment. Moore and Brook (66) reported two cases of young girls who had received NLs and/or anticonvulsive drugs over an extended period of time and who were found dead without any preceding acute illness. The outstanding pathologic finding was a segmental nodular, occasionally annular intraadventitial lymphomonocytic infiltration of the meningeal and intracerebral veins without arterial and parenchymatous involvement or extracerebral vascular disease. Similar inflammatory reaction of cerebral veins was mentioned in an epileptic who had been "allergic" to antiepileptic drugs (66). We observed this type of *"cerebral segmental nodular phlebitis"* in four patients, three of whom had received long-term NL treatment. A man aged 65 with organic psychosis who developed

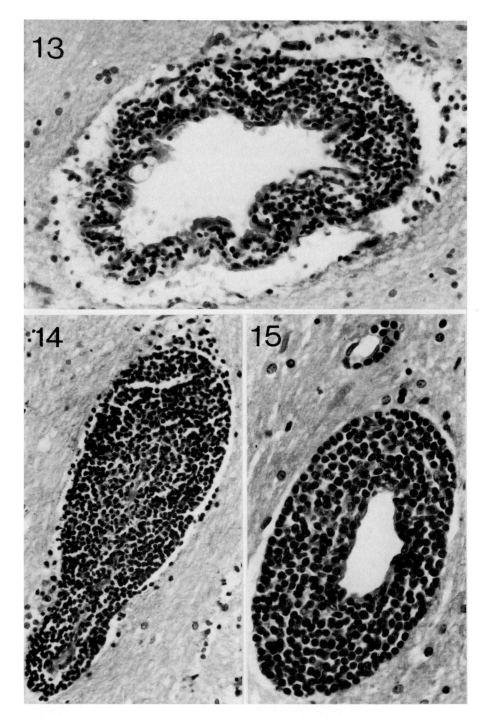

FIG. 13. Adventitial monocytoid infiltration in striatal vein. H. & E. ×250.
FIGS. 14 and 15. Mural and adventitial lymphoid infiltration of small veins in thalamus (**Fig. 14**) and globus pallidus (**Fig. 15**). H. & E. Fig. 14, ×250. Fig. 15, ×360.

dyskinesia after 8 years of intermittent administration of phenothiazines died from myocardial infarction. The brain, in addition to a small old cystic infarction in the striatum, disclosed disseminating lymphocytic infiltration of the cerebral veins without meningeal or parenchymal involvement. In a schizophrenic woman aged 30 who for at least 10 years received combined NL treatment without dyskinesia and who died in acute catatonia, disseminated phlebitis was seen in the striatum, thalamus, hypothalamus, amygdaloid nucleus, and medulla oblongata (Figs. 13,14,15). Similar phlebitic lesions in the white matter and basal ganglia were observed in a 52-year-old schizophrenic woman who, after several years of treatment with NL and antiepileptic drugs, died in an acute coma. Thorough histologic review of other tissues of the body failed to uncover any lesions of the extracerebral vasculature or of the cerebral arteries. The explanation for the singular involvement of the brain (the spinal cord was not available for study), with the escape of other tissues of the body, is not forthcoming, nor is there any manifest explanation for the sole attack on the veins to the exclusion of the arteries. No definite conclusion about the type of cerebral phlebitis observed after prolonged treatment with phenothiazines and anticonvulsive drugs being a form of sensitization to autoimmune reaction can be reached. However, the appearance of intramural segmental or annular phlebitis in the brain and meninges has been observed in other conditions, e.g., in demyelinating disorders including multiple sclerosis (62), indicating immune activity on the CNS. A study of similar cases could assist in clarifying the relationship between the clinical data and pathology findings.

The same applies for the pathogenetic elucidation of other neuropathologic findings after long-term NL therapy including the reported changes in the caudate nuclei that may or may not repre-sent some morphologic substrates for drug-induced dyskinesia. We can guess that, under certain circumstances, NL treatment primarily causes reversible structural and ultrastructural changes in certain extrapyramidal systems that later progress to irreversible damage, particularly in caudate nucleus. However, this guess can only be proved if these findings are reproduced in larger autopsy material and correlated with experimental ultrastructural and biochemical data.

SUMMARY

Biochemical and experimental electron microscope data on the effects of NL drugs indicating a blockage of the postsynaptic DA receptors or of the presynaptic DA release in the striatum and electron microscope data on synaptic changes probably resulting from partial blockage of glycolysis and of rapid axonal transport with disorders of the physiologic remodeling of synaptosomes suggest the possibility of permanent structural CNS lesions following prolonged administration of phenothiazines and tranquilizers. Changes in the glioneuronal ratio and degeneration of boutons in brainstem are tentatively related to chronic biochemical denervation. The majority of changes described in human brains after long-term NL treatment with or without dyskinesia are nonspecific or related to normal aging (nigral lesions, axonal dystrophy) and lethal disease. A neuropathologic study of 28 cases following prolonged NL treatment, with persistent hyperkinesia in 14, disclosed damage to large neurons in the caudate nuclei with increased satellitosis and slight glial reaction in 46%. The incidence of these changes was higher in the dyskinesia group (57%) than in cases without extrapyramidal disorders (37.5%), but there was no correlation between the intensity of the morphologic changes and the clinical syndromes. The pathogenesis of the caudate lesions and their relation to the biochemical effects and clinical side effects of NLs are obscure. A rare type of isolated cerebrovascular lesion observed after prolonged NL and anticonvulsive treatment is cerebral segmental nodular phlebitis which may represent some form of autoimmune reaction to these drugs.

REFERENCES

1. Alksne, J. F., Blackstadt, R. W., Walberg, F., and White, L. E., Jr. (1966): Electron microscopy of axon degeneration. A valuable tool in experimental neuroanatomy. *Ergebn. Anat. Entwickl.-Gesch.*, 39:6–39.
2. Andén, N. E. (1972): Dopamine turnover in the corpus striatum and the limbic system after treatment with neuroleptic and antiacetylcholine drugs. *J. Pharm. Pharmacol.*, 24:905–906.
3. Anzil, A., Herrlinger, H., and Blinzinger, K. (1975): Lamellar and crystalloid inclusions in central and peripheral nervous tissues of chlorphentermine-treated mice. In: *Proc. VIIth Int. Congr. Neuropathol.*, edited by St. Környey, St. Tariska, and G. Gosztonyi, pp. 395–398. Excerpta Medica, Amsterdam, and Akademiai Kiado, Budapest.
4. Arefolov, V. A., and Raevsky, M. (1973): Electron microscopic study of the neurons in the reticular formation and mesencephalon of rats exposed to the action of triftazine (trifluoperazine). *Farmakol. Toksikol.*, 36:5–8.
5. Arseni, C., Nereantiu, F., Nicolescu, P., and Horvath, L. (1976): Encephalopathy subsequent to accidental poisoning with chlorpromazine. *Eur. Neurol.*, 14:29–38.
6. Ayd, F. J. (1956): Fatal hyperpyrexia during chlorpromazine therapy. *J. Clin. Exp. Psychopathol.*, 17:189–195.
7. Bak, I. J., Choi, W. B., Hassler, R., Usunoff, K. G., and Wagner, A. (1975): Fine structural synaptic organization of the corpus striatum and substantia nigra in rat and cat. In: *Advances in Neurology*, Vol. 9, edited by D. B. Calne, T. N. Chase, and A. Barbeau, pp. 25–41. Raven Press, New York.
8. Bernheimer, H., and Hornykiewicz, O. (1973): Brain amines in Huntington's chorea. In: *Advances in Neurology*, Vol. 1, edited by A. Barbeau, T. N. Chase, and G. W. Paulson, pp. 525–531. Raven Press, New York.
9. Bom, F. (1958): Über die Wirkung von Chlorpromazin und verwandten Stoffen auf die Ganglienzellen, insbesondere im Hypothalamus. *Nord. Psykiatr. Medlemsbl.*, 12:261–270.
10. Brosnan, C. F., Bunge, M. B., and Murray, M. R. (1970): The response of lysosomes in cultured neurons to chlorpromazine. *J. Neuropathol. Exp. Neurol.*, 29:337–353.
11. Bruyn, G. W. (1968): Huntington's chorea. In: *Handbook of Clinical Neurology*, Vol. 6, edited by P. J. Vinken and G. W. Bruyn, pp. 298–378. North-Holland Publ., Amsterdam.
12. Calne, D. B., Chase, T. N., and Barbeau, A. (editors) (1975): *Dopaminergic Mechanisms. Advances in Neurology*, Vol. 9, Raven Press, New York.
13. Cares, R. M. (1971): Tranquilizers, sedatives and hypnotics. In: *Pathology of the Nervous System*, Vol. 2, edited by J. Minckler, pp. 1682–1685. McGraw-Hill, New York–London.
14. Carlsson, A. (1972): Biochemical and pharmacological aspects of parkinsonism. *Acta Neurol. Scand. [Suppl.]*, 51:11–42.
15. Cazzullo, C. L., Goldwurm, G. F., and Vanni, F. (1966): Correlations between chemical structures of psychotropic drugs and histological features experimentally induced in the central nervous system. In: *Proc. Vth Int. Congr. Neuropathol.*, edited by F. Lüthy and A. Bischoff, pp. 842–853. Int. Congr. Ser., No. 100. Excerpta Medica, Amsterdam.
16. Cervos-Navarro, J., Ebhardt, G., and Schneider, H. (1972): Morphologie des Rückenmarks und Hirnstammes bei 90 jährigen. In: *Gerontopsychiatrie 2*, Janssen Symposien, Vol. 9, edited by S. Kanowski, pp. 42–55. Janssen, Düsseldorf.
17. Christensen, E., Møller, J. E., and Faurbye, A. (1970): Neuropathological investigation of 28 brains from patients with dyskinesia. *Acta Psychiatr. Scand.*, 46:14–23.
18. Christian, S. T. (1974): The interaction of phenothiazine derivatives with synaptosomal membranes. *Int. J. Neurosci.*, 6:57–66.
19. Crane, G. E. (1973): Persistent dyskinesia. *Br. J. Psychiatry*, 122:395–406.
20. Dom, R. (1967): Local glial reaction in the CNS of albino rats in response to the administration of a neuroleptic drug (butyrophenone). *Acta Neurol. Belg.*, 67:755–762.
21. Duffy, O. (1972): Discussion. *Neurology (Minneap.)*, 22/II:66–70.
22. Duvoisin, R. C. (1968): Neurological reaction to psychotropic drugs. In: *Psychopharmacology: A Review of Progress*, edited by A. H. Efron, pp. 29–53. US Govt. Printing Office, Washington, D.C.
23. Edström, A., Hansson, H.-A., and Norström, A. (1973): Inhibition of axonal transport *in vitro* in frog sciatic nerves by chlorpromazine and lidocaine. A biochemical and ultrastructural study. *Z. Zellforsch.*, 143:53–69.
24. Edström, A., Hansson, H.-A., and Norström, A. (1973): The effect of chlorpromazine and tetracaine on the rapid axonal transport of neurosecretory material in the hypothalamo-neurohypophysial system of the rat. A biochemical and ultrastructural study. *Z. Zellforsch.*, 143:71–91.
25. Eijk, R. van, and Bots, G. Th. A. M. (1970): Morfologische veranderingen in manselijke hersenen bij gebruik van psychopharmaca. *Ned. Tijdschr. Geneeskd.*, 114:1253–1258.
26. Eijk, R. van, and Bots, G. Th. A. M. (1972): Psy-

chopharmacological agents and brain edema. *Psychiatr. Neurol. Neurochir. (Amsterdam)*, 75:61–67.

27. Forrest, F. M., Forrest, I. S., and Roizin, L. (1963): Clinical, biochemical and postmortem studies in a patient treated with chlorpromazine. *Agressologie*, 4:259–267.

28. Fyro, B., Nyback, H., and Sedvall, G. (1972): Tyrosine hydroxylation in the rat striatum *in vivo* and *in vitro* after nigral lesion and chlorpromazine treatment. *Neuropharmacology*, 11:531–537.

29. Glowinski, J. (1975): Effects of neuroleptics on nigroneostriatal and mesocortical dopaminergic systems. In: *Biology of the Major Psychoses*, edited by D. X. Freedman, pp. 233–246. Raven Press, New York.

30. Greiner, A. C., and Nicolson, G. A. (1964): Pigment deposition in viscera associated with prolonged chlorpromazine therapy. *Can. Med. Assoc. J.*, 91:627–631.

31. Gross, H., Jellinger, K., and Kaltenbäck, E. (1970): Neuropathologische Befunde bei persistierenden Hyperkinesen nach neuroleptischer Langzeittherapie chronischer Psychosen. In: *Proc. VIth Int. Congr. Neuropathol.*, edited by J. E. Gruner, pp. 148–149. Masson, Paris.

32. Gross, H., and Kaltenbäck, E. (1968): Neuropathological findings in persistent hyperkinesia after neuroleptic long-term therapy. In: *The Present Status of Psychotropic Drugs, Proc. VIth Int. Congr. C.I.N.P.*, pp. 474–476. Int. Congr. Ser., No. 180. Excerpta Medica, Amsterdam.

33. Gross, H., and Kaltenbäck, E. (1970): Zur Neuropathologie der persistierenden choreiformen Hyperkinesen unter neuroleptischer Langzeittherapie. *Psihofarmakalogija (Zagreb)*, 2:195–204.

34. Grünthal, E., and Walther-Bühl, H. (1960): Über Schädigung der Oliva inferior durch Chlorperphenazin (Trilafon). *Psychiatr. Neurol. (Basel)*, 140:248–257.

35. Grunnet, M. L. (1973): The effects of exposure of neurons *in vitro* to nortriptyline and mesoridazine. *Trans. 49th Ann. Mt. Am. Assoc. Neuropathol. 1973.* (Abstr.)

36. Grunnet, M. L. (1977): The effects of nortriptyline and other psychotropic drugs on neurons and glia *in vitro:* An ultrastructural study. In: *Neurotoxicology (This volume).*

37. Guyeniseman, Y. Y. (1962): Les modifications morphologiques du cerveau chez les animaux par l'action de l'aminazine et de l'imizine (Russian). *Zh. Nevropatol. Psikhiatr.*, 62:190–196.

38. Hackenberg, P., and Lange, E. (1975): On the problem of irreversible brain damage due to neuroleptic long-term therapy. *Exp. Pathol. (Jena)*, 10:132–142.

39. Hökfelt, T. and Ungerstedt, U. (1969): Electron and fluorescence microscopical studies on the nucleus caudatus putamen of the rat after unilateral lesions of ascending nigro-neostriatal dopamine neurons. *Acta Physiol. Scand.*, 76: 415–426.

40. Hornykiewicz, O. (1972): Dopamine and its physiological significance in brain function. In: *The Structure and Function of Nervous Tissue,* Vol. 4, edited by G. Bourne, pp. 367–415. Academic Press, New York and London.

41. Hunter, R., Blackwood, W., Smith, M. C., and Cumings, J. N. (1968): Neuropathological findings in three cases of persistent dyskinesia following phenothiazine medication. *J. Neurol. Sci.*, 7:263–273.

42. Jellinger, K. (1973): Neuroaxonal dystrophy: Its natural history and related disorders. In: *Progress in Neuropathology*, Vol. 2, edited by H. M. Zimmerman, pp. 129–180. Grune & Stratton, New York.

43. Jellinger, K. (1975): Neuropathologische Befunde bei Neuroleptika-Langzeittherapie. In: *Probleme der Langzeittherapie mit Depot-Neuroleptika*, edited by W. Solms-Rödelheim, and H. Gross, pp. 124–140. Facultas Verlag, Wien.

44. Karobath, M., and Leitich, H. (1974): Antipsychotic drugs and dopamine-stimulated adenylcyclase prepared from corpus striatum of rat brain. *Proc. Natl. Acad. Sci. USA*, 71:2915–2918.

45. Kemali, D., Scharlato, G., and Pariante, F. (1958): Aspetti istologici ed istochemici del sistema nervoso dopo somministrazione di chlorpromazina, reserpina e rauwolfia serpentina. *Acta Neurol. (Napoli)*, 13:414–422.

46. Kemp, J. M., and Powell, T. P. S. (1971): The site of termination of afferent fibres in the caudate nucleus. *Trans. R. Soc. Lond. (B)*, 262:413–427.

47. Kim, J.-S., and Hassler, R. (1975): Effects of acute haloperidol on the gamma-aminobutyric acid system in rat striatum and substantia nigra. *Brain Res.*, 88:150–153.

48. Klawans, H. L., Jr., Bergen, D., and Bruyn, G. W. (1973): Prolonged drug-induced parkinsonism. *Confinia Neurol.*, 35:368–377.

49. Klinghardt, G. W. (1974): Experimentelle Schädigungen von Nervensystem und Muskulatur durch Chlorochin: Modelle verschiedenartiger Speicherdystrophien. *Acta Neuropathol. (Berl.)*, 28:117–141.

50. Koizumi, J., and Shiraishi, H. (1970): Glycogen accumulation in dendrites of the rabbit pallidum following fluoperazine administration. *Exp. Brain Res.*, 11:387–391.

51. Koizumi, J., and Shiraishi, H. (1970): Ultrastructural appearance of glycogen in the hypothalamus of the rabbit following chlorpromazine administration. *Exp. Brain. Res.*, 10:276–282.

52. Koizumi, J., and Shiraishi, H. (1970): Glycogen accumulation in astrocytes of the striatum and pallidum of the rabbit following administration of psychotropic drugs. *J. Electron Micrsc. (Tokyo)*, 19:182–187.

53. Koizumi, J., and Shiraishi, H. (1972): Synaptic alterations in the rabbit hypothalamus following long-term administration of haloperidol. *Folia Psychiatr. Neurol. Jpn.*, 26:319–326.

54. Koizumi, J., and Shiraishi, H. (1973): Synaptic alterations in the hypothalamus of the rabbit fol-

lowing long-term chlorpromazine administration. *Folia Psychiatr. Neurol. Jpn.*, 27:59–67.

55. Koizumi, J., and Shiraishi, H. (1973): Synaptic changes in the rabbit pallidum following long-term haloperidol administration. *Folia Psychiatr. Neurol. Jpn.*, 27:51–57.

56. Korczyn, A. D. (1972): Pathophysiology of drug-induced dyskinesias. *Neuropharmacology*, 11:601–607.

57. Lampert, P. W. (1967): A comparative electron microscopic study of reactive, degenerating, regenerating, and dystrophic axons. *J. Neuropathol. Exp. Neurol.*, 26:345–368.

58. Liebaldt, G. (1970): Zur Frage des Hirnödems bei kombinierter psychopharmakologischer Therapie. *Arzneimittelforsch.*, 20:879–882.

59. Liles, S. L., and Davis, G. D. (1969): Athetoid and choreiform hyperkinesis produced by caudate lesions in the cat. *Science*, 164:195–197.

60. Lüllmann-Rauch, R. (1974): Lipidosis-like alterations in spinal cord and cerebellar cortex of rats treated with chlorphentermine or tricyclic antidepressants. *Acta Neuropathol. (Berl.)*, 29:237–249.

61. Lüllmann-Rauch, R. (1976): Retinal lipidosis in albino rats treated with chlorphentermine and with tricyclic antidepressants. *Acta Neuropathol. (Berl.)*, 35:55–67.

62. Lumsden, C. E. (1970): The neuropathology of multiple sclerosis. In: *Handbook of Clinical Neurology*, Vol. 9, edited by P. J. Vinken, and G. W. Bruyn, pp. 217–309. North-Holland Publ., Amsterdam.

63. Mackiewicz, J., and Gershon, S. (1964): An experimental study of the neuropathological and toxicological affects of chlorpromazine and reserpine. *J. Neuropsychiatr. (Chic.)*, 5:159–169.

64. Matsuki, A., Oyama, Y., Izai, S., and Zsigmond, E.-K. (1972): Excessive mortality in schizophrenic patients on chronic phenothiazine treatment. *Agressologie*, 13:407–418.

65. Mettler, F. A. (1964): Selective vulnerability of the large cells of the corpus striatum. *Acta Neurol. Lat. Am.*, 10:100–114.

66. Moore, M. T., and Brook, M. H. (1966): Cerebral segmental nodular phlebitis. *J. Neuropathol. Exp. Neurol.*, 25:269–282.

67. Nauta, W. J. H. (1973). Quoted in: Stevens, J. R. (1973): An anatomy of schizophrenia. *Arch. Gen. Psychiatry*, 29:177–189.

68. Nybäck, H., and Sedvall, G. (1972): Effect of chlorpromazine and some of its metabolites on synthesis and turnover of catecholamines formed from ¹⁴C-tyrosine in mouse brain. *Psychopharmacologie*, 26:155–160.

69. Orthner, H., Sabuncu, N., Tolppanen, L., and Friedrich, H. (1972): Maschinelle Zählung der pigmentierten Neurone in der Substantia nigra beim Parkinsonsymdrom im Vergleich zur Norm. *Deutsch-Schweizerische Neuropathologen-Tagung Gstaad, 1972*.

70. Palmer, A. C., and Noel, P. R. (1963): Neuropathological effects of prolonged administration of some hydrazine monoamine oxidase inhibitors in dogs. *J. Pathol. Bacteriol.*, 86:463–476.

71. Paulson, G. W. (1975): Tardive dyskinesia. *Ann. Rev. Med.*, 26:75–82.

72. Peters, G. (1972): Arzneimittelschäden und ZNS. Pathologische anatomie. *Verh. Dtsch. Ges. Pathol.*, 56:112–126.

73. Pozos, R. S., and Holbrook, J. R. (1971): Tremorogenesis: Effects of reserpine on the substantia nigra. *Exp. Neurol.*, 32:317–330.

74. Rees, S. (1976): A quantitative electron microscopic study of the aging human cerebral cortex. *Acta Neuropathol. (Berl.)*. (*In press.*)

75. Roizin, L., True, C., and Knight, M. (1959): Structural effects of tranquilizers. The effect of pharmacologic agents. *Proc. Assoc. Res. Nerv. Ment. Dis.*, 37:285–324.

75a. Roizin, L., Kaufman, M., and Casselman, B. (1961): Structural changes induced by neuroleptics. *Rev. Can. Biol.*, 20:221–229.

76. Roizin, L., Schneider, J., Willson, N., Liu, J. C., and Mullen, C. (1974): Effects of prolonged LSD-25 administration upon neurons of spinal cord ganglia tissue cultures. *J. Neuropathol. Exp. Neurol.*, 33:212–225.

77. Romasenko, V. A., and Jacobson, I. S. (1969): Morpho-histochemical study of the action of trifluoperazine on the brain of white rats. *Acta Neuropathol. (Berl.)*, 12:23–32.

78. Seeman, P. (1972): The membrane actions of anesthetics and tranquilizers. *Pharmacol. Rev.*, 24:583–655.

79. Seeman, P., and Lee, T. (1975): Antipsychotic drugs: Direct correlation between clinical potency and presynaptic action on dopamine neurons. *Science*, 188:1217–1219.

80. Shenker, D. M., Grossman, H. J., and Klawans, H. L., Jr. (1973): Treatment of Sydenham's chorea with haloperidol. *Dev. Med. Child. Neurol.*, 15:19–24.

81. Sommer, H., and Quandt, J. (1970): Langzeitbehandlung mit Chlorpromazin im Tierexperiment. *Fortschr. Neurol. Psychiatr.*, 38:466–491.

82. Sotelo, C. (1968): Permanence of postsynaptic specialization in the frog sympathetic ganglion cells after denervation. *Exp. Brain Res.*, 6:294–305.

83. Sotelo, C., and Palay, S. L. (1971): Altered axons and axon terminals in the lateral vestibular nucleus of the rat. Possible example of axonal remodelling. *Lab. Invest.*, 25:633–671.

84. Tennyson, V. M., Mythilineou, C., Heikkila, R., Barrett, R. E., Cohen, G., Cote, L., Duffy, P. E., and Marco, L. (1975): Dopamine-containing neurons of the substantia nigra and their terminals in the neostriatum. In: *Brain Mechanisms in Mental Retardation*, edited by N. Buchwald, and M. A. B. Brazier, pp. 227–264. Academic Press, New York.

85. Tischner, K. (1974): Effects of chloroquine on neurons on long-term cultures of peripheral and central nervous system. A light and electron microscopic study. *Acta Neuropathol. (Berl.)*, 38:233–242.

86. Ungerstedt, U. (1971): Stereotaxic mapping of the monoamine pathways in the rat brain. *Acta Physiol. Scand. [Suppl.]*, 367:1–48.

87. Ungerstedt, U., Ljungberg, T., Hoffer, B., and Siggins, G. (1975): Dopaminergic supersensitivity in the striatum. In: *Advances in Neurology, Vol. 9: Dopaminergic Mechanisms*, edited by D. B. Calne, T. N. Chase, and A. Barbeau, pp. 57–66. Raven Press, New York.

88. Utyurin, B. V., and Tumanov, V. P. (1971): The ultrastructure of the synaptic apparatus after the injection of phenamine and haloperidol (Russian). *Biull. Eksp. Biol. Med.*, 72:108–110.

89. Van Putten, T., and Menkes, J. H. (1973): Huntington's disease masquerading as chronic schizophrenia. *Dis. Nerv. Syst.*, 34:54–56.

90. Van Rossum, J. M. (1966): The significance of dopamine receptor blockade for the action of neuroleptic drugs. In: *Neuro-Psycho-Pharmacology, Proc. Vth Int. Congr. C.I.N.P.*, edited by H. Brill, pp. 25–37. Excerpta Medica, Amsterdam.

91. Worden, A. N., Palmer, A. C., Noel, R. P. B., and Mawdesley-Thomas, L. E. (1967): Lesions in the brain of the dog induced by prolonged administration of mono-amine oxidase inhibitors and isoniazid. In: *Neurotoxicology of Drugs*, Vol. 8, edited by S. J. Alcock, pp. 149–161. Int. Congr. Ser., No. 118. Excerpta Medica, Amsterdam.

92. Yahr, M. D., Wolf, A., Antunes, J. L., Miyoshi, K., and Duffy, P. (1972): Autopsy findings in parkinsonism following treatment with L-dopa. *Neurology (Minneap.)*, 22/II:56–71.

93. York, D. H. (1972): Dopamine receptor blockade — a central action of chlorpromazine on striatal neurones. *Brain Res.*, 37:91–100.

Neurotoxicology, edited by L. Roizin, H. Shiraki, and N. Grčević. Raven Press, New York © 1977.

Neuropathology of "Grumose Degeneration" of the Cerebellar Dentate Nucleus With Special Reference to Certain Neurotoxic Disorders and Other Pathological Processes

*H. Shiraki, *A. Okumura, and **Sh. Oyanagi

*Department of Neuropathology, Institute of Brain Research, Tokyo University Medical School; and **Division of Neuropathology, Psychiatric Research Institute of Tokyo, Tokyo, Japan*

In an autopsy case of progressive supranuclear palsy (PSP) Steele et al., who first reported it in 1964 (15), described alterations of the cerebellar dentate nucleus as an unusual form of degeneration of nerve cells of the cerebellar dentate nucleus, including swelling of cytoplasms, granular and fragmented cytoplasms, and disintegration of Nissl bodies. Anzil (1), on the other hand, termed those alterations "grumose degeneration" (GD), and he emphasized the presence of granular degeneration of the cytoplasms of nerve cells.

The reason why we have been concerned with GD of the cerebellar dentate nucleus particularly during recent several years is because GD of this nucleus has been found not only in PSP but also in other presenile neuropsychoses complicated with parkinsonian features. In addition, GD was also encountered in cases of Ramsay-Hunt's syndrome and simulated Ramsay-Hunt's syndrome as well as in certain neurotoxic disorders, such as intoxication with phenothiazine derivatives and ethylmercury compound. In all of them, except for certain examples of presenile neuropsychoses, involuntary hyperkinetic and/or dyskinetic movements were always found. Thus far, GD has never been associated with cer-

tain specific neurological disorders but has disclosed a neuropathological syndrome associated with various other disease processes such as pathological aging, systemic degenerations, reactions to neurotoxic agents, etc. (6, 12–14).

From our routine stainings and electron microscopic examinations, the most important neuropathological finding of GD of this nucleus was that it was essentially related to certain alterations of perineuronal and/or peridendritic terminals and/or preterminals presumably originating from Purkinje cells and projecting to dentate nerve cells, whereas it was never involved with dentate nerve cells themselves. In addition, a time-dependent shift of the common metamorphosis of GD could be identified irrespective of a variety of different disease processes.

ESSENTIAL NEUROPATHOLOGY OF GD OF THE CEREBELLAR DENTATE NUCLEUS IN DIFFERENT DISEASE GROUPS

The essential clinical features of different disease groups showing the presence of GD in the cerebellar dentate nucleus are summarized in Table 1.

TABLE 1. *Summarized clinical features of disease group with common neuropathology in cerebellar dentate nucleus (GD)*

Case no. Age Sex	Total duration of illness (Family history)	Main clinical features
Progressive supranuclear palsy		
#1 65 M	11 years (Sporadic)	Rigidity of all limbs, backward prevention of head, nuchal rigidity, loss of ocular movement, slurred speech, dysphagia, hypersalivation, delusions, dementia *Note:* No description of hyperkinetic movements
Parkinsonism-dementia complex in Guam		
#2 53 M	Over 3 years & 4 months (Sporadic)	Parkinsonian gait, station, & speech, cog-wheel in upper limbs, flattened affect, dementia *Note:* No description of hyperkinetic movements
Idiopathic parkinsonism of IANT type		
#3 67 F	15 years (Sporadic)	Rigidity of all limbs, hunched posture, oculogyric crisis ?, dysphagia, dysarthria, finger deformity, pes equinus, hypersalivation, hyperhidrosis, irritability, euphoria, amnesia *Note:* Tremor of tongue
Simulated or genuine Ramsay-Hunt's syndrome		
#4 47 F	22 years (Positive)[a]	*Choreatic movement of neck since age 25,* stumbled easily, *choreatic movement in whole body, clonic convulsion 1x,* inability to coordinate, dysarthria, psychomotor excitement, euphoria, emotional incontinence, impaired orientation in time
#5 31 F	12 years & 9 months (Positive)[b]	*General tonic convulsions at age 19, myoclonic jerks of fingers, myoclonic jerks in whole body, clonic convulsions,* psychomotor excitement, euphoria
Phenothiazine intoxication with tardive dyskinesia in schizophrenia		
#6 70 M	7½ years since onset of schizophrenia 2½ years since onset of dyskinesia	*Note:* Long-term administration of neuroleptics including phenothiazine derivatives *Tardive dyskinesia:* Initial onset of unnatural movements of perioral region, coarse involuntary movement of bilateral shoulders, involuntary movement in whole body, tremor of fingers, rigor of upper limbs
Ethylmercury intoxication with intravenous injection of LHP		
#7 13 M	13 years since onset of protein-losing enteropathy 6 years & 11 months since onset of SMON: *10 days* since onset of Hunter-Russell's syndrome (Sporadic)	*Protein-losing enteropathy:* From age of 7 months until death *SMON:* From age of 7 years until death *Hunter-Russell's syndrome at terminal stage:* Administered 9,000 ml of LHP containing 0.01% of ethylmercury sodium salcylate for 29 days, numbness of fingers, hands, & lips, itching feeling of whole body, tetraplegia, dysarthria, dyspnea, hyperhidrosis, hypersalivation, psychomotor excitement, comatose *Note:* Involuntary movement of hands, intention tremor

[a] *One sib,* slightly euphoric & dysarthric; *another sib,* slightly mentally retarded; *another sib,* low intelligence, convulsions after head trauma.

[b] *Father,* myoclonus, cerebellar ataxia, impaired intelligence & emotion but abortive; *another sib,* same myoclonic jerks as propositus.

IANT, intracytoplasmic Alzheimer's neurofibrillary tangles; LHP, liquid human plasmanate; SMON, subacute myeloopticoneuropathy.

Presenile Neuropsychoses Complicated with Parkinsonian Features

PSP; Case 1 (5,10,11)

In a 65-year-old male patient with 11 years of typical clinical features of PSP, a different type of ordinary itracytoplasmic Alzheimer's neurofibrillary tangles (IANT) (8) was widespread from the brainstem to the cerebral cortices, whereas the disintegration of nerve cells was predominant and bilateral mostly in the substantia nigra and then in the subthalamus. In addition, typical GD of the cerebellar dentate nucleus could be visualized clearly. It was characterized by moderately-to-severely disintegrated nerve cells (Fig. 1A), and an exceedingly large number of faintly stained, finely fibrillary and/or granular structures attached mainly to the apical dendrites of remaining nerve cells and, less conspicuously, to their cytoplasms, which were occasionally degenerated severely (Fig. 1B). With Bodian preparation, these structures revealed deeply argyrophilic, roundly shaped, large-sized solid bodies and ring-shaped, smaller ones, both of which were more or less connected with slender-calibered axonal structures. These bodies were visualized around the nerve cells and their apical dendrites (Fig. 1C). The Purkinje cells, however, were almost completely preserved and disclosed no particular alterations, although a few of them were focally disintegrated and torpedoes were occasionally encountered.

Parkinsonism-Dementia Complex in Guam; Case 2 (9–14)

In a 51-year-old, Guam-born, Chamorro man with over 3 years and 4 months' duration of clinical features of parkinsonism-dementia complex (P-D-C), the typical neuropathology of the disease was identified: nerve cells of hippocampal cortices, substantia nigra, and locus ceruleus were severely disintegrated due to the IANT formation, and thus, corresponded with the manifestation of dementia and parkinsonian neurological impairments. Nerve cells of the cerebellar dentate nucleus were moderately disintegrated, and the IANT formation actually was one of the causes of their cell deaths. GD was also numerous, but the deeply argyrophilic bodies seen in case 1 were far less evident or even absent, whereas the faintly argyrophilic, amorphous masses were pronounced particularly around the apical dendrites of nerve cells

(Fig. 2). There were no remarkable changes of the Purkinje cell layer, except for a few torpedoes.

Idiopathic Parkinsonism of IANT Type; Case 3 (9–14)

In a 67-year-old female patient with about 15 years' duration of parkinsonian features complicated with certain psychic impairments, the typical IANT were widespread from the brainstem and diencephalon to the cerebral cortices. Disintegration of nerve cells was particularly predominant in the substantia nigra, oculomotor nucleus, and locus ceruleus. Nerve cells of the cerebellar dentate nucleus, on the other hand, were disintegrated moderately, and the cause of those cell deaths may in part be ascribed to IANT formation (Fig. 3). The two bodies of GD seen in Case 1 were again identified here, whereas the atypical but faintly argyrophilic, amorphous masses seen in case 2 comprised the background for these two bodies (Fig. 3). No remarkable alterations were found in the Purkinje cell layer.

Comments

The essential neuropathology of GD of the dentate nucleus in the present disease group was comprised of two types of deeply argyrophilic bodies and faintly argyrophilic background masses. However, there were no outstanding clinical descriptions of hyperkinetic involuntary movements, except for case 3 with tremor of the tongue. The reason for this clinicopathological dissociation is discussed later.

Multisystemic Degenerations of Simulated Ramsay-Hunt's Syndrome and of Genuine Ramsay-Hunt's Syndrome
Case 4 (4,6,12,14)

In a 47-year-old female patient with approximately 22 years of conspicuous in-

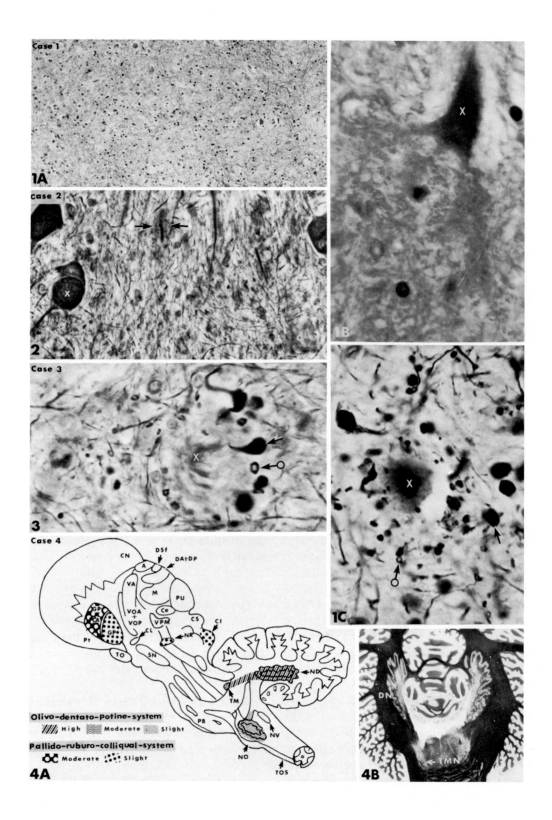

voluntary hyperkinesia on the whole body simulating Huntington's chorea and with a positive family history, multisystemic degenerations of simple atrophic process of nerve cells were symmetric and bilateral and found in certain basal ganglia, brainstem, and cerebellum. There were moderately disintegrated nerve cells in the external segment of globus pallidus, while slight one in its internal segment, well-preserved nerve cells but diffuse astrocytosis in the red nucleus, slightly disintegrated caudal colliculus, diffuse astrocytosis with well-preserved nerve cells of olivary nucleus accompanied by a few spheroid bodies, slightly-to-moderately disintegrated nerve cells of the trigeminal motor nucleus, and pronounced demyelination of hilus of the cerebellar dentate nucleus (Fig. 4B). Thus, this patient indicated multisystemic degenerations of the olivodentatopontine and pallidoruburocollicular systems simulating the neuropathology of Ramsay-Hunt's syndrome, although the nature of hyperkinesia in the present example differed from myoclonic jerks (Fig. 4A).

GD of the dentate nucleus was exceedingly conspicuous and showed all the characteristics of GD mentioned above, and the nerve cells were also moderately to severely disintegrated. The Purkinje cells, combined with a very few torpedoes, were well-preserved, however.

Case 5 (7)

In a 31-year-old female patient with myoclonic jerks and certain cerebellar in-

volvements of approximately 12 years' duration and with a positive family history, symmetric bilateral multisystemic degenerations were again found in the basal ganglia, brainstem, and cerebellum, and as in case 4 there was degeneration in the pallidorubural system, demyelination of hilus of the dentate nucleus, and moderate gliosis in the olivary nucleus. Some ways in which the degenerations in the present example differed from case 4, however, were the slight astrocytosis in the striatum and tegmentum of the brainstem, the moderate gliosis and nerve cell degeneration of the rostral colliculus, and the slight but diffuse nerve cell loss in cerebral cortices.

Summarizing the clinicopathological features, the present example could belong in the same category as the original descriptions of Ramsay-Hunt's syndrome (dyssynergia cerebellaris myoclonica; 2).

As far as GD of the dentate nucleus was concerned, the neuropathology of this case was identical to that of case 2 of P-D-C, in that the peridendritic and/or perineuronal, faintly argyrophilic amorphous masses were mostly outstanding, whereas the two deeply argyrophilic bodies were present but not conspicuous (Fig. 5A–C). No remarkable alterations were found in the Purkinje cell layer.

Comments

Although the nature of involuntary hyperkinesia in this group was different in each, i.e., Huntington's chorea-like hyperkinesia in case 4 and myoclonic jerks in

FIG. 1. Cerebellar dentate nucleus. PSP; *case 1* in Table 1. **A:** Severely disintegrated nerve cells. ×110. **B:** Magnified area in **A**. Abundant peridendritic grumose structures and darkly shrunken nerve cell (*cross*). ×900. **C:** Centrally located darkly shrunken nerve cell (*cross*), and perineuronal deeply argyrophilic large-sized solid bodies (one example, *arrow*), and similar but ring-shaped tiny bodies (one example, *arrow with zero*). ×1,150. **A,** Luxol fast blue with cresylviolet; **B,** PAS; **C,** Bodian method.
FIG. 2. Cerebellar dentate nucleus. P-D-C in Guam; *case 2* in Table 1. Advanced IANT (*zero*) and recent IANT (*cross*). Arrows indicate one example of the abundant faintly argyrophilic peridendritic amorphous substances. ×575. Hirano's simple silver.
FIG. 3. Cerebellar dentate nucleus. Idiopathic parkinsonism of IANT type; *case 3* in Table 1. Centrally located nerve cell with advanced IANT (*cross*). Otherwise, similar to Fig. 1C. ×1,000. Hirano's simple silver.
FIG. 4. Ramsay-Hunt's syndrome; *case 4* in Table 1. **A:** Schematic diagram of systemic degenerations from diencephalon and brainstem to cerebellum. **B:** Cerebellar hemispheres and midpons. ×1.2. Luxol fast blue with cresylviolet. DN, dentate nucleus; TMN, trigeminal motor nucleus.

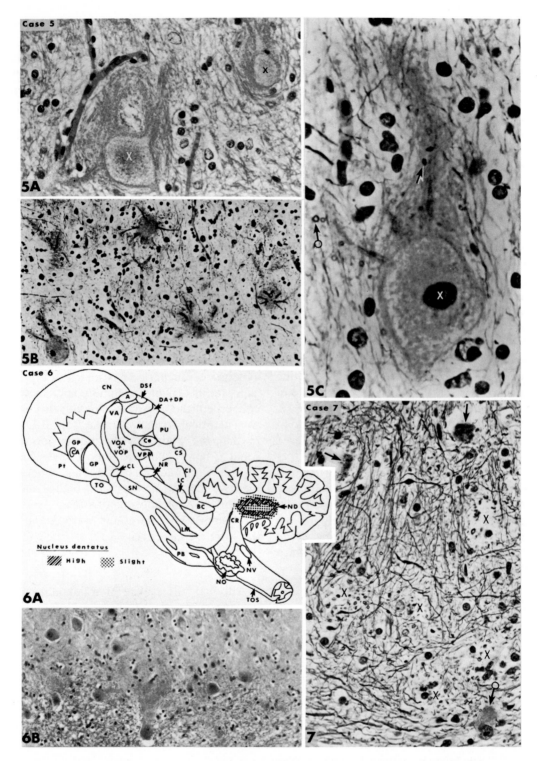

FIG. 5. Cerebellar dentate nucleus. Ramsay-Hunt's syndrome; *case 5* in Table 1. **A:** Magnified abundant grumose structures around the swollen cytoplasm and dendrites of nerve cells (*crosses*). H. & E. stain. **B:** Abundant faintly argyrophilic amorphous structures around dendritic processes of nerve cells. Bodian method. **C:** Magnified one of similar nerve cells as in **B.** Similar to Figs. 1C, 2, 3, and 5B. Bodian method.

FIG. 6. Cerebellar dentate nucleus. Phenothiazine intoxication; *case 6* in Table 1. **A:** Schematic diagram of cerebellar degeneration. **B:** Similar to Figs. 1B and 5A. H. & E. stain.

FIG. 7. Cerebellar dentate nucleus. Ethylmercury intoxication; *case 7* in Table 1. Darkly shrunken nerve cells (*arrows*), intact one (*arrow with zero*), and disintegrated nerve cells (crosses) surrounded by multiple ring-shaped argyrophilic tiny bodies. ×476. Bodian method.

case 5, the neuropathology of both the cerebellar dentate nucleus and other systemic degenerations was quite close or could even have fallen into the same category of the disease process. In the present group as well as the former group with presenile neuropsychoses, no remarkable alterations or disintegration occurred in the Purkinje cell layer. Thus far, one of the necessary conditions for the development of GD of the dentate nucleus seems to be less or no involvement of Purkinje cells themselves. Since nerve cells of the dentate nucleus receive a considerable number of centrifugal axons from Purkinje cells and detailed neuropathology even at the photo-microscopic level suggests the alteration of terminals and/or preterminals of axodendritic and/or axosomatic synapses, it may be that GD involves alterations of most distal endings and/or adjacent axons originating from Purkinje cells but never those originating from dentate nerve cells themselves.

In addition, one can cautiously suggest that the involuntary hyperkinesia in the present disease group is closely associated with the development of GD of the dentate nucleus, although there existed other systemic degenerations that could be associated more or less with the manifestation of involuntary hyperkinesia.

Certain Neurotoxic Disorders

Phenothiazine Intoxication; Case 6 (3,6,12,13,14)

A 70-year-old male patient had been diagnosed as schizophrenic at the age of 57 years and medicated with neuroleptics including phenothiazine derivatives for 10 years or more. At the age of 67 years, approximately 9 years after the first medication of neuroleptics, unnatural movement of the perioral region, coarse involuntary movement of the shoulders bilaterally, and involuntary movements on the whole body

occurred one after another, and persisted until death, even when the medication of neuroleptics was stopped. One year after the first symptoms, rigor of the upper limbs and tremor of the fingers appeared. Subsequently, he became emaciated and dysarthric, and died in an unconscious state at the age of 70. The total duration of involuntary hyperkinesia was approximately 2 years and 6 months.

GD of the dentate nucleus that was completely identical to the GD in the above-mentioned cases comprised the only outstanding neuropathological feature in this example (Fig. 6A and B), and thus, the pathomorphological basis for the outbreak of the long-lasting, pronounced involuntary movements can be ascribed exclusively to GD of the dentate nucleus for the following reasons: (a) since there was a long-term incubation from the first medication of neuroleptics to the onset of hyperkinesia, i.e., 9 years, the hyperkinesia coincided well with the beginning of the tardive dyskinesia that occurs not infrequently in schizophrenic patients treated with long-term administration of phenothiazine derivatives; such dyskinetic movements are never associated with the essential schizophrenic process; and (b) the possibility that the cingulectomy conducted when he was 60 years old could have caused tardive dyskinesia can be ruled out, since movement having the character of a lobotomy or cingulectomy can occur even in non-operated schizophrenic patients.

The present example, therefore, is the most favorable and pure case of a positive relationship between the developmental mechanism of dyskinetic movement and GD of the dentate nucleus.

Ethylmercury Intoxication; Case 7 (14, Chapter 24)

A 13-year-old boy began experiencing protein-losing enteropathy at the age of 7 months. At the age of 7 years, he was treated intensively with quinoform for severe diarrhea, and subacute myelooptico-neuropathy (SMON) developed and was identified postmortem at the most chronic stage. At the age of 13 years on account of general weakness, he received intravenous injections totaling 9,000 ml of "liquid human plasmanate" containing 0.01% sodium ethylmercury thiosalcylate as an antiseptic agent. Consequently, he developed Hunter-Russell's syndrome for 10 days at his terminal stage. Actually, the total mercury content in fresh tissues after the autopsy ranged in very high values, i.e., 17.0 to 20.8 ppm in brain, 43.3 ppm in liver, and 12.5 to 21.2 ppm in kidney.

The essential neuropathology of the ethylmercury intoxication in the present example is described in another presentation of alkylmercury intoxications in this volume (see Chapter 24, by Shiraki et al., *this volume*). The cerebellar cortices disclosed only minor changes, whereas the dentate nucleus demonstrated severe alterations that can be summarized as follows: at low power magnification, severe disintegration of nerve cells seemed to have occurred; the higher-power magnification, however, disclosed that the nerve cells were still preserved, but a great majority of them were degenerated severely, showing ischemic and/or homogeneous change and conspicuous shrinkage. With the Bodian preparation, the deeply argyrophilic, ring-shaped, small bodies connected with extremely slender-calibered axons were shown in great numbers around both the cytoplasms and the dendrites of severely degenerated nerve cells or at places of disintegrated nerve cells. The similar but larger-sized solid bodies as well as the faintly argyrophilic amorphous background masses were almost absent (Fig. 7).

Therefore, these features indicated GD at the most initial stage, because while features similar to the aforementioned cases were few in number, they certainly did exist, and the total duration of apparent illness in the present example was only 10 days.

Comments

It now became clear that certain neurotropic or neurotoxic agents, such as phenothiazine derivatives and/or alkylmercury compound, can cause GD of dentate nucleus, and thus, there exists the possibility that certain experimental models can reproduce GD of the dentate nucleus.

ELECTRON MICROSCOPIC FINDINGS OF GD OF THE CEREBELLAR DENTATE NUCLEUS

GD of the dentate nucleus in two cases, cases 5 and 6, was analyzed from the electron microscopic standpoint. Case 5 was recovered from formol-fixed material, whereas case 6 was fixed immediately and adequately at autopsy 1 hr after death. Even when both cases were of human materials and thus had inevitably a certain, perhaps great, limitation, it was assumed that the following findings could contribute more or less to an understanding of morphopathogenesis of GD of the dentate nucleus.

1. It at least is a convincing finding that the remarkable alterations never happened in postsynapses either of an axosomatic or of an axodendritic nature, but were restricted exclusively to presynapses (Figs. 8, 9A, and B). Some presynapses were enlarged; some became atrophic, and they contained the normal and/or degenerated mitochondria, certain electron-dense different-sized fine structures, small vacuoles, etc. They were, as a rule, surrounded by holo spaces the nature of which was difficult to determine.

2. Deeply argyrophilic, ring-shaped, small bodies comprised centrally located, aggregated multiple mitochondria and concentrically proliferated neurofilaments pe-

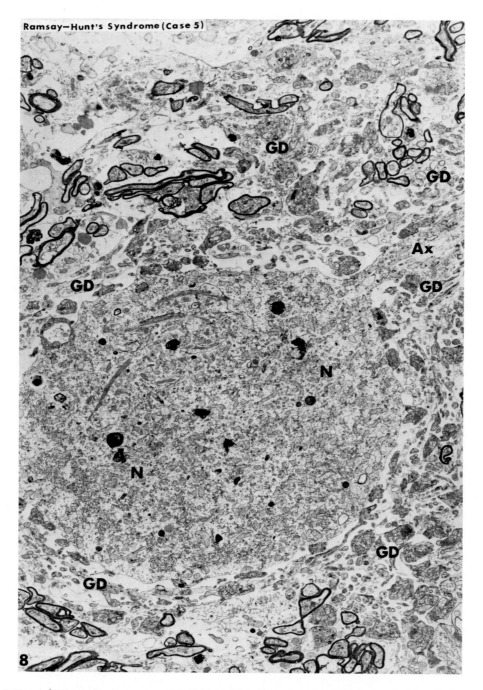

FIG. 8. Ramsay-Hunt's syndrome; case 5 in Table 1. Magnified nerve cell of the cerebellar dentate nucleus and adjacent areas. Electron microscope from fresh tissue. ×4,000. N; cytoplasm of nerve cell. Ax, axonal dendrite; GD, grumose structures.

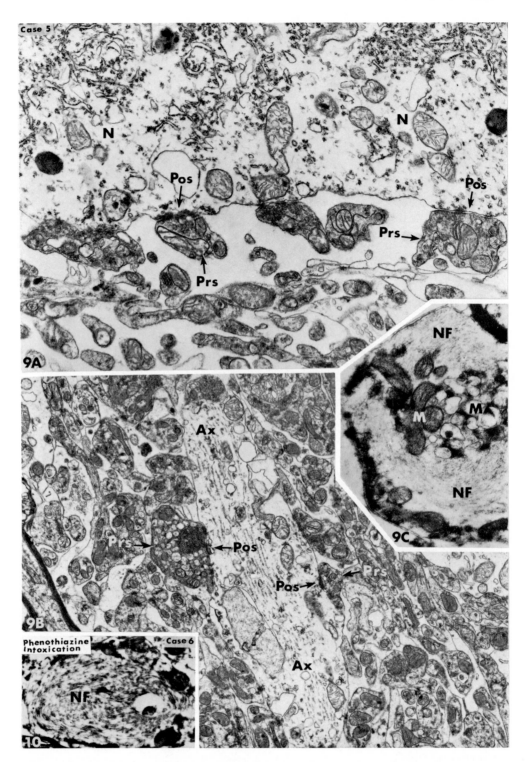

FIG. 9. Ramsay-Hunt's syndrome (Case 5 in Table 1). Cerebellar dentate nucleus. **A:** Magnified cytoplasm of the nerve cell (N) and closely adjacent areas. ×10,000. Prs, presynapse; Pos, postsynapse. **B:** Magnified axonal dendrite (Ax) of the nerve cell and adjacent grumose structures. ×6,000. Prs, presynapse; Pos, postsynapse. **C:** Highly magnified axonal structure corresponding to the above-mentioned ring-shaped deeply argyrophilic tiny body. Electron microscope from fresh tissue. M, mitochondria; NF, neurofilament.

FIG. 10. Phenothiazine intoxication (Case 6 in Table 1). Magnified axonal structure corresponding to the above-mentioned deeply argyrophilic solid body. Electron microscope from formalin-fixed tissue. NF, neurofilament.

ripherally (Fig. 9C). Similar but larger-sized solid bodies, on the other hand, comprised almost exclusively concentrically proliferated neurofilaments alone (Fig. 10). Both bodies disclosed enlarged unmyelinated axonal structures and were presumably of a preterminal and/or more proximal axonal structure.

3. Analysis of the faintly argyrophilic, amorphous background masses was most difficult. These broad-dimensioned masses consisted of normal or degenerated numerous mitochondria, some membranous structures, holo spaces of unknown origin, numerous synapses or simulating synapse-like structures whose close connection to dendrites and cytoplasms of nerve cells remained equivocal, etc. And they surrounded the two above-mentioned bodies as well as the cytoplasms and unmyelinated dendrites of nerve cells of the dentate nucleus (Figs. 8 and 9B). The presence of the neuro- and gliofilaments in those masses was very uncertain, but some did exist although they were very few in number. The question whether these masses are associated mainly with axonal structure or not, suggesting some proliferative and/or hypertrophic disease process, arises. In any case, one can cautiously suggest that these observations correspond with the photomicroscopic findings of these masses, i.e., faint argyrophilia with the Bodian preparation and much less or even negative gliosis with the Holzer preparation.

In summary, it at least is reasonable to assume that GD of the dentate nucleus effects alterations of the most distal endings of centrifugal axons, in other words, those of presynapses either of an axosomatic or of an axodendritic nature, as well as the preterminal and/or more proximal axons but that GD never or much less frequently involves the nerve cells of the dentate nucleus. And thus, these findings coincide well with those at the level of photomicroscopic examination.

SUMMARIZED NEUROPATHOLOGY OF GD OF THE DENTATE NUCLEUS AND ITS CLINICOPATHOLOGICAL SIGNIFICANCE

Now it has become clear that GD never occurs in certain specific central nervous system (CNS) disorders but is commonly found in various other CNS diseases and, thus, discloses a neuropathological syndrome. GD begins at the most distal endings and/or their closest parts of centrifugal axons presumably originating from the Purkinje cell but is less involved or never involved with dentate nerve cells themselves. In addition, one of the necessary conditions to the onset of GD is well preserved Purkinje cells. Further, there exists a series of pathomorphological varieties of GD that actually indicate a time-dependent shift of its metamorphosis depending on tempo, intensity, and continuity of each disease process. However, the question whether GD discloses a proliferative, hypertrophic, regenerative, or regressive process and/or combination of them remains open.

A positive relationship between GD and the onset of involuntary hyperkinesia was precisely identified in a schizophrenic patient with tardive dyskinesia derived from long-term administration of neuroleptics including phenothiazine derivatives. In this regard, this experience may reasonably indicate a positive clinicopathological relationship between the two in other examples mentioned above.

CONCLUDING REMARKS

The involuntary hyperkinesias in the above-mentioned cases disclosed, as a rule, a certain topographical predominancy in each, i.e., perioral dyskinesia alone, predominant head shaking, choreic movements predominantly in the upper body half or the whole body, myoclonic jerks predominantly in different areas of the body, etc. In addition, these hyperkinesias revealed their shift and/or progression in time, space, quality, and quantity even in the same example. Therefore, a question can arise whether the topographical predominancy of hyperkinesias may correspond with certain selective topography of GD foci in different regions of the dentate nucleus itself, or whether this predominancy could be associated with the selective involvement of other deep nuclei of the cerebellum, such as nucleus fastigi, emboliformis, and globosus. It, however, is to our regret that the results of our examinations at present cannot reply to this question.

Although the typical GD of the dentate nucleus was found in the disease group of presenile neuropsychoses complicated with parkinsonian features, involuntary hyperkinesias were absent, except for tremor of the tongue in case 3. With regard to reasons for this clinicopathological dissociation, two possibilities exist: (a) the degeneration and/or disintegration of dentate nerve cells partly ascribed to the IANT formation in this group were more severe in quality and quantity than in other disease groups; and (b) it is noted that the cerebellar signs and symptoms became equivocal or even suppressed in cases of parkinsonian syndrome of multisystemic degenerative character in which the nigral, striatal, nigrostriatal, and/or pallidonigral degenerations existed concurrently (12,13). Actually, in all cases of this group, the compact zone of substantia nigra was moderately to severely disintegrated bilaterally. And the dentate nucleus actually comprises one of the deep nuclei of the cerebellar system in both ontogenetical and anatomical senses.

The dentate nerve cells themselves in all cases examined were degenerated and/or disintegrated, and thus, the question arises whether the main cause of these alterations is of a primary nature or can be ascribed to a secondary process. Several possibilities exist: (a) GD is secondary to damage of dentate nerve cells themselves; (b) since GD seems to involve primary alterations of distal endings of centrifugal axons from Purkinje cells, dentate nerve cells are degenerated secondarily in a transsynaptic way (if it is true, it is possible that the pronounced demyelination of hilus of the dentate nucleus found only in the two cases of Ramsay-Hunt's syndrome and allied disorder is caused secondarily by the severe disintegration of dentate nerve cells during exceedingly long-term clinical courses, i.e., 22 years in case 4 and 12 years in case 5); and (c) a combination of the two possibilities mentioned above.

The above-mentioned electron microscopic findings that alterations occurred selectively in presynapses but not in postsynapses seem to favor the second possibility. This, however, remains a matter of conjecture, at least at present.

ACKNOWLEDGMENTS

The author gratefully acknowledges the generous cooperation of Dr. M. Iwase, Instructor of Psychiatry, Nagoya University Medical School, Nagoya, and Dr. Y. Toyokura, Professor of Neurology, Institute of Brain Research, Tokyo University Medical School, Tokyo.

REFERENCES

1. Anzil, A. P. (1969): Progressive supranuclear palsy: Case report with pathological findings. *Acta Neuropathol. (Berl.),* 14:72–76.
2. Hunt, J. R. (1921): Dyssynergia cerebellaris myoclonica—primary atrophy of the dentate system. A contribution of the pathology and symptomatology of the cerebellum. *Brain,* 44:490–538.
3. Iwase, M. (1974): An autopsy case of tardive dyskinesia. *Saishin Igaku,* 29:306–312.
4. Kobayashi, H., Kosaka, K., Hoshino, T., and Shibayama, H. (1975): An autopsy case of the characteristic degeneration of the dentate nucleus with choreic movement and psychic symptoms. *Clinical Neurol. (Tokyo),* 15:724–730.
5. Mannen, T., Toyokura, Y., Tsukakoshi, H., and Miyatake, T. (1972): Progressive supranuclear

paly: Report of autopsied case. *Adv. Neurol. Sci.,* 16:497–503.

6. Okumura, A., Oda, M., Iwase, S., and Shiraki, H. (1975): Pathomorphological and clinicopathological study of so-called grumose degeneration in the cerebellar dentate nucleus. *Adv. Neurol. Sci.,* 19:483–492.

7. Oyanagi, Sh., Tanaka, M., Naito, H., Shirakawa, K., Saito, K., Nakamura, N., and Ohama, E. (1976): A neuropathological study of 8 autopsy cases of degenerative type of myoclonus epilepsy. With special reference to latent combination of degeneration of the pallido-luysian system. *Adv. Neurol. Sci.,* 20:410–424.

8. Roy, S., Datta, C. K., Hirano, A., Ghatak, N. R., and Zimmerman, H. M. (1974): Electron microscopic study of neurofibrillary tangles in Steele-Richardson-Olszewski syndrome. *Acta Neuropathol. (Berl.),* 29:175–179.

9. Shiraki, H. (1968): Essential questions for idiopathic parkinsonism from neuropathological viewpoint. *Adv. Neurol. Sci.,* 12:874–876.

10. Shiraki, H. (1971): The neuropathology of idiopathic parkinsonism and parkinsonian syndrome. With special reference to a relationship of clinical features and criticism for clinical classification and therapeutic evaluation. *Shinryo,* 24:569–619.

11. Shiraki, H. (1972): Diagnosis and treatment for extrapyramidal motor diseases from neuropathological viewpoint. With special reference to diagnosis and L-dopa treatment for idiopathic parkinsonism and allied disorders. *Yakubutsu Ryoho,* 5:123–147.

12. Shiraki, H. (1974): The neuropathology of cerebellar disease groups. With special reference to their clinical features. *Adv. Neurol. Sci.,* 17:941–985.

13. Shiraki, H. (1974): Mechanism of motor ataxia from the neuropathological viewpoint. With special reference to the cerebellar involvements and hyperkinesia. *Sogo Rinsho,* 23:791–829.

14. Shiraki, H. (1975): The neuropathology of alkylmercury intoxication in humans with special reference to cerebellar involvement. In a comparison with wholebody autoradiographic studies in experimental animals. In: *Studies on the Health Effects of Alkylmercury in Japan,* edited by T. Tsubaki, pp. 71–128. Environment Agency, Japan.

15. Steele, J. C., Richardson, J. C., and Olszewski, J. (1964): Progressive supranuclear palsy. *Arch. Neurol.,* 10:333–359.

Neurotoxicology, edited by L. Roizin, H. Shiraki, and N. Grčević. Raven Press, New York © 1977.

Alternative Diagnoses to Tardive Dyskinesia: Neuropathologic Findings in Three Suspected Cases

Mavis A. Kaufman

New York State Psychiatric Institute, Department of Neuropathology, New York, New York 10032

Although the clinical syndrome of tardive dyskinesia associated with phenothiazine medication has become fairly well defined, the histopathologic substrate remains unknown. The few autopsy reports that have appeared have shown either no specific, consistent lesion to account for the syndrome or lesions characteristic of other organic brain syndromes (2,3). It appears important therefore to record the histopathologic findings in as many suspected cases as possible. The following three cases illustrate the wide range of lesions simulating tardive dyskinesia.

CASE 1

This 47-year-old man had been in difficulty with the law repeatedly since his teens for offenses such as burglary and, later, public intoxication and vagrancy. He was in the Navy briefly but received a less than honorable discharge. He was one of five siblings, the rest of whom lived in another state. His marriage ended in divorce after the birth of two sons. A family history of mental or neurologic disease was denied. The patient had had three prior hospitalizations beginning in 1954, when he was 29, with successive diagnoses of psychosis with psychopathic personality without mental disorder, psychopathic personality with asocial and amoral trends, and schizophrenia, undifferentiated type. The final hospitalization in 1966, when he was 41, was from the county home where he exhibited increasingly bizarre behavior.

On admission on March 25, 1966 his affect was flat. He was slow in answering questions but cooperative and oriented. Paranoid trends, suicidal ideas, and hallucinations were denied. His gait was described as spastic, slow, and shuffling. The Romberg test was negative. Finger-nose and finger-to-finger coordination was poor. His head and muscles of his face moved continually. Muscle tone was increased throughout the body. Deep tendon reflexes were equal bilaterally. Biceps and triceps 3+, patellar 4+, and Achilles 2+. Bilateral Babinski signs were present. Speech was slightly slurred. When asked to write, he had to position his arm first, and his arms moved slowly and jerkily.

Course

He continued to have involuntary movements of the head and to some extent of the hands and arms with a peculiar shuffling, hesitant gait. In 1971 examination also revealed slight tremor of the tongue and slight cogwheel rigidity at the elbows. His voluntary movements were very slow. The coordination became progressively poorer; he became more rigid and had urinary incontinence at times. He developed bronchopneumonia and died on April 24, 1973 at the age of 47.

Comment

The medications received in the earlier hospitalizations are unknown, but neurologic abnormalities were present before trifluoperazine hydrochloride, 10 mg b.i.d., was begun in 1966.

An autopsy revealed the gross and microscopic features of Huntington's chorea. The brain was reduced in weight (1,150 g). The lateral ventricles were symmetrically enlarged. The caudate nucleus and putamen were reduced in size bilaterally and showed extensive loss, particularly of small neurons with diffuse astrocytosis (Fig. 1). There was slight diffuse loss of cortical neurons. Some of those remaining contained excessive lipofuscin. In spite of the absence of a positive family history, the clinical story is typical of the rigid type of Huntington's chorea (1). The neurologic symptoms were preceded in this case by the mental manifestations.

CASE 2

This 84-year-old woman had several hospital admissions for paranoid schizophrenia, the first in 1939 at the age of 49, but was said to have been ill for many years before that. During the final hospitalization in 1958 (at age 69), her mental state vacillated considerably but her paranoid delusions persisted. No notes were made about her gait or balance, but she had numerous falls from 1962 on, resulting in fractures of an arm and both hips. She showed progressive mental deterioration eventually becoming incoherent, totally disoriented, confused, and doubly incontinent. Death was due to volvulus of the sigmoid colon about a month after surgical pinning of a fractured hip.

Comment

The basis for the diagnosis of tardive dyskinesia is unknown. She had received phenothiazines, with rest periods, for many years.

At autopsy the brain was found to be reduced in weight (950 g). The cerebral gyri were diffusely narrowed and the lateral and third ventriculoes enlarged. There was a small area of superficial old encephalomalacia in the right cerebellar hemisphere. Microscopically, the characteristic lesions of Alzheimer's disease involved not only the cerebral cortex and hippocampus, but also the central gray masses, cerebellum, and midbrain (Fig. 2).

CASE 3

This patient was hospitalized for the first time at his own request in May, 1936 when he was 28. The diagnosis was paranoid schizophrenia. He was discharged in 6 weeks but attempted suicide several times and was readmitted on September 21, 1936. He admitted vague auditory hallucinations and ideas of persecution. Examination revealed him to be cooperative and oriented, but overproductive, manneristic, silly, and he grimaced without provocation. Patellar reflexes were increased, and there was slight bilateral ankle clonus. In November, 1937 he was hit on the head by another patient and sustained a hematoma of the right occipital scalp. A skull X-ray revealed no fracture, but he appeared confused for several days. Thereafter he steadily improved and was released on May 29, 1939. Readmission in February, 1941 was because of sudden hyperactivity and confusion with rambling, unintelligible speech. He was uncooperative, evasive, silly, and grimaced in a peculiar childish fashion. He was treated with ambulatory insulin and electroconvulsive therapy without much improvement. He became mute and underactive. In October, it was noticed that he walked on his toes with a stiff jerky gait that was later described as slow, uncertain, and broad-based. Cerebrospinal fluid contained no cells, total protein was 130 mg%, colloidal gold 0, and pressure was not recorded. Neurological examination revealed no impairment of position or vibratory sense; pinprick sensation was normal, and there were no involuntary movements. The lower extremities offered some resistance to passive movement, but not the upper. Possibly some reduction of muscle power in the lower extremities was present. The upper extremities showed no ataxia or adiadokokinesia. There was heel to knee dysmetria. All deep tendon reflexes markedly increased bilaterally. Hoffman signs were present bilaterally. There were no Babinski signs, but plantar flexion was slight to absent. No clonus was elicited. Abdominal reflexes were equally diminished. Pneumoencephalogram in January, 1942 revealed fairly marked dilatation of the ventricular system, including third, fourth, and aqueduct, and large collections of air in cisterna magna. The cerebral sulci appeared normal. Repeat cerebrospinal fluid examination in August, 1942 revealed two lymphocytes and a total protein of 75 mg%. Because of the unsteady gait, he was confined to a wheelchair. He continued to be mute, smiled in a silly fashion and stared into space. At times he appeared to understand what was going on around him, but did not respond to questions. Occasionally he cried out a few unintelligible words, and it was decided that his speech was dysarthric. The lower extremities were increasingly spastic. A Babinski sign appeared on the right. A coarse tremor of the head was noted in 1948 and a slight intention tremor on finger-nose testing in 1972. The deep tendon reflexes in the lower extremities continued to be exaggerated. It was believed he understood questions and obeyed commands when able but remained mute. He finally died of bronchopneumonia in 1974 at the age of 66.

Comment

This patient's neurologic signs appeared many years before the advent of phenothiazine therapy.

Autopsy revealed a brain reduced in weight (1,000 g) with an old contusion of the left gyrus rectus. The entire brain had been sectioned prior to fixation and numerous areas removed, so the gross examination was limited. There appeared to be moderate diffuse enlargement of the lateral ventricles with rounding of the lateral angles.

Microscopically, there was slight nerve cell loss in the frontal cortex and a parenchymatous cerebellar degeneration (Fig. 3) (5). The Purkinje cell loss was most severe in the dorsal vermis. At some levels of the medulla, the dorsal laminae of the inferior olives, and the accessory olivary nuclei showed a patchy neuron loss and gliosis, interpreted as secondary to the cerebellar changes. The pneumoencephalographic findings and the pyramidal tract signs in the absence of appropriate anatomic lesions suggest that this patient might also have had the syndrome of normal pressure hydrocephalus (4).

SUMMARY

Three cases of suspected tardive dyskinesia were presented. Two were diagnosed schizophrenia, with durations of 35 and 38 years. Another patient, considered to have undifferentiated schizophrenia or psychosis with psychopathic personality, was hospitalized several times over a period of 19 years.

At autopsy, each brain revealed definite lesions consistent with the neurologic symptoms and characteristic of well-known pathologic entities. The areas most severely involved differed from one case to another. The only common pathologic feature was lateral ventricle enlargement. This was clearly secondary to the primary

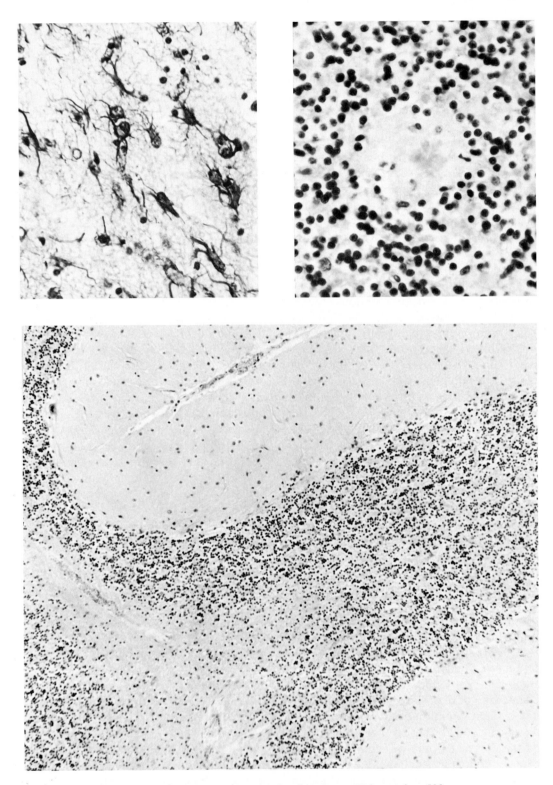

FIG. 1. Diffuse astrocytosis and neuron loss in striatum. Holzer stain. ×500.
FIG. 2. Senile plaque in granular layer of cerebellum. H. & E. stain. ×550.
FIG. 3. Diffuse loss of Purkinje cells in cerebellar cortex. H. & E. stain. ×160.

disease in cases 1 and 2 and of obscure etiology in case 3.

The remote possibility that tardive dyskinesia coexisted in these patients cannot be ruled out until sufficient instances uncomplicated by other neurologic disease have been examined at autopsy.

REFERENCES

1. Bittenbender, J. B., and Quadfasel, F. A. (1962): Rigid and akinetic forms of Huntington's chorea. *Arch. Neurol., 7:275–288.*
2. Crane, G. E. (1973): Tardive dyskinesia and Huntington's chorea: Drug-induced and hereditary dyskinesias. In: *Advances in Neurology, Vol. 1: Huntington's Chorea, 1872–1972,* edited by A. Barbeau, T. N. Chase, and G. W. Paulson, pp. 115–122. Raven Press, New York.
3. Hunter, R., Blackwood, W., Smith, M. C., and Cumings, J. N. (1968): Neuropathological findings in three cases of persistent dyskinesia following phenothiazine medication. *J. Neurol. Sci., 7:263–273.*
4. Messert, B., and Baker, N. H. (1966): Syndrome of progressive spastic ataxia and apraxia associated with occult hydrocephalus. *Neurology (Minneap.),* 16:440–452.
5. Parker, H. L., and Kernohan, J. W. (1933): Parenchymatous cortical cerebellar atrophy (chronic atrophy of Purkinje's cells). *Brain,* 56:191–212.

Neurotoxicology, edited by L. Roizin, H. Shiraki, and N. Grćević. Raven Press, New York © 1977.

Biochemical Effects of the Use of Narcotic Analgesic Drugs

Doris H. Clouet

New York State Office of Drug Abuse Services, Testing and Research Laboratory, Brooklyn, New York 11217

The consumption or administration of narcotic analgesic drugs by man or by experimental animals leads to a sequence of biochemical events in the central nervous system and in other tissues. Some metabolic events that precede the interaction of the opiate with its specific receptor in nervous tissue (i.e., absorption of the drug, distribution in tissues, and, possibly, the catabolism of the drug or events that relate to the route of administration, dose, and physiochemical characteristics of the drug) may be important in quantifying the drug–receptor interaction in terms of the extent and the duration of drug–receptor binding. The sites of specific receptor binding of opiates have been localized in the central nervous system (5,34) and spinal cord (63) and in neuromuscular junctions (32,49). The pharmacological effects produced by opiates can be classed as changes in pain perception, in overt behavior, in thermoregulation, in some vegetative functions, and in pituitary hormone systems (13). The distinguishing characteristics of narcotic analgesic drugs, however, are that chronic use leads to tolerance and dependence and that drug discontinuation leads to an abstinent state (23).

Although important events occur outside the central nervous system (e.g., drug detoxication and elimination, tolerance at neuromuscular junctions, and secondary responses in target tissue for pituitary hormones), this chapter emphasizes biochemical events in the central nervous system. The synaptic junction between the cell processes of two neurons has been identified as the subcellular site of opiate-receptor interaction (11). This chapter describes some neurochemical systems in which opiates effect alterations that may affect synaptic function.

NEUROTRANSMITTERS

Catecholamines

The administration of morphine or other opiates to laboratory animals induces alterations in the content of catecholamines in brain. A depletion of brain catecholamines in the hypothalamus and midbrain of the cat was described by Vogt in 1954 (79). Both dopamine and norepinephrine levels fall after morphine administration to mice (71). The magnitude of the effect was shown to be dose dependent with maximal depletion at intermediate doses of morphine (26,28). Not only morphine but also codeine, methadone, etorphine, levorphanol, meperidine, and pentazocine produced transient falls in brain catecholamine levels after an initial dose of drug (1,59). In tolerant subjects, brain catecholamine levels are either at normal or slightly above normal values and depletion is not found (28,59). The most common effect of withdrawal from chronic opiate use is a further depletion of brain catecholamines (31).

The multiphasic nature of the responses in brain catecholamine levels after opiate administration suggests that the drug may induce alterations in the turnover as well as the levels of the biogenic amines. The most prominent effect is a sharp rise in the rate of dopamine biosynthesis in the caudate nucleus of the striatum after a single moderate dose of morphine (14,17). Tolerance develops in this biochemical parameter as morphine or other opiates are used chronically (66).

The administration of nonopiate drugs to experimental animals may have an effect on the action of opiates. Amphetamine, cocaine, iproniazid, and apomorphine generally enhance the effects of opiates, whereas chlorpromazine, haloperidol, 6-hydroxydopamine, and tetrabenazine antagonize opiate responses (12). Drugs that tend to increase the levels of catecholamines, particularly dopamine at the receptor, tend to enhance opiate action, whereas drugs that lower receptor levels inhibit opiate action (12). It is obvious that some of the pharmacological responses to opiate administration are effected via adrenergic mechanisms.

Serotonin

An antagonism to morphine-induced responses by *p*-chlorophenylalanine, an inhibitor of serotonin biosynthesis, has been shown in several laboratories (4, 72,81). The importance of the serotonin-to-catecholamine ratios has been indicated for analgesia (68), temperature regulation (25,51), and oxytremorine analgesia (9). In these studies norepinephrine antagonized morphine effects, and serotonin potentiated them.

Morphine has been reported to accelerate the rate of serotonin turnover in brain (84). Changes in serotonin levels,

however, have not been uniformly observed.

Not only depressant effects of opiates but also excitant effects are antagonized by the administration of *p*-chlorophenylalanine to opiate-treated animals. Locomotor activity, which is depressed in rats by opiates, is enhanced if the administration of the inhibitor of serotonin biosynthesis precedes that of the opiate (50). Thus, the participation of this biogenic amine in the manifestation of pharmacological responses to opiate administration is indicated.

Acetylcholine

In 1957, two investigators reported that morphine and other opiates prevented the release of acetylcholine from guinea pig ileum preparations (53,61). This neuromuscular preparation has been very useful in assaying morphine-like activity recently discovered in brain (41). In the central nervous system also, morphine has been shown to have antirelease action (48). This effect is antagonized by naloxone and other narcotic antagonists and is not seen in tolerant animals (44). However, this is not a direct effect of opiates on acetylcholine release (22). An interaction between dopamine and acetylcholine has been demonstrated in experiments in which an increase in acetylcholine output followed the blockade of the dopamine receptor by haloperidol (69). In rat striatum, however, the effect of morphine on dopamine turnover is accomplished without a change in the rate of acetylcholine turnover (10).

Other Neurotransmitters

The involvement of the neurotransmitter γ-aminobutyric acid (GABA) in pharmacological responses to opiates has been suggested. In subcortical areas of the brains of morphine-tolerant rats, the levels of GABA are significantly higher than in control animals (47). However, if the levels of GABA in brain are increased by the administration of GABA or an inhibitor of its catabolism aminooxyacetic acid, the response to acute morphine is reduced (35). Tolerance and dependence are enhanced in animals treated with the same agents (35). GABA neurons in the substantia nigra modify the nigrostriatal pathway (2) that has been implicated in some responses to opiate administration. It is interesting that whereas GABA increases the turnover of striatal dopamine by blocking impulse flow in the nigrostriatal pathway, stimulation of the pathway also increases striatal dopamine turnover (60). In rats, the rate of impulse flow in nigrostriatal neurons is increased by the systemic or direct administration of morphine into the caudate nucleus (38).

Histamine is released peripherally by morphine administration (62). In rat brain, the acute administration of morphine has no effect on brain histamine levels (33). However, in animals treated chronically with morphine, there is a significant decrease in histamine levels in the hypothalamus (33). Histamine levels are even lower in naloxone-induced withdrawal. It may be that morphine effects on histamine are detectable because in this tissue histamine has the highest concentration and rate of turnover (21).

Conclusion

The evidence, briefly reviewed above, that all neurotransmitters are involved in the expression of various pharmacological responses to opiate administration forces the conclusion that none of the conventional neurotransmitters is uniquely involved in the mechanism of action of narcotic analgesic drugs.

NEUROREGULATORS

Prostaglandins

In guinea pig ileum, morphine is known to inhibit the contractions evoked by PGEs (prostaglandins of the E series) (39). Collier and Roy have reported that opiates inhibit the stimulation of cyclic AMP formation by E prostaglandins in rat brain homogenates (16). Similar effects have been found in cultured hybrid neuroblastoma x glioma cells *in vitro* (40,77). The ratio of cyclic AMP to cyclic GMP in these cells is important in determining the effect that opiates have on PGE-stimulated adenylate cyclase activity. At low-opiate concentrations, the responsiveness of adenylate cyclase to PGE is enhanced, whereas at high-drug concentrations, the enzyme is inhibited (77). PGE hyperpolarizes neuronal cells, thereby inhibiting neuronal activity (78). If opiates act on inhibitory neurons, a reversal of PGE-induced hyperpolarization by the opiates would lead to activation of an inhibitory pathway and thus selective depression of neuronal activity.

Peptide Hormones

Peptides are known to play a role in neuronal excitability (3,58). The possibility that some peptides act as neurotransmitters in the central nervous system is supported by studies in which peptides such as thyrotropin releasing hormone (TRH), somatostatin, or substance P are localized in synaptosomes (7,54) and are released on nerve stimulation (24). However, there is a difference in length of action between neurotransmitters and peptides: neuropeptides have long-lasting effects.

Many behavioral parameters are altered by the administration of peptides to experimental animals, especially hypophyseal trophic hormones and hypothalamic releasing factors. TRH produces euphoria (7). TRH and melanocyte-stimulating hormone release-inhibiting factor (MIF) have antisedative activity (57), whereas vasopressin antagonizes the amnesia produced in mice by puromycin (80). It is pertinent to note that the administration of narcotic analgesic drugs to man or laboratory animals has significant effects on the release of trophic hormones from the pituitary gland (30).

Responses to morphine are altered by the simultaneous administration of peptides. An analog of vasopressin increases the analgesic response to morphine in mice (42), and somatostatin antagonizes the increased release of growth hormone induced by morphine (27). β-Melanocyte-stimulating hormone (β-MSH) and adreno-corticotropic hormone 1–24 (ACTH$_{1-24}$) antagonize the actions of morphine in spinal cats (85), and substance P abolishes the abstinence syndrome (70). It is interesting that the microinjection of TRH into brain areas produces shaking behavior in rats that is similar to abstinence shaking and that the brain areas positive for TRH-shaking are the same as those in which naloxone microinjection produces shaking in morphine-tolerant animals (83).

In a following section, the naturally occurring morphine-like factors isolated from brain that are peptides with sequences of amino acids common to the polypeptide hormone of the anterior pituitary β-lipotropin are discussed.

OPIATE RECEPTORS

The presence of specific opiate receptors in nervous tissue was suggested by the structural specificity required for opiate action. In 1973, three groups of investigators independently demonstrated that radiolabeled opiates are bound stereospecifically in brain homogenates *in vitro* (55,64,73). The binding affinities of a large number of the narcotic drugs are related to their potency *in vivo,* either as narcotic agonists or antagonists (20). One interesting difference between the binding of agonists and that of antagonists is that sodium ions inhibit the binding of agonists and enhance the binding of antagonists (56,65). The ratio of binding in the presence and absence of sodium ions

is actually indicative of the proportion of agonist and antagonist activity in narcotic drugs (67).

Opiate receptors are distributed heterogeneously in brain with the highest levels in the limbic system and in hypothalamus in both human and monkey brain (34,43). Other tissues such as the guinea pig ileum and neuronal cells in culture also contain opiate receptors (40,74).

ENDORPHINS

The presence in nervous tissue of 'endogenous ligands,' substances that bind stereospecifically to opiate receptors, was suggested by the unique characteristics of the receptors. The discovery of possible endogenous ligands was first reported by Terenius and Wahlström (75) and by Hughes (36). Other groups described the partial isolation of substances with morphine-like activity from brain (52) and from the pituitary gland (70). The chemical identification of the brain morphine-like factors as pentapeptides of the sequence: tyr.gly.gly.phe.metOH or tyr.gly.gly.phe.leuOH and the recognition that the first sequence is amino acid 61 to 65 of the pituitary polypeptide hormone β-lipotropin were made by Hughes and Kosterlitz and their colleagues (37). These investigators called the pentapeptides enkephalins (met-enkephalin and leu-enkephalin). The general term for endogenous morphine-like substances is endorphins (19). The common amino acid sequences of enkephalin and β-lipotropin are not fortuitous since other fragments of β-lipotropin, or more exactly, of the C fragment of β-lipotropin (amino acids 61–91) also have morphine-like activity (6,45,46). In most of these studies morphine-like activity is defined as the ability to bind stereospecifically to opiate receptors in brain. In addition, the activity of the peptide endorphins has been assayed on the neuromuscular junction in isolated guinea pig ileum (37,45).

The evocation of opiate-like effects on the administration of endorphins was not successful at first, until it was recognized that the peptides are rapidly destroyed by tissue enzymes (63). Endorphins such as the C fragment or smaller peptides produce pharmacological responses when injected into animals (8,18). Morphine-tolerant animals are tolerant to endorphins (82), and endorphin-tolerant animals are tolerant to morphine (82). The effects of the endorphins are antagonized by naloxone and other narcotic antagonists (29). Therefore, the endorphins are endogenous substances with all of the specific biological properties of the narcotic analgesic drugs.

The question arises whether the endorphins, found throughout brain (63), derived from β-lipotropin synthesized in the anterior pituitary gland or are biosynthesized in brain tissue. We have injected H^3-glycine into the cerebrospinal fluid (CSF) of rats and isolated enkephalins with the labeled amino acid in the peptide 30 min later (15). This result shed more light on the speed of enkephalin biosynthesis than on the site of its formation.

CONCLUSIONS

The biochemical changes produced by the administration of narcotic analgesic drugs to experimental animals that are narcotic specific (i.e., stereospecific and antagonized by antagonists) represent several phases of the addiction process:

1. an opiate 'metabolic' stage that includes all of the changes undergone by the drug after its introduction into the body (activation or detoxication) and all of the factors that determine the amount of drug reaching the central nervous system (route of injection, physical characteristics of the drug, elimination, etc.);

2. the 'initial' drug–tissue interaction or the stereospecific binding of opiate to receptor;

3. the 'transduction' stage, wherein the activity of the opiate receptor binding is transferred to a connected biochemical action;

4. the 'initial biochemical' response, in which immediate alterations in membrane permeability, ion flux, impulse flow, neurotransmitter metabolism, etc., are found;

5. homeostatic response in which biochemical systems respond to the insult introduced by the presence of the drug to preserve function;

6. tolerance or adaptation to the chronic presence of opiates in brain, in which the initial biochemical responses are diminished by the homeostatic 'set' established during stage 5;

7. acute withdrawal stage in which the sudden reversal of the homeostatic 'set' is produced by opiate withdrawal;

8. abstinence, a stage that includes stage 7, but mainly is concerned with the slow return to the predrug state. Long-term tolerance, described as altered pharmacological responses to opiate administration months after last drug use, is an extension of this stage.

These stages, which are much more complex than their descriptions, also have behavioral correlates. The role of endorphins in this series of events is the challenge for this generation of opiatologists.

REFERENCES

1. Ahtee, L. (1973): Catalepsy and stereotyped behavior in rats treated chronically with methadone: Relation to brain homovanillic acid levels. *J. Pharm. Pharmacol.,* 25:649–651.
2. Anden, N. E., and Stock, G. (1973): Inhibitory effect of GABA and γ-hydroxybutyric acid on dopamine cells in the substantia nigra. *Naunyn Schmiedebergs Arch. Pharmacol.,* 279:88–92.
3. Barker, J. L. (1976): Peptides: Roles in neuronal excitability. *Physiol. Rev.,* 56:435–452.

4. Berney, S. A., and Buxbaum, D. M. (1973): The effect of morphine on catecholamine turnover and its relationship to morphine-induced motor activity. *Pharmacologist,* 15:202.

5. Borison, H. L. (1971): Sites of action of narcotic analgesic drugs in the nervous system. In: *Narcotic Drugs: Biochemical Pharmacology,* edited by D. H. Clouet, pp. 342–365. Plenum Press, New York.

6. Bradbury, A. F., Smyth, D. G., and Snell, C. R. (1976): C-fragment of lipotropin has a high affinity for brain opiate receptors. *Nature,* 260: 793–795.

7. Burt, D. R., and Snyder, S. H. (1975): TRH: An apparent binding in rat brain membranes. *Brain Res.,* 93:309–328.

8. Büscher, H. H., Hill, R. C., Romer, D., Cardinaux, F., Closse, A., Hauser, D., and Pless, J. (1976): Evidence for analgesic activity of enkephalin in the mouse. *Nature,* 261:423–425.

9. Calcutt, C. R., Doggett, N. S., and Spencer, P. S. J. (1971): Modification of the antinociceptive effect of morphine by centrally administered ouabain and dopamine. *Psychopharmacologia,* 21:111–114.

10. Carenzi, A., Cheney, D. L., Costa, E., Guidotti, A., and Racagni, G. (1975): Action of opiates, antipsychotics, amphetamine and apomorphine on dopamine receptors in rat striatum. *Neuropharmacology,*14:927–939.

11. Clouet, D. H. (1972): Theoretical biochemical mechanisms for drug dependence. In: *Chemical and Biological Aspects of Drug Dependence,* edited by S. J. Mulé and H. Brill, pp. 545–561. CRC Press, Cleveland.

12. Clouet, D. H. (1975): Catecholamines in the action of narcotic drugs. In: *Catecholamines and Behavior,* Vol. 2, edited by A. J. Friedhoff, pp. 167–196. Plenum Press, New York.

13. Clouet, D. H., and Iwatsubo, K. (1975): Mechanisms of tolerance to and dependence on narcotic analgesic drugs. *Annu. Rev. Pharmacol.,* 15:49–71.

14. Clouet, D. H., and Ratner, M. (1970): Catecholamine biosynthesis in brains of rats treated with morphine. *Science,* 168:854–856.

15. Clouet, D. H., and Ratner, M. (1976): The incorporation of H³-glycine into enkephalins in the brains of morphine treated rats. In: *Opiates and Endogenous Opioid Peptides,* edited by H. W. Kosterlitz, pp. 71–78. North Holland, Amsterdam.

16. Collier, H. O. J., and Roy, A. C. (1974): Morphine-like drugs inhibit the stimulation by E prostaglandins of cyclic AMP formation by rat brain homogenates. *Nature,* 248:24–27.

17. Costa, E., Carenzi, A., Guidotti, A., and Revuelta, A. (1973): Narcotic analgesics and the regulation of neuronal catecholamine stores. In: *Frontiers in Catecholamine Research,* edited by E. Costa and E. Usdin, pp. 833–840. Pergamon Press, New York.

18. Cowan, A., Doxey, J. C., and Metcalf, G. (1976): A comparison of the pharmacological effects produced by leu-enkephalin, met-enkephalin, morphine and ketocyclazocine *in vivo.* In: *Opiates and Endogenous Opioid Peptides,* edited by H. W. Kosterlitz, pp. 95–102. North-Holland, Amsterdam.

19. Cox, B. M., Goldstein, A., and Li, C. H. (1976): Opioid activity of a peptide, β-lipotropin-(61–91), derived from β-lipotropin. *Proc. Natl. Acad. Sci. USA,* 73:1821–1823.

20. Creese, I., and Snyder, S. H. (1975): Receptor binding and pharmacological activity of opiates in the guinea-pig intestine. *J. Pharmacol. Exp. Ther.,* 194:205–219.

21. Dismukes, K., and Snyder, S. H. (1974): Histamine turnover in rat brain. *Brain Res.,* 78:467–481.

22. Domino, E. F. (1975): Role of central cholinergic mechanisms in the specific actions of narcotic agonists. In: *Cholinergic Mechanisms,* edited by P. G. Waser, pp. 356–453. Raven Press, New York.

23. Eddy, N. B., Halbach, H., Isbell, H., and Seevers, M. H. (1965): Drug dependence — its significance and characteristics. *Bull. WHO,* 32:721–735.

24. Edwardson, J. A., and Bennet, G. W. (1974): Modulation of corticotropin releasing factor release from hypothalamic synaptosomes. *Nature,* 251:425–427.

25. Feldberg, W., and Sherwood, S. L. (1954): Injection of drugs into the lateral ventricles of the cat. *J. Physiol. (Lond.),* 107:372–381.

26. Fennessey, M. R., and Lee, J. R. (1972): Comparison of the dose-response effects of morphine on brain amines, analagesia and activity in mice. *Br. J. Pharmacol.,* 45:240–247.

27. Ferland, L., Labrie, F., Coy, D. H., Arimura, A., and Schally, A.V. (1976): Inhibition by somatostatin analogs of plasma GH levels stimulated by morphine in the rat. *Mol. Cell. Endocrinol.,* 4:79–88.

28. Fukui, K., and Takagi, H. (1972): Effect of morphine on cerebral contents of metabolites of dopamine in normal and tolerant mice: Its possible relation to analgesic action. *Br. J. Pharmacol.,* 44:45–51.

29. Gent, J. P., and Wolstencraft, J. H. (1976): Effects of met-enkephalin and leu-enkephalin compared with those of morphine on brainstem neurons in cat. *Nature,* 261:426–427.

30. George, R. (1973): Drug effects on endocrine regulation. *Prog. Brain Res.,* 39:339–346.

31. Gunne, L. M. (1963): Catecholamines and 5-hydroxytryptamine in morphine-tolerance and withdrawal. *Acta Physiol. Scand. [Suppl.],* (204) 58:1–91.

32. Henderson, G., Hughes, J., and Kosterlitz, H. W. (1972): A new example of a morphine-sensitive neuro-effector junction: Adrenergic transmission in the mouse vas deferens. *Br. J. Pharmacol.,* 46:764–766.

33. Henwood, R. W., and Mazurkiewicz-Kwilecki, I. M. (1975): Possible role of brain histamine in morphine addiction. In: *The Opiate Narcotics,*

edited by A. Goldstein, pp. 209–210. Pergamon Press, New York.

34. Hiller, J. M., Pearson, J., and Simon, E. J. (1973): Distribution of stereospecific binding of the potent narcotic analgesic etorphine in the human brain. *Res. Commun. Chem. Pathol. Pharmacol.*, 6:1052–1062.

35. Ho, I. K., Loh, H. H., and Way, E. L. (1973): Influence of GABA on morphine analgesia, tolerance and physical dependence. *Proc. West. Pharmacol. Soc.*, 16:4–7.

36. Hughes, J. (1975): Isolation of an endogenous compound from the brain with pharmacological properties similar to morphine. *Brain Res.*, 88:295–308.

37. Hughes, J., Smith, T., Kosterlitz, H. W., Fothergill, L. A., Morgan, B. A., and Morris, H. R. (1975): Identification of two related pentapeptides from brain with potent opiate agonist activity. *Nature*, 258:577–579.

38. Iwatsubo, K., and Clouet, D. H. (1976): Electrical activity of nigrostriatal neurons after morphine or haloperidol. *Pharmacologist*, 18:178.

39. Jacques, R. (1969): Morphine as inhibitor of prostaglandin E-1 in the isolated guinea pig intestine. *Experientia*, 25:1059–1060.

40. Klee, W. A., Sharma, S. K., and Nirenberg, M. (1975): Opiate receptors as regulators of adenylate cyclase. In: *The Opiate Narcotics*, edited by A. Goldstein, pp. 111–122. Pergamon Press, New York.

41. Kosterlitz, H. W., and Hughes, J. (1975): Some thoughts on the significance of enkephalin, the endogenous ligand. In: *The Opiate Narcotics*, edited by A. Goldstein, pp. 245–250. Pergamon Press, New York.

42. Krivoy, W. A., Zimmerman, E., and Lande, S. (1974): Facilitation of the development of resistance to morphine analgesia by desglycinamide lys-vasopressin. *Proc. Natl. Acad. Sci. USA*, 71:1852–1856.

43. Kuhar, M. J., Pert, C. B., and Snyder, S. H. (1973): Regional distribution of opiate receptor binding in monkey and human brain. *Nature*, 245:447–450.

44. Labrecque, G., and Domino, E. F. (1974): Tolerance to and physical dependence on morphine. *J. Pharmacol. Exp. Therap.*, 191:189–200.

45. Lazarus. L. H., Ling, N., and Guillemin, R. (1976): β-Lipotropin as a prohormone for the morphinomimetic peptides, endorphins, and enkephalins. *Proc. Natl. Acad. Sci. USA*, 73:2156–2159.

46. Li, C. H., and Chung, D. (1976): Isolation and structure of an untriakontapeptide with opiate activity. *Proc. Natl. Acad. Sci. USA*, 73:1145–1148.

47. Lin, S. C., Sutherland, V. C., and Way, E. L. (1973): Brain amino acids in morphine tolerant and nontolerant rats. *Proc. West. Pharmacol. Soc.*, 16:8–13.

48. Matthews, J. D., Labrecque, G., and Domino, E. F. (1973): Effect of morphine, nalorphine and naloxone on neocortical release of acetylcholine

in the rat. *Psychopharmacologia*, 29:113–120.

49. North, R. A., and Henderson, G. (1975): Action of morphine on guinea pig myenteric plexus and mouse vas deferens. In: *The Opiate Narcotics*, edited by A. Goldstein, pp. 217–220. Pergamon Press, New York.

50. Oka, T., and Hosoya, E. (1976): The effect of *p*-chlorophenylalanine on the pethidine- or methadone-induced decrease in locomotor activity of rats. *Eur. J. Pharmacol.*, 37:393–395.

51. Oka, T., Nozaki, M., and Hosoya, E. (1972): The effect of cholinergic antagonists on the increases of spontaneous motor activity and body weight induced by the administration of morphine to tolerant rats. *Psychopharmacologia*, 23:231–238.

52. Pasternak, G. W., Goodman, R., and Snyder, S. H. (1975): An endogenous morphine-like factor in mammalian brain. *Life Sci.*, 16:1765–1769.

53. Paton, W. D. M. (1957): The action of morphine and related substances on contraction and on acetylcholine output of coaxially stimulated guinea-pig ileum. *Br. J. Pharmacol.*, 12:119–127.

54. Pelletier, G., Labrie, F., Arimura, A., and Schally, A. V. (1974): Electron microscope immunohistochemical localization of LH-RIF in rat median eminence. *Am. J. Anat.*, 140:445–450.

55. Pert, C. B., and Snyder, S. H. (1973): Opiate receptor: Demonstration in nervous tissue. *Science*, 179:1011–1014.

56. Pert, C. P., and Snyder, S. H. (1974): Opiate receptor binding of agonists and antagonists affected differentially by sodium. *Mol. Pharmacol.*, 10:868–879.

57. Plotnikoff, N. P., and Kastin, A. J. (1976): Neuropharmacology of hypothalamic releasing factors. *Biochem. Pharmacol.*, 25:363–365.

58. Renaud, L. P., Martin, J. P., and Brazeau, P. (1975): Depressant action of TRH, LH-RH and somatostatin on the activity of central neurons. *Nature*, 225:233–235.

59. Rethy, C. R., Smith, C. B., and Villarreal, J. (1971): Effects of narcotic analgesics upon locomotor activity and brain catecholamine content of the mouse. *J. Pharmacol. Exp. Ther.*, 176:472–479.

60. Roth, R. H., Walters, J. R., and Aghajanian, G. K. (1973): Effect of impulse flow on the release and synthesis of dopamine in the striatum. *Life Sci.*, 13:139–146.

61. Schaumann, W. (1957): Inhibition by morphine of the release of acetylcholine from the intestine of the guinea-pig. *Br. J. Pharmacol.*, 12:115–118.

62. Schmidt, C. F., and Livingston, A. E. (1933): The action of morphine on mammalian circulation. *J. Pharmacol. Exp. Ther.*, 47:411–420.

63. Simantov, R., Kuhar, M. J., Pasternak, G. W., and Snyder, S. H. (1976): The regional distribution of morphine-like factor enkephalin in monkey brain. *Brain Res.*, 106:189–197.

64. Simon, E. J., Hiller, J. M., and Edelman, I. (1973): Stereospecific binding of the potent

narcotic analgesic H³-etorphine to rat brain homogenate. *Proc. Natl. Acad. Sci. USA,* 70: 1947–1949.

65. Simon, E. J., Hiller, J. M., Groth, J., and Edelman, I. (1975): Further properties of stereospecific opiate binding sites in rat brain: On the nature of the sodium effect. *J. Pharmacol. Exp. Ther.,* 192:531–537.

66. Smith, C. B., Sheldon, M. I., Bednarczyk, H. J., and Villarreal, J. (1972): Morphine-induced increases in the incorporation of C^{14}-tyrosine into C^{14}-dopamine and C^{14}-norepinephrine in the mouse brain. *J. Pharmacol. Exp. Ther.,* 180: 547–557.

67. Snyder, S. H. (1975): Opiate receptor in normal and drug altered brain function. *Nature,* 257: 185–189.

68. Sparkes, C. G., and Spencer, P. S. J. (1971): Antinociceptive activity of morphine after injection of biogenic amines in the cerebral ventricles of the conscious rat. *Br. J. Pharmacol.,* 42:230–241.

69. Stadler, H., Lloyd, K. G., Gadea-Ciria, M., and Bartholini, G. (1973): Enhanced striatal acetylcholine release by chlorpromazine and its reversal by apomorphine. *Brain Res.,* 55:472–480.

70. Stern, P., and Hadzovic, S. (1973): Pharmacological analysis of central actions of substance P. *Arch. Intern. Pharmacodyn.,* 202:259–262.

71. Takagi, H., and Nakama, M. (1968): Studies on the mechanism of action of tetrabenazine as a morphine antagonist. *Jpn. J. Pharmacol.,* 18: 54–58

72. Tenen, S. S. (1968): Antagonism of the analgesic effect of morphine and other drugs by *p*-chlorophenylaline, a serotonin depletor. *Psychopharmacologia,* 12:278–285.

73. Terenius, L. (1973): Stereospecific interaction between narcotic analgesics and a synaptic plasma membrane fraction of rat cerebral cortex. *Acta Pharmacol. Toxicol. (Kbh.),* 32:317–320.

74. Terenius, L. (1973): Stereospecific uptake of narcotic analysis by a subcellular fraction of the guinea-pig ileum. *Ups. J. Med. Sci.,* 78:150–152.

75. Terenius, L., and Wahlstrom, A. (1974): Inhibitor(s) of narcotic receptor binding in brain extracts and cerebrospinal fluid. *Acta Pharmacol. Toxicol. (Kbh),* 35:55

76. Teschemacher, H., Opheim, K., Cox, B. M., and Goldstein, A. (1975): A peptide-like substance from pituitary that acts like morphine. *Life Sci.,* 16:1771–1776.

77. Traber, J., Gullis, R., and Hamprecht, B. (1975): Influence of opiates on the levels of adenosine 3′-5′-cyclic monophosphate in neuroblastoma x glioma hybrid cells. In: *The Opiate Narcotics,* edited by A. Goldstein, pp. 111–116. Pergamon Press, New York.

78. Traber, J., Reiser, G., Fisher, K., and Hamprecht, D. (1975): Measurements of AMP and membrane potential in neuroblastoma glioma hybrid cells; opiates and adrenergic agonists cause effects opposite to those of prostaglandin E-1. *FEBS Lett.,* 52:327–333.

79. Vogt, M. (1954): The concentration of sympathin in different parts of the CNS under normal conditions, and after the administration of drugs. *J. Physiol. (Lond.),* 123:451–481.

80. Walter, R., Hoffman, P. L., Flexner, J. B., and Flexner, L. B. (1975): Neurohypophyseal hormones, analogs and fragments: Their effect on puromycin-induced amnesia. *Proc. Natl. Acad. Sci. USA,* 72:4180–4184.

81. Way, E. L. Loh, H. H., and Shen, F. H. (1968): Morphine tolerance, physical dependence and the synthesis of brain serotonin. *Science,* 162: 1290–1292.

82. Wei, E. and Loh, H. H. (1976): Chronic intracerebral infusion of opiates and peptides with osmotic minipumps and the development of physical dependence. In: *Opiates and Endogenous Opioid Peptides,* edited by H. W. Kosterlitz, pp. 303–310. North-Holland, Amsterdam.

83. Wei, E., Sigal, S., Loh, H. H., and Way, E. L. (1975): TRH and shaking behavior in the rat. *Nature,* 253:739–740.

84. Yarborough, G. G., Buxbaum, D. M., and Sanders-Bush, E. (1973): Biogenic amines and narcotic effects. *J. Pharmacol. Exp. Ther.,* 185: 328–334.

85. Zimmermann, E., and Krivoy, W. A. (1973): Antagonism between morphine and the polypeptides ACTH, $ACTH_{1-2-4}$ and MSH in the N.S. *Prog. Brain Res.,* 39:383–392.

Neurotoxicology, edited by L. Roizin, H. Shiraki, and N. Grčević. Raven Press, New York © 1977.

Methadone Maintenance in the Treatment of Heroin Addicts in New York City: A Ten Year Overview

Frances Rowe Gearing

Division of Epidemiology, Columbia University School of Public Health, Methadone Maintenance Evaluation Unit, New York, New York 10032

HISTORICAL BACKGROUND

The methadone maintenance "experiment" started at Rockefeller University in 1964 with six heroin addicts (three of Spanish extraction and three non-Spanish whites) under the supervision of Dole and Nyswander.

In the intervening 10 years this "experiment" has escalated in the greater New York area so that as of December 31, 1974 there were approximately 40,000 patients known to be in methadone maintenance treatment programs either in one of the five boroughs of New York City or in Nassau, Suffolk, or Westchester County. These patients were receiving treatment in 168 separate treatment units scattered throughout these eight counties. As methadone maintenance treatment has expanded, the criteria for admission with reference to age, duration of addiction, and previous criminal behavior have changed. The induction phase has changed from a period of 6 weeks on an inpatient basis to complete ambulatory induction, and the Dole–Nyswander or Beth Israel program has been supplemented by four other publicly supported programs including Bronx State, New York City Health Services Administration, Westchester County, and the Van Etten Tuberculosis Unit. In addition, a group of treatment programs has developed under separate funding either on a fee-for-service or on a Medicaid-reimbursement basis. These will be referred to in this report as unaffiliated and private clinics. The number of patients admitted to each of these programs through December 31, 1974, as well as the increase during 1974 is shown in Table 1. It should be noted that 41% (16,450 of 39,910) of

TABLE 1. *Change in census from December 31, 1973 through December 31, 1974*

	December 31, 1973 cumulative		December 31, 1974 cumulative	
	Adm.	In Rx	Adm.	In Rx
Beth Israel & affiliates	10,000	7,170	10,700	7,370
Bronx State & affiliates	3,270	2,400	3,500	2,430
Van Etten	460	265	490	290
Health Services Administration	16,290	11,380	17,700	11,640
Westchester	2,460	1,300	2,700	1,730
Subtotal	32,480	22,515	35,090	23,460
Unaffiliated & private clinics	25,240	16,070	29,280	16,450
Total	57,720	38,585	64,370	39,910

the patients in treatment as of the end of last year were under treatment in unaffiliated or private clinics. This proportion in 1972 was 27%. This change is of interest for this evaluation, because *none* of the private clinics has been under follow-up surveillance and only two of the unaffiliated clinics were included during the first 3 years of study.

RETENTION RATES

One measure of the effectiveness of a program for a chronic illness that requires long-term treatment is its acceptability to the patients and their willingness to continue medication and remain under observation for an indefinite period of time. We have measured this by looking at retention rates over time in each of the various program units in each admission cohort.

Table 2 shows the distribution of patients admitted to each program unit by date of first admission, as well as the percentage from each cohort who were in treatment as of the end of 1974. This table shows that of all the patients with a date of first admission between 1964 and 1968, 63% (834 out of 1,345) were under observation as of December 31, 1974. Of those admitted to Beth Israel, 66% were in treatment. This is after a period of 7 years or

more. In this cohort, the proportion in continuous treatment is 78% (651).

Among patients admitted in 1971, 59% were in treatment as of the end of last year. In the Beth Israel group, the retention rate was 67% after a period of 4 years. These changes in retention rate probably reflect a combination of the relaxation of the admission criteria and the change in ethnic mix, since the retention rates are lowest for the age cohort under 20 at time of admission and for the black cohort. This is not shown in this table but has been reported previously (1).

It further shows that the retention rate for the Beth Israel, Bronx State, and Health Services Administration units are remarkably similar. In Westchester County the retention rates are consistently lower than in the first three units and tend to resemble the Van Etten Tuberculosis unit where patients are admitted with the double problem of tuberculosis and addiction. (The retention rates for the patients in the unaffiliated and private sector are consistently lower than either Beth Israel, Bronx State, or Health Services Administration.)

A treatment program that requires daily medication and clinic visits two to three times each week that can sustain retention rates of this magnitude (approximately two out of three on the average) must be doing

TABLE 2. *Retention rates in percentages as of December 31, 1974 among six methadone maintenance treatment units by date of first admission*

	Beth Israel	Bronx State	HSA*	Van Etten	Westchester	Total
1964–1968	66	63		26	65	63
1969	66	60		44	68	63
1970	67	63	61	48	49	64
1971	67	62	54	39	50	59
1972	64	63	62	54	51	61
1973	71	80	67	51	71	68
1974**	89	94	90	94	81	89
Total	70	67	64	53	56	65
N	10,700	3,500	17,700	490	2,700	35,090

* HSA, Health Services Administration.
** January to August admissions only.

something right for the patients who request methadone maintenance treatment.

SOCIAL PRODUCTIVITY

One of the major goals of the Methadone Maintenance Treatment Program in New York City has been to assist patients in becoming employable and in obtaining meaningful jobs. Data on changes in social productivity through December 31, 1974, for a sample of approximately 12,000 patients admitted through December 31, 1972, is shown in Fig. 1 for each admission cohort for men. Social productivity here is measured by employment, vocational training, or school attendance. (For this analysis the category of homemaker for women was omitted in order to make the comparison between men and women as meaningful as possible.)

The slopes of the curves in this figure for successive admission cohorts are very similar. However, each successive admission cohort shows a slightly lower rate of increased social productivity. This figure also shows a leveling off or a slight decrease in the rate of social productivity during the last year of observation.

Figure 2 shows that for women, the rate of increase in social productivity is greater than for men in the early years, although the proportion of women who become

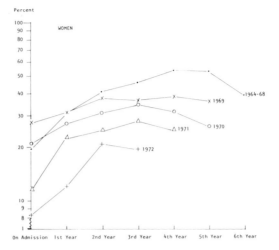

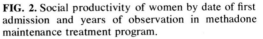

FIG. 2. Social productivity of women by date of first admission and years of observation in methadone maintenance treatment program.

socially productive is consistently lower than men (50 versus 85%) and the "fall off" in the last year of observation is noted for each cohort of women. This fall off undoubtedly is a reflection of the general employment problem in the New York area, and this impact is even more dramatically demonstrated for women than for men. To substantiate this observation, we have noted a considerable increase in the number of patients both men and women who are currently collecting unemployment insurance.

Table 3 converts the percentages in the preceding graphs into numbers for each year of observation to demonstrate the magnitude of this change in social productivity. It shows that among the 35 patients who have been under observation for at least 10 years, 30 (85%) are currently socially productive as compared with 12 (35%) who were considered socially productive at the time of admission to treatment. This is an increase of 18 or 50%. This may not be impressive because the numbers are small. However, if we look at the fifth year where the change is from

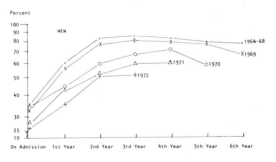

FIG. 1. Social productivity of men by date of first admission and years of observation in methadone maintenance treatment program.

TABLE 3. *Increase in social productivity by years of observation*

Years under observation	Social productivity				
	As of December 31, 1974			On admission	
	N	No.	%	No.	%
10	35	30	85	12	35
9	155	130	84	55	35
8	370	305	82	150	41
7	610	475	78	200	33
6	1,205	795	66	505	42
5	2,485	1,555	63	945	38
4	7,565	4,365	60	2,320	31
3	14,140	7,495	53	4,125	29
2	21,710	10,315	48	6,265	29
1	25,870	9,400	36	7,335	28

38% to 63%, an increase of 25%, the number of patients who have become newly productive is 610. For the total population of 25,870 admitted through 1972 who were in treatment at the end of December 1974, the change from 28% to 36% in the first year involves a change in social productivity for 2,165 patients.

Increasing the social productivity of this sizeable group of former heroin addicts, most of whom had previously been incapable of obtaining or retaining a job that allowed them to be self-supporting, must be considered a positive feature of the Methadone Maintenance Treatment Program in New York City.

ANTISOCIAL BEHAVIOR

In attempting to measure changes in antisocial behavior we have used *reported* arrests and incarcerations as an indicator. This has come under criticism, because arrests are not considered an accurate measure of criminal activity, since illicit activities for which arrests are not made are excluded. However, for lack of a more accurate index it provides useful information not otherwise available. Besides this was something that could be counted, and there is no information that indicates that

methadone on a daily basis gives the patients an ability to evade the law that they did not have when they were using heroin.

Patients in methadone maintenance treatment have access to legal counsel *after* arrests. This has allowed the majority of the arrested patients to remain under treatment while awaiting trial rather than being incarcerated prior to conviction. Despite an almost universal history of previous criminal activity as measured by reported arrests and incarcerations in the cohorts admitted through 1972, a marked change in the arrest pattern has been noted. Arrests following admission are confined to less than 15% of patients. The remaining 85% have no record of involvement with the law while in treatment.

It has been suggested that the decrease in arrests is the result of "bad patients" leaving the program and "good patients" remaining in treatment. However, among 600 arrested patients from a sample of 4,000 from the early cohorts, 245 (41%) were in treatment as of December 31, 1974. Of these 76 (31%) have been in continuous treatment, and the remaining 169 (69%) left but have subsequently returned to treatment.

It has been suggested further that the marked decrease in arrests observed in

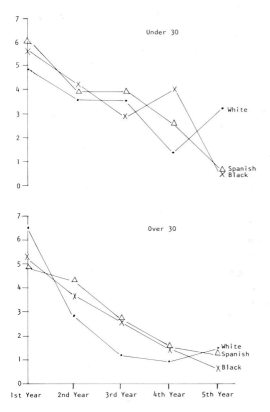

FIG. 3. Number of arrests per 100 person-years in methadone maintenance treatment program by age, ethnic group, and years of observation.

year is greater in the over-30 group than in the under-30 group.

For the over-30 group, the white cohort shows the most consistent decrease. The number of arrests for the black and Spanish cohorts decreases at similar rates. However, the overall number of arrests is higher than that for the whites. The under-30 cohort shows similar rates of arrests for the three ethnic groups.

Changes in antisocial behavior of this magnitude as measured by involvement with the law in a population of mostly "hard core" addicts with previous histories of consistent criminal activity has to be considered another positive feature of methadone maintenance treatment.

PROBLEMS OF POLYDRUG AND ALCOHOL ABUSE

It has been said that depriving an addict of the heroin "highs" to which he is accustomed leads him to seek alternative sources of drug-induced satisfaction. Among patients in methadone maintenance in New York, excessive use of alcohol remained unchanged as compared with pretreatment use (about 20%), as did use of amphetamines (5 to 10%) among patients admitted prior to 1972. Use of barbiturates, which was initially 20%, declined to 6%.

Continued use of drugs such as barbiturates, amphetamines, and cocaine has been a problem in approximately 5% of the patients, whereas problems related to alcohol involve about 20%. Despite these figures, 45% of the patients with continuing alcohol problems have remained gainfully employed, and 38% of the patients who continue to use drugs have been either gainfully employed or in a training program.

In the early admission cohorts (1965 to 1971) attempts were made to identify and reject patients who admitted to alcohol or polydrug problems during the initial interview.

the patients under our surveillance is due to the preponderance of older patients in this population (older is defined as over 30 at time of admission).

In order to respond to this question, we look at the arrests per 100 person-years of observation in our sample among those who were *30 and under* at time of admission compared with those *over 30*. The results are shown graphically in Fig. 3 for each ethnic group. The slopes of the curves are very similar indicating that in both groups there is a decrease in arrests with time in treatment. This trend is steady and constant in the group over 30, but a bit more erratic in the group under 30. The drop in the number of arrests after the first

Among the cohorts admitted in 1972 and 1973, an increased proportion of patients present either serious medical problems or problems with multiple drug abuse including alcohol. This has been noted both in New York and in other areas.

Alcohol problems were more common among black patients, and drug abuse was more commonly a factor among white and hispanic patients.

DETOXIFICATION TO METHADONE-FREE

Methadone maintenance treatment for heroin addicts has been characterized by some as either "substituting one addictive drug for another" or "a lifetime dependency on a crutch."

When the methadone maintenance treatment program started in New York, no specific time period of treatment was envisioned, and patients were detoxified and became methadone free only on demand or when the unit director, in consultation with his staff, decided that the patient could no longer be retained in the program.

As a result of the 1972 federal guidelines with reference to both the number of days of "take-home" methadone allowed and the recommendation that patients on methadone maintenance be "encouraged" to attempt detoxification after 2 years in treatment, two new cohorts have been generated. One is a *low-dose* methadone group in the process of very slow detoxification, and another *no-methadone* or *methadone-free* group.

Among the 35 patients who have been in treatment for 10 years or longer 20% were on low dose and 26% were methadone free as of the end of last year. Among approximately 2,000 patients who had been in treatment 5 years or more, 21% were on low dose and 12% were methadone free. Of those who had completed at least 3 years of treatment (5,250), 23% were on

low dose and 11% were methadone free as of December 31, 1974.

The methadone-free cohort includes patients who have been off methadone for periods of a few months to a year or more. It should be noted that this is a status report at one point in time, namely December 31, 1974. This is important to bear in mind because previous experience has shown that in the methadone-free cohort, approximately one-half may request return at least to low-dose methadone.

Patients who are deemed ready for slow detoxification are encouraged to reduce their dosage gradually enough for them to remain *comfortable*. This detoxification process may take from several months to a year or more. Patients who become methadone free have the option of returning to low dose or build up to high dose on request.

The fact that the timing and the rate of detoxification is a mutual decision between the doctor and the patient, and the "open door" policy for the methadone-free group for reentry into treatment must be considered another positive aspect of these methadone maintenance treatment programs.

CHANGES IN MORTALITY

In order to examine the effect of methadone maintenance treatment in changing the mortality experience of patients, both death rates and causes of death were examined.

Death Rates

Data were collected on four groups, as shown in Table 4.

Group I. Deaths reported to have occurred over a 5-year period among 3,000 patients in methadone maintenance treatment programs while they were in treatment.

Group II. Deaths reported to have oc-

TABLE 4. *Observed death rate/1,000 and the expected death rates based on deaths in New York City in 1969–1971 in the population 20–54 years of age*

	Deaths/1,000 population		95% Confidence limits	Number in group
	Observed	Expected		
Group I (In Rx)	7.6	6.6	1.4------11.8/1000	3,000
Group II (Left Rx)	28.2	7.6	2.2------13.0/1000	850
Group III (Detox. group)	82.5	7.8	4.4------11.2/1000	109
Group IV (New York City)	5.6		3.3-------7.9/1000	1,875,000

curred in the same time span among 850 patients who had been on methadone maintenance, but who had left treatment alive.

Group III. Deaths over the same period of time in a contrast group of 109 selected from patients admitted to Morris Bernstein Institute *only* for detoxification during the year 1965.

Group IV. Deaths in the general New York City population in 1969–1971 in the age range 20 to 54 years.

Group IV was selected to give an expected figure against which to compare each of the other groups, and Group III was chosen to give an approximate figure to reflect the impact of death in this age group of untreated heroin addicts.

Using a life-table technique and postulating a Poissant distribution, the expected deaths for each group and the 95% confidence limits were calculated, using the deaths in Group IV as the norm.

The similarity between the death rate in the methadone maintenance treatment program population and the New York City population is striking (7.6 versus 5.6), but the differential between this rate and each of the other two groups is even more dramatic (7.6 versus 28.2 and 7.6 versus 82.5). These differences persist when deaths among the white and nonwhite populations are looked at separately in each group.

Causes of Death

The causes of 153 deaths for which data were available from the Medical Examiner's Office as of December 31, 1972 have been grouped into three categories.

1. *Probably drug associated* including: a) acute intravenous narcotism or overdose; b) pulmonary edema, visceral congestion, or pending chemical investigation; c) infections such as hepatitis, tetanus, and subacute bacterial endocarditis.
2. *Possibly drug associated* including: a) violence including assault and homicide, suicide, and falls from height; b) alcoholism or fatty cirrhosis.
3. *Probably not drug associated* including: a) chronic diseases including cancer, myocardial infarction, tuberculosis, cerebral hemorrhage, nephritis, etc.; b) infections such as bronchopneumonia, and others not included in category 1c; c) accidents such as fires, traffic accidents, etc.

This classification, although arbitrary, permits comparisons between patients continuing in treatment with those discharged from treatment (for whatever cause) and with a small target group of heroin addicts who have not been involved

TABLE 5. *Causes of death*

	% of deaths		
Cause of death	Group 1 (N = 110)	2 (N = 33)	3 (N = 10)
Probably drug associated	30	65	68
Possibly drug associated	20	15	22
Total drug associated	50	80	90
Probably not drug associated	50	20	10

in methadone maintenance treatment. Table 5 shows the distribution of causes of death in each group.

Fifty percent of the deaths among 110 patients in the group who died while in a methadone treatment program were considered probably not drug associated, compared with 20% of the 33 who died after leaving treatment, and with 10% of the 10 deaths in the group from the detoxification unit.

It is apparent that there is a gradient in mortality among untreated heroin addicts. Two-thirds of all their deaths are probably drug associated, and 90% are either probably or possibly drug associated.

These data support the position that patients who accept and remain in methadone maintenance treatment tend to die at a rate very similar to the general New York City population in the same age group, in sharp contrast to those who leave treatment or the patients from the detoxification unit.

The causes of death likewise show a

TABLE 6. *Percentage distribution of deaths during methadone maintenance treatment in early and later cohorts by cause of death*

	A. % of deaths during first year		
	Date of admission		
Cause of death	1964–1970 Total	1971–1973 Total	Total
Probably drug associated	28	35	33
Possibly drug associated			
Violence	17	37	31
Alcohol & other	11	10	10
Probably not drug associated	44	18	26
Total	100	100	100
N	54	117	171

	B. % of deaths during second year		
	Date of admission		
Cause of death	1964–1970 Total	1971–1972 Total	Total
Probably drug associated	32	29	30
Possibly drug associated			
Violence	11	23	18
Alcohol & other	13	15	14
Probably not drug associated	44	33	38
Total	100	100	100
N	38	73	111

marked contrast when looked at with reference to drug involvement. It would appear that methadone maintenance has prolonged the productive lives of a substantial number of previous heroin addicts.

As a result of what appeared to be an increase in mortality during the first 2 years of treatment in the more recent admissions (1971–1973), and of an impression gained from studying the causes of death as reported (there seemed to be an increase in the number of patients who were recorded as victims of violent death, including gunshot wounds, stabbings, suicide, fires, pedestrian accidents, and falls under subways or from tall buildings), causes of death were looked at separately for the three early cohorts (1964–1970) and compared with three later cohorts (1971–1973), classifying this group of violent deaths in the category of "possibly drug associated." The results for deaths in the *first year* are shown in Table 6A. The shift in the proportion of deaths by violence from 17% in the early group to 37% in the later group is significant and was much greater among men than among women.

Distribution of causes of death during the *second year* for the same two groups are shown in Table 6B. The increase in the proportion of violent deaths in the later admission group has continued.

SUMMARY

Our response to the question "What's good about methadone maintenance after 10 years?" can be summarized as follows:

1. Methadone maintenance treatment in the New York City area has been effective in maintaining relatively high retention rates over extended periods of treatment in most treatment programs.

2. Substantial increases in social productivity have been achieved for the majority of patients who have remained in methadone maintenance treatment.

3. Effecting changes in patients' social productivity has broken the chain of antisocial behavior for a large majority of patients.

4. A permissive readmission policy for patients who leave treatment either voluntarily or by administrative decision can result in converting "failure" into "success" in a large proportion of the first time "losers."

5. For selected patients who have been on methadone maintenance at high dosage levels for periods from 2 to 10 years, a lowering of their dosage can be achieved with the mutual cooperation of the doctor and the patient, and for those who achieve a methadone-free state, there is the option of reentry into treatment on request.

6. Methadone maintenance has prolonged the productive lives of a substantial number of former heroin addicts.

REFERENCES

1. Gearing, F. R. (1970): Successes and failures in methadone maintenance treatment of heroin addiction in New York City. *Proc. 3rd. Natl. Conf. Methadone Maintenance,* NIMH, Public Health Service Publication No. 2172; pp. 2–16.

Neurotoxicology, edited by L. Roizin, H. Shiraki, and N. Grčević. Raven Press, New York © 1977.

Drugs-of-Abuse Detection in Biological Specimens

Richard L. Stiller and David Pierson

Neurotoxicology Research Unit, Bronx, New York 10461; and Psychiatric Institute, New York City, New York 10032

The field of toxiocology has expanded rapidly in the last decade, and as a result of this situation, a large portion of the toxicologist's work schedule requires him to keep abreast of new methods. He must be able to detect toxic and therapeutic levels of drugs, and since intake of more than one drug is common among drug abusers, multiple drug analyses may be required for each specimen screened.

An effective screening (24,52) should include the techniques necessary for identification of both the commonly used and the newly introduced drugs of abuse, and one must ensure high accuracy for each determination followed by positive confirmation of the suspected drugs. There is no single toxicological examination that can be employed in screening all the pharmacological agents, and specific analyses are required for so many drugs that it is impossible, with the current methodologies, to accomplish a complete drug screen on one specific specimen. The number of compounds that could have some pharmacological effect is unknown, and with each new drug, new or modified methods for detection must be devised or revised to detect these drugs in biological specimens.

ANALYTICAL PROCEDURES

The isolation and identification of drugs from biological specimens have advanced greatly in the past 10 years. The current routine procedures for drugs of abuse are thin-layer chromatography (TLC), gas chromatography (GC), and immunoassay. All of these methods can be used for routine screenings.

TLC and GC are not limited assays techniques, whereas the immunoassay techniques are limited to specific compounds and are not available for many drugs of abuse as indicated in the following.

1. Radioimmunoassay (RIA): morphine (opiates), amphetamine, barbiturates, cocaine (benzoylecgonine), and methadone

2. Enzyme multiplied immunoassay technique (EMIT): morphine (opiates), amphetamine, barbiturates, cocaine (benzoylecgonine, methadone, benzodiazepines, and propoxyphene)

3. Hemagglutination inhibition technique (HIT): morphine (opiates), barbiturates, methadone, and cocaine (benzoylecgonine).

The cost of immunochemicals is expensive, and they have a limited shelf life. In the case of RIA and EMIT expensive spectrometric instrumentation is needed. The least expensive assay is TLC, and then GC.

EXTRACTION AND DRUG MOLECULAR STRUCTURES

Drug assay methodology is based on the molecular structures of the drugs to be analyzed, in particular their functional groups, which divide drugs generally into four categories. The four categories are designated by the functional group of a drug and its partition coefficient at a certain pH between an immiscible organic solvent and an aqueous solvent. The designations are acidic, neutral, basic, and amphoteric. The partition coefficients are reflective of the hydrogen ion concentration in the aqueous medium that changes the ionic state of the drug molecule. This places the molecular structure in an un-ionized or less polar state that helps to extract the drug from a physiological specimen into an organic solvent (15).

Acidic drugs, such as barbiturates and salicylates, are extractable into a particular organic solvent at a pH of less than 7.

Basic drugs, such as amphetamines, propoxyphene, and imipramine, are cationic and are extractable into an organic solvent at pH of greater than 7 (10).

Neutral drugs, such as meprobamate and glutethimide, because of their functional groups, are non-ionizable and nonpolar and are extracted into organic solvents at any pH (Table 1).

Amphoteric drugs, such as morphine and catecholamines, have more than one functional group that is ionizable at different hydrogen ion concentrations. Therefore, one must find the isoelectric point of that particular drug: that is, the pH when the molecular structure exists in the most nonpolar or un-ionizable state. Narcotic drugs that possess a tertiary aliphatic amino group and an aromatic with phenolic hydroxyl are weak bases with some amphoteric tendencies and a pK_a between 6.6 to 9.5 that results in the formation of salts with acids and depends on the tendency of the salts to form ion pairs that can be extracted in organic solvents. Solubility and extraction procedures have been described by Curry (18) and Freimuth (30).

Many drug metabolites are not easily extracted from an aqueous medium. The conjugates, such as glucuronides, are as

TABLE 1. *TLC drug separation*

Drug	Development system R_f		
	1st[a]	2nd[b]	3rd[b]
Acidic fraction			
Phenobarbital	0.38	0.26	
Secobarbital	0.72	0.60	
Pentobarbital	0.75	0.63	
Glutethimide	0.93	0.90	
Basic fraction			
Methadone metabolite	0.99		0.91
Methadone	0.96	0.99	0.70
Diazepam	0.95		
Cocaine	0.95	0.97	0.85
Thorazine	0.94	0.98	0.75
Amphetamine	0.70		
Chlordiazepoxide	0.68	0.86	
Methamphetamine	0.65		
Guinine	0.60	0.70	
Codeine	0.45	0.54	0.40
Morphine	0.30	0.32	0.20
Neutral fraction			
Methaqualone	0.99		0.95

Conditions: [a]Chloroform: n-butanol: ammonia (70:40:5) (25% ammonia). [b]Ethyl acetate: methanol: conc. ammonia (85:10:5). 1st develop in [a]; 2nd develop in [b] then [a] to one-half plate height.

soluble as amino acids. Therefore, in order to be extracted, their molecular structure must be changed. Acidic hydrolysis splits the conjugate and liberates the free drug, which falls into one of the four categories for extraction. An example is morphine glucoronide, which on acidic hydrolysis at elevated temperatures splits into a sugar moeity and free morphine that can be extracted into an organic solvent at its isoelectric point (21).

There have been many approaches cited in the literature describing the extraction of drugs of abuse and their metabolites from biological specimens. There is no single pH or solvent procedure that will efficiently recover all drugs from different types of biological materials. The multiple pH–multiple solvent extraction procedures result in the highest recovery of a large range of drugs. These procedures have been widely described and used. We have found all the procedures cited to be effec-

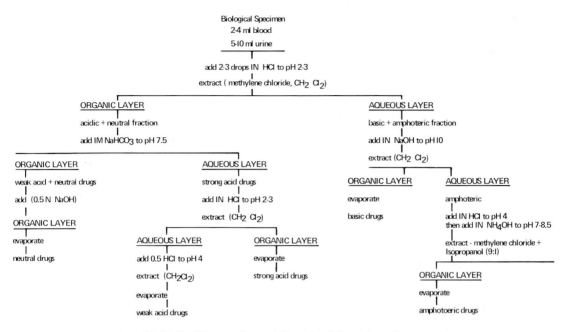

FIG. 1. Multiple pH extraction technique for GC confirmation procedure.

tive, and we have devised an extraction procedure that has a high reliability (Fig. 1) (3,15,37,38,50,57).

In some cases where rapid screening utilizing extraction is needed, we use a slightly varied Davidow procedure, as shown in Fig. 2, of a single pH–single solvent extraction procedure (21,26).

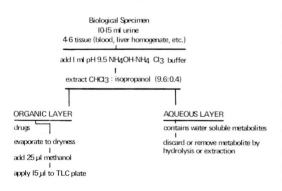

FIG. 2. Single pH–single extraction procedure.

CHROMATOGRAPHY

Chromatography is the separation, using many type of phenomena, of components by physical means. Gas and solution chromatography are two major subdivisions of chromatography, and we discuss here the partition and absorption phenomena as they pertain to these two subdivisions.

In partition the components are distributed between two phases: a stationary phase and a mobile phase. In the case of gas-liquid chromatography the stationary phase is liquid, and the mobile phase is gas. The mobile phase moves along the stationary phase by gas pressure and is sometimes termed the carrier gas. The vaporized components, as they are carried along the stationary phase by the mobile phase, are separated. The separations are the result of their differences in distribution coefficients, random migration, sorption, and desorption. Each component follows a random migration, a stop-and-go path, as it is sorbed and desorbed, and its distribution between phases is rapid. Basically, the mobile phase carries the vaporized component mixture through the column, and during transport, portions of it are sorbed according to their affinity for the stationary phase. The higher the affinity, the more tightly they are sorbed and the longer is their column's retention time. Retention time is a physical characteristic related to a component's molecular structure and column factors. The retention time can be used for identification: it is the time elapsed between a sample's introduction on to the column and its maximum peak emergence. The individual components are separated, emerge from the column, and are continually monitored by various detection means.

In absorption chromatography the stationary phase is the surface of an active solid such as silica gel. In TLC the silica gel is supported as a thin layer upon a glass, plastic, or other plate surface. The mobile phase is a solvent composed of one or more organic liquids and possibly some inorganic compounds. The separation of compounds is the result of a differential absorption by each component on the surface of the stationary phase. The strongly absorbed components migrate more slowly than the weakly absorbed components. Thus, the strongly absorbed components move the least up the plate, and the weakly absorbed moves the furthest (34,38).

The absorption phenomena is the result of weak molecular interaction forces such as hydrogen bonding, charge transfer, electrostatic forces, and London forces.

The solvent or mobile phase elutes the sample and moves up the plate by capillary force, and the solvent competes with the sample for absorption sites on the surface of the stationary phase. The strong eluents (polar) decrease absorption, whereas weak elements (nonpolar) increase the absorption.

The retention value of a component on a TLC plate is the distance the component travels in relation to the solvent front (R_f) or a standard substance (R_x). The migration distance of the component is usually measured to the center of the component zone or area of maximum concentration. Therefore, the R_f of a component is equal to the distance a component (d_c) travels divided by the distance the solvent front (S_f) travels (34,38).

$$R_f = \frac{d_c}{S_f} \quad \text{or} \quad R_x = \frac{d_c}{d_x}$$

DRUG ANALYSIS BY TLC

For screening of drugs of abuse by TLC, it is usually sufficient that the extraction removes enough of the drugs present for a qualitative indication of their presence to be obtainable. In this situation one can use a simple extract at a pH 9 to 9.5 (59). Sample size is an important factor, for one needs an adequate amount of material (10 to 15 ml of urine or 5 ml of blood) to extract a sufficient amount of drug for assay. The acidic fraction has a poor recovery, but this type of procedure is helpful as a preliminary screen or where there are large work loads and a knowledge of the drugs of abuse. In all other situations, we prefer one of the multiple extraction techniques for TLC as shown in Fig. 3.

We have found that a silica gel-G TLC developed in either (a) chloroform:n-butanol:ammonia (70:40:5) (25% ammonia) (54) or (b) ethyl acetate:methanol: concentrated ammonia (85:10:5) (25) produces a workable resolution of many drugs (Table 2).

If one uses a double-development system (i.e., first develop in solvent system 2 for total plate height, remove TLC plate, dry in a vacuum, and rerun in system 1 to one-half the plate height), there will be a

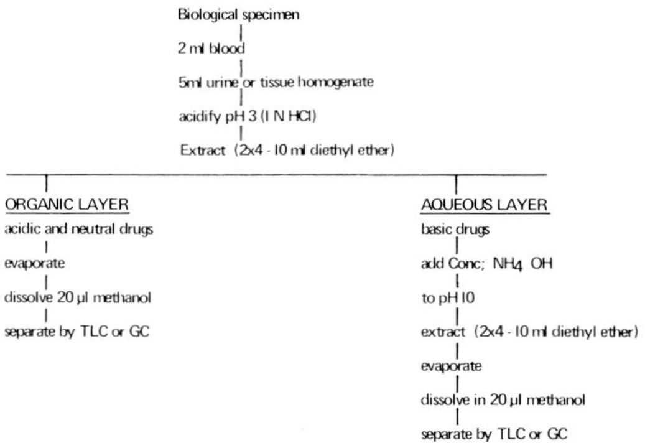

FIG. 3. Abridged multiple pH extraction technique.

better resolution of basic fraction (see Table 1).

There are many development systems that work equally well on drugs (6,8,20, 42,45,48,49,59), and there are specific systems for barbiturates (33,36), amphetamines (12,25,33), methadone and metabolite (73), basic fraction (10,25), nonbarbiturate hypnotics (17), and morphine and narcotics (21,33,35,44).

Visualization techniques of drugs by various chromatogenic spray reagents have been described in detail by Davidow (21,29), Dole (25), or Clarke (15).

DRUG ANALYSIS BY GAS CHROMATOGRAPHY

TLC provided the toxicology laboratories with an absorption chromatography procedure. With the introduction of gas chromatography, another means of separation and identification was added: partition chromatography. This made available a better resolution of drugs and their metabolites from biological artifacts (4,17,27,28, 40,42,44,51).

The sensitivity of gas chromotography approaches that of immunoassay. Flame ionization detection levels are about 100 ng/1 ml because of naturally interfering components (8). In our own experience with a flame alkaline nitrogen detector, we have found that the lower limit from blood samples is about 20 to 40 ng/ml. This means that a smaller sample for analysis is needed with gas chromatography, less than 1 ml of blood or 4 ml of urine. We utilize a multiple pH extraction (Fig. 2,3) for most analysis. When a specific drug is to be confirmed from a TLC-positive identification, we use the specific pH and solvent for ease and high recovery.

The type of columns and conditions used for separation is extremely important for drugs. These can encompass a wide range of techniques for individual drugs, such as routine detection (8,9,27,28,31,48,51), amphetamine (12,40), morphine (29,35,44,61, 67), cocaine (29,63), barbiturate (19,36,41), glutethimide (41), propoxyphene (43), nonbarbiturate hypnotics (17,64), and methadone (7).

We have found for general free drug analysis that 3% OV-17 on 100–120 mesh gas chrom Q, 3% S.E. 30 on 80–100 mesh chromosorb W (HP), and 3% OV-1

TABLE 2. *Types of drug fractions*

Acidic	Basic	Neutral	Amphoteric
Strongly	Propoxyphene	Meprobamate	Morphine
Diphenylhydantoin	Amphetamine	Phenglycol	Phenylephrine
Salicylates	Methamphetamine	Glutethimide	Catecholamines
	Imipramine	Ethylchlorvynol	
Weakly	Ephedrine	Methadone	
	Benzodiazepines	Acetaminophen	
Barbiturates	Cocaine	Meperidine	
	Nicotine	Carbromal	
	Quinine	Caffeine	

TABLE 3. *Gas chromatography drug separations*

Drug	Retention time (R_t) (in minutes)	Relative retention (R_r)
Amphetamine	1.2	0.50
Methamphetamine	1.7	0.71
n-n-Propylamphetamine (IS)	2.4	1.00
Methadone	11.5	4.80
Propoxyphene	12.1	5.00
Cocaine	12.6	5.25
Codeine	13.8	5.75
Quinine	16.6	6.9
Morphine	18.1	7.4

Conditions: column 3% OV-17 on 100–120 mesh gas chrom Q. n-n-Propylamphetamine is the internal standard (IS). Used basic fraction from Figs. 1,7. Flow-rate: 40 to 50 ml/min. Temperature program: 120 to 250 °C at 8° C/min with initial delay of 5 min.

$$\text{Relative retention} = \frac{\text{Retention time of a component}}{\text{Retention time of the internal standard or marker}} \text{ or } R_r = \frac{R_{tc}}{R_{tIS}}$$

on 80–100 mesh chromosorb W (HP) are very effective. In special situations we use columns cited in above references.

We use a temperature program of 120 to 250°C at 8° C/min with a 5-min initial delay, and our flow rate is 40 to 50 ml/min with a maximum analysis time of 25 min and an average of approximately 15 min (Table 3).

In certain analyses we derivatize our free drugs for better resolution and to prevent absorption losses as follows: methylation of the barbiturates (36), acetylation of the morphine (35) and amphetamines (40), and, in general, for phenyl alkylamines we form the trimethyl silyl ether (8).

IMMUNOASSAY

Immunoassay can be used as an analytic procedure for a qualitative or quantitative determination of compounds in a biological specimen. In the formation of an antigen–antibody complex, there is a competitive displacement of a labeled compound from the complex by an unlabeled compound in the specimen. The concentration of the compound can be evaluated by the amount of displaced labeled compound. There are two types of assays techniques used:

the homogeneous and the heterogeneous. The homogeneous technique requires no separation steps, whereas the heterogeneous requires separation of the displaced labeled compound from the complex fraction (60,68,69).

EMIT is a homogeneous technique (11). It is a microassay for specific drugs of abuse in urine. A specific drug (antigen) is labeled with an enzyme and the enzyme–drug complex when bound to the antibody against this drug reduces the enzymatic activity. If the drug is contained in a specimen, it competes with the enzyme–drug complex for the antibody with a commensurate increase in enzyme activity. The increase in enzyme activity is directly proportional to the drug concentration.

In the case of drugs of abuse detected in a urine specimen, the EMIT system has the drug labeled to an active lysozyme. This lysozyme has the ability to break down a bacteria cell wall. The antibody against this drug causes steric hindrance and prevents the lysozyme from acting on the cell wall, and the unlabeled drug displaces the enzyme–drug-labeled complex, thereby increasing the enzymatic activity. Urine, a drug-labeled lysozyme, antibody, and bacteria are added and mixed together. An initial turbidity measure is made, and after 40 sec another measurement is made. The difference between readings is calculated. A decrease in the turbidity is proportional to drug concentration in urine, and a clear solution is a positive result (53,62,66).

EMIT can be automated (150 samples/hr) for rapid screening of drugs such as total morphine opiates, barbiturates, amphetamines, methadone, cocaine, diazepam, and propoxyphene in urine. The major advantages of EMIT are that minimal technical skill is needed, and homogeneous solution eliminates the need for a separation step. Some of the disadvantages are that false-positive detections occur due to endogenous lysozome in some urines, that it cannot readily be used on other biological materials, that it is less sensitive than other immunoassays, and that the instrumentation and reagents are expensive (46).

HIT is an immunoassay in which tanned red cells are coated with a drug-carrier protein complex (antigen). If no drug is present, the antibodies against the antigen will agglutinate, and these red cells will appear as a diffused pattern in the titer tray well. If the drug is present, it will bind with the antibody, and when the antibody is bound, it cannot react with the red cell antigen. In this case the agglutination is inhibited, and the red cells will precipitate and form a distinct pellet in the titer tray well.

A drop of urine is added to the antiserum-containing antibody in a titer tray well. The red cells labeled with the drug complex are added to this well. In 1 to 2 hr the reaction is completed forming either a pellet if the drug is present or a diffused pattern if the drug is not present. This method can be semiquantitative by dilution of urine until reaction is negative, and it can be a parallel standard to determine concentration (1,2,13).

This is a homogeneous analysis, and no instrumentation is needed. The reagents are inexpensive and highly sensitive at the 10-ng level. It can detect free and bound morphine, barbiturates, methadone, and cocaine, and the analysis can be adjusted for sensitivity. Assay time is lengthy; interpretation is highly skilled and subjective. It can be confused by various sediments in certain urines. Quality of reagents can vary. The method is fatiguing, and it cannot be automated (46).

In RIA a drug is labeled with a radioactive isotope, such as iodine[125], carbon[14], or tritium. RIA is based on a competitive reaction between the unlabeled drug and the labeled drug for specific antibodies against the drug present in the antisera.

A mixture of unlabeled drug, labeled drug, and antibody is allowed to equilibrate. The antibody–drug complex is precipitated, and the amount of free labeled drug is determined by measuring the radioactivity level in the supernate or the precipitate. The counts per minute are compared to positive and negative controls, and by comparing the counts to a standard curve (a series of known concentrations), the concentration of drug present can be evaluated (16,32,47,55,56).

The advantages of RIA are that it can be quantitative for drug concentration ranging from 40 ng/ml. It has a low level of detection, 10 ng/ml, and is objective. It detects bound and free morphine and the metabolites of methadone and cocaine. The disadvantages of this assay are the high cost of reagents and instrumentation, high technical skills needed for analysis, and the handling of radioactive materials. The completion of analysis is lengthy (46).

In our situation RIA has proved to be the most reliable when confirming a drug that is suspected or shown to be positive on a TLC screening procedure. It is highly specific for amphetamine, barbiturates, cocaine, benzoylecgonine, and methadone with little cross-reaction with other drugs. It produces few false-positive or negative results. In the case of morphine, RIA cross-reacts with other opiates (codeine, hydromorphine, etc.) and must be identified by other methods such as GC or TLC (21).

All of the immunoassay techniques offer a major advantage over all other methods: that is, a small (50 to 250 μl) native sample can be analyzed directly without any separation steps.

ERRONEOUS RESULTS

Even in an ideal analytical laboratory mistakes can occur. Quality control begins with the introduction of the biological specimen to be analyzed. Blind samples should be introduced along with the unknowns as a parallel analysis at both a therapeutic and toxic level for drugs commonly abused or requested (5,65). Many factors can produce erroneous results such as pH, specimen storage, temperature, extraction solvents, glassware contamination, or plastecizers from plastic collect containers (22,23). These plastecizers can give false positives for drugs such as diazepam and pentobarbital. Barbiturates, cocaine, and amphetamine are not stable in stored specimens or at elevated temperatures, but morphine, methadone and codeine are stable.

Many invalid analytical results are obtained for a variety of reasons, but poor quality control over samples and analysis is a major factor (50). One positive result is not necessarily sufficient proof that a drug is present; additional analyses may be needed to prove it is not an artifact. A negative result also does not mean a drug is absent; many drug metabolites are not easily extracted from an aqueous medium and give a negative result on a drug screen. When a positive has been determined by a TLC screen, it must be confirmed by another method. If we have a positive amphetamine, barbiturate, methadone, opiate, cocaine, or proproxyphene, we do a direct assay of the native specimen via one of the several immunoassay techniques. If one of the above is positive or if the drug cannot be assayed by this technique, we do a second extraction for GC.

DISCUSSION

We have examined only a few areas of drug analysis and mainly on topics that we have found effective in the development of our laboratory procedures. We have utilized the pH–solvent extraction techniques to give us the best recoveries regardless of the nature of the specimen received and whether or not specific drugs are suspected. We depend on the TLC system as our main screening tool because it is reliable, sensitive, rapid, and inexpensive. We have used other screening tools such as GC and immunoassay but have found in our laboratory environment and type and amount of samples received that these procedures are too expensive, complex, and time-consuming. GC we have found to be more effective and economical as a confirmation and quantitation instrument. RIA and EMIT proved the most expensive to operate and can only detect a limited number of drugs. These procedures are mainly suited for secondary confirmation. Since most drug screening performed by this unit proved to be negative, it has not been necessary to change our drug screening procedures. We use either an abridged multiple pH extraction or a single extraction technique.

SUMMARY

Less than 15 drugs account for 90% of drug abuse, and a simple, rapid drug screening procedure suffices for these identifications. The procedure is flexible and may be altered to expand the screening scope for inclusion of newer drugs of abuse and confirmation of suspected positive drugs. The system contains three steps: (a) extraction-isolation of drugs;

(b) TLC drug screening; and (c) GC drug confirmation.

There are many excellent review articles on these procedures (14,15,30,31,34,37, 38,39,58,60,61,68,69).

REFERENCES

1. Adler, F., and Liu, C. T. J. (1971): Detection of morphine by hemagglutination inhibition. *J. Immunol.,* 196:1684–1685.
2. Adler, F., Liu, C. T. J., and Catlin, P. H. (1972): Immunological studies on heroin addiction. I. Methodology and application of a hemagglutination inhibition test. *Clin. Immunol. Immunopathol.,* 1:53–68.
3. Aggarwal, V., Bath, R., and Sunshine, I. (1974): Technique for rapidly separating drugs from biological specimens. *Clin. Chem.,* 20:307–311.
4. Barrett, M. J. (1971): An integrated gas chromatographic program for drug screening in serum and urine. In: *Clin. Chem. Newsletter,* Vol. 3, p. 1. Perkin-Elmer Corp., Norwalk, Conn.
5. Basselt, R. C., Wright, J. A., and Cravey, R. H. (1975): Therapeutic and toxic concentration of more than 100 toxicologically significant drugs in blood plasma and serum: A tabulation. *Clin. Chem.,* 22:44–62.
6. Bastos, M. C., Kannen, G. E., Young, R. M., Monforte, J. R., and Sunshine, I. (1970): Detection of basic organic drugs and their metabolites in urine. *Clin. Chem.,* 16:931–940.
7. Beckett, A. H., Taylor, J. F., Casy, A. F., and Hassan, M. M. A. (1968): The biotransformation of methadone in man: Synthesis and identification of a major metabolite. *J. Pharm. Pharmacol.,* 20:754–762.
8. Beckett, A. H., Tucker, G. T., and Moffat, A. C. (1967): Routine detection and identification in urine of stimulants and other drugs, some of which may be used to modify performance in sport. *J. Pharm. Pharmacol.,* 19:273–294.
9. Bloomer, H. A., Maddock, R. K., Sheehe, J. B., and Adams, E. J. (1970): Rapid diagnosis of sedative intoxication by gas chromatography. *Ann. Intern. Med.,* 72:223–228.
10. Brodie, B. B., and Udenfriend, S. (1945): The estimation of basic organic compounds and a technique for the appraisal of specificity. *J. Biol. Chem.,* 158:705–714.
11. Bidanset, J. H. (1974): Drug analysis by immunoassay. *J. Chromatogr. Sci.,* 12:293–296.
12. Bost, R. O., Sutheimer, C. A., and Sunshine, I. (1976): Relative merits of some methods for amphetamine assay in biological fluids. *Clin. Chem.,* 22:789–801.
13. Catlin, D. H. (1973): A guide to urine testing for drugs of abuse. In: *Special Action Office Monograph,* Series B, No. 2, Executive Office of the President, Washington, D.C.
14. Clarke, E. G. C. (1962): Isolation and identification of alkaloids. In: *Methods of Forensic Science,* Vol. 1, edited by F. Lundquist, pp. 1–241. Wiley (Interscience), New York.
15. Clarke, E. G. C. (1969): *Isolation and Identification of Drugs.* Pharmaceutical Press, London.
16. Cleeland, R., Christenson, J., Usatequi-Gomez, M., Heveran, J., Davis, R., and Grunberg, E. (1976): Detection of drugs of abuse by radioimmunoassay: A summary of published data and some new information. *Clin. Chem.,* 22:712–725.
17. Cravey, R. H., and Jain, N. C. (1974): The identification of nonbarbiturate hypnotics from biological specimens. *J. Chromatogr. Sci.,* 12:237–245.
18. Curry, A. S. (1959): *Methods of Biochemicals Analysis,* Vol. 7, edited by D. Glick, pp. 39–76. Wiley (Interscience), New York.
19. Curry, A. S., and Fox, R. H. (1968): Thin layer chromatography of the common barbiturates. *Analyst,* 93:834.
20. Davidow, B., Petri, N. L., and Quame, B. (1968): A thin layer chromatographic screening procedure for detecting drug abuse. *Am. J. Clin. Pathol.,* 50:714–719.
21. Davidow, B., Petri, N. L., Quame, B., Searle, B., Fastlich, E., and Savitzky, J. (1966): A thin layer chromatographic screening test for detection of users of morphine or heroin. *Am. J. Clin. Pathol.,* 46:58–62.
22. Deome, A. J. (1974): Interference from serum separators in gas chromatographic drug analysis. *Clin. Chem.,* 20:1383.
23. de Zeeuw, R. A., Jonkman, J. H. G., and Van Mansvelt, F. J. W. (1975): Plasticers as contaminants in high-purity solvents: A potential source of interference in biological analysis. *Anal. Biochem.,* 67:339–341.
24. Dinovo, E. C., Gottschalk, L. A., McGuire, F. L., Birch, H., and Herser, J. F. (1976): Analysis of results of toxicological examinations performed by Coroners, or Medical Examiners' Laboratories in 2,000 drug-involved deaths in nine major U.S. cities. *Clin. Chem.,* 22:847–850.
25. Dole, V. P., Kim, M. K., and Eglitis, I. (1966): Detection of narcotic drugs, tranquilizers, amphetamines and barbiturates in urine. *JAMA,* 198:115–118.
26. Ehrsson, H., and Knapp, D. (1974): Rapid, efficient procedure for extraction of drugs for toxicological analysis. *Clin. Chem.,* 20:1366–1367.
27. Finkle, B. S., Cherry, E. J., and Taylor, D. M. (1970): A GLC based system of the detection of poisons, drugs and human metabolites encountered in forensic toxicology. *J. Chromatogr. Sci.,* 9:393–419.
28. Finkle, B. S., Foltz, R. C., and Taylor, D. M. (1974): A comprehensive G.C.-M.S. reference data system for toxicological and biomedical purposes. *J. Chromatogr. Sci.,* 12:304–328.
29. Fish, F., and Wilson, W. D. C. (1969): Gas chromatographic determination of morphine and

cocaine in urine. *J. Chromatogr.,* 40:164–168.

30. Freimuth, H. C. (1960): Isolation and separation from biological material. In: *Toxicology: Mechanisms and Analytical Methods,* Vol. 1, edited by C. P. Steward and A. Stolman, pp. 285–302. Academic Press, New York.

31. Gudzinowicz, B. J. (1967): *Gas Chromatographic Analysis of Drugs and Pesticides.* Marcel Dekker, New York.

32. Harwood, C. T. (1974): Radioimmunoassay: Its application to drugs of abuse. *Pharmacology,* 11:52–57.

33. Heaton, A. M., and Blumberg, A. G. (1969): Thin layer chromatographic detection of barbiturates, narcotics, and amphetamines in urine of patients receiving psychotropic drugs. *J. Chromatogr.,* 41:367–370.

34. Heftmann, E. (1967): *Chromatography,* Reinhold Publ. New York.

35. Jain, N. C., Sneath, T. C., Budd, R. D., and Leung, W. J. (1975): Gas chromatographic and thin-layer chromatographic analysis of acetylated codeine and morphine in urine. *Clin. Chem.,* 21:1486–1489.

36. Jain, N. C., and Cravey, R. H. (1974): The identification of barbiturates from biological specimens. *J. Chromatogr. Sci.,* 12:228–236.

37. Jones, C. R. (1976): Assay of drugs and trace organics, in biological fluids. In: *Methodological Developments in Biochemistry,* Vol. 5, edited by E. Reid, pp. 337–349. Biological and Medical Press, Amsterdam.

38. Karger, B. L., Snyder, L. R., and Horvath, C. (1973): *An Introduction to Separation Science,* Wiley, New York.

39. Law, N. C. (1973): A modern approach for drug identification. *Am. J. Med. Technol.,* 39:237–243.

40. Lebish, P., Finkle, B. S., and Brack, J. W. (1970): Determination of amphetamine, methamphetamine, and related amines in blood and urine by gas chromatography with hydrogen flame ionization detector. *Clin. Chem.,* 16:195–200.

41. MacGee, Joseph (1971): Rapid identification and quantitative determination of barbiturates and glutethimide in blood by gas-liquid chromatography. *Clin. Chem.,* 17:587–591.

42. Machata, G. (1967): TLC in systematic toxicological analysis. *Dtsch. Z. Ges. Gericht Med.,* 59:181–185.

43. McBay, A. J. (1976): Propoxyphene and norpropoxyphene concentrations in blood and tissue in cases of fatal overdose. *Clin. Chem.,* 22:1319–1321.

44. Mulé, S. J. (1964): Determination of narcotic analgesics in human biological materials—application of ultraviolet spectrophotometry, thin-layer and gas-liquid chromatography. *Anal. Chem.,* 36:1907–1914.

45. Mulé, S. J. (1969): Identification of narcotics, barbiturates, amphetamines, tranquilizers, and psychotominetrics in human urine. *J. Chromatogr.,* 39:302–311.

46. Mulé, S. J., Bastos, M. L., and Jokofsky, D. (1974): Evaluation of immunoassay methods for detection in urine, of drugs subjected to abuse. *Clin. Chem.,* 20:243–248.

47. Mulé, S. J., Whitlock, E., and Jukosky, P. (1975): Radioimmunoassay of drugs subject to abuse: Critical evaluation of urinary morphine-barbiturate morphine, barbiturate, and amphetamine assay. *Clin. Chem.,* 21:81–86.

48. Peat, M. A. (1976): Screening for drugs of abuse in urine samples from a drug addiction center. *Clin. Toxicol.,* 9:203–219.

49. Raudonat, H. W. (1967): The importance of TLC in chemical toxicological analysis. *Dtsch. Z. Ges. Gericht Med.,* 59:175–180.

50. Reid, E. (1976): Sample preparation in the micro-determination of organic compounds in plasma or urine. *Analyst,* 101:1–18.

51. Reid, R. W., Katzen, R., and Clinger, J. M. (1970): Analysis of blood and other body fluids by gas chromatography. *Am. J. Clin. Pathol.,* 53:462–467.

52. Robinson, A. E., and Holder, A. T. (1974): Chemical evaluation of drug cocktails in autopsy specimens. *J. Chromatogr. Sci.,* 12:281–284.

53. Rubenstein, R. E., Schneider, S. S., and Ullman, E. F. (1972): Homogeneous enzyme immunoassay. A new immunochemical technique. *Biochem. Biophys. Res. Commun.,* 47:846–851.

54. Schweda, R. (1967): Thin layer chromatography of toxicologically significant substances of silica gel-coated plates and polyester sheets. *Anal. Chem.,* 39:1019–1022.

55. Spector, S. (1971): Quantitative determination of morphine in serum by radioimmunoassay, *J. Pharmacol. Exp. Ther.,* 178:253–258.

56. Skelley, D. S., Brown, L. P., and Besch, P. K. (1973): Radioimmunoassay. *Clin. Chem.,* 19:147–186.

57. Stoner, R. E., and Parker, C. (1974): Single pH extraction procedure for detecting drugs of abuse. *Clin. Chem.,* 20:309–311.

58. Sunshine, I. (1969): *Handbook of Analytical Toxicology,* CRC Press, Cleveland.

59. Sunshine, I. (1967): Drug analysis by TLC. In: *Brinkmann Bulletin Br. 207.* Brinkmann Instrument, Inc., Westbury, New York.

60. Sunshine, I., Mulé, S. J., Braude, M., and Willette, R. E. (1974): *Immunoassay for Drugs Subject to Abuse,* CRC Press, Cleveland.

61. Taylor, J. F. (1971): Methods of chemical analysis. In: *Narcotic Drugs Biochemical Pharmacology,* edited by D. H. Clouet, pp. 17–88. Plenum Press, New York.

62. Van der Slooten, E. P. J., and Van der Helm, H. J. (1976): Comparison of the EMIT (Enzyme Multiplied Immunoassay Technique) opiate assay and a gas-chromatographic-mass spectrometric determination of morphine and codeine in urine. *Clin. Chem.,* 22:1110–1111.

63. Wallace, J. E., Hamilton, H. E., King, D. E., Bason, D. J., Schwertner, H. A., and Harris, S. C. (1976): Gas-liquid chromatographic determination of cocaine and benzoylethylecgonine in urine. *Anal. Chem.,* 48:34–38.

64. White, J. M., and Graves, M. H. (1974): The

detection of sedative/hypnotic drugs in the impaired driver. *J. Chromatogr. Sci.*, 12:219–224.

65. Winek, C. L. (1976): Tabulation of therapeutic, toxic and lethal concentration of drugs and chemicals in blood. *Clin. Chem.*, 22:833–836.

66. Wisdom, G. B. (1976): Enzyme-immunoassay. *Clin. Chem.*, 22:1243–1255.

67. Wilkinson, G. R., and Way, E. L. (1969): Submicrogram estimation of morphine in biological fluids by gas-liquid chromatography. *Biochem. Pharmacol.*, 18:1435–1439.

68. Zettner, A. (1973): Principles of competitive binding assays (saturation analyses). I. Equilibrium techniques. *Clin. Chem.*, 19:699–705.

69. Zettner, A., and Dale, P. E. (1974): Principles of competitive binding assays (saturation analyses). II. Sequential saturation. *Clin. Chem.*, 20:5–14.

Neurotoxicology, edited by L. Roizin, H. Shiraki, and N. Grčević. Raven Press, New York © 1977.

Drug Detection and Identification: Direct Immunoassay of Urinary Specimens Adsorbed on Papers Loaded with Ion Exchange Resins

George J. Alexander, Sandra M. Machiz, and Stanley Marynowski

Neurotoxicology Research Unit, New York State Department of Mental Hygiene, New York State Psychiatric Institute, and Bronx Psychiatric Center, Bronx, New York 10461

The current trend in drug abuse toxicology favors large centralized laboratories possessing expensive equipment and highly skilled personnel. Most of the screening is currently performed in a limited number of large organizations. Specimens that are collected in many scattered points are, therefore, routinely shipped out for processing. In addition to reliability and economy, the ease and safety of the shipment are among the decisive factors considered in selection of a method for drug screening. Adsorption of drugs on papers loaded with ion exchange resin presents the most convenient method of specimen transfer (6). After adsorption, dry specimens can be sent by regular mail without risk of spoilage or spillage. The treatment has the additional advantage of partially purifying the specimen through removal of water-soluble urinary pigments and salts (9). Unfortunately, the procedure is not efficient and leads to losses of a large portion of the material (2). For this reason, although widely used, it has been severely criticized (8).

As long as thin-layer chromatography (TLC) followed by color development (5) was the method employed for detection of drugs, interpretation of data after adsorption on ion exchange paper required extreme caution (7). However, the introduction of reliable and sensitive procedures utilizing several variants of immunochemical methodology altered the picture. By being able to detect picogram quantities of the drugs, these later techniques compensated for losses during adsorption on ion exchange paper. Therefore, use of immunochemical detection procedures made it possible to return with renewed confidence to the ion exchange paper for preliminary treatment of specimens.

As originally proposed by Dole et al. (6), the procedure called for adsorption of the drugs from urine on the ion exchange paper followed by elution off the paper into solvents for TLC analysis. For either hemagglutination inhibition test (HIT) (1) or radioimmunoassay (RIA) (10), eluted specimens had to be reconstituted after evaporation of solvents in either water or saline (2). We obtained reliable results after reconstitution of the specimens from SA-2 resin ion exchange papers in aqueous media, bypassing the solvent extraction of papers (3). Even more directly, we used pieces of dry SA-2 paper in either the HIT (4) or the RIA (G. J. Alexander, *unpublished information*).

Drug detection with HIT has the advantage of not requiring extensive and expensive instrumentation. The necessary reagents are commercially available. Unlike HIT, RIA requires expensive equipment. Laboratory personnel at times hesitate to work with radioisotopes. The advantages, however, are obvious — RIA is very reliable and very sensitive. Reagents are commercially available either as complete kits, or separately from different suppliers.

Preliminary Treatment of Urines with Ion Exchange Papers

A specimen of urine, 20 ml, is diluted 1:1 with distilled or deionized water in the field, on the ward, or at a local clinic. One 6 cm × 6 cm square of SA-2 ion exchange paper (Reeve Angel Co., Clifton, N. J.) is placed in the specimen and swirled for 30 min. The "spent" urine is discarded. The paper is rinsed briefly with distilled water and dried in the air. Once adsorbed on paper and dried, the specimen is stable and can be stored in the dark for future use. It can be shipped in a letter; it occupies little space, needs no refrigeration, does not smell, and does not spoil.

Shipped to a central laboratory, the specimen is available without delay for use in drug detection. Small disks, 0.7 cm in diameter (0.38 cm^2 in area), are punched out for any of the immunochemical assays. We have used such disks directly to inhibit agglutination of coated erythrocytes or to adsorb radioactive antigen eluted off drug specific antibodies. There is no reason why they could not be also used to modify ultraviolet (UV) adsorption in an enzyme-multiplied immunoassay. The remainder of the paper is available for further screening or confirmatory procedures as desired. Among the procedures that we have selected for such further treatment after solvent extraction in the presence of salt were TLC, gas–liquid chromatography, and spectrophotofluorimetric or UV analyses.

HIT

The test is performed in conical wells in a disposable plastic tray. We have used commercially available plastic trays with 96 wells for 22 quadruplicate assays along with one known positive and one known negative urine standard. One drop (50 μl) of a commercially available drug specific antiserum is equilibrated in each well for 10 min with a disk (0.38 cm^2) of SA-2 paper, the disk is then removed and 50 μl of a suspension of tanned sheep erythrocytes bonded to the specific hapten is added (4). In the absence of a drug, antiserum removes the hapten molecules from the cells and thereby allows them to agglutinate. When the specific drug from a urine specimen is present on the paper, approximately half of it transfers from resin to antibodies, thus occupying antiserum sites. Antiserum being unavailable to remove cell-bound haptens, the latter remain bound, agglutination is inhibited, and the cells precipitate in the well within 1 to 2 hr as a dark pellet. We found the results easy to interpret. The reliability and sensitivity of the detection step is excellent. This method can be applied to any drug or chemical for which reagents are either commercially available (currently, opiates, barbiturates, methadone, and cocaine, among others) or for which they can be produced locally.

RIA

The procedure calls for a 30-min equilibration in a small test tube of 1 to 5 nCi of radioactive drug (50 μl of the commercial preparation), a sufficient amount of specific antiserum to bind all labeled molecules (50 μl of the commercial antiserum should suffice), and one small disk (0.38 cm^2) of SA-2 ion exchange paper previously saturated with a urine specimen. An exchange of labeled and unlabeled hapten takes place, the rate depending on the ratio of the two. The amount of labeled drug being negligible, the rate is largely controlled by the amount of drug that has been adsorbed from the urine specimen. Originally, the labeled drug is all bound to the antibody molecules. The unlabeled drug molecules, if any, are bound to the sites on the ion exchange resin attached to the SA-2 paper. With time, some radioactive molecules become displaced from the antibody by the nonradioactive ones and become bound to the sites on paper. The main difference between the two types of site lies in the fact that the antibody sites are specific for a given hapten, whereas the resin sites on paper are not specific but adsorb any cation present, as well as many anions such as barbiturates, through nonionic attraction. After equilibration, the paper disks are removed and rinsed briefly, and the amount of radioactivity retained on them is assayed in an appropriate counter. The counts on papers derived from positive urines are much higher than the counts from negative urines.

PERSONAL INVESTIGATIONS

Treatment of urine specimens with ion exchange papers leads to adsorption of the drugs, if present, onto the papers. The yields, however, are poor, and losses of a large proportion of drugs occur. Mulé who studied these yields in 1969 (8) recovered as little as 2% of some of the drugs. When we reexamined the recoveries recently using paper that is now manufactured under careful product control, we found considerably better yields, although the losses remained large (2). A thorough study of the efficiency of each step in the treatment with trace amounts of labeled drugs diluted with nonlabeled carriers, proved the adequacy of the procedure. Each drug was added individually to control urine. Portions of each urine were diluted with deionized water and in one case with saline for comparison. The amounts of drugs adsorbed and held on the washed and dried ion exchange papers ranged from 25% for a barbiturate to 84% for methadone (Table 1). Of the approximately 30,000 cpm added to the original urine specimen, 86 to 92% were recovered either on the ion exchange paper or in the solvent extract of urine after ion exchange treatment. Not surprisingly, dilution of urine with saline decreased significantly the recovery of methadone on paper and increased the amount left behind. We recommend, therefore, that specimens be diluted with distilled or deionized water, never with saline.

TABLE 1. *Preliminary treatment of urines with ion exchange papers — adsorption of drugs*

| | Total in urine | | Percent adsorption on ion exchange paper | | | |
| | | | Urine diluted with deionized water | | Urine diluted with saline | |
Drug	μg	mμCi	Adsorbed	Left in urine	Adsorbed	Left in urine
Dihydromorphine–7,8–^{3}[H]	10	100	68.1	18.6	—	—
Methadone–1–^{3}[H]	20	150	84.1	7.6	61.6	37.9
Amphetamine–^{3}[H]–sulfate	40	200	51.4	35.5	—	—
Pentobarbital–2–^{14}[C]	40	20	25.3	65.3	—	—
Chlorpromazine	40	0	30.4[a]	12.6	—	—

A trace amount of labeled drug and unlabeled carrier added to 20 ml urine, diluted with 20 ml deionized water (or 4% saline), and adsorbed on one 6 cm × 6 cm square of ion exchange paper.

[a] Chlorpromazine calculated from fluorescence in urine before and after ion exchange treatment.

TABLE 2. *Increased elution of drugs from ion exchange papers into solvents in presence of NaCl*

Drug	Total on paper (μg)	Percent elution in presence of NaCl			
		0	2	4	10
Dihydromorphine-7,8-^{3}[H]	6.8	62.8	64.9	68.7	75.6
Methadone-1-^{3}[H]	16.8	58.6	59.6	64.1	68.1
Amphetamine-^{3}[H]–sulfate	20.6	51.2	–	68.9	–
Pentobarbital-2-^{14}[C]	10.1	58.9	59.7	59.7	59.7
Chlorpromazine	30.4	68.0	79.9	94.7	38.0

In our laboratory the yield during extraction of drugs from ion exchange papers with chloroform isopropanol (3:1) was 51 to 68% (Table 2). Addition of 2% NaCl to the buffer prior to extraction raised the yields to 60 to 80%. Increasing the amount of NaCl increased the yield, but salt concentrations of 10% and over interfered with subsequent immunoassays. Based on our overall experience we recommend, therefore, use of 4% NaCl for optimum yield compatible with further detection techniques. NaCl did not enhance the yield of barbiturates, because they were held not by ionic forces but through adherence to the paper, and they were washed off by agitation.

Addition of NaCl also had a striking effect on reconstitution of specimens in aqueous media. Although the fractions of drugs eluted from the paper into regular aqueous buffers ranged from 1/30 to 1/8 of the totals, the presence of NaCl raised the proportions considerably (Table 3).

The yield of opiate increased most dramatically (almost fourfold). The yield of barbiturates did not change.

Reliable results can be obtained by incubating a segment of the ion exchange paper directly with the immunoassay reagent without prior extraction of drugs into either organic or aqueous phase. We have checked this by adding a trace amount of labeled opiate to urine and determining the radioactivity adsorbed on paper and eluted by antibodies in HIT. In this case 63.3% of the approximately 30,000 cpm added to 20 ml urine was adsorbed on the paper, and 56.7% of that amount was removed from the paper by opiate specific antiserum (Table 4). Thus, of the total 5 μg in urine, 35.9% or 1.8 μg was available to the antibodies. Inasmuch as in HIT a fraction of a nanogram can be detected (1), it is obvious that use of a small piece of paper (approximately 1% of the area) is quite adequate to provide a large excess of detectable antigen.

TABLE 3. *Elution of drugs from ion exchange papers with buffers and saline*

Drug	Amount (μg)		Percent elution	
	In urine	On paper	Buffer	Buffer + 4% NaCl
Dihydromorphine-7,8-^{3}[H]	10.0	6.8	3.7	14.2
Methadone-1-^{3}[H]	20.0	16.8	4.0	8.6
Amphetamine-^{3}[H]–sulfate	40.0	20.6	4.3	11.7
Pentobarbital-2-^{14}[C]	40.0	10.1	11.9	11.5
Chlorpromazine	40.0	30.4	5.7	9.9

TABLE 4. *Direct use of opiates adsorbed on ion exchange papers to inhibit agglutination*

	cpm	ng
Added to urine	29,700	5,000
Adsorbed on ion exchange paper	18,800	3,160
Present in a 0.38-cm² circle	202.3 ± 11.4	34.1
Eluted by antibodies	114.7 ± 14.2	19.3

Proportion of opiate available to bind antibodies determined through the use of 0.1 μCi of 7,8–[H]³ dihydromorphine and 4.3 μg carrier in a 20-ml urine specimen.

Optimum Conditions for Drug Detection by Hemagglutination Inhibition

The small disks with drugs adsorbed on them which had been punched out from ion exchange papers were equilibrated in plastic test wells with antibodies prior to addition of coated cells. Among the variables examined in our search for optimum conditions were: concentration of drugs in the original urine, volume of urine, dilution, area of ion exchange paper placed in the urine, area in the detection step, period of equilibration, temperature of equilibration, amount of added antibody, amount of coated cells, and time to interpret the results.

The test proved to be more sensitive for opiates than for methadone or barbiturates. At a concentration of 62.5 ng/ml, morphine was detected in eight of 10 specimens, whereas neither methadone nor barbiturates gave any positive responses (Fig. 1). At 0.25 μg/ml of original urine, all 10 opiates and methadone but only four of 10 barbiturates gave a positive test. At 0.5 μg/ml all specimens were positive.

A standard volume of urine, 20 ml, diluted with an equal volume of deionized water and a standard size piece (6 cm × 6 cm) of ion exchange paper gave satisfactory results. Modifications of these parameters within a wide range were equally satisfactory. Volumes could be varied from 5 to 50 ml, dilution from 1:1 to 1:5, and area of paper from 4.5 to 72.0 cm². In all cases 100% of morphine (0.5 μg/ml), methadone (1.0 μg/ml), and phenobarbital (1.0 μg/ml) was detected. The area of paper during equilibration with antibodies could be varied from 0.095 to 0.76 cm², except that the smallest size proved too difficult to handle. There was no obvious advantage to controlled temperatures (between 25 and 40°C), and ambient temperature was found satisfactory. The amount of drug to be bound dictated the amount of antibodies. Given the need for a visible size pellet of cells at the end of the test, 50 μl of reconstituted antiserum and an equal volume of cell suspension were found optimal. The amounts could be halved, and the results were generally

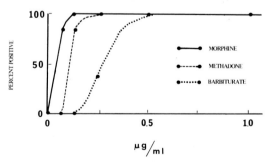

FIG. 1. Use of ion exchange papers in drug detection through inhibition of hemagglutination. The test was 80% positive for $^1/_{16}$ μg of morphine and $^1/_8$ μg of methadone per ml of original urine but was less sensitive for barbiturates ($^1/_4$ μg was detected in only four of 10 cases and $^1/_2$ μg was needed for 100% detection).

satisfactory, although a little more difficult to read. There was no advantage to increased amounts of either cells or antiserum.

Equilibration time between antiserum and the disk of ion exchange paper was varied from 10 min to 2 hr. Results were satisfactory after 10 min, and equally satisfactory after 20 or 30 min. At 1 hr some negative specimens began to appear slightly positive. Perhaps a deterioration of antiserum had set in. Papers were removed after equilibration and prior to addition of cells. Agglutination took place 1 to 3 hr later. Results could be interpreted after 90 min and were usually satisfactory even 24 hr later.

RIA: Drug Recovery Data

Segments of ion exchange paper with drugs, if any, adsorbed on them were equilibrated directly with mixtures of antibody and labeled antigen, then, removed, rinsed, and counted. All had adsorbed labeled drugs, but positive papers adsorbed more than negative ones. The ratio of positive-to-negative counts varied from 1.16 in the case of methadone to 2.15 in the case of morphine (Table 5). Not surprisingly, use of tritiated morphine led to higher positive:negative ratios than use of conjugated morphine labeled with

$^{25}[I]$, but the advantage was more theoretical than real — tritiated specimens had to be corrected for quenching and $^{125}[I]$ was easier to assay accurately. Opiate antiserum was as satisfactory for heroin or codeine as for morphine. Amphetamine antiserum was more specific for amphetamine than methamphetamine, but adequate for the detection of both.

The method led to detection of 0.125 μg/ml morphine, barbiturate, or amphetamine, and 0.25 μg/ml methadone in the original urine. Again, as in the hemagglutination test, there was no obvious difference when the amount of urine used in the test was varied from 10 to 40 ml, the area of ion exchange paper in urine varied between 9.0 and 36 cm², or the dilution with deionized water varied from 2:1 to 1:2. There was also no obvious advantage to altering the size of the segment of paper used in the detection step. Increasing the size from 0.09 to 1.14 cm² led to a proportional increase in the amount of radioactivity adsorbed in papers derived from negative specimens as well as those from morphine, methadone, or secobarbital (Table 6). The correlation coefficients for these increases were reliably high (0.974 to 0.998), indicative of the general reliability of the procedure. The ratios, however, of positive:negative specimens were, with few exceptions, not affected

TABLE 5. *Direct use of ion exchange papers in RIA for drug abuse*

Drug	Conc. (μg/ml)	Isotope	Radioactivity		Ratio Pos./Neg.	P(%)
			Positive cpm ± SD	Negative cpm ± SD		
Morphine	0.5	$^{125}[I]$	1,732 ± 130	1,231 ± 81	1.41	< 0.5
Morphine	0.5	$^{3}[H]$	659 ± 42	306 ± 13	2.15	< 1.0
Heroin	1.0	$^{3}[H]$	586 ± 112		1.91	< 1.0
Methadone	1.0	$^{125}[I]$	1,138 ± 25	979 ± 12	1.16	< 2.5
Secobarbital	1.0	$^{125}[I]$	845 ± 86	536 ± 58	1.57	< 0.5
Amphetamine	2.0	$^{125}[I]$	649 ± 130	341 ± 43	1.90	< 0.5
Methamphetamine	2.0	$^{125}[I]$	529 ± 57		1.55	< 0.5

Ten positive (enriched) and ten negative (control) urines, each tested in quadruplicate. Statistical analysis by Student's *t*-test.

TABLE 6. *Drug RIA — effect of altering the area of ion exchange paper in the detection step*

Area	Morphine		Methadone		Barbiturates	
(cm²)	Positive	Negative	Positive	Negative	Positive	Negative
0.09	487.2 ± 88.2	149.7 ± 35.5	—	—	257.9 ± 14.5	10.9 ± 6.4
0.19	661.8 ± 177.4	395.5 ± 198.9	560 ± 44	444 ± 31	484.0 ± 43.1	277.9 ± 43.1
0.28	969.5 ± 197.4	726.5 ± 141.0	—	—	770.5 ± 127	538.4 ± 137.9
0.38	1,229.2 ± 284.6	811.0 ± 100.5	1,158 ± 18	907 ± 48	860.8 ± 99.5	580.2 ± 32.5
0.76	—	—	2,041 ± 194	1,741 ± 191	—	—
1.14	—	—	2,934 ± 201	2,400 ± 175	—	—

by the size of the paper. The exception was the smallest size, 0.09 cm² which was difficult to cut accurately and which was perhaps subject to saturation of available ion exchange sites by ordinary urinary cations in the absence of specific drugs. This latter effect was evident in the case of morphine and was particularly noticeable in the case of barbiturates — during equilibration of 0.09 cm² of a negative ion exchange paper with labeled secobarbital, practically no labeled material was attracted to the paper. Except for those two cases, the ratios varied from 1.14 to 1.27 for methadone and 1.33 to 1.67 for morphine to 1.43 to 1.74 for barbiturates.

Varying the amount of antigen and antibody from 20 to 200 μl had opposite effects on the amount of radioactivity adsorbed on the ion exchange papers. Increase in labeled antigen led to a proportional increase in the count in papers containing either negative or positive samples (correlation coefficient 0.986 to 0.998) (Fig. 2 A and C). Increase in antiserum, on the other hand, led to proportional decreases in radioactivity adsorbed on the ion exchange papers; the increased number of antibody sites bound greater numbers of labeled antigen molecules, leaving fewer to attach themselves to the ion exchange sites on the paper (Fig. 2 B and D). However, inasmuch as both positive and negative specimens were affected, no obvious advantage in terms of positive:negative

ratios was obtained. The recommended amount, 50 μl of each reagent, was selected because it was the minimum that we could handle accurately and conveniently.

Variation in the equilibration temperature between 25 and 50°C did not increase the positive:negative ratio, although the

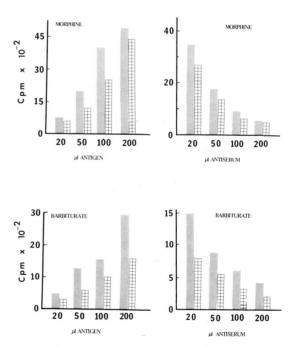

FIG. 2. Use of varying amounts of antigen and antibody in morphine and barbiturate detection through ion exchange disk RIA. Increased amounts of labeled antigen led to increased adsorption of radioactivity (cpm) on disks saturated with either positive (*stippled bars*) or negative (*lattice bars*) specimens. Increased amounts of antibody led to decreased adsorption of radioactivity on disks from both positive and negative specimens.

TABLE 7. *RIA equilibration time*

Time	Morphine		Methadone		Barbiturate	
	Positive	Negative	Positive	Negative	Positive	Negative
10 min	—	—	711 ± 45	635 ± 37	—	—
20 min	—	—	932 ± 71	830 ± 88	—	—
30 min	1,687 ± 163	1,152 ± 182	1,230 ± 90	994 ± 81	564 ± 37	329 ± 126
1 hr	2,003 ± 208	1,592 ± 305	1,527 ± 141	1,191 ± 47	685 ± 68	382 ± 89
2 hr	2,562 ± 247	1,779 ± 86	—	—	688 ± 35	517 ± 89
3 hr	2,246 ± 675	2,079 ± 269	—	—	736 ± 72	410 ± 113
24 hr	—	—	3,740 ± 189	2,119 ± 265	—	—
1 week	—	—	3,355 ± 212	2,477 ± 114	—	—

higher temperatures speeded up the process and during any given time interval led to an increase in the amount of label transferred to the ion exchange papers containing either negative or positive samples. At room temperature (25.5°C) the duration of equilibration could be varied from 10 to 60 min. Beyond that time, the antibodies tended to deteriorate, and between 2 and 3 hr the actual counts decreased in several cases (Table 7). Up to 1 hr in the case of methadone and 2 hr in the case of morphine, the correlation coefficient between radioactivity transferred to the paper and equilibration time ranged from 0.960 to 0.996. The ratios, however, were not significantly altered.

Specificity of the Immunoassays

The specificity of the assays depends, of course, on the antisera. In general, commercial antisera are specific not for individual drugs but for classes such as opiates or barbiturates. Methadone antiserum is essentially specific for that drug only. Depending on the source, amphetamine antiserum can be specific either for amphetamine only or for the entire class of amphetamines and their metabolites. The distinction is more important in the case of standards and enriched specimens than in the case of patient urines, because methamphetamine and other members of the group are metabolized in the body and appear in the urine, at least in part, as the primary amine.

When control urines were enriched with opiates, methadone, amphetamines, and barbiturates, singly or in combination, 0.5 to 1.0 μg/ml, both immunoassay procedures utilizing ion exchange paper to adsorb the drugs and to react with the antibodies gave 100% reliable results in the

TABLE 8. *Screening for drugs added to control urines and adsorbed on ion exchange papers*

Compound added	Amount (μg/ml)	No. of Specimens	Results of screening	
			HIT	RIA
Morphine	0.5	40	40	40
Codeine	1.0	20	20	20
Methadone	1.0	40	39	38
Amphetamine	2.0	20	—	21
Methamphetamine	2.0	17	—	17
Pentobarbital	1.0	35	35	35
Phenobarbital	1.0	35	35	35
Secobarbital	1.0	35	35	35
Amobarbital	1.0	35	34	34
None of above	—	100	100	102

TABLE 9. *Screening for drugs in field urines after adsorption on ion exchange papers*

| | \multicolumn{4}{c}{Results of screen} | | | |
| | \multicolumn{2}{c}{TLC} | HI | RIA |
	Pos.	Neg.	Pos.	Pos.
Opiates	21	439	21	21
Methadone	18	442	19	18
Barbiturates	23	437	24	25
Amphetamines	8	452	–	8

case of opiates and 95 to 98% reliable results in the case of methadone (Table 8). Amobarbital gave one false negative and amphetamine one false positive in the RIA. These results were considerably more accurate than those obtained on the same specimens by TLC (3) where several barbiturates and an occasional opiate gave negative readings. Similarly, in 460 largely negative urines obtained from patients and employees, HIT and RIA led to detection of more drugs than TLC (Table 9).

Most of our enriched specimens contained, in addition to the specific drug tested for, other drugs of abuse as well as nicotine, caffeine, and occasionally acetylsalicylic acid, or other common therapeutic agent. These did not interfere with proper identification of the specific drug. A typical series of enriched urines screened for the presence of amphetamines, but containing a variety of opiates, barbitu-

rates, and other agents, is shown in Table 10. One of 32 samples positive for amphetamine gave a positive:negative ratio lower than 1.3, and was therefore deemed negative, as was one of 16 methamphetamine samples. One negative specimen in 40 did have a ratio of 1.49 and would have been judged positive had it been an unknown. Similar results were obtained in enriched urines tested for opiates or barbiturates in the presence of phenothiazine tranquilizers, diphenylhydantoin, oxazepines, cocaine, meprobamate, or propoxyphene, and in patient urines that also contained a variety of drugs in addition to the one being tested.

ACKNOWLEDGMENTS

We wish to thank Sheryl Britton and Lillian Dean for technical assistance and Frances Henning for secretarial help. This work would not have been possible without Dr. Leon Roizin, Director of the Neurotoxicology Unit, Chief of Psychiatric Research in Neuropathology at the New York State Psychiatric Institute, and Professor of Neuropathology at the College of Physicians and Surgeons of Columbia University.

REFERENCES

1. Adler, F. L., and Liu, C. T. (1971): Detection of morphine by hemagglutination-inhibition, *J. Immunol.,* 106:1684–1685.

TABLE 10. *RIA screen for amphetamine and methamphetamine in enriched urines—no interference from other drugs*

Antigen present	Other drugs present	Number of specimens	Correct result (%)
Amphetamine	Pentobarbital, methadone, chlorpromazine	16	93.7
Amphetamine	Aprobarbital, codeine	8	100.0
Amphetamine	Butabarbital	8	100.0
Methamphetamine	Secobarbital, heroin, thioridazine	12	100.0
Methamphetamine	Amobarbital, morphine, fluphenazine	4	75.0
None	Secobarbital, morphine, methadone, cocaine	16	100.0
None	Chlorpromazine, nicotine, salicylate	8	100.0
None	None	16	93.7

2. Alexander, G. J. (1975): Screening for drug abuse: Use of NaCl to increase drug recovery from papers coated with ion-exchange resins. *Clin. Chem.,* 21:1803–1804.

3. Alexander, G. J. (1976): A procedure for drug screening without the need to transport urines: Use of ion-exchange papers and hemagglutination inhibition. *Clin. Toxicol.,* 9:435–446.

4. Alexander, G. J. (1976): Direct use of ion-exchange papers in hemagglutination inhibition test for drug abuse. *Clin. Chem.,* 22:1105–1106.

5. Davidow, B., Petri, N. L., and Quame, B. (1968): A thin-layer chromatographic screening procedure for detecting drug abuse. *Am. J. Clin. Pathol.,* 50:714–719.

6. Dole, V. P., Kim, W. K., and Eglitis, I. (1966): Detection of narcotic drugs, tranquilizers, am-phetamines, and barbiturates in urine. *JAMA,* 198:349–352.

7. Kaistha, K. K., and Jaffe, J. H. (1971): Extraction techniques for narcotics, barbiturates, and central nervous system stimulants in a drug abuse urine screening program. *J. Chromatogr.,* 60:83–94.

8. Mulé, S. J. (1969): Identification of narcotics, barbiturates, amphetamines, tranquilizers and psychotomimetics in human urine. *J. Chromatogr.,* 39:302–311.

9. Sohn, D., Simon, J., Hanna, M. A., and Ghali, G. (1972): Preparatory procedures in screening for drugs of abuse: "Clean-up" methods in current use. *J. Chromatogr. Sci.,* 10:294–296.

10. Spector, S., and Parker, C. W. (1970): Morphine: Radioimmunoassay. *Science,* 168:1347–1348.

Neurotoxicology, edited by L. Roizin, H. Shiraki,
and N. Grčević. Raven Press, New York © 1977.

Certification of Deaths from Drug Addiction

Milton Helpern*

Retired Chief Medical Examiner, City of New York; Department of Forensic Medicine, New York University School of Medicine, New York, New York 10022

The complexity of the problem of death certification is well illustrated by the large number of deaths from narcotism in the United States. These deaths, when correctly determined, are an important indication of the overall increase or decrease of narcotic and other drug addiction and provide evidence of changes in the prevalence and pattern of drug abuse.

In most jurisdictions, the investigation and certification of these deaths are the responsibility of an official medicolegal agency, either the office of coroner or that of medical examiner. The coroner system is considerably older and was brought from England when the Colonies were established. Coroners in this country are *elected* officials of the county and, with the exception of the states of Ohio and Louisiana, are not required to be physicians. Medical examiners are *appointed* officials of a county, municipality, or state. In jurisdictions adopting a medical examiner system after 1915, medical examiners, in addition to a medical requirement, must be qualified pathologists in order to perform autopsies. This last important requirement varies considerably in different places (2).

Coroners and medical examiners have the same authority regarding the investigation of deaths that are reported to them, but the lay or nonpathologist coroner, in order to do his work effectively (no matter how well-intentioned he may be), may or may not call on a physician to assist him with the medical aspects of a death and may or may not employ the services of a pathologist, who even so does not have primary responsibility in evaluating the death, if an autopsy is indicated. There may not be the necessary rapport between a lay or physician coroner and a pathologist available to the coroner. The coroner may not call on the pathologist, and the pathologist may not provide the necessary interpretation and evaluation of the findings or may omit observations that would have been suggested by a scene investigation (which may or may not have been carried out) or by a careful perusal of the medical history of a death in a hospital many days after admission.

In an effort to improve this unsatisfactory situation, the National Board of Medical Examiners (4) has issued standards of performance for official medicolegal investigative agencies to provide a basis for their accreditation.

The careful and meaningful certification of the cause of death is a responsibility that may have to be undertaken by a physician who has been in medical attendance on the deceased person. In many jurisdictions, the physician can exercise this function only when death has resulted entirely from natural causes, that is, from disease, and when the physician was in attendance long enough to make such a diagnosis. If the circumstances preceding or surrounding the death are indicative of violence or otherwise unusual, or if the death has been sud-

---

* Deceased.

den and unexpected, without medical attention, in whole or part the result of traumatic injury or poisoning, or has occurred during official custody, a physician, who may or may not have been in attendance, cannot certify the death but must report it to a medical examiner or coroner for official investigation and certification. Unfortunately not all deaths without medical attention or of obvious suspicion are reported or accepted for investigation as they should be. What should be mandatory requirement in practice is too often optional and not much is done to compel compliance with the law in many jurisdictions.

Whether or not the postmortem investigation includes an autopsy and other indicated examinations is at the discretion of the medical examiner or coroner. Further, the fact that an autopsy is included does not imply that determination and certification of cause of death can be based on its findings exclusively, although such an impression exists in the minds of many physicians and most laymen.

The fallacy persists that the correct answer can always be obtained from the autopsy alone, but in many cases this is far from true. In many postmortem investigations the autopsy, although essential for what it does reveal in a positive or negative sense, does not provide the complete answer. The absence of chance information from an available source may result in failure to discover a subtle traumatic injury without which the nature of an evident homicide would be obscured and gross findings of brain hemorrhage and meningitis misinterpreted as natural. Without knowledge of circumstances, the autopsy may be incomplete in a toxicological sense; or due to the fact that it has to be done after the body has been embalmed or exhumed after a variable postmortem interval or after decomposition has set in, or the fact that it is inexpertly done by an inexperienced pathologist, or completely done by a

pathologist who uncovers all findings but misinterprets them, the autopsy may lead to an erroneous conclusion or to no conclusion about the cause and manner of death.

It is surprising how often during an autopsy the pathologist is content to take a body apart quite thoroughly and, after cataloguing his findings, arrive at a definite conclusion as to the cause of death despite the fact that his findings are incomplete, or if complete, subject to several interpretations, dependent on the knowledge of prior circumstances, which he fails to determine or take into consideration.

The autopsy does not always reveal evident unequivocal causes of death. It is very comforting for the medical examiner and forensic pathologist to encounter a case of spontaneous rupture of a fresh myocardial infarction into the pericardial sac with massive hemopericardium or a case of a ruptured aneurysm in various parts of the body, or of stab or gunshot wounds or other gross traumatic injuries involving vital organs.

Many examples are available of how serious error can be committed in the determination, certification, and classification of the cause of death in cases in which an autopsy has been included as part of the postmortem investigation but the circumstances have been disregarded. These examples, in addition to addiction deaths and those following episodes of acute psychosis with exhaustion in which tranquilizing drugs have been therapeutically administered, include deaths during surgery, anesthesia, and diagnostic and therapeutic procedures when investigation is difficult and often handicapped because in most instances autopsy findings in themselves do not provide the answer, but depend in large part on accurate knowledge of the circumstances preceding death, information available at the scene to a knowledgeable investigator.

Autopsy can demonstrate overt findings, such as the effects of an explosion of an anesthetic, gross inadvertent injury to a large blood vessel during a difficult surgical procedure, perforation of the esophagus during esophagoscopy followed by fulminating suppurative mediastinitis, air embolism during uterine insufflation, and perforation of the pericardium and right ventricle with hemopericardium during diagnostic sternal puncture. But such cases are relatively rare and in most deaths during surgery and anesthesia, the pathologist does not find an anatomical cause of death. In some cases, the prior condition for which surgery and anesthesia were heroically undertaken may be so obvious as to explain that they are only a circumstance during which death occurred and not a cause of death. Examples would be cases when the victim of a shooting or stabbing is operated upon for profusely bleeding perforated wounds and dies during the procedure or when a person who is already exsanguinated from a bleeding ulcer, carcinoma, or esophageal varix dies during surgery and anesthesia carried out in an attempt to save his life. Then there are cases in which highly complicated and difficult surgery is undertaken electively in an attempt to repair or correct what is an imminently dangerous condition, like congenital or acquired valvular disease of the heart or great vessels.

Take the case of the bedridden patient with advanced carcinomatosis and clinical evidence of painful hydrothorax. Suppose a thoracentesis is performed as a palliative measure, during which there is inadvertant, clinically unsuspected perforation of the enlarged elevated adherent liver largely replaced by metastatic cancer, the puncture of which causes a large hemorrhage into the peritoneal cavity so that the dying patient is speeded on his way. Certification of this type of case can be done in such a way as to convey the impression that the neo-plastic disease was not immediately dangerous to life and that the thoracentesis caused death by puncturing the liver just as a stab wound of a normal liver might do. Improper certification of the cause of death after autopsy in such a case might very well convey the impression of malpractice. The language used on death certificates must be considered very carefully. It must not conceal and prejudice anyone's rights if a surgical, anesthetic, diagnostic, or therapeutic misadventure has occurred, but neither should it be casual or suggest negligence that never took place. The responsibility of the forensic pathologist, the medical examiner, and the coroner in certifying the cause of death is extremely important in such situations.

A history of prior illness and medical care no matter how well documented does not establish that a death was natural. Where the death occurred or the circumstances under which the body was found are more important in a medically unattended and unwitnessed death than the fact that there had been a prior medical history. If the death is considered likely to be a natural one, the required investigation should include a complete autopsy to confirm and establish this. The autopsy must be more than perfunctory, for obviously if a history of heart disease was reliable but misleading, evidence of prior occlusive coronary artery disease and myocardial infarction would be found at autopsy but would not rule out the possibility of concealed violence, like choking on a bolus of food, strangulation, electrocution, a fractured upper cervical spine, or poisoning.

Deaths from narcotism and drug abuse are easily overlooked. Corroborative autopsies, to be such, must be thoroughly performed and subtle competitive causes considered and looked for. A recent fatal unlabeled acute amphetamine poisoning of a middle-aged man would have been overlooked if the spurious history of rheumatic heart disease had been believed by the medical examiner and had an autopsy not been performed. The death led to investigation of the physician's practice and revocation of his medical license.

Any reasonable possibility of violence must be explored by the forensic pathologist, who should be skilled and experienced in his work. Too often such autopsies, if they are undertaken at all, have been delegated to the least experienced pathologist on the staff who has only just begun his training. It is not possible to review such autopsies satisfactorily the following day, for subtleties and omissions of the autopsy are not available. An autopsy is not a simple technical procedure but one that requires experience and skill for a correct interpretation and an awareness of indications for additional studies, including toxicological, histological, microbiological, and serological examinations. X-ray facilities should be available when needed. Good photography of significant findings should be carried out at the autopsy table and, when indicated, at the scene. A poorly performed incomplete autopsy by an inexperienced, unsupervised pathologist in a sense is worse than none at all, for in the latter situation the limitations of the investigation are not recognized; a poorly performed autopsy provides the erroneous impression that the cause of death has been determined, which may be far from fact.

Another need for the meaningful investigation of deaths is a better understanding of what the cause of death is in a given case. Usually with gunshot wounds and other penetrating or blunt force injuries or with unequivocal poisoning or natural death, the cause of death can be pinpointed. This type of case offers no problems. But there are many deaths in which the cause cannot be designated in this manner.

This is particularly true nowadays when an unexpected death occurs and the clinical records reveal an illness best illustrated by the acutely disturbed maniacal patient who is confined in a psychiatric hospital for treatment. What happens when death occurs? And they do occur unexpectedly in such disturbed subjects or patients. Formerly before the days of tranquilizers such disturbed catatonic patients were treated palliatively with hydrotherapy by immersion in a tub of cool water and restraints. After a period of time most patients would improve and quiet down. Some, however, developed persistent fever and died. A thorough autopsy would disclose no anatomical cause of death. Toxicology was also negative. The cause of such deaths was certified as acute psychosis with exhaustion or exhaustive psychosis. Death was physiological, and the mechanism was not clear and not evident in the autopsy. Without knowledge of the history, the cause of death would have to be listed as undetermined. With the history and negative autopsy the death was designated as having resulted from an exhaustive psychosis. But the fact remains that such unexpected deaths of acutely disturbed and maniacal patients occurred, and the cause of death could not be pinpointed. The difficulties of certifying the cause of such deaths were appreciated by everyone.

During the past few years, with the advent of tranquilizers and more recently in the case of narcotic addicts, such disturbed patients continue to be admitted to psychiatric hospitals, and instead of the cold tub therapy they are given tranquilizers such as glutethimide (Doriden®), chlorpromazine (Thorazine®), phenothiazine, and, more recently, in the case of addicts if these other substances are not effective, methadone. Without any indication (anymore than in the former unmedicated disturbed patient) that these substances were producing a toxic effect, unexpected deaths of such persistently resistant disturbed patients occur.

Again the autopsy is negative for an

anatomical cause of death. Now the toxicologist is called in, and his sophisticated complete analysis can reveal the drugs that had been used in treatment. Can the cause of such a death be pinpointed any more than it was in the more psychotic patient who did not receive such tranquilizing medications? I believe not, and I believe that it is incorrect and an oversimplification to state the cause of death as acute glutethimide, and/or phenothiazines or methadone poisoning. Yet this is being done in many instances by forensic pathologists who do not understand what a cause of death is and whose experience has mainly been with "pin-point" causes of death, such as gunshot or stab wounds, which are easily found on and in the body and retained as evidence in a bag or jar. Such deaths are easy to certify as to cause although there may be some difficulty in classification of the manner of death, about whether it was homicidal, suicidal, accidental, or undetermined.

The determination and certification of the cause of death, as much as vital statistical divisions would like it so stated for ease of coding and classification, cannot always be clearly pinpointed. At times, the cause of death must be drawn or described within a framework of circumstances and clinical history rather than one of several toxicological findings alone.

The value and need of the "framework" certification of the cause of death are shown in the following two cases. The first case is somewhat similar to the unexpected death of an acutely disturbed person who has not received any tranquilizers. The second case is a disturbed former heroin addict who was committed to a prison ward, and treated with tranquilizers, including methadone, and who died unexpectedly.

Case 1: Case one illustrates the complexity of certification of the cause of death and why it is not possible to provide a pin-

point cause. It did not involve the discovery or history of the use of drugs. There was no addiction factor, rather a sudden onset of maniacal and antisocial behavior.

The deceased was an 18-year-old athletic, strongly built black man who excelled in track and football and was the recipient of a college scholarship. He was apparently doing well but unexpectedly decided to give up his college career and return home to the disappointment of his parents.

He then developed an acute personality disorder including an interest in voodooism followed by unusual, aggressive, violent, antisocial criminal behavior manifested by the commission of assault and robbery necessitating forceful arrest, which he violently resisted, receiving multiple contusions of the scalp, neck, shoulders and wrists, and an exposure to tear gas. His sudden death following arrest was not explicable on the basis of traumatic injuries, which were absent at autopsy. There was no demonstrable evidence of tear gas exposure. It was concluded that death was caused by a combination of all the circumstances. This sudden death is somewhat analogous to those resulting from acute exhaustion following the extreme hyperactivity of an acute mentally disturbed patient with or without minor physical injuries and with an otherwise negative autopsy.

Case 2: The clinical history in this death of a disturbed narcotic addict remanded to the prison ward of a large hospital by the court on complaint of his mother whom he attempted to stab, illustrates the importance and necessity of an inclusive framework certification of the cause of death with none of the significant facts omitted. An attempt to pinpoint the cause of death in such a case, selecting only one of the many findings, may inadvertently or deliberately attribute death erroneously to only one drug with complete disregard for the circumstances and the mentally disturbed condition of the patient, in this instance a known intravenous heroin addict. The unsuccessful use of other tranquilizers, such as phenothiazine and glutethimide, prior to the use of methadone and the calming effect of methadone immediately after it was given indicate that the situation is a complex one. When this death was first investigated, the medical examiner concluded that death was caused by acute methadone poisoning, which did not take into consideration all the clinical facts. The certification suggested that the medication was routinely and carelessly given to the patient and that the fatal poisoning was an immediate consequence.

When the patient was first admitted in a disturbed state he was given chlorpromazine at 12 noon, 3, and 9 P.M.. Forty milligrams of methadone was administered at 3:40 P.M. on December 26, 1972. The first two of three doses of chlorpromazine (Thorazine®) did not control the patient's antagonistic, disturbed behavior. The methadone was administered in a 40-mg dose because the chlorpromazine had not had any calming effect on the patient's hostility. After it was given the patient became more tractable and manifested a more cooperative relationship with those around him on the ward. At no time when he was given the third dose of chlorpromazine was there any indication of an adverse reaction from any of the medication. The deceased was up and around and described as active and alert during his dinner meal and afterwards. He was observed entering his bed at 11:30 P.M., at which time his gait was steady and he was in no apparent distress.

In the 12 P.M. to 8 A.M. nurses' rounds he appeared to be asleep. At 6:45 A.M. on December 27, 1972 he was found dead by the nurses and at 7 A.M. was pronounced dead by a physician. The death was reported to the medical examiner's office.

There was evidence clinically and in previous admissions that the deceased had been a narcotic addict and had used heroin and cocaine. Old needle-track scars were noted in the hospital and confirmed at autopsy.

Autopsy revealed pulmonary edema, acute bronchopneumonia, and other evidences of drug addiction. Toxicological examination of urine by thin-layer chromatography revealed evidence of methadone and chlorpromazine. Toxicological examination of the organs, urine, and bile in the medical examiner's office revealed a small amount of methadone in the liver and a faint amount in the brain, a small amount of methadone in the urine, and a chlorpromazine derivative in the stomach with a trace amount in urine and bile. Opiates were absent in the bile and urine. Acidic drugs were absent in the brain, stomach, and urine.

In view of the clinical report, the long period of time after the administration of methadone during which the deceased ex-

hibited no evidence of an untoward reaction to any of the medication, including chlorpromazine and glutethimide followed by a single 40-mg dose of methadone, and the knowledge that the deceased had been an intravenous heroin addict and had admittedly taken cocaine on occasions make the determination of the precise cause of death uncertain.

The death was unexpected and unusual. The autopsy findings of pulmonary edema, acute pneumonitis, and hyperplasia of lymph nodes corroborate the fact that the deceased was an addict with small amounts of methadone and chlorpromazine in the tissues. The previously disturbed condition of the patient must also be considered. There is no basis for the conclusion that death resulted from an error in the therapy of methadone for a disturbed narcotic addict, who was also mentally deranged.

When deaths from intravenous heroin addiction were rampant in New York City (3), the pattern of circumstances, with the simple improvised devices for intravenous injection, multiple needle punctures and their scars, and other almost characteristic postmortem and chemical findings of heroin derivatives, made it easy to pinpoint the cause of death as an acute reaction to an intravenous injection of heroin or as an infectious reaction to injections of heroin with contaminated syringes and needles. It is important to recognize and trace cases of infectious endocarditis, generalized sepsis, and viral hepatitis to direct complications of intravenous narcotism in heroin addicts. Endocarditis is not primary but secondary to a primary site of thrombophlebitis in an infected vein. Tetanus, more common in females than in males, is a complication of subcutaneous narcotism (skin poppers). The gross appearance of the cutaneous addict with deep subcutaneous abscesses and phlegmons is usually characteristic when tetanus is a fatal complication.

In recent years in New York City there has been a striking change in the pattern of narcotic addiction. This dates back to the introduction of methadone as a treatment by Vincent Dole at Rockefeller University, using a group of hospitalized carefully controlled intravenous heroin addicts, and later at larger methadone maintenance centers set up throughout the city and elsewhere.

Methadone, a synthetic substitute for morphine introduced during World War II, has been found to block the intense craving of addicts for heroin and to maintain them when it is administered as a substitute. It is given orally usually in orange juice in gradually increasing doses starting with about 10 mg increasing to 100 or 120 mg/day after tolerance has been developed.

Carelessness has resulted in children finding and drinking methadone solution left in a refrigerator by the addict. Some fatalities have occurred in this manner and also when it was surreptitiously administered in large doses to a nonaddict without tolerance. Heroin addicts who have gone on a supervised program of methadone maintenance have been able to function and return to work without reverting to heroin. Some addicts who have not cooperated in the program have been found to use a variety of drugs including methadone obtained illicitly. The large variety of illicit drugs available to addicts has enabled them to get along with an occasional indulgence in heroin but without the intense craving for it that formerly existed among all heroin addicts. With substitute drugs including alcohol, barbiturates, methaqualone (Quaalude®), diazepam (Valium®), methadone, amphetamines, and other substances all obtained illicitly, former heroin addicts, even though not in a supervised methadone program, are able to use heroin without continuous addiction. In other words, with the use of methadone and other drugs, the heroin addict has developed a facultative ability rather than a firm addiction to heroin.

In a critical review of a group of autopsy-negative deaths of mentally ill patients attributed to phenothiazines during the 15-year period prior to 1973 when this drug was used extensively as a tranquilizing agent, Peele and Von Loetzen (5) pointed out that these unexpected deaths were reported as long ago as 1849 by Luther Bell (1) of the McLean Asylum in Massachusetts to the Association of Medical Superintendants of American Institutions for the Insane. Bell's paper concerned 10 patients who died suddenly, in whom autopsies failed to reveal an adequate explanation for their deaths. His report gave rise to the term "Bell's mania," to describe this entity, which later was more commonly designated as "lethal catatonia." It was also called "exhaustive death" and "deadly catatonia" or "exhaustive psychosis." The author also pointed out that after 1956 such unexpected deaths were designated as "phenothiazine deaths" and not "lethal catatonia." He questioned attributing these deaths to phenothiazines and suggested that these mentally ill patients who died unexpectedly after a period of agitation, disturbed behavior, and fever with negative autopsy findings were dying from the "lethal catatonia" described by Bell rather than from the effects of medication with phenothiazines. The administration of a tranquilizer and its recovery in the body during life or after death does not establish it as a cause of death.

Deaths of addicts in New York City from intravenous injection of heroin mixtures have diminished from 100 to 10%. Deaths of addicts in which methadone alone was found according to complete toxicological analysis were 11% in the first half of 1973, cases which the author personally reviewed. The remainder and majority of deaths of addicts revealed multiple drugs including mixtures of methadone, heroin, alcohol, amitriptyline (Elavil®), barbiturates, propoxyphene (Darvon®), and benzodiazepine (Valium®). Other drugs now encountered less frequently in fatal cases include phenothiazines (chlorpromazine), glutethimide, cocaine, and methaqualone. The importance of complete toxicological analysis in all fatalities from addiction is evident. With the multiplicity of drugs encountered, it is no longer sufficient for the toxicologist to confirm the presence of a single drug considered as the most likely substance to have caused death. Alcohol or its effect on the liver occurs more often than it is found by the toxicologist. In addicts surviving more than 24 hr after its ingestion, alcohol cannot be demonstrated chemically, and its presence must be determined from the autopsy and history.

None of the other drugs produces any characteristic anatomical changes in the addicted person except for occasional irregular cystic degenerations in the basal ganglia, hyperplasia of lymph nodes at the hilum of the liver, and hyperplasia of lymphoid tissue in the thymus. Repeated intravenous heroin injections over a prolonged period of time produce characteristic scars over the injection sites.

The total number of deaths of narcotic and heroin addicts in New York City has diminished since 1971.

Framework causes of death that include circumstances underlying an acute psychosis with an exhaustion component require considerable deliberation, now confounded by the use of therapeutic tranquilizers easily detected by modern sophisticated methods of toxicology available today in large centers and subject to unintentional and at times deliberate misinterpretation and distortion and wrongful designation as the cause of death. All these cases require careful analysis of the clinical record and manifestations, the mental state of patient, a complete chemical analysis, and no discontinuance of the analysis when a substance is found. It is easy to detect metha-

done and to misinterpret its presence. The medical examiner and coroner are to provide reasonable interpretation to assist the modalities of treatment of narcotic addiction. They are not supposed to, deliberately or through lack of understanding, color the interpretation of the results to the advantage of one modality and the disadvantage of another, something that has happened in recent years and has reflected discredit to official agencies concerned with the investigation of deaths of narcotic addicts.

CONCLUSION

The cause of death of present-day drug addicts cannot be pinpointed but must be derived from a careful study of history and circumstances and a complete autopsy, including toxicological analysis. It is not sufficient to consider any single chemical finding as the cause of death. It is necessary in many of the deaths to describe the cause within a framework.

REFERENCES

1. Bell, L. V. (1849): On a form of disease resembling mania and fever. *Am. J. Insanity,* 6:97–127.
2. Helpern, M. (1965): Official medicolegal investigation in the United States. *NY State J. Med.,* 65:1261–1268.
3. Helpern, M., and Rho, Y. M. (1966): Deaths from narcotism in New York City: Incidence, circumstances and postmortem findings. *NY State J. Med.,* 66:2391–2408.
4. National Association of Medical Examiners (1974): *Standards for Inspection and Accreditation of a Modern Medicolegal Investigative System.* October.[1]
5. Peele, R., and Von Loetzen, I. S. (1973): Phenothiazines deaths: A critical review. *Am. J. Psychiatry,* 130:306–309.

[1] Copies of this report may be obtained from Dr. Ali Hameli, Chief Medical Examiner, State of Delaware, Wilmington, Delaware 19801.

Neurotoxicology, edited by L. Roizin, H. Shiraki, and N. Grčević. Raven Press, New York © 1977.

Ultrastructural Investigation of the Hypothalamus in Chronically Heroin Addicted Monkeys

L. Roizin and J. C. Liu

Departments of Neuropathology and Neurotoxicology, New York State Psychiatric Institute, New York, New York 10032

Heroin was first synthesized from morphine by Wright in 1874 (136). Subsequently, Dresser (30) evaluated its potency, and the Bayer Pharmaceutical Company of Germany introduced it to the public in 1898 (124). Since then, it has been abused in Egypt and China. Now, this narcotic is abused by addicts all over the world, particularly in the United States.

Heroin is diacetylmorphine. It is rapidly hydrolyzed to 6-monoacetylmorphine which, in turn, is hydrolyzed to morphine in the animal body (131,137).

In the normal adult, both human and animal, the blood-brain barrier tends to prevent the entry of morphine into the brain, but the barrier is considerably less effective for monoacetylmorphine and heroin, since both are more lipid soluble than is morphine. Therefore, most evidence suggests that morphine is responsible for the pharmacological actions of heroin (80,131).

Compared to morphine, heroin has greater analgesia and antitussis potency, weaker emetic, milder constipation, and less respiratory depressant activities. It has faster onset, shorter duration, greater euphorogenic, and stronger addictive properties (32,33,68).

The mechanisms by which morphine and heroin affect the central nervous system (CNS) have recently been explored by a variety of biochemical procedures (18,28, 40,69,85,111,128). Morphine and heroin in experimental animals influence several metabolic processes of the CNS including protein synthesis (19,25), which has been implicated in the development of tolerance to morphine. It has been experimentally demonstrated that the development of morphine tolerance is blocked by the following protein synthesis inhibitors — actinomycin D (23a,23b), cycloheximide (65), 8-azaquanine (114), puromycin (110), and *p*-chlorophenylalanine (53).

Experiments have also determined that morphine may affect the metabolic functions of serotonin (65,105,121,132), acetylcholine (29,104), dopamine (17,49), and norepinephrine (70).

It has been pointed out that: (a) "there is no substance in the animal body that would neutralize the poison of morphine" (55), (b) "morphine and other narcotic analgesics act at all levels of the central nervous system and whatever their mode of action, it is on a very fundamental basic and widespread neuronal process" (69), and (c) the tolerance of animals to morphine could remain altered for months, perhaps for a lifetime, after a single injection of this drug (21,60).

However, much less information is available about the effects of morphine and heroin on the structural (55,67,73,84,91,

92) and ultrastructural aspects of the CNS (9,10,38) compared with biochemical studies.

Our studies[1] aim to determine the possible effects of prolonged administration of heroin on the ultrastructural constituents of the hypothalamus, since its nuclei play an essential role in the emotional, behavioral, and neurochemical mechanisms of the CNS. These experiments have been carried out in *Macacus* rhesus monkeys addicted to "street heroin" for purposes of closer comparison with human heroin addicts.

MATERIAL AND METHODS

Nine young female *Macacus* rhesus monkeys, ages three- to four-and-a-half-years-old, weighing 3.5 to 6.8 kg were selected. Of these, six monkeys received a heroin mixture containing 20% heroin, 20% quinine, and 60% mannitol. The composition of this mixture approximately corresponds to one commonly used street heroin (92,116). The heroin was obtained from the Office of the Medical Examiner of New York City (Helpern and Baden) and the National Institute on Drug Abuse, Rockville, Maryland (J. R. Bryant). The powder was dissolved in physiological saline solution. The initial dose was 0.1 mg mixture/kg body weight, and it was administered intravenously 6 days per week. The dosage was progressively increased every week for 6 months up to 3.5 mg/kg body weight (32, 130). The animals were maintained at this level for 14 months, then the dosage was increased to 5 mg mixture/kg body weight at the end of 21 months. At this dosage, the urine samples of all six monkeys showed a positive reaction for morphine.

Three control monkeys received 0.5 cc of saline solution by the same schedule as the

___

[1] This is part of a multidisciplinary research program on short and prolonged effects of neuropsychotropic agents upon the CNS.

heroin-treated animals. Twenty-three to 24 months from the initial heroin injection, the animals were sacrificed under mild ether anesthesia 24 hr after the last injection. For electron microscopic studies, small pieces of specimens from different areas were removed from the CNS, chopped into very small pieces, and directly immersed in cold 1% buffered osmium tetroxide for $1\frac{1}{2}$ hr at 4°C (71). After fixation all specimens were dehydrated through graded ethanol and propylene oxide and finally embedded with Epon 812. The blocks were cut on an LKB ultramicrotome, Model 8800; sections were double stained with uranyl acetate and lead nitrate. The stained sections were examined with an RCA electron microscope, Model EMU-3G. The electron micrographs were measured and reexamined with a Bausch and Lomb stereo-zoom microscope, Model 7.

RESULTS

The following review is limited to the ultrastructural constituents of the ventromedial and paraventricular nuclei of the hypothalamus.

Nucleonucleolar System

Some nuclei showed the presence of nucleolar segregation, an increase of nucleolar-associated chromatin, and intranucleolar twisted chromatin fibrils of 230 to 250Å thickness (Fig. 1). The ribonucleoprotein granules and chromatin fragments appeared dispersed throughout the whole nucleus. Nuclear matrix extended into the interstices of the nucleolus. In these instances, the nucleolar fibrillary component assumed the appearance of "rod-like" or ribbon-like features (Fig. 1B). In addition, oval and round granulofibrillary bodies were randomly noted. Their diameters ranged from 0.4 to 1.0 μm and, at times, they were surrounded by a halo. Some of these bodies contained a dense core, other granules, and still other variants

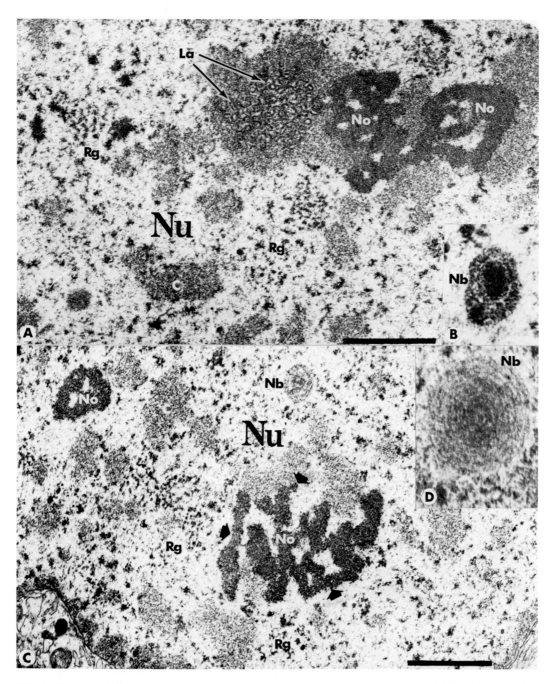

FIG. 1. Chronic administration of heroin. Hypothalamus. Monkey. **A:** Reveals segregation of the nucleolar-associated chromatin-containing twisted chromatin lamellae (La), measuring 230 to 250Å in thickness; dispersion of ribonucler protein granules (Rg) and chromatin fragments (C). Note also in the right corner (**B**) a nuclear granulofibrillary body (Nb) with a diameter of 0.35 µm and dense core of 0.14 µm. **C:** Shows in particular rod-like features (*short arrows*), splitting and segregation of the pars fibrosa of the nucleolus, irregular distribution and concentration of ribonuclear protein granules (Rg) and presence of nuclear granulofibrillary bodies (Nb). The largest (*right upper corner*) has a concentrically arranged structure with a diameter of 1 µm. **A:** ×28,300; **B:** ×56,600; **C:** ×26,000; **D:** ×33,900. Scale = 1.0 µm. No, nucleolus; Nu, nucleus.

were composed principally of fibrils (Fig. 1C and D).

Endoplasmic Reticulum and Lamellar Bodies

The smooth endoplasmic reticulum (SER) or the Golgi apparatus (GA) exhibited various degrees of proliferation in the perikaryon region (Fig. 2A). In some instances, however, the cananicular system appeared disorganized and disintegrated (Fig. 2B). The rough endoplasmic reticulum (RER) displayed irregular enlargements of the cisternae with well-preserved membrane profiles. Free ribosome of the rosette type and the ribosomes anchored to the surface of the RER were often irregularly distributed and, at times, diminished. In several instances, the endoplasmic reticulum (ER) assumed a circular or oval configuration with parallel channels or whorl-like patterns (Fig. 3) like the so-called "ER lamellar body" (5,51b, 62). In these instances, the smooth surfaced canaliculi of the ER communicated directly with the cisternae of the RER. The latter frequently contained amorphous or dense fine granules. Along some segments, membranes of two or three adjacent channels fused together as indicated in Fig. 3 (*arrows*). The fused membranes measured 200 to 400Å in thickness.

Lipofuscin and Pigment Bodies

Lipofuscin products, in early stages of degeneration, appeared increased in many neurons, occupying, at times, large portions of the cytoplasm (Fig. 4). Within the areas affected by lipofuscin, the ER and the ribosomes frequently appeared condensed. The lipofuscin material, in the more advanced stages of degradation, was composed of numerous electron-dense and electron-lighter lipid granules or large lipid droplets with preserved or disrupted limiting membranes (Fig. 4C). In the same areas lysosomes appeared increased in number and intermixed with "pigment bodies" ranging from 1.0 to 1.2 μm in diameter. Their matrix contained a variety of closely packed straight or curved bands or lamellae (Fig. 4B) with a width of 60 to 80Å. At other times crystalline-like features were also encountered.

Membranous Bodies and Astrocytic Lamellar Processes (Fig. 5).

Membranous bodies measuring 1 to 4 μm were detected in neuronal cytoplasm and various cellular processes where they were associated with mitochondria, vesicles, tubules, and some unidentified structures. They were mostly particle free, membrane paired, and concentric. In the same specimens, astrocytic lamellar processes, arranged in concentric patterns, were found around synapses containing vesicles, mitochondria, tubules, and multivesicular bodies (Fig. 6). Such astrocytic lamellar processes, in some instances, also surrounded the whole synapic complex including the postsynaptic structures (Fig. 6).

Mitochondria or Pleometabolosomes

These organelles show both qualitative and quantitative variations. Fig. 7 illustrates marked alterations of the matrix and cristae. Some pleometabolosomes (PMS) contained various amounts of lipid-like products (Fig. 7D and F). Congregations of large numbers of PMS were observed in particular in some degenerating neurites or neurodystrophic processes, as illustrated in Fig. 8A.

Degenerating Neurites or Neurodystrophic Processes

Of variable size, many of these reach dimensions up to 5 μm (in our material). In the initial stages they contain mainly

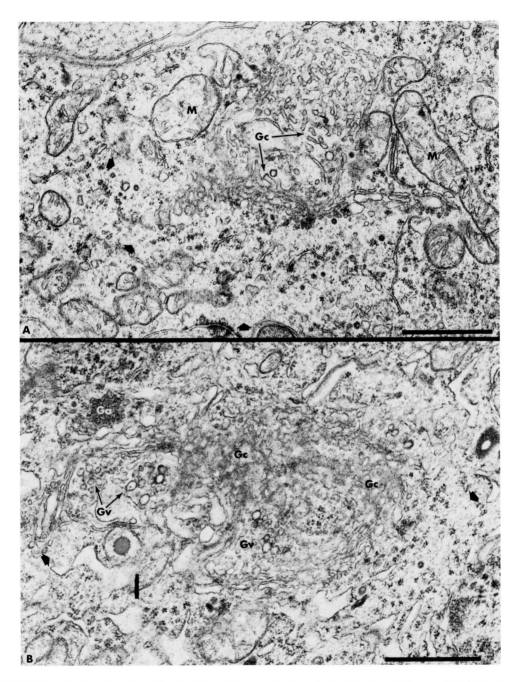

FIG. 2. Chronic administration of heroin. Hypothalamus. Monkey. **A:** Proliferation of the canaliculi of the Golgi complex (Gc) and some irregular distribution and depletion of ribosomes (*short arrow*). Note also some pleomorphism of mitochondria (M). **B:** Shows, in particular, disorganization and dissolution of the Golgi complex (Gc) with some fine changes of the Golgi vesicles (Gv) and a granular aggregation (Ga). **A:** ×35,000; **B:** ×38,400. Scale = 1.0 μm.

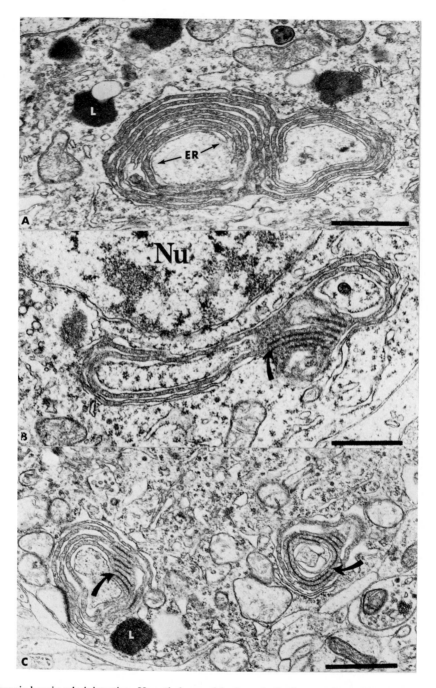

FIG. 3. Chronic heroin administration. Hypothalamus. Monkey. **A–C:** Concentric or whorl patterns of the ER or "ER lamellar body." Arrows point out fusion of membranes. **A:** Shows also increase in lysosomes (L). **A:** ×28,700; **B** and **C:** ×27,100. Scale = 1.0 μm. Nu, nucleus.

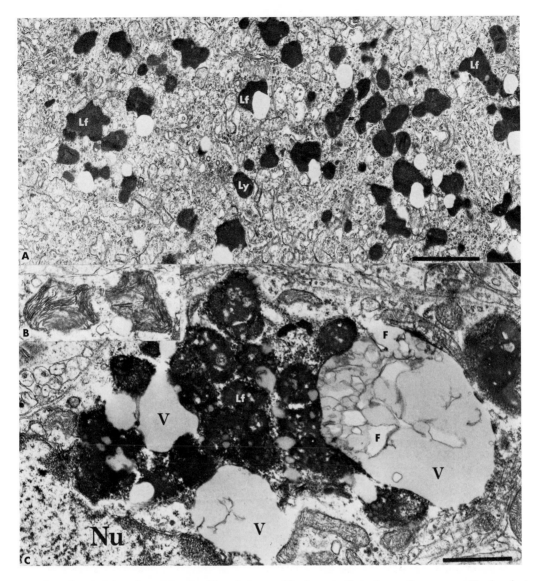

FIG. 4. Chronic administration of heroin. Hypothalamus. Monkey. **A:** Cytoplasm of a neuron with abundant lipofuscin (Lf) degenerative products, and increased lysosomal reaction (Ly). Note also condensation of the ER and ribosomal granules. **B:** Shows pigment body with lamellar structures. **C:** Composite lipofuscin products with multiple digestive vacuoles (V) and fenestrations (F) in more advanced stages of digestion. **A:** ×27,400; **B** and **C:** ×28,300. Scale = 1.0 µm. Nu, nucleus.

well-preserved organelles (Fig. 8A). Subsequently, in a second or intermediary stage (Fig. 8B), the neural processes appear laden with mitochrondria intermixed with granules, broken membranes, amorphous material, and other unidentified structures. In a more advanced or third stage (Fig. 8C), the contents of the degenerating neurite or neural processes consist principally of heteromorphic organelles in severe stages of degeneration. In these conditions the degenerating organelles

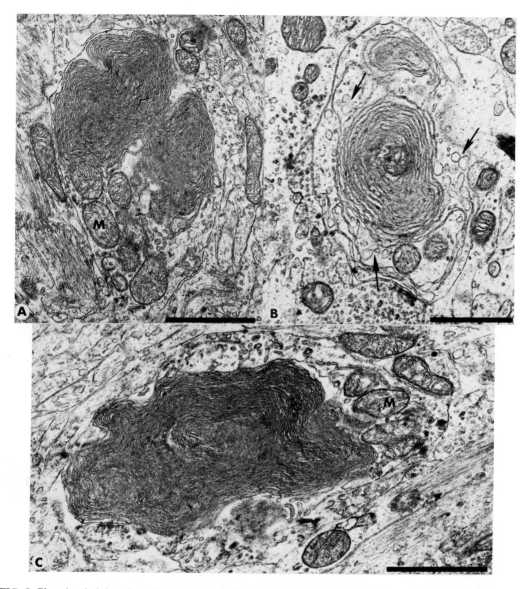

FIG. 5. Chronic administration of heroin. Hypothalamus. Monkey. **A–C:** Demonstrate membranous bodies with concentric arrays of paired membranes and free of granules. **A** and **C** are associated predominantly with congregation of mitochondria (M) and **B** with vesicles (*arrows*). **A:** ×26,600; **B:** ×28,300; **C:** ×32,900. Scale = 1.0 μm.

show the presence of various concentrations of acid phosphatase reaction products (Fig. 8D).

Amyloid Bodies

Such bodies of variable structural configuration (Fig. 9A–D) appeared randomly scattered in the neuropil, and some were located in the presynaptic terminals (Fig. 9B). Their size ranged from 1 to 5 μm. The largest (in our specimens) measured 10 μm in length and 5 μm in width.

Synapses

Various degrees of ultrastructural changes of the synaptic terminal contents,

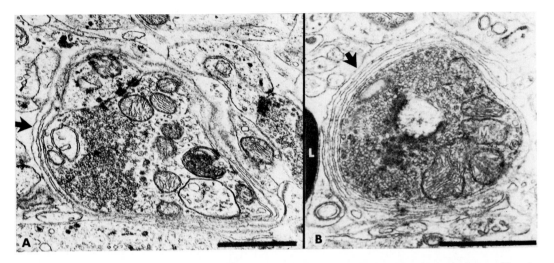

FIG. 6. Chronic administration of heroin. Hypothalamus. Monkey. **A** and **B** disclose, in particular, proliferation of astrocytic processes (*arrows*) around synaptic terminals containing packed vesicles and organelles consisting predominantly of mitochondria. **A:** ×27,100; **B:** ×33,900. Scale = 1.0 μm.

synaptic vesicles, and synaptic cleft have been observed in the ventromedial and paraventricular nuclei of the hypothalamus.

The most common changes were manifested by an increase in concentration of the clear (cholinergic) and dense-core (aminergic) types of vesicles (Fig. 10A, B, and D). A significant number of synaptic terminals also showed clumping and reduction of the synaptic vesicles (Fig. 10C and E).

The synaptic vesicles appeared, at times, enlarged and evacuated. These features were assumed on the basis of the translucid appearance of the matrix of the synaptic vesicles (Fig. 11A, B, and D). In other instances, the synaptic vesicles lost their individuality through the fragmentation or disintegration of their membranes (Fig. 11B, D, and E). In addition, the synaptic terminals, on several occasions, contained organelles undergoing various stages of degeneration, dense membrane-bound osmiophilic bodies, and some lamellar structures (Fig. 11E).

The synaptic clefts displayed variable amounts and extensions of heavy deposits of osmiophilic material at both the pre- and postsynaptic sides. A significant number of synaptic clefts appeared disrupted (Figs. 10C and 11C).

Many giant synapses have also been encountered; one of the largest measured 4μm by 6 μm. Most of them had average content and fine morphological features of the vesicles and cleft. But, some of these synaptic terminals also revealed various phases of vesicle degeneration, fine granular material, neurofilaments, and clumping of vesicles (Fig. 12). We detected similar findings in the basal ganglia of rats subjected to chronic administration of prochlorperazine (99).

DISCUSSION

Nucleonucleolar System (Fig. 1)

The functional activity of the nucleolus and its characteristic structure appear to be interdependent. When its structural integrity is disturbed, nucleic acid synthesis is impaired, and, conversely, when a drug or a chemical or a virus binds to or acts on the DNA of the nucleus and interferes with DNA-dependent RNA synthesis, then the normal organization of the

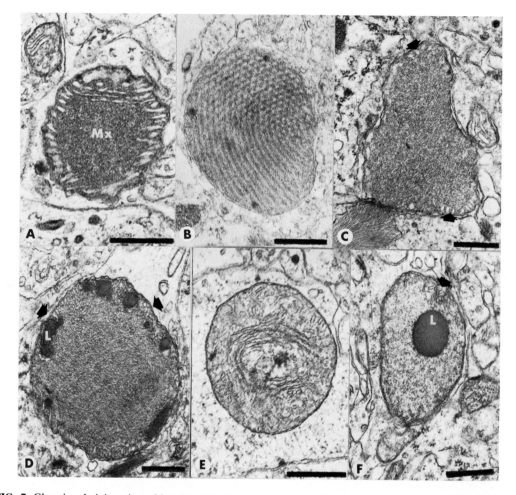

FIG. 7. Chronic administration of heroin. Hypothalamus. Monkey. Demonstrative example of mitochondrial (PMS) changes: **A, C,** and **D:** PMS with dense matrix (Mx) consisting of dense granulofilamentous material with peripheral distribution of cristae. **B:** PMS with paracrystalline-like arrangements of the cristae. **E:** PMS with disorganization and some concentrically patterned cristae. **F** and **D:** PMS with almost complete absence of cristae, except a few residuals (*arrow*). Note also lipid-like (L) inclusions. **A:** ×41,100; **B:** ×33,900; **C** and **F:** ×30,900; **D:** ×28,100; **E:** ×37,700. Scale = 0.5 μm.

nucleolus is affected and expressed by various structural changes (37,108).

It has been reported that the nuclear dry mass was changed in the neurons of rat hypothalamus after 12 to 19 daily injections of heroin (64) and that the nuclear fraction of rat brain homogenate could bind with ^{3}H-haloxane, an opiate antagonist (87). It has been demonstrated that morphine inhibits RNA synthesis in the rat brain for up to 2 hr, but after a fifth daily injection of morphine, RNA synthesis is increased (19). These facts imply that heroin acts on or binds with the nucleolus after acute or chronic administration.

The formation of "intranucleolar chromatin lamellae" in the nucleolus (Fig. 1A) is similar to the fibroblast of monkey kidney cell culture treated with hydroxyurea, an inhibitor of protein and DNA synthesis (6). The nucleolar segregation and fragmentation shown in Fig. 1A and B appear similar to nucleolar changes induced by 5-fluorouracil, a DNA synthesis inhibitor

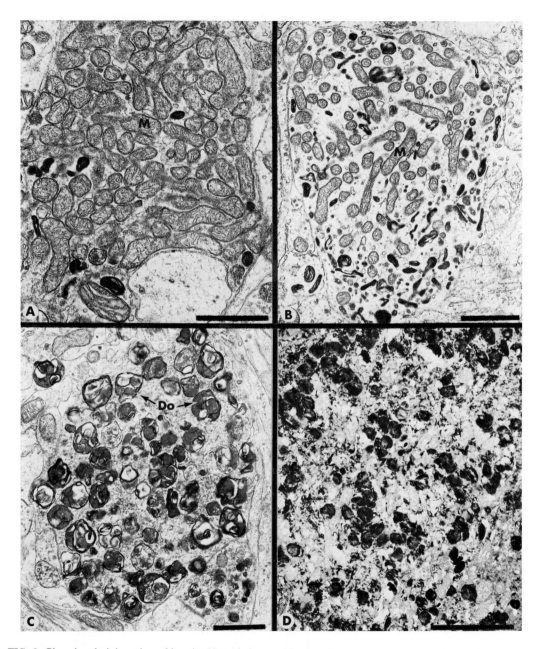

FIG. 8. Chronic administration of heroin. Hypothalamus. Monkey. Neurodystrophic processes containing predominantly **A:** packing of a large number of well-preserved PMS (M); **B:** large number of preserved PMS and degenerating organelles; **C:** predominantly pleomorphic degenerated organelles (Do) in various stages of metamorphosis; and **D:** acid phosphatase reaction products in degenerating organelles (Gomori's acid phosphatase method, 1-hr incubation). **A:** ×22,600; **B:** ×19,000; **C:** ×17,000; **D:** ×26,600. Scale = 1.0 μm.

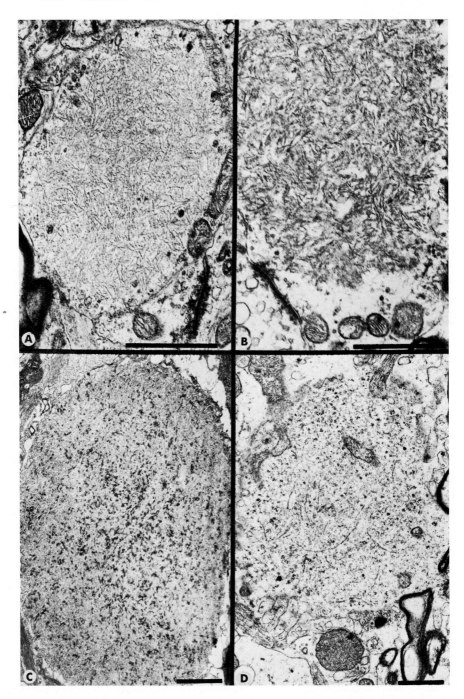

FIG. 9. Chronic administration of heroin. Hypothalamus. Monkey. Amyloid bodies consisting of variable fibrillary or granulofilamentous (**A** and **B**) or tubular (**C** and **D**) and floculent structures intermixed, in various amounts, with electron-dense material and probably glycogen granules. At times, they are surrounded or in contact, or contain PMS with well-preserved ultrastructures or undergoing various stages of degeneration. **A** and **B:** ×34,300; **C** and **D:** ×17,000. Scale = 1.0 μm.

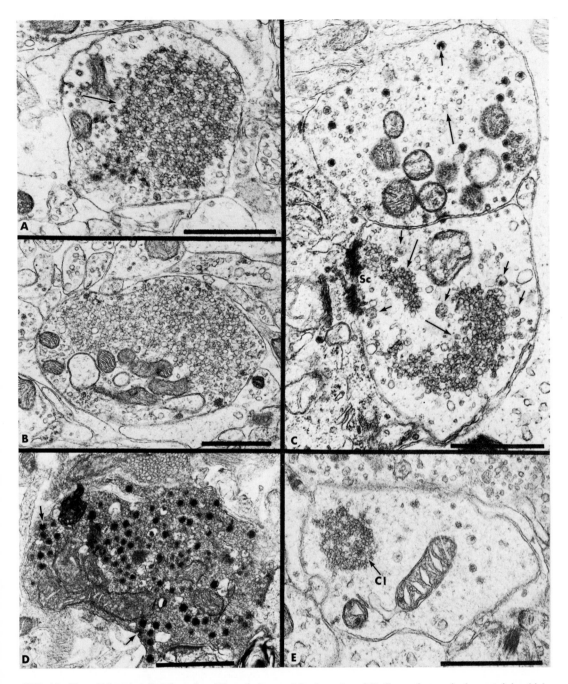

FIG. 10. Chronic heroin administration. Hypothalamus. Monkey. **A** and **B**: Synaptic terminals containing high concentration of predominantly cholinergic (*long arrows*) type of vesicles. **C**: Synaptic terminal with densely packed cholinergic (C) and bioaminergic or dense core (*short arrows*) vesicles. **D**: Synaptic terminal with marked reduction and some alterations of the cholinergic type of vesicles (*upper side of illustration*). In contact with the above, notice also a synaptic terminal with tendency of clumping of C type of vesicles (Cl). Some of these appear also of variable dimensions and translucid. **E**: Illustrates clumping of the cholinergic type of vesicles. **A**: ×33,900; **B**: ×26,600; **C**: ×35,600; **D**: ×29,400; **E**: ×38,500. Scale = 1.0 μm. Sc, synaptic cleft.

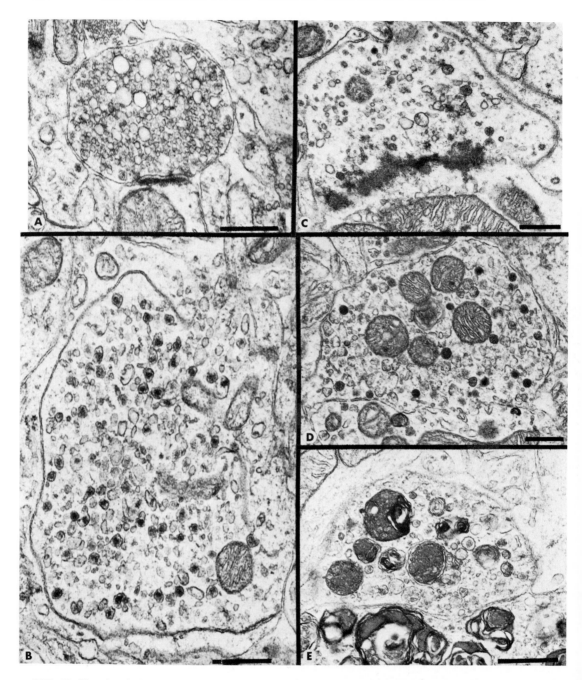

FIG. 11. Chronic administration of heroin. Monkey. Hypothalamus. **A:** Synaptic terminal containing cholinergic types of vesicles of various dimensions; some of these appear markedly enlarged with translucid matrix. **B:** Large synapse with very pronounced abnormal dimensions and osmiophilic character, particularly of the dense core vesicles, including some breaking or disintegration of the membranes. **C:** Reveals variations in size of the synaptic vesicles. Note also dense deposits of osmiophilic material at the pre- and postsynaptic levels of the cleft (CL). **D:** Presynaptic terminal with mixed clear and dense core vesicles undergoing various degrees of disruptions. **E:** Synaptic terminal with various types of vesicles intermixed with an abnormal number of pleomorphic organelles in various stages of degeneration. **A:** ×43,600; **B:** ×43,900; **C:** ×29,300; **D:** ×28,300; **E:** ×44,600. Scale = 0.5 μm.

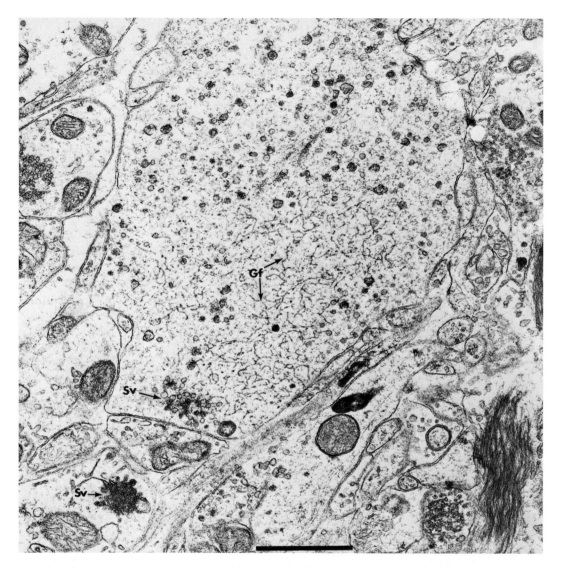

FIG. 12. Chronic administration of heroin. Hypothalamus. Monkey. A giant synapse with mixed type of synaptic vesicles undergoing various degrees of alteration. Note also tendency to clumping of synaptic vesicles (Sv), presence of granulofilamentous-like structures (Gf), and fine osmiophilic granules dispersed throughout the synaptic matrix. ×33,000. Scale = 1.0 µm.

(6), and some antimetabolites, such as nagalamycin, echinomycin, chromomycin A3, actinomycin D, proflavin (108), and ethionine (106,107).

The abnormal nuclear granulofibrillar bodies in Fig. 1B have been found in the nuclei of human bronchial mucosa, in the human placenta, and in the liver of phenobarbitone-treated hamster (41), but they are quite rare in the CNS.

Review of the literature did not yield any studies on the effect of narcotic drugs on DNA in the animal brain (19).

Our findings seem to indicate that the ultrastructural alterations of the nuclei and nucleoli in the heroin-treated monkey hypothalamus are due to the interaction of heroin with the chemical constituents and some metabolic processes of the nucleonucleolar system.

Endoplasmic Reticulum and Lamellar Bodies (Figs. 2 and 3)

It is known that the RER is primarily associated with protein synthesis (11,81, 88), whereas the SER shows a close relationship with glycogenesis and glycolysis (72,77,88). It has also been demonstrated that pretreatment of animals with inhibitors of protein synthesis blocks the development of tolerance to morphine (23a,23b). It seems, therefore, that studies of these organelles in addicted animals might shed some light on the mechanisms of action of morphine on the cytometabolism and structural correlates of the affected CNS.

The GA of neurons in acute morphine experiments in rats showed hypertrophy and fragmentation (55,67). It was also reported that the GA in spinal ganglion of guinea pigs treated with morphine for 11 days appeared to be loosened and swollen. After 16 daily injections it became fragmented, and after 19 daily injections the GA was disorganized. However, the GA returned to normal after a month recovery period (73).

The fine structural changes of the GA and SER in Fig. 2A are similar to those of the hypothalamus of rats treated with methadone, as we reported previously (98).

The ER lamellar bodies (62) appeared as special patterns of the ER, and they were connected to the RER. Similar changes of the GA and ER were observed following administration of lithium (96), ethionine, some antimetabolites (2), and cycloheximide (*unpublished personal observations*). The development of ER lamellar bodies (whorls) was also reported in the neurons of cats after spino-rubral tractotomy (5) and axon section (27) and in ovariectomized-androgenized rat females (59).

It has been suggested that the alteration and disorganization of the GA and ER is associated with shifts in protein production (63), as for instance, morphine decreases the uptake of leucine into the protein of rat brain (16) but exhibits a marked increase in its ability to incorporate P^{32} into the brain of the guinea pig. It has also been considered that morphine could alter phospholipid metabolism within intracellular organelles (75,76).

Lipofuscin and Pigment Bodies (Fig. 4)

It has been suggested and demonstrated that the GA and ER are the source of lysosomes (26,54,78), and that lipofuscin is derived from lysosomes by secondary modification of lysosomal residual bodies that represent the insoluble autooxidized residuum of material accumulated during a process of autophagocytosis (36,79). Furthermore, experiments have established that lipofuscin forms when there is a deficiency of antioxidants such as vitamin E, and it has been suggested that lipid peroxidation leads to damage of unsaturated lipid membranes with their final disintegration into lipofuscin granules (14). However, the details of the mechanism involved in this degenerative metamorphosis are not fully understood.

The increase of lipofuscin and its ultrastructural variations in the CNS have been reported also in Huntington's chorea (100,120), in heroin-methadone addicts (97), in aged animals (3,103,135a,135c), in Alzheimer's disease, and in Pick's disease (135b).

The pigment bodies have been reported mainly in aged animals, and it is believed that they were derived from lysosomes. The crystalline-like structures present inside of the pigment suggest a particular stage in the transportation of phospholipids (103).

Thus, the increase of lipofuscin (Fig. 4A), the formation of pigment bodies (Fig. 4B), and the metamorphosis in multiple digestive vacuoles (Fig. 4C) may be attributed to the effects of heroin on the: (a) protein-lipid and phospholipid metabolism and/or (b) lysosomal enzymatic processes causing reduced ability for digesting the phagocytosed lipid or phospholipid products, or (c) mechanisms of exocytosis (100) and possibly various combinations of the above.

Membranous Whorls and Astrocytic Processes (Figs. 5 and 6)

The formation of membrane whorls (bodies) in the cellular cytoplasm and in its processes has been observed in a variety of pathological conditions in the CNS, as for instance, in aged mouse brain (126), in degenerated neurons (113), in castrated rats (12), in morphine-treated rats (38), and in hepatic cells stimulated by dioxane (1), dimethylnitrosamine (35), ethionine (107,115), cycloheximide, and emetine (56). Whorl formations in our material (Fig. 5) were present principally in neuronal processes and neurons in the basal ganglia (99). They were similar in configuration to those reported by Ford et al. (38) in morphine-treated rats and by Vaughan (126) in aged mice. The source of these membranous bodies is uncertain and much debated (126). They have been experimentally induced by inhibitors of protein synthesis (56), and we have confirmed these findings in experiments with cycloheximide (*unpublished personal observations*). These findings seem to support the contention that heroin acts as an inhibitor of some protein synthesis. However, the astrocytic processes (Fig. 6) wrapped around the synapses were connected to an astrocyte process (Fig. 6, *arrow*). Its origin may be different from the membranous whorls, but the formation mechanism could be similar although the pathogenesis remains unclear.

The astrocytic processes surrounding the synapses in the CNS have also been observed in retrograde degeneration (4), hypoxia (138), and in adult staggerer (52), and we found this type of astrocytic reaction in rat basal ganglia following prolonged treatment with prochlorperazine (Compazine®, ref. 99).

Mitochondria or PMS (Fig. 7)

Both numerical and qualitative changes were detected in our material. Numerical changes were observed more frequently with the development of neurodystrophic processes. These were expressed by marked changes of the matrix and cristae (Fig. 7). In addition, some PMS contained lipid products or lipid droplets (Fig. 7D and F) and, at times, granular material. Paracrystalline-like arrangement of the cristae was only occasionally detected (Fig. 7B). Enlarged, giant, and pleomorphic PMS with variable number of cristae were detected both in the cellular cytoplasm and in a variety of processes in the neuropil. Similar PMS changes have been reported in animals maintained on vitamin E- and essential fatty-deficient diets (117,118, 134) and oxygen deprivation (138). In addition, these types of PMS alterations have been observed after administration of puromycin (39), lead poisoning (129), alcoholism (74,125), Huntington's chorea (100,120), and Warthin's tumor (119).

It is particularly significant, in considering some pathological processes, that PMS membranes are quite different from other biochemical membranes in their functions and chemical compositions. They contain a large amount of phospholipids, which are significantly high in unsaturated fatty acryl chains (13). It has been reported that the lipid peroxidation of PMS gives fluorescent products having the fluorescence and excitation spectra similar to lipofuscin (14). This does not imply that lipofuscin is derived from mitochondria, but that lipid peroxidation contributes to the development of some chemical and ultrastructural changes in PMS.

The mitochondrial changes we observed in the hypothalamus of the chronic heroin-treated monkeys may, on the basis of a review of the literature and our observations, be attributed to several factors, including the effects of heroin on the PMS metabolism, increase of the process of lipid peroxidation, reduction in the oxygen supply (depression of the respiratory center), and some dietary deficiency (diminished or changed appetite or digestive disorders).

Degenerating Neurites or Neurodystrophic Processes (Fig. 8)

These degenerative processes also occur in a variety of pathological conditions in animals—in senile animals (135a); after nerve transections in rats, rabbits, and cats (123); following administration of acrylamide (42); and in humans—in Alzheimer's disease (61,122), Pick's disease (135b), and Huntington's chorea (100). However, the cause of accumulation and degeneration of the PMS in the neurodystrophic processes is uncertain.

Amyloid Bodies (Fig. 9)

Such bodies of variable ultrastructural organizations are frequently observed in senile brains (135a), some cases of epilepsy (89), Pick's disease (135a), Huntington's chorea (*unpublished personal observation*), and a variety of chronic degenerative conditions commonly associated with aging.

Amyloid bodies were experimentally induced in laboratory animals by various chemicals, such as casein in mice (51a) and rabbits (22), ribonucleate in rabbits (90), and methylcholanthrene in ducks (93).

The pathogenesis of the amyloid bodies is still obscure. They may be the expression of: (a) polymerized products from the precursors expelled by histocytes (48), (b) a disturbance of intracellular carbohydrate metabolism (50a), (c) a disorder of protein metabolism (86), and (d) antibody-antigen process, since the amyloid could be produced by stimulating the production of antibodies to various antigens (58,102).

Since heroin can affect different metabolic processes in the CNS, it may be that amyloid bodies also represent degradation by-products resulting from disorders of carbohydrate or protein metabolism.

Synapses (Figs. 10, 11, and 12)

Structurally, the initial synaptic degeneration has been demonstrated following enucleation of one eye in monkeys. It showed both shrinkage and enlargements of the synaptic terminals with decrease in the number of synaptic vesicles. The PMS within synaptic terminals displayed pleomorphism with disorganization of the cristae (44,66). During this stage, proliferation of astrocytic processes around the synaptic terminals was also reported (7). In a second stage, the degeneration of synapses was manifested by the enlargement of and closed packing or clumping of synaptic vesicles, and increase of the density of the matrix. The synaptic vesicles were also undergoing disintegration, fragmentation, and loss of individual differentiation. The third stage of synaptic degeneration was demonstrated by vacuolization and fragmentation of degenerating mitochondria and disintegration of the synaptic vesicles beyond recognition (24,127).

Synaptic degeneration has also been observed in Alzheimer's disease (47,61), psychomotor retardation (46), mental retardation and cortical blindness (45), infantile neuroaxonal dystrophy (50b), Pick's disease (95), and Huntington's chorea (100,120). Synaptic degeneration has been induced also by methionine sulfoximine (94), lithium (96), prochlorperazine (199), and morphine (38).

In recent years extensive studies have been carried out about the effects of morphine on the brain biochemistry in drug dependence (15,20,28,43,109,112). In reference to our discussion it is of interest to note that: (a) narcotic drugs affect synaptic transmission, and (b) all four major neurotransmitters are involved in the following manner: (i) morphine increases serotonin turnover in the brain of rodents (105,132) and reduces its level in mice (121); (ii) morphine increases dopamine turnover in rat hypothalamus and striatum (17) and decreases dopamine synthesis in rat brain (49); (iii) morphine increases synthesis of norepinephrine (49) and raises its content level in the rat brain (70); and (iv) morphine inhibits the release of acetylcholine from the cerebral cortex of rat (104) and decreases acetylcholine utilization in the rat brain (29).

As to the pathogenic significance of the synaptic ultrastructural changes it is pertinent to recall that: (a) the synaptic complex and its subunits (including the axonal or presynaptic terminals, synaptic vesicles, presynaptic membrane, synaptic cleft, and postsynaptic membrane) are uniquely specific organelles of the nervous system, (b) they are principally related to transmission or communication of neural activity (action potentials and related integrative functions), (c) they compartmentalize the metabolic processes concerned with the storage, transport, release, and reuptake of neurochemical transmitters (8,31,57,82,83), and (d) the postsynaptic membrane has been designated "opiate receptor" (20,34,87) and probably the target of interaction with many other neuropsychotropic agents (101). It would be presumptious to pinpoint, only on electron microscope observations, which of the above-listed neurofunctional mechanisms is affected by the ultrastructural changes illustrated in Figs. 10,11, and 12. However, on the basis of comparative controls, it could be assumed that since in normal conditions the synaptic complex is the anatomical substrate of the above-indicated neurophysiological activities, its ultrastructural alterations should also directly or indirectly affect the essential biophysical and neurochemical processes related to CNS neurogenic mechanisms.

CONCLUDING REMARKS

Prolonged administration of street heroin to *Macacus* rhesus monkeys affected, in variable manners and in different degrees, the ultracellular constituents of the ventromedial and paraventricular nuclei of the hypothalamus.

On the basis of the electron microscope examinations it is assumed that:

1. The disorganization of the nucleonucleolar ultrastructural constituents and the presence of intranucleolar chromatin lamellae and granulofibrillary bodies are probably the result of some metabolic disorders of DNA and RNA metabolism.

2. Changes of the ER, particularly those of the granular or rough component, the irregular distribution and, at times, depletion of ribosomes, and the formation of the lamellar structures may be due to the effects of the drug on the synthesis of some proteins and ribonucleic acids. Similar changes have been observed following the administration of inhibitors of protein synthesis. The fragmentation and disintegration of the canalicular profiles as well as of the related subunits of the smooth component of the ER (Golgi complex) have been observed in various degenerative processes and may be related to disorders of the intracytoplasmic transport mechanisms.

3. The fine alterations of the matrix and cristae of the mitochondria or PMS, formation of multilamellar bodies (or structures), clumping of the synaptic vesicles, and proliferation of astrocytic processes around the synaptic terminals may be attributed to a certain degree to tissue oxygen deficit. This assumption is based on the facts that heroin depresses the respiratory centers and that

analogous ultrastructural changes have been induced by experimental chronic hypoxia.

4. The numerical variations of the synaptic cholinergic and biogenic amine type of vesicles, the alterations of their content (based on the osmiophilic reaction), the enlargement (swelling) or ballooning of the vesicles, the disruption or disintegration of the vesicles' membrane, and changes of the cleft (including distribution of the osmiophilic products) could be the expression of direct or indirect effects of the drug on the synaptic ultrastructural-metabolic correlates, which, in the final analysis, would affect also their neurochemical and biophysical communication mechanisms. Some of the ultrastructural changes of the synapses and their subunits are not uniquely associated with the chronic heroin administration, but they have also been observed in various pathological processes of the CNS including the retrograde degeneration.

5. Irregular distribution in the neuronal cytoplasm and neuropil and qualitative and quantitative changes of the "dense core vesicles" or the bioaminergic type are discussed in the chapter on "chemogenic lesion."

6. The presence of neurodystrophic processes or degenerating neurites and increased numbers of organelles undergoing degenerative changes not only in axons, but also in the synaptic terminals, may be related to some disorders of the axonal flow or intracellular transport mechanisms.

7. The lipofuscin deposits and the formation of pigment and amyloid bodies, frequently associated with increase in number and metamorphosis of lysosomes, seem to be the by-products of degenerative processes of a metabolic character with coparticipation of possible nutritional disorders and aging factors.

These ultrastructural findings indicate that the pharmacodynamic properties of street heroin, also in experimental conditions, interact in variable manners and different degrees with multiple targets or bioreceptors even in very circumscribed areas such as the hypothalamic nuclei.

ACKNOWLEDGMENTS

The authors gratefully acknowledge the assistance and cooperation of K. M. Wu and S. Avrin for electron microscopy procedures, V. Bystron for illustrations, W. Rivers for bibliography, and M. Van Cleef for secretarial work.

REFERENCES

1. Argus, M. F., Schal, R. S., Bryant, G. M., Hogh-Ligeti, C., and Arcos, J. G. (1973): Dose response and ultrastructural alterations in dioxine carcinogenesis. *Eur. J. Cancer*, 9:237–243.
2. Arstila, A. U. (1972): Ethionine induced alterations in the Golgi apparatus and in the endoplasmic reticulum. *Virchows Arch. Cell Path.*, 10:344–353.
3. Barden, H. (1970): Relationship of Golgi thiaminepyrophosphatase and lysosomal acid phosphatase to neuromelanin and lipofuscin in cerebral neurons of the aging Rhesus monkeys. *J. Neuropathol. Exp. Neurol.*, 29:225–240.
4. Barron, K. D., and Doolin, P. F. (1968): Ultrastructural observations on retrograde atrophy of lateral geniculate body. II. The environs of neuronal soma. *J. Neuropathol. Exp. Neurol.*, 27:401–420.
5. Barron, K. D., Dentinger, M. P., Nelson, L. R., and Mincy, J. E. (1975): Ultrastructure of axonal reaction in red nucleus of rat. *J. Neuropathol. Exp. Neurol.*, 34:222–248.
6. Bernard, W. (1969): Drug-induced changes in the interphase nucleus. In: *Advances in Cytopharmacology, Vol. 1: 1st Int. Symp. Cell Biology and Cytopharmacology*, edited by F. Clementi and B. Ceccarelli, pp. 49–67. Raven Press, New York.
7. Blackstad, T. W., Walberk, F., and White, L. E. (1965): Early stages of terminal axonal degeneration in the fascia dentata. *J. Ultrastruct. Res.*, 12:236.
8. Bloom, F. E., and Costa, E. (1974): The effects of drugs on sexotonergic nerve terminals. In: *Advances in Cytopharmacology, Vol. 1: 1st Int. Symp. Cell Biology and Cytopharmacology*, edited by F. Clementi and B. Ceccarelli, p. 379. Raven Press, New York.
9. Borowicz, J. W., Gajkowska, B., and Jurkiewiez, J. (1974): Electron microscope studies of the supraoptic nucleus and paraventricular nucleus of the rat hypothalamus in acute and chronic

morphine poisoning. *Ann. Med. Sect. Pol. Acad. Sci.,* 19:97–98.

10. Borowicz, J. W., Jurkiewicz, J., and Olszewoka, K. (1974): Electron microscopic changes in acute morphine poisoning of the rat brain. *Ann. Med. Sect. Pol. Acad. Sci.,* 19:99–100.

11. Braunsteiner, H. K., Fellinger, K., and Pakesch, F. (1955): Elektronenmikroskopishce Untersuchungen ueber Zellstruktur und Zellfunktion. *Klin. Wochenschr.,* 33:4–8.

12. Brawer, J. O. R. (1971): The role of the arcuate nucleus in the brain-pituitary-gonad Axis. *J. Comp. Neurol.,* 143:411–446.

13. Chapman, D., and Leslie, R. B. (1970): Structure and function of phospholipids in membranes. In: *Membranes of Mitochondria and Chloroplasts,* edited by E. Racker, pp. 91–126. Van Nostrand-Reinhold, New York.

14. Chio, K. S., Reiss, U., Fletcher, B., and Tappel, A. L. (1969): Peroxidation of subcellular organelles: Formation of lipofuscin-like fluorescent pigments. *Science,* 166:1535–1536.

15. Christian, S. T. (1972): Enzymes. In: *Chemical and Biological Aspects of Drug Dependence,* edited by S. J. Mulé and H. Brill, p. 449. CRC Press, Cleveland.

16. Clouet, D. H., and Ratner, M. (1968): The effect of morphine administration on the incorporation of ^{14}C-leucine into protein in cell-free system from rat liver and brain. *J. Neurochem.,* 15:17–23.

17. Clouet, D. H., and Ratner, M. (1970): Catecholamine biosynthesis in brain of rats treated with morphine. *Science,* 168:854–856.

18. Clouet, D. H. (editor) (1971): *Narcotic Drugs: Biochemical Pharmacology.* Plenum Press, New York.

19. Clouet, D. H. (1971): Protein and nucleic acid metabolism. In: *Narcotic Drugs: Biochemical Pharmacology,* edited by D. H. Clouet, pp. 216–228. Plenum Press, New York.

20. Clouet, D. H. (1972): Theoretical biochemical mechanisms for drug dependence. In: *Chemical and Biological Aspects of Drug Dependence,* edited by S. J. Mulé and H. Brill, p. 545. CRC Press, Cleveland.

21. Cochin, J., and Kornetsky, C. (1964): Development and loss of tolerance to morphine in the rat after single and multiple injections. *J. Pharmacol. Exp. Ther.,* 145:1–10.

22. Cohen, A. S., Calkins, E., and Levene, C. I. (1959): Studies on experimental amyloidosis. I. Analysis of histology and staining reactions of casein-induced amyloidosis in rabbit. *Am. J. Pathol.,* 35:971–990.

23a. Cohen, M., Keats, A. S., Krivoy, W., and Ungar, G. (1965): Effect of actinomycin D on morphine tolerance. *Proc. Soc. Exp. Biol. Med.,* 119:381–384.

23b. Cox, B. M., Ginsburg, M., and Osman, O. M. (1968): Acute tolerance to narcotic analgesic drugs in rats. *Br. J. Pharmacol.,* 33:245–256.

24. Cuenod, M., Sandri, C., and Akert, K. (1970): Enlarged synaptic vesicles as an early sign of secondary degeneration in the optic nerve terminals of the pigeon. *J. Cell Sci.,* 6:605–613.

25. Datta, R. K., and Antopol, W. (1973): Effect of chronic administration of morphine on mouse brain aminoacyl-t-RNA synthetase and t-RNA-amino acid binding. *Brain Res.,* 53:373–386.

26. de Duve, C., and Wattaux, R. (1966): Functions of lysosomes. *Annu. Rev. Physiol.,* 28:435–492.

27. Dixon, J. S. (1968): Changes in the fine structure of neurons after axon section. *J. Anat.,* 103:396–397.

28. Dole, V. D. (1970): The biochemistry of addiction. *Annu. Rev. Biochem.,* 39:821–840.

29. Domino, E. F., and Wilson, A. E. (1975): Decreased rat brain acetylcholine utilization after heroin and cross tolerance to L-methadone. *Biochemistry,* 24:927–928.

30. Dresser, H. (1898): Pharmacologisches über einige morphinderivate. *Deut. Med. Wochenschr.,* 24:185–186.

31. Ecles, J. C. (1964): *The Physiology of Synapses.* Academic Press, New York.

32. Eddy, N. B., and Howes, H. A. (1935): Studies of morphine, codeine and their derivatives. VIII. Monoacetyl- and diacetylmorphine and their hydrogenated derivative. *J. Pharmacol. Exp. Ther.,* 53:430–439.

33. Eddy, N. B. (1953): Heroin (diacetylmorphine): Laboratory and clinical evaluation of its effectiveness and addiction liability. *Bull. Narc.,* 5:39–44.

34. Ehrenpreis, S., and Teller, D. N. (1972): Interaction of drugs of dependence with receptors. In: *Chemical and Biological Aspects of Drug Dependence,* edited by S. J. Mulé and H. Brill, p. 177. CRC Press, Cleveland.

35. Emmelot, P., and Benedetti, E. L. (1960): Changes in the fine structure of rat liver cells brought about by dimethylnitrosamine. *J. Biophys. Biochem. Cytol.,* 7:393–395.

36. Essner, E., and Novikoff, A. B. (1960): Human hepatocellular pigments and lysosomes. *J. Ultrastruct. Res.,* 3:374–391.

37. Fawcett, D. W. (1966): Nucleolus. In: *The Cell: Its Organelles and Inclusions,* by D. W. Fawcett, p. 26. Saunders, Philadelphia.

38. Ford, D. H., Voeller, K., Callergari, B., and Gresik, E. (1974): Changes in neurons of the eminence arcuate region of rats induced by morphine treatment: An electron microscopic study. *Neurobiology,* 4:1–11.

39. Gambetti, P., Gonatas, N. K., and Flexner, L. B. (1968): The fine structure of puromycin-induced changes in mouse entorhinal cortex. *J. Cell Biol.,* 36:379–390.

40. George, R., and Lomaz, P. (1965): The effects of morphine, chlorpromazine and reserpine on pituitary-thyroid activity in rats. *J. Pharmacol.,* 150:129.

41. Ghadially, F. N. (editor) (1975): *Ultrastructural Pathology of the Cell,* pp. 1–84. Butterworths, Boston.

42. Ghetti, B., Wisniewski, H. M., Cook, R. D., and Schaumburg, H. (1973): Changes in the CNS

after acute and chronic acrylamide intoxication. *Am. J. Pathol.,* 70:78a.

43. Ginsburg, M., and Cox, B. M. (1972): Proteins and nucleic acids. In: *Chemical and Biological Aspects of Drug Dependence,* edited by S. J. Mulé and H. Brill, p. 465. CRC Press, Cleveland.

44. Glees, P., and Hasan, M. (1968): The signs of synaptic degeneration—a critical appraisal. *Acta Anat. (Basel),* 69:153–167.

45. Gonatas, N. K., and Goldensohn, E. S. (1965): Unusual neocortical presynaptic terminals in a patient with convulsions, mental retardation and cortical blindness: An electron microscopic study. *J. Neuropathol. Exp. Neurol.,* 24:539–562.

46. Gonatas, N. K., Evengelista, I., and Walsh, G. O. (1967): Axonic and synaptic changes in a case of psychomotor retardation. *J. Neuropathol. Exp. Neurol.,* 26:179–199.

47. Gonatas, N. K., Anderson, W., and Evengelista, I. (1967): The contribution of altered synapses in the senile plaque: An electron microscopic study in Alzheimer's dementia. *J. Neuropathol. Exp. Neurol.,* 26:25–39.

48. Gueft, B., and Ghidosi, J. J. (1963): The site of formation and ultrastructure of amyloid. *Am. J. Pathol.,* 43:837–854.

49. Gunne, L. M., Jonsson, J., and Fuxe, K. (1969): Effects of morphine intoxication on brain catecholamine neurons. *Eur. J. Pharmacol.,* 5:338–342.

50a. Harriman, D. G. F., Millar, J. H. D., and Stevenson, A. C. (1955): Progressive familial myoclonic epilepsy in three families: Its clinical features and pathological basis. *Brain,* 78:325–349.

50b. Hedley-White, E. T., Gilles, F. H., and Uzman, B. J. (1968): Infantile neuroaxonal dystrophy. A disease characterized by altered terminal axons and synaptic endings. *Neurology, (Minneap.),* 18:891–906.

51a. Heefner, W. A., and Sorenson, G. D. (1962): Experimental amyloidosis. I. Light and electron microscopic observations of spleen and lymph nodes. *Lab. Invest.,* 11:585–593.

51b. Herndon, R. M. (1964): Lamellar bodies, an unusual arrangement of granular endoplasmic reticulum. *J. Cell Biol.,* 20:338–342.

52. Hirano, A., and Dembitzer, H. M. (1976): The fine structure of astrocytes in the adult staggerer. *J. Neuropathol. Exp. Neurol.,* 35:63–74.

53. Ho, I. K., Lu, S. E., Stolman, S., Loh, H. H., and Way, E. L. (1972): Influence of p-chlorphenylalanine on morphine tolerance and physical dependence and regional brain serotonin turnover studies in morphine tolerant-dependent mice. *J. Pharmacol. Exp. Ther.,* 182:155–165.

54. Holtzman, E., and Novikoff, A. B. (1965): Lysosomes in the rat sciatic nerve following crush. *J. Cell Biol.,* 27:651–669.

55. Horning, E. S. (1934): Cytopathological studies of morphine poisoning and chronic morphinism in the albino rat with reference to subsequent lecithin treatment. *Am. J. Pathol.,* 10:219–252 (Citation p. 225).

56. Hwang, K. M., Yang, L. C., Carrico, C. K., Schulz, R. A., Schenkman, J. B., and Sartorelli, A. C. (1974): Production of membrane whorls in rat liver by some inhibitors of protein synthesis. *J. Cell Biol.,* 62:20–31.

57. Iversen, L. L. (1971): Role of transmittent uptake mechanisms in synaptic neurotransmission. *Br. J. Pharmacol.,* 41:571–591.

58. Janigan, D. T., and Duret, R. L. (1966): Experimental amyloidosis, role of antigenicity and rapid induction. *Am. J. Pathol.,* 48:1013–1026.

59. King, J. C., and Gerall, A. A. (1976): Localization of luteinizing hormone-releasing hormone. *J. Histochem. Cytochem.,* 24:829–845.

60. Kornetsky, C., and Bain, G. (1968): Morphine: Single-dose tolerance. *Science,* 162:1011–1012.

61. Krigman, M. R., Feldman, R. G., and Bensch, K. (1965): Alzheimer's presenile dementia. A histochemical and electron microscopic study. *Lab. Invest.,* 14:381–396.

62. LeBeux, Y. J. (1972): Subsurface cisterns and lamellar bodies: Particular forms of endoplasmic reticulum in the neurons. *Z. Zellforsch.,* 133:327–352.

63. Lieberman, A. R. (1971): The axon reaction: A review of principle features of perikaryal responses to axon injury. *Int. Rev. Neurobiol.,* 14:49–124.

64. Lloyd, O. L. (1973): Effects of diamorphine on various neurons in the rat central nervous system. *Nature [New Biol.],* 243:153–155.

65. Loh, H. H., Shen, F., and Way, E. L. (1969): Inhibition of morphine tolerance and physical dependence development and brain serotonin synthesis by cycloheximide. *Biochem. Pharmacol.,* 18:2711–2721.

66. Lund, R. D. (1972): Synaptic patterns in the superficial layers of the superior colliculus of the monkey Macaca Mulatta. *Exp. Brain Res.,* 15:194–211.

67. Ma, W. C. (1931): A cytopathological study of acute and chronic morphinism in albino rat. *Chin. J. Physiol.,* 5:251–278.

68. Martin, W. R., and Fraser, H. F. (1961): A comparative study of physiological and subjective effects of heroin and morphine administered intravenously in postaddicts. *J. Pharmacol. Exp. Ther.,* 133:388–399.

69. Martin, W. R. (1967): Opioid antagonists. *Pharmacol. Rev.,* 19:463–521 (Citation p. 509).

70. Maynert, E. W., and Klingman, G. I. (1962): Tolerance to morphine. I. Effects on catecholamines in the brain and adrenal glands. *J. Pharmacol. Exp. Ther.,* 135:285–295.

71. Millonig, G. (1961): Advantages of a phosphate buffer for OsO₄ solution in fixation. *J. Appl. Physiol.,* 32:1637.

72. Millonig, G., and Porter, K. R. (1960): Structural elements of rat liver cells involved in gly-

cogen storage. *Proc. Eur. Conf. Electron Microscopy Delft.*, 11:655–659.

73. Moussa, T. A., and El-Beih, Z. M. (1972): Effects of morphine on the Golgi apparatus and mitochondria of mammalian neurons. *La Cellule*, 60:191–203.

74. Mugnaini, E. (1964): Filamentous inclusion in the matrix of mitochondria from human livers. *J. Ultrastruct. Res.*, 11:525–544.

75. Mulé, S. J. (1967): Morphine and the incorporation of P^{32} into brain phospholipids of nontolerant, tolerant and abstinent guinea pigs. *J. Pharmacol. Exp. Ther.*, 156:92–100.

76. Mulé, S. J. (1971): Phospholipid metabolism. In: *Narcotic Drugs: Biochemical Pharmacology*, edited by D. H. Clouet, pp. 190–215. Plenum Press, New York.

77. Novikoff, A. B., and Essner, E. (1960): The liver cell. Some new approaches to its study. *Am. J. Med.*, 29:102–131.

78. Novikoff, A. B., Essner, E., and Quintana, N. (1964): Golgi apparatus and lysosomes. *Fed. Proc.*, 23:1010–1022.

79. Novikoff, A. B. (1967): Lysosomes in nervous cells. In: *The Neuron*, edited by H. Hyden, pp. 319–377. Elsevier, Amsterdam.

80. Oldendorf, W. H., Syman, S., Braun, L., and Oldendorf, S. Z. (1972): Blood-brain-barrier: Penetration of morphine, codeine, heroin and methadone after carotid injection. *Science*, 178: 984–986.

81. Palade, G. E., and Siekevitz, P. (1955): A correlated structural and chemical analysis of microsomes. *Anat. Rec.*, 121:347–348.

82. Pappas, G. D., and Purpura, D. P. (1972): *Structure and Function of Synapses*. Raven Press, New York.

83. Pappas, G. D., and Waxman, S. G. (1972): Synaptic fine structure-morphological correlates of the chemical and electronic transmission. In: *Structure and Function of Synapses*, edited by G. D. Pappas, and D. F. Purpura, p. 1. Raven Press, New York.

84. Pearson, J., Baden, M. B., and Richter, R. W. (1975/76): Neuronal depletion in the globus pallidus of heroin addicts. *Drug Alc. Dpend.*, 1:349–356.

85. Pearson, J., Hiller, J., and Simon, E. (1975): Anatomic localization of narcotic analgesic binding in the brain. *J. Neuropathol. Exp. Neurol.*, 34:101.

86. Pease, A. G. E. (editor) (1968): *Histochemistry: Theoretical and Applied*, 3rd ed., Vol. 1, p. 382. Little Brown, Boston (Citation p. 382).

87. Pert, C. B., and Snyder, S. H. (1973): Opiate receptor: Demonstration in nervous tissue. *Science*, 179:1011–1014.

88. Porter, K. R. (1961): The ground substance: Observations from electron microscopy. In: *The Cell*, Vol. II, edited by J. Brachet and A. E. Mirsky, pp. 621–675. Academic Press, New York/London.

89. Ramsey, H. J. (1965): Ultrastructure of corpora amylacea. *J. Neuropathol. Exp. Neurol.*, 24:25–39.

90. Richter, G. W. (1954): The resorption of amyloid under experimental conditions. *Am. J. Pathol.*, 30:239–262.

91. Richter, R. W., and Rosenberg, R. N. (1968): Transverse myelitis with heroin addiction. *JAMA*, 206:1255–1257.

92. Richter, R. W., Pearson, J., Bruun, B., Challenor, Y. B., Brust, J. C. M., and Baden, M. M. (1973): Neurological complications of addiction to heroin. *Bull. NY Acad. Med.*, 49:3–21.

93. Rigdon, R. H. (1960): Amyloidosis–experimental production in ducks with methylcholanthrene. *Tex. Rep. Biol. Med.*, 18:93–102.

94. Rizzuto, N., and Gonatas, N. K. (1974): Ultrastructural study of effect of methionine sulfoximine on developing and adult rat cerebral cortex. *J. Neuropathol. Exp. Neurol.*, 3?:237–250.

95. Roizin, L., Kaufman, M. A., Wharton, R., Housepian, E., Keosian, S., and Liu, J. C. (1967): Synaptic changes in Pick's disease (correlated histochemical and electron microscope studies). *2nd Pan Am. Congr. Neurol.*, edited by P. Bailey and R. E. Fiol, p. 499. Impreso por los Talleres de Artes Graficas del Departamento de Instruccion Publica, San Juan, P. R.

96. Roizin, L., Akai, K., Lawler, H. C., and Liu, J. C. (1970): Lithium neurotoxicologic effects. 1. Acute phase (preliminary observations). *Dis. Nerv. Syst.*, 31: (*Suppl.*):38–44.

97. Roizin, L., Helpern, M. M., Baden, M., Kaufman, M. A., Hashimoto, S., Liu, J. C., and Eisenberg, B. (1972): Neuropathology of drug dependence. In: *Chemical and Biological Aspects of Drug Dependence*, edited by S. J. Mulé and H. Brill, p. 389. CRC Press, Cleveland.

98. Roizin, L., Liu, J. C., Hashimoto, S., and Avrin, S. (1972): Methadone effects on central nervous system Golgi complex. *Fed. Proc.*, 31:665A.

99. Roizin, L., Liu, J. C., and Akai, K. (1975): Electron microscopy of basal ganglia in chronic prochlorperazine administration. *Fed. Proc.*, 34:849.

100. Roizin, L., Kaufman, M. A., Willson, N., Stellar, S., and Liu, J. C. (1976): Neuropathologic observation in Huntington's chorea. In: *Progress in Neuropathology*, Vol. III, edited by H. M. Zimmerman, pp. 447–488. Grune & Stratton, New York.

101. Roizin, L. (1977): Chemogenic lesion. In: *Neurotoxicology*, edited by L. Roizin, H. Shiraki, and N. Grčević. (*This volume.*)

102. Rothbard, S., and Watson, R. F. (1954): Amyloidosis and renal lesion induced in mice by injection with Freund-type of adjuvant. *Proc. Soc. Exp. Biol. Med.*, 85:133–137.

103. Samorajski, T., Ordy, J. R., and Keefe, J. R. (1965): The fine structure of lipofuscin age pigment in the nervous system of aged mice. *J. Cell Biol.*, 26:779–795.

104. Sharkawi, J., and Schulman, M. P. (1969): Inhibition by morphine of the release of ^{14}C-acetylcholine from rat brain cortex slices. *J. Pharm. Pharmacol.*, 21:546–547.

105. Shen, F. H., Loh, H. H., and Way, E. L. (1970): Brain serotonin turnover in morphine tolerance and dependent mice. *J. Pharmacol. Exp. Ther.*, 175:427–434.

106. Shinozuka, H., Goldblast, P. J., and Farber, E. F. (1968): The disorganization of hepatic cell nucleoli induced by ethionine and its reversal by adenine. *J. Cell Biol.*, 36:313–328.

107. Shinozuka, H., Reid, I. M., Shull, K. H., Liang, H., and Farber, E. (1970): Dynamics of liver cell injury and repair. Spontaneous reformation of the nucleolus and polyribosomes in the presence of extensive cytoplasmic damage induced by ethionine. *Lab. Invest.*, 23:253–267.

108. Simard, R. (1966): Specific nuclear and nucleolar ultrastructural lesions induced by proflavin and similarly acting antimetabolites in tissue culture. *Cancer Res.*, 26:2316–2328.

109. Simon, E. J. (1972): Lipids. In: *Chemical and Biological Aspects of Drug Dependence*, edited by S. J. Mulé and H. Brill, p. 505. CRC Press, Cleveland.

110. Smith, A. A., Karmin, M., and Gavitt, J. (1967): Tolerance to the lenticular effects of opiates. *J. Pharmacol. Exp. Ther.*, 156:85–91.

111. Smith, C. B., Villarreal, J. E., Bednarczyk, J. H., and Sheldon, M. I. (1970): Tolerance to morphine-induced increases in (^{14}C) catecholamine synthesis in mouse brain. *Science*, 170:1106.

112. Smith, C. B. (1972): Neurotransmitters and narcotic analgesics. In: *Chemical and Biological Aspects of Drug Dependence*, edited by S. J. Mulé and H. Brill, p. 495. CRC Press, Cleveland.

113. Sotelo, C., and Palay, S. L. (1971): Altered axons and axon terminals in the lateral vestibular of rat. *Lab. Invest.*, 25:653–671.

114. Spoerlein, M. Y., and Scrafini, J. (1967): Effects of time and 8-azaguanine on the development of morphine tolerance. *Life Sci.*, 6:1549–1564.

115. Steiner, J. W., Miyai, K., and Philips, M. J. (1964): Electron microscopy of membrane-particle arrays in liver cells of ethionine-intoxicated rats. *Am. J. Pathol.*, 44:169–214.

116. Stimmel, B. (1975): Getting off and coming down. In: *Heroin Dependency*, edited by B. Stimmel, p. 99. Stratton Int., New York.

117. Sulkin, N. M., and Sulkin, D. (1962): Mitochondria alterations in liver cells following vitamin E deficiency. In: *5th Int. Congr. Electron Microscopy*, Vol. 2, pp. 228–229. Academic Press, New York.

118. Svoboda, D. J., and Higginson, J. (1963): Ultrastructural hepatic changes in rats on a necrogenic diet. *Am. J. Pathol.*, 43:477–496.

119. Tandler, B., and Shipkey, F. H. (1964): Ultrastructure of Warthkin's tumor. II. Crystalloids. *J. Ultrastruct. Res.*, 11:306–314.

120. Tellez-Nagel, I., Johnson, A. B., and Terry, R. D. (1974): Studies on brain biopsies of patients with Huntington's chorea. *J. Neuropathol. Exp. Neurol.*, 33:308–332.

121. Tenen, S. S. (1968): Antagonism of analgesic effect of morphine and other drugs by p-chlorophenylalanine, a serotonin depletor. *Psycopharmacologia*, 12:278–285.

122. Terry, R. D., Gonatas, N. K., and Weiss, M. (1964): Ultrastructural studies in Alzheimer's presenile dementia. *Am. J. Pathol.*, 44:269–298.

123. Thomas, P. K. (1974): Nerve injury. In: *Essays on the Nervous System*, edited by R. Bellairs, and E. G. Gray, pp. 44–70. Clarendon Press, Oxford.

124. United Nations Department of Social Affairs (1953): History of heroin. *Bull. Narcot.*, 5:3–16.

125. Vaelz, H. (1968): Structural comparison between intramitochondrial and bacterial crystalloids. *J. Ultrastruct. Res.*, 25:29–36.

126. Vaughan, D. W. (1976): Membranous bodies in the cerebral cortex of aging rats: An electron microscope study. *J. Neuropathol. Exp. Neurol.*, 35:152–166.

127. Walberg, F. (1965): An electron microscopic study of terminal degeneration in the inferior olive of the cat. *J. Comp. Neurol.*, 125:205–222.

128. Walsh, F. O'F. (1972): Carbohydrates. In: *Chemical and Biological Aspects of Drug Dependence*, edited by S. J. Mulé and H. Brill, p. 477. CRC Press, Cleveland.

129. Watrach, A. M. (1964): Degeneration of mitochondria in lead poisoning. *J. Ultrastruct. Res.*, 10:177–181.

130. Way, E. L., Kemp, J. W., Young, J. M., and Grassetti, D. R. (1960): The pharmacologic effects of heroin in relationship to its rate of biotransformation. *J. Pharmacol. Exp. Ther.*, 129:144–151.

131. Way, E. L., Young, J. M., and Kemp, J. W. (1965): Metabolism of heroin and its pharmacologic implications. *Bull. Narc.*, 17:25–33.

132. Way, E. L., Loh, H. H., and Shen, F. H. (1968): Morphine tolerance, physical dependence, and synthesis of brain 5-hydroxytryptamine. *Science*, 162:1290–1292.

133. Webster, H. de F. (1962): Transient focal accumulation of axonal mitochondria during the early stages of Wallerian degeneration. *J. Cell Biol.*, 12:361–383.

134. Wilson, J. W., and Leduc, E. H. (1963): Mitochondrial changes in the liver of essential fatty acid-deficient mice. *J. Cell Biol.*, 16:281–296.

135a. Wisniewski, H., Johnson, A. B., Raine, C. S., Kay, W. J., and Terry, R. D. (1970): Senile plaques and cerebral amyloidosis in aged dogs: A histochemical and ultrastructural study. *Lab. Invest.*, 23:287–296.

135b. Wisniewski, H. M., Coblentz, J. M., and Terry, R. D. (1972): Pick's disease, a clinical and ultrastructural study. *Arch. Neurol.*, 26:97–108.

135c. Wisniewski, H. M., and Terry, R. D. (1973): Morphology of the aging brain, human and animal. *Prog. Brain Res.*, 40:167–186.

136. Wright, C. R. A. (1874): On the action of organic acids and their anhydrides on the nature alkaloids. *J. Chem. Soc. (London)*, 27:1031–1043.

137. Wright, C. I. (1942): The deacetylation of heroin and related compounds by mammalian tissues. *J. Pharmacol. Exp. Ther.*, 75:328–337.

138. Yu, M. C., Bakey, L., and Lee, J. C. (1973): Effects of hypoxia and hypercapanic hypoxia on the ultrastructure of central nervous system. *Exp. Neurol.*, 40:114–125.

Neurotoxicology, edited by L. Roizin, H. Shiraki, and N. Grčević. Raven Press, New York © 1977.

Review of Effects of Chronic Exposure to Low Levels of Halothane

†Alden W. Dudley, Jr., ††Louis W. Chang, †Mary A. Dudley, *Robert E. Bowman, and **Jordan Katz

*Departments of Pathology, *Psychology, and **Anesthesiology, University of Wisconsin, Madison, Wisconsin 53706*

The stated purpose of this volume is to collate and interpret data from the entire spectrum of science. This chapter reviews the results within our laboratories of both acute and chronic exposure to high and low concentrations of inhaled halothane. The studies performed include learning experiments, biochemical assays, and both light and electron microscopy of the liver and kidney as well as brain. We attempt to show that prolonged exposure to trace levels of the anesthetic gas commonly occurring in operating suites has the potential of injuring all operating room personnel at least slightly and unborn children greatly.

Halothane was introduced for clinical use in 1956. Because it is nonexplosive, nonflammable, and less nauseating, it quickly gained worldwide popularity and displaced ether as the anesthetic of choice. Its chemical structure (1,1,1-trifluoro-2,2-chlorobromoethane) resembles carbon tetrachloride, so that it was not difficult to relate cases of idiopathic hepatitis to halothane intoxication if it occurred postoperatively. An increasing frequency of such allegations prompted the *National Halothane Study* published in 1969 (17). The incidence of hepatitis following surgery with a variety of anesthetics was sufficiently low as to prohibit statistical significance. The absence of an animal model lent further credence to halothane supporters, and two groups of philosophy evolved.

Anesthesiologists became concerned about the possibility that trace or contamination levels induce disease after prolonged exposure (14). A survey of the causes of death in anesthetists from 1947 to 1956 and from 1957 to 1966 showed an increasing incidence of chronic renal disease, lymphomas, and liver disease (1,15). The early 1970s were characterized by sporadic reports of liver disease, spontaneous abortion, severe headaches, and personality changes in anesthetists. Hepatitis was successfully induced in both rats and guinea pigs (13). Finally, evaluation for subliminal signs of tissue injury during halothane anesthesia revealed moderate but definite and repeatable elevation of liver function tests in man (19).

Once the question of hepatitis was settled, the next concern was whether the fivefold increase in spontaneous abortion in anesthetists presaged the induction of congenital malformations or of mental retardation in the offspring of operating room nurses, women surgeons, anesthetists, or anesthesiologists (8). Prospective studies of first-year residents in anesthesiology showed progressive loss of motivation,

---

† Present address: Department of Pathology, University of South Alabama, Mobile, Alabama 36688; †† National Center for Toxicologic Research, Jefferson, Arkansas 72709.

respect for authority, and other features not uncommon for residents. However, there also was suggested the occurrence of measurable organic brain degeneration.

The anesthetizing level of halothane is 1.25% of the inspired air or 12,500 ppm. Leaks around the face mask and permeation of the rubber tubing create levels of 100 ppm (10 to 500 ppm) in the working area of the anesthetist and of 10 ppm (1 to 85 ppm) throughout the surgical suite. The spouse readily detects halothane in the expired air of an anesthetist returning home 4 hr after a shower and change of clothes following the administration of anesthetics. The scrub nurse at the foot of the operating table still has measurable levels of halothane on forced expiration when returning to work after a 2-day leave (9).

The purpose of this project has been to identify the minimal exposure necessary to cause injury and the mechanism responsible. Part of the study relates to the major organs of detoxification: the liver and the kidney. Secondary effects of injury to these organ systems could contribute to or even be the sole cause of lesions of the nervous system. Yet to be performed are studies with metabolites. For example, the release of bromine to form a radical could lead to bromism as well as provide a radical that could bind to essential molecules to become toxic itself.

METHODS

Acute experiments were conducted at 12,500 ppm for 2 hr on nonpregnant and pregnant adult Sprague-Dawley rats. The pregnant rats had timed pregnancies so that the fetal age of the exposed pups would be known. Chronic studies involved exposure for 8 hr per day, 5 days a week to trace levels of halothane at 10 ppm and 500 ppm.

In experiment A, pregnant rats were divided into eight groups, half exposed to 10 ppm and the other half to 500 ppm as follows: UU = control, conception through age 330 days; UD = exposed after weaning at age 60 days; DU = exposed during pregnancy and weaning only; DD = exposed throughout 50-week experiment.

Twelve naive pups age 135 days from each group were tested for shock avoidance in a Y-shaped maze where a 10-sec margin after a buzz permitted the pup to move to the lighted arm to avoid a shock. Success was 90% correct responses in a 30-trial session given every other day. A second test involved 10 naive pups from each group seeking to run a maze for food reward. Four of 5 consecutive responses during a 48-trial session met the criterion. All animals were sacrificed at 330 days.

In experiment B, several F_1 pups were permitted to mature and breed. Their progeny, F_2, were encouraged to produce F_3. Records of viability, resorption, and malformations were maintained on both exposed and control animals.

For experiment C, the effect and critical period for toxic results of acute exposure to narcotizing levels at 12,500 ppm were tested with 2 hr of anesthesia at days 3, 10, and 17 of pregnancy (normal gestation 20 days). Some pups were sacrificed at birth; others were weaned at age 30 days, tested beginning at 100 days, and terminated at varying intervals up to 200 days.

Animals were sacrificed according to the intended use of their tissues. A portion of each group was sacrificed with a guillotine and the brain and liver rapidly removed for biochemical studies. The organs were rapidly chilled, sliced, and frozen for enzyme histochemistry or minced in a cold room and processed for biochemical assays. The biochemical assays were for DNA, RNA, protein, glucose-6-phosphatase, N-demethylase, nitroreductase, and aniline hydroxylase.

Most animals were narcotized with phenobarbital and rapidly perfused by intracardiac injection of 15% body weight of saline and then 15% body weight of formalin for light microscopy or Karnovsky's fixative for electron microscopy (EM). Stains for light microscopy included hematoxylin and eosin (H&E), Luxol Fast Blue–H&E, period acid-Schiff, trichrome, Oil Red O, or modified silver stains, and enzyme histochemistry of reduced nicotinamide adenine dinucleotide (NADH), succinic dehydrogenase, adenosine triphosphatase, and phosphorylase.

RESULTS

In experiment A, there were two levels of educability. Pups exposed after weaning (UD) performed the shock-avoidance test on a par with the controls, whereas both groups treated during pregnancy (DU, DD) revealed a statistically significant 30% increase in error trials before reaching the criterion (Fig. 1). The food-maze test repeated the group distribution with a 32% learning deficit in those animals exposed during pregnancy and weaning. Learning deficits persisted unchanged at least 100 days after exposure (18).

Complete autopsies yielded few alterations on routine H&E preparations. Particular attention was paid the central nervous system (CNS), liver, and kidney. Because of the antecedent history of halothane hepatitis, it was anticipated that minor changes might be detected in the liver but that the kidney and brain would not be affected by such low concentrations, especially in rats with a 270-day recovery period.

However, the kidneys were found to have the lumen of the proximal convoluted tubules (PCT) occupied totally or in part by cellular debris derived from sloughed epithelial cells. There was essentially no leukocytic response. The tubular epithelium contained lipid droplets but otherwise appeared to be continuous without obvious defects created by the sloughing of cells. All treated animals

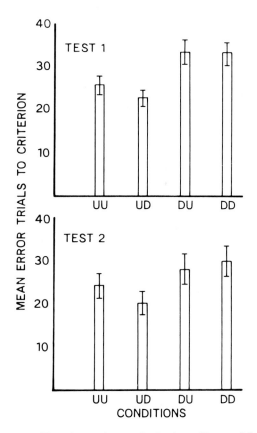

FIG. 1. Experiment A, test 1: shock avoidance trials revealing greater numbers of errors by pups exposed during pregnancy and weaning. Experiment A, test 2: maze mastery trials confirming a greater number of errors by pups exposed during pregnancy and weaning.

showed this response. A silver stain devised in our laboratory for detecting the presence of excessive aldehydes in degenerating cells showed a positive uptake by the PCT. The liver showed occasional lipid accumulation and leukocyte infiltration of hepatic cords at central sites that were positive by the silver stain.

The CNS showed no overt signs of degeneration on gross examination and no significant alteration by light microscopy. However, electron microscopy of the pups showed focal weakening and disruption of the nuclear envelope of cortical neurons. Vacuolation, myelin figure formation, and vesicular structures were seen

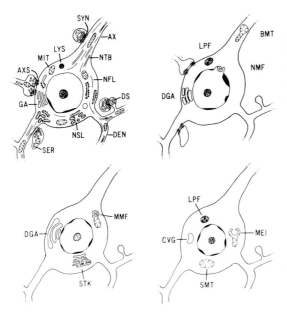

(RER). The lysosomes were increased in number and size. There was a C-shaped transformation and membranous degeneration of the mitochondria sometimes leading to myelin figure formation. Dilation of the Golgi complex and vacuole formation were common within cortical neurons. Intracellular edema in oligodendrocytes

FIG. 2. Drawing of normal neuron in upper left shows the nucleus (NUC), nucleolus (NCL), Golgi apparatus (GA), mitochondrion (MIT), and smooth endoplasmic reticulum (SER). The rough endoplasmic reticulum (RER) is referred to as Nissl substance (NS); lysomes (LYS), neurofilaments (NFL), and neurotubules (NTB) are added. Cell processes are the axon (AX), dendrite (DEN), and dendritic spine (DS). Synapses (SYN) can occur most anywhere including axosomatic (AXS) connections. Such connections show a discontinuous synaptic density, commonly present in up to 30% of synapses of control animals. Reactions to chronic exposure *in utero* are depicted in the upper right and include disrupted nuclear membranes forming myelin figures (NMF), lipofuscin (LPF), distended Golgi (DGA), drumstick or ballooned mitochondria (BMT), and a suggested increase in discontinuous synaptic densities. (Adapted from Chang et al., ref. 3.) Reactions seen in adults receiving 10 to 500 ppm halothane are depicted in the lower drawings. These reveal DGA, stacked RER, or stacked endoplasmic reticulum (STK), mitochondrial myelin figures (MMF), LPF, swollen mitochondria (SMT), mitochondrial endoplasmic inclusions (MEI), and swollen, curvilinear fragments of Golgi (CVG) or of SER. (Adapted from Chang et al., ref. 2.)

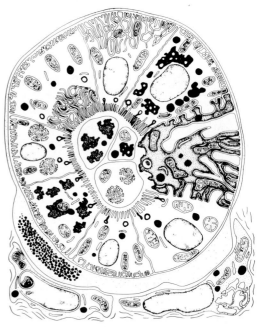

FIG. 3. Stylized drawing of PCT, normal epithelial cell at 6 o'clock. Proceeding clockwise we see irregular, dense, membranous bodies apparently formed by autophagy of mitochondria. At 9 o'clock is the proliferation of relatively large spheres of SER covered by RER. Such spheres are generally hyperplastic but hypoactive. The next epithelial cell shows infolding of the apical villi, and 12 o'clock has proliferation of the basal feet. The following cell has increased formation and coalescence of lysosomes with some having electron-lucid defects. The next cell is pyknotic and being extruded to the lumen by foot processes and lateral buds from neighboring cells. When assuming a void created by a sloughed cell, the new epithelial cell may not have basal feet. The basement membrane is normal over the top of the tubule but markedly thickened at the bottom and contains spheroid microparticles on the left. The interstitial cells show a defect in the nuclear membrane on the lower left and distended endoplasmic reticulum on the lower right. (Adapted from Chang et al., refs. 5 and 6, and Dudley et al., ref. 10.) (See Fig. 2 for abbreviations.)

in the cytoplasm of some neurons. Neuronal necrosis and glial edema were not infrequent. These changes persisted through adulthood. The mother rat with 12 weeks of exposure showed collapse of the neuronal rough endoplasmic reticulum

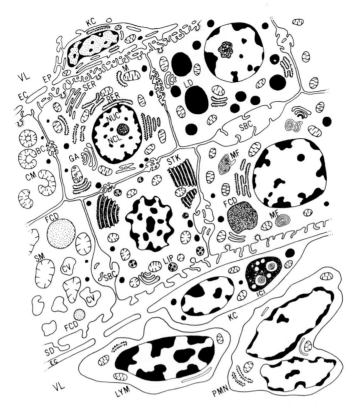

FIG. 4. Composite diagram of effects of low levels of halothane on a hepatic cord bounded on the upper left and lower margins by vascular channels (VL) and lined by Kupffer cells (KC) and endothelial cells (EC). The upper left KC and complete hepatocyte are normal with proliferation of villi into the sinusoidal space of Disset (SD) plus the formation of occasional pinocytotic vesicles. Normal organelles include the NUC with NCL, mitochondria (M), the GA, SER, RER, and bile canaliculi (BC) between hepatocytes. The small hepatocyte fragment to the left of the normal cell contains enlarged mitochondria that become C-shaped (CM) or, when cut appropriately, appear to be donut forms. The upper right has an accumulation of lipid deposits (LD). The lower right hepatocyte has a swollen nucleus, several myelin figures (MF), and a dense focal cytoplasmic degradation (FCD). It is bordered by swollen bile canaliculi (SBC). The lower middle cell has a crenated, dark nucleus, lipofuscin granules (LIP), condensed or STK, and reduced numbers of villi. The lower left hepatocyte shows extreme swelling of the mitochondria (SM), cytoplasmic vacuoles (CV) presumed to be from distended SER, pale FCD, and edematous villi. The lower right KC has an intracytoplasmic inclusion (ICI) of debris from dead hepatocytes and has lost its villi. The vessel lumen shows reacting polymorphonuclear leukocytes (PMN) and lymphocytes (LYM). (Adapted from Chang et al., refs. 4 and 7, and Dudley et al., ref. 11.) (See Fig. 2 for abbreviations.)

has been noted (2). A composite of these changes is provided by Fig. 2.

Electron microscopy of the kidney showed changes of almost every organelle in the PCT (Fig. 3). There was enlargement of the apical vacuoles, increase in number and density of lysosomes, disorientation and swelling of the mitochondria, formation of clusters of smooth endoplasmic reticulum (SER), elongation and curling of the apical villi, marked proliferation of plasma membrane increasing the basal infolding and lateral digitations, thickening of the basement membrane, and fracturing of the epithelial cells, of interstitial cells, and of collections of spheroid microparticles in the interstitial space. Focal areas of necrosis of epithelial cells led to sloughing of the pyknotic cell as a replacement epithelial cell took its place

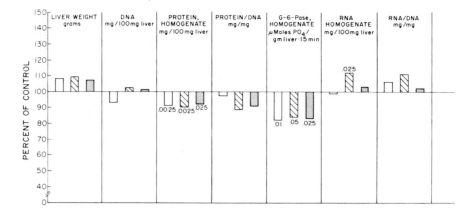

FIG. 5. Effects of chronic exposure to 10 ppm halothane on rat liver homogenates expressed as percentage of control with p value. □, 20 to 90 days; ▧, 20 to 330 days; ■, 90 to 330 days.

initially with minimal basal infolding (5,6, 10,11).

The ultrastructure of the liver showed: scalloped nuclear membranes an increase in mitochondrial matrical electron density, swelling, and C-shaped transformation; myelin figures; dilatation or condensation of RER; floccular precipitates around and between the stacked RER; vacuole formation; lysosomal accumulation within hepatocytes around dilated biliary canaliculi; loss of canalicular villi; extrusion of debris into the biliary system; occasional hepatocyte necrosis; and leukocyte infiltration (Fig. 4) (4,7,11).

Biochemical studies were initiated on the liver because of the clinical halothane hepatitis, rapid access to liver, and larger volume in small animals. The DNA and RNA levels were normal, but the homogenate and microsomal protein values were depressed in all groups (Figs. 5 and 6). All enzyme activity values were depressed, particularly in those rats exposed *in utero*, except for N-demethylase, which has a complete reversal with the greatest elevation ($p = 0.01$) in the animals exposed only through weaning (12) (Fig. 7).

Experiment B on teratology showed no mortality or detectable morbidity effects on the first two generations of rats bred under the influence of halothane. The F_3

generation did show fetal wastage without other external evidence of malformations (3).

Experiment C revealed that pups exposed to anesthetic levels of halothane during the third trimester had no appreciable difficulty in learning new tasks, whereas those treated on days 3 or 10 of pregnancy had fully twice as many errors as controls before mastering learning experiments (Fig.

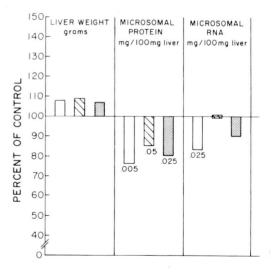

FIG. 6. Effects of chronic exposure to 10 ppm halothane on rat liver weight and microsomal protein and RNA content expressed as percentage of controls with p value. □, 20 to 90 days; ▧, 20 to 330 days; ■, 90 to 330 days.

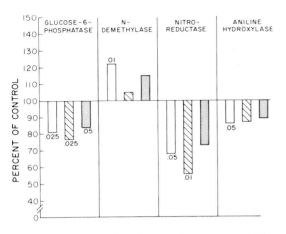

FIG. 7. Changes in microsomal enzyme activities (per mg microsomal protein) of 10 ppm-halothane rats as percentage of controls with p value. □, 20 to 90 days; ▨, 20 to 330 days; ■, 90 to 330 days.

8). DNA assays are being prepared to determine whether or not marked losses of neurons are occurring in rats exposed *in utero* during the early phase of pregnancy.

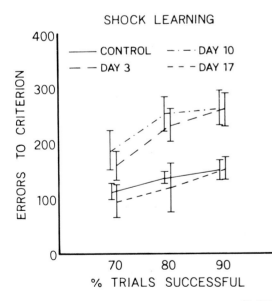

FIG. 8. Preliminary data on acute exposure to 12,500 ppm halothane for 2 hr during different trimesters of timed pregnancy. Shock learning is delayed markedly in groups exposed at fetal ages of 3 to 10 days. Control, ——; day 3, — —; day 10, —·—·; day 17, ----.

DISCUSSION

That halothane can be toxic to the nervous system in acute, high doses is obvious simply by the fact that it is an anesthetic. However, these effects have always been believed to be reversible. Evidence presented here suggests that the unborn may be subjected to permanent injury with learning disabilities if the mother is anesthetized with halothane.

Chronic exposure to trace amounts of halothane and nitrous oxide in the operating room ambient air has been shown recently to affect mentation and motor agility within 4 hr. Thus patient management by an intoxicated staff can be avoided only by replicating operating room personnel and rotating teams unless fastidious collection systems are developed to trap the contaminating gases. No evidence is available to suggest serious mental impairment of a permanent nature in adult humans. Our adult rats behaved similarly.

An unexpected finding in our study was the degree of learning disability and cellular reaction provoked and sustained in pups exposed *in utero* to trace levels of halothane alone for 40 hr per week. Although exposure was discontinued with weaning at age 60 days, alterations in cell morphology and biochemistry were easily demonstrated at age 330 days after a 9-month recovery period. Persistence in tissue of toxins such as mercury has long been accepted. Recent evidence suggests that polychlorinated biphenyls can be retained for long periods as well. However, halothane was considered to be a volatile anesthetic largely excreted through the lungs unchanged or through the kidneys as harmless metabolites.

Halothane is now believed to be broken down to a collection of metabolites including radicals (20) (Fig. 9). Most of the products, like halothane, are fat soluble. Proliferation of hypoactive SER by the kidney is a nonspecific mechanism of

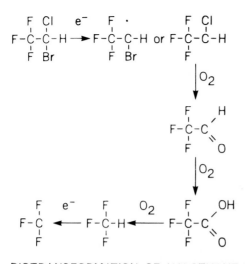

BIOTRANSFORMATION OF HALOTHANE

FIG. 9. Biodegradation of halothane by electron donors to form active halide ethane radicals. Oxidation to trifluoracetaldehyde and trifluoracetic acid permit the formation of a trifluormethane radical.

detoxification also seen in poisoning by methyl mercury, dieldrin, etc. One can easily imagine halothane binding the lipids in the SER or the proliferating cytoplasmic membrane. Interference in membrane function may explain the mitochondrial changes, stacking of the RER, and even fracturing of the nuclear envelope.

The depressed hepatic microsomal enzyme levels are believed to be a reflection of the impact of halothane or its metabolites, or both, on cell membranes. Selective enhancement of the demethylase system suggests that trifluormethane or a related radical may be one of the metabolic products. This conclusion is supported by work by Mansury et al. (16) showing that the effect of halothane on the cytochrome P450 system parallels exactly the effect of methane.

The uniquely high ratio of plasma membrane to nuclear size in neurons with their lengthy cell processes and intricate synapses may help to explain both the anesthetic action and toxicity of halothane to the CNS. However, localization of the

site of action on the neuron remains incomplete. It is evident that many organelles can be involved as reflected by the condensation of neuronal RER, dilatation of the Golgi complex with vacuole formation, proliferation of large lysosomes, swelling and C formation of mitochondria, myelin figure formation, and weakening of the nuclear envelope.

CONCLUSION

One fact is abundantly clear. There is a great likelihood that halothane has deleterious effects on the embryo and fetus. Extrapolation to man cannot be done casually nor would we encourage waiting for prospective studies. Retrospective, epidemiologic surveys can relate the exposure time of operating room personnel during pregnancy to the health of progeny adequately to determine the critical period of susceptibility as well as the likelihood of injury. Until such studies are conducted, personnel contemplating pregnancy should transfer to support roles elsewhere in the hospital at least 1 month before conception.

It is also evident that aggressive scavenging equipment should be installed in all operating rooms.

ACKNOWLEDGMENT

This work was supported by NIH grant GM 22685–01A1.

REFERENCES

1. Bruce, D. L., Eide, K. A., Linde, H. W., and Eckenhoff, J. E. (1968): Causes of death among anesthesiologists—20 year survey. *Anesthesiology,* 29:565–569.
2. Chang, L. W., Dudley, A. W., Jr., Lee, Y. K., and Katz, J. (1974): Ultrastructural changes in the nervous system after chronic exposure to low levels of halothane. *Exp. Neurol.,* 45:209–219.
3. Chang, L. W., Dudley, A. W., Jr., Martin, H. A., and Katz, J. (1974): Nervous system development following *in utero* exposure to trace amounts of halothane. *Teratology,* 9:(Abstr.)15.
4. Chang, L. W., Dudley, A. W., Jr., Lee, Y. K.,

and Katz, J. (1975): Ultrastructural changes of hepatocytes following chronic exposure to low levels of halothane. *Exp. Mol. Pathol.,* 23:35–43.

5. Chang, L. W., Dudley, A. W., Jr., Lee, Y. K., and Katz, J. (1975): Ultrastructural changes in the kidney following chronic exposure to low levels of halothane. *Am. J. Pathol.,* 78:225–242.

6. Chang, L. W., Dudley, A. W., Jr., Lee, Y. K., and Katz, J. (1975): Ultrastructural studies on the pathological changes in the neonatal kidney following *in utero* exposure to halothane. *Environ. Res.,* 10:174–189.

7. Chang, L. W., Lee, Y. K., Dudley, A. W., Jr., and Katz, J. (1975): Ultrastructural evidence of hepatotoxicity of halothane in rats following *in utero* exposure. *Can. Anaesth. Soc. J.,* 22: 330–338.

8. Corbett, T. H. (1972): Anesthetics as a cause of abortion. *Fertil. Steril.,* 23:866–869.

9. Corbett, T. H. (1973): Retention of anesthetic agent following occupational exposure. *Anesth. Analg.,* 52:614–618.

10. Dudley, A. W., Jr., Chang, L. W., and Katz, J. (1974): Ultrastructural changes in the kidney following chronic exposure to low levels of halothane. *Am. J. Pathol.,* 74:21a–22a.

11. Dudley, A. W., Jr., Chang, L. W., and Katz, J. (1974): Ultrastructural evidence of hepatic and renal changes in neonatal rats following *in utero* exposure to low levels of halothane. *Fed. Proc.,* 33:625.

12. Dudley, A. W., Jr., Allen, J. R., Chang, L. W., and Dudley, M. A. (1975): Effect of chronic low level exposure to halothane on hepatic micro-somal enzyme activity. *Am. J. Pathol.,* 78:142.

13. Hughes, H. C., and Lang, C. M. (1972): Hepatic necrosis produced by repeated administration of halothane to guinea pigs. *Anesthesiology,* 35: 466–471.

14. Jenkins, L. C. (1973): Chronic exposure to anesthetics — toxicity problem? *Can. Anaesth. Soc. J.,* 20:104–120.

15. Linde, H. W., and Bruce, D. L. (1968): Occupational exposure of anesthetists to halothane, nitrous oxide and radiation. *Anesthesiology,* 30:363–386.

16. Mansury, D., Nastainczyk, W., and Ullrich, V. (1974): The mechanism of halothane binding to microsomal cytochrome P450. *Arch. Pharmacol.,* 285:315–324.

17. Ngai, S. H. (1969): Hepatic effects of halothane — reviews of the literature. In: *National Halothane Study,* edited by J. P. Bunker, W. H. Forrest, F. Mosteller, and L. D. Vandam, pp. 11–18. NIH, NIGMS, Bethesda, Maryland.

18. Quimby, K. L., Aschkenase, L. J., Bowman, R. E., Katz, J., and Chang, L. W. (1974): Enduring learning deficits and cerebral synaptic malformation from exposure to 10 ppm halothane. *Science,* 185:625–627.

19. Thompson, D. R., and Greifenstein, F. E. (1975): Enzyme patterns reflecting hepatic response to anesthesia and operation. *South. Med. J.,* 67: 69–74.

20. Van Dyke, R. A. (1973): Biotransformation of volatile anesthetics with special emphasis on the role of metabolism in the toxicity of anesthetics. *Can. Anaesth. Soc. J.,* 20:21–33.

Neurotoxicology, edited by L. Roizin, H. Shiraki, and N. Grčević. Raven Press, New York © 1977.

Drug Interactions: Methylphenidate

Lester C. Mark, *James M. Perel, and Leonard Brand

*Departments of Anesthesiology and *Psychiatry, Columbia University; and the New York State Psychiatric Institute, New York, New York 10032*

INTERACTION 1: INHIBITION OF DRUG METABOLISM

The subject of drug interactions has aroused much interest in recent years. Most examples studied have involved acceleration of the biotransformation of one drug in the presence of another, with consequent shortening of action of the first drug. Although the opposite effect, inhibition of drug metabolism, seems less common, it may be clinically more significant.

Methylphenidate (Ritalin®) is a sympathomimetic agent with stimulant effects on the central nervous system. Its molecule possesses two asymmetric carbon atoms, hence can exist in four different stereoisometric configurations. Most potent is the 2R:2′R, (+) threo isomer reported by Maxwell et al. (5) to be approximately 400 times more potent than the 2R:2′S, (+) erythro isomer (the designations "threo" and "erythro" are derived from carbohydrate chemistry and refer to the spatial configurations of the sugars threose and erythrose, respectively). The remainder of this chapter is concerned solely with threo-methylphenidate, marketed as Ritalin® hydrochloride. Clinical uses of this preparation have included treatment of psychiatric depression, narcolepsy, hyperactivity in children, and even (formerly) barbiturate poisoning. Another property — the ability to inhibit the action of drug metabolizing enzymes in the liver — was recognized more recently by Garrettson et al. (1), who first demonstrated the phenomenon in a hyperkinetic child also receiving primidone, diphenylhydantoin, and phenobarbital. In this patient, diphenylhydantoin levels rose from therapeutic to toxic, resulting in ataxia. To study this apparent inhibition of drug metabolism, experiments were performed in four adult male volunteers receiving daily doses of the anticoagulant ethyl biscoumacetate. Methylphenidate administered for 3 to 5 days slowed the rate of disappearance of the anticoagulant from the blood stream, an effect which, in patients on anticoagulant therapy, could be disastrous. Methylphenidate-induced inhibition of drug metabolism was also demonstrated by Wharton et al. (7) in patients receiving imipramine, with concomitant therapeutic improvement.

INTERACTION 2: ALTERATION IN VOLUME OF DISTRIBUTION

Another type of interaction may result in marked change in apparent volume of distribution of a drug, with potentially significant clinical implications. Circulatory changes may be involved. For example, Levy (4) found the apparent volume of distribution of penicillin G significantly lower in adult human males when ambulatory than during bed rest. Gibaldi and

Schwartz (2) reported decreased volumes of distribution of various penicillins in man caused by probenecid administration. Since many psychoactive agents have large apparent volumes of distribution because of their considerable lipid solubility, a decrease in these values would presumably yield higher blood levels, making more drug available to highly perfused organs such as the brain. Perel et al. (6) observed such an interaction with the combination of thiopental and methylphenidate, previously advocated by Hoagland (3) to treat barbiturate depression. In three of four human volunteers pretreated with methylphenidate by mouth for 3 days who then received a sleep dose of thiopental intravenously, plasma thiopental concentrations during the early distribution phase were significantly higher than in previous control studies without methylphenidate. The values returned to control slopes within 45 to 180 min. In other studies, six mongrel dogs received thiopental, 25 mg/kg, intravenously, followed 35 to 75 min later by methylphenidate, 5 mg/kg, or an equivalent volume of saline. In all cases where methylphenidate was superimposed on thiopental, significant increases in thiopental plasma levels were observed within 10 min of methylphenidate administration; thiopental levels returned to the original slope within 20 to 40 min. The data suggest a reduction in apparent volume of distribution of thiopental produced by methylphenidate, resulting in higher blood levels of the barbiturate being presented to the brain and seemingly discrediting the rationale for the use of methylphenidate as a barbiturate antagonist.

SUMMARY

Methylphenidate has been demonstrated capable of exerting two different kinds of interaction with other drugs—one associated with chronic administration of methylphenidate, the other with acute dosage. Chronic administration can inhibit drug metabolizing enzymes in the liver, resulting in the accumulation to potentially toxic levels of other drugs (e.g., diphenylhydantoin, primidone) being prescribed simultaneously. Acute administration can result in seemingly more transient but nevertheless marked changes in apparent volume of distribution of another drug (e.g., a barbiturate). Both may present hazards to the patients of unwary physicians.

ACKNOWLEDGMENT

The work presented in this chapter has been supported in part by National Institutes of Health grants GM-09069 and MH-17044.

REFERENCES

1. Garrettson, L. K., Perel, J. M., and Dayton, P. G. (1969): Methylphenidate interaction with both anticonvulsants and ethyl biscoumacetate. *JAMA,* 207:2053–2056.
2. Gibaldi, M., and Schwartz, M. A. (1968): Apparent effect of probenecid on the distribution of penicillins in man. *Clin. Pharmacol. Ther.,* 9:345–349.
3. Hoagland, R. J. (1965): Pharmacologic treatment of coma of diverse origins. *Am. J. Med. Sci.,* 249: 623–635.
4. Levy, G. (1967): Effect of probenecid on blood levels and urinary recovery of ampicillin. *Am. J. Med. Sci.,* 250:174–176.
5. Maxwell, R. A., Chaplin, E., Eckhardt, S. B., Soares, J. R., and Hite, G. (1970): Conformational similarity between molecular models of phenylethylamine and of potent inhibitors of the uptake of tritiated norepinephrine by adrenergic nerves in rabbit aorta. *J. Pharmacol. Exp. Ther.,* 173:158–165.
6. Perel, J. M., Brand, L., Heiber, S., and Mark, L. C. (1972): Effect of methylphenidate on rate of disappearance of thiopental from plasma. *Clin. Res.,* 20:411.
7. Wharton, R. M., Perel, J. M., Dayton, P. G., and Malitz, S. (1971): Potential clinical use for methylphenidate with tricyclic antidepressants. *Am. J. Psychiatry,* 127:1619–1625.

Neurotoxicology, edited by L. Roizin, H. Shiraki, and N. Grčević. Raven Press, New York © 1977.

Cortical Atrophy Caused by Long-Term Therapy with Antidepressive and Neuroleptic Drugs: A Clinical and Experimental Study

*N. Sabuncu, *S. Salacin, R. Saygill, †K. Kumral, and ‡T. Örnek

*Departments of *Pathology, †Neurology, and ‡Psychiatry, Ege University Medical School, Bornova-Izmir, Turkey*

Reports on the neurotoxic effects of antidepressive and neuroleptic drugs are scarce. Greiner and Nicolson (5,6) detected pigment deposits in the viscera and neurons. Rifkin et al. (11) observed an organic brain syndrome after treatment with lithium carbonate, although the blood level did not exceed therapeutic levels. Lüllmann-Rauch (9) was able to produce lipidosis-like alterations after treatment with tricyclic antidepressants. There are reports on sudden death during the course of therapy with phenothiazine derivatives (3,7,8,10). It remains in the dark whether a nonspecific depression of autonomic regulation of circulation or medullary control of respiration is in question as has been suggested by Feldman (3) and Reinert and Hermann (10).

An incidental pneumoencephalography (PEG) brought to light a case of cortical atrophy after prolonged treatment with tricyclic antidepressants. There followed two more such observations. This fact caused us to perform a PEG in chronic schizophrenic patients. An experimental research project was added. The three observations are presented here, followed by the results of the serial examination and the experimental research.

CLINICAL OBSERVATIONS

Case 1

A fifty-year-old housewife born in 1920 was never seriously ill. In 1961 her menopause began. Menopausal complaints lasted until 1966. Then she became extremely frightened, suffered from insomnia, and developed depressive ideas. With all these complaints she was entered for treatment in our psychiatric clinic in that same year. The diagnosis was involutional depression. For 2 months she was under inpatient treatment in our clinic. Initially four electroconvulsive treatments (ECT) were applied. In addition to this she received 200 mg of imipramine (Tofranil®) and 75 mg of levomeprosamine (Nozinan®). After some improvement, she was released. Up to 1970 she was treated mainly with 100 to 200 mg of imipramine, 150 mg of amitriptyline (Laroxyl®), and 75 to 150 mg of levomeprosamine. Toward the end of 1970 the PEG showed cortical atrophy (Fig. 1).

Case 2

The second case is a 43-year-old businessman, born in 1928. In 1948,

149

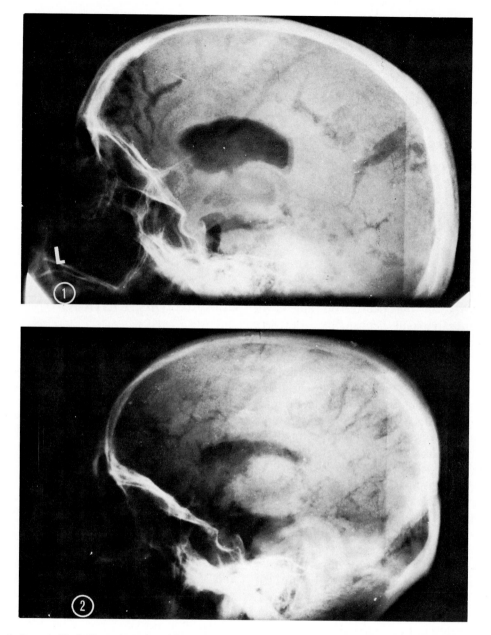

FIG. 1. *Case 1:* Skull X-ray, lateral position. Air collections localized especially at frontal and parieto-occipital regions.
FIG. 2. *Case 2:* Skull X-ray, lateral position. Minimal cortical atrophy.

according to his own statement, he had been treated with nine ECTs because of a psychotic reaction. He was free of complaints until 1965. At that time he suffered from tuberculosis of the lungs. In this case antitubercular drugs [isonicotinic acid hydrazide (INAH) and streptomycin] had been applied for a year and a half. In 1967 there followed outpatient treatment with 150 mg of amitriptyline, 150 mg of imipramine (alternately), and 200 mg of thioridazine (Mellaril®). At the end of 1971, in the PEG cortical atrophy was evident (Fig. 2).

Case 3

Our third observation was a manic depressive patient born in 1927. He was hospitalized in 1963 during his manic phase and was under treatment as an in- and outpatient until 1970. Once or twice a year he was for 2 to 3 months either manic or depressive. According to this he got 300 mg of chlorpromazine (Largactil®) during his manic phase and, alternately, 150 mg of imipramine or 150 mg of amitriptyline and 75 to 150 mg of levo-meprozamine. Once during his stay in the clinic, he received lithium acetate for 2 weeks. Thereafter, this treatment was discontinued since the patient was not able to present himself for blood examination. In this case also atrophy appeared on PEG (Fig. 3).

Schizophrenic Series

The cases of this series originate from the Psychiatric Hospital at Manisa. The series consisted of 20 males and 10 females 20 to 50 years of age who had been hospitalized for 5 to 20 years because of schizophrenia. They received chiefly 300 mg of chlorpromazine/day. In addition, 11 males underwent an ECT. A PEG was applied under the same conditions. (After lumbar puncture 45 to 50 cc of air was given fractionally. Thereafter the ventricular system subarachnoidal space was completely filled.)

Results

Out of 20 males nine presented atrophies. In six cases more or less distinct cortical atrophy was revealed (Fig. 4). In four cases this cortical atrophy was localized

at the parietooccipital region, and in two cases it was diffuse. The other three cases showed cerebral atrophy (Fig. 5). Out of 10 females two showed cerebral atrophy.

The distribution of the cases with or without atrophy according to age and duration of disease has been classified in Table 1. In the age group 20 to 30, none of three studied cases revealed atrophies. In the age group 30 to 40, three out of 12 cases and, in the age group from 40 to 50, eight out of 15 cases presented atrophies. The distribution according to the duration of disease is similar: in the group of 5 to 10 years duration three out of 12; in that of 10 to 15 years duration two out of eight, and in that of 15 to 20 years duration six out of 10 cases showed cerebral atrophy. None of these cases was pneumoencephalographically controlled before treatment. Six out of the nine males with atrophy had received a series of ECTs, and of the 11 without atrophy, five had ECTs. None of these cases has developed organic brain syndrome.

DISCUSSION

It is neither necessary nor customary to apply a PEG to depressive or schizophrenic patients. As the husband of our first case is a physician, he asked us to perform a PEG because he was thinking of organic damage. The result aroused our interest and led us to carry out all the other examinations. The results are conspicuous. More than a third of the cases show atrophy, minimal, yet present. It seems unlikely that there was atrophy before the beginning of the therapy. At first sight the correlation with age is striking, but it has to be considered that the patients are not very old. All of them are under 50 years of age, and in this period of age a purely age-bound atrophy is unthinkable, not to mention as high a rate of occurrence as one-third of the cases.

From Table 1 also another fact may be

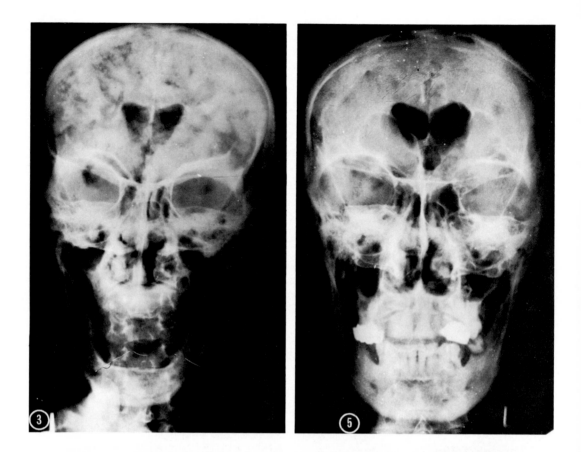

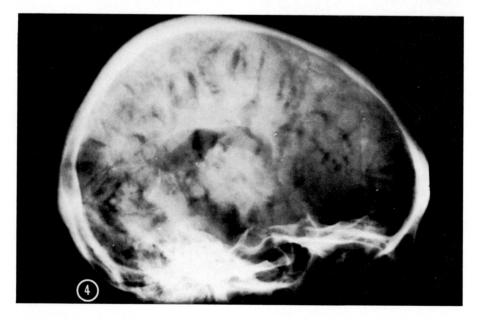

FIG. 3. *Case 3:* Skull X-ray, A-P view. Brow up position. Minimal cortical atrophy is seen.
FIG. 4. Skull X-ray, lateral position. Minimal cortical atrophy.
FIG. 5. Skull X-ray, A-P view. Brow up position. Cerebral atrophy predominantly on the left side.

TABLE 1. *Incidence of atrophy depending on age and duration of illness and/or therapy*

| | Years of illness and/or therapy | | | | | |
| | 5–10 | | 10–15 | | 15–20 | |
Age	N	A	N	A	N	A
20–30	3	–	–	–	–	–
30–40	3	3	4	–	2	–
40–50	3	–	2	2	2	6

N, normal; A, atrophy.

seen: the atrophy shows a correlation with the duration of treatment. Out of 11 cases with atrophy six had been treated for 15 to 20 years, and this group consists only of 10 patients. Therefore, in 60% of the cases of this group atrophy developed. This percentage diminishes in the groups with shorter duration of treatment, i.e., 20 and 25%. In this sense the correlation with age seems to be a natural coincidence. It is clear: the longer the treatment, the higher the age.

All patients are free from cardiovascular diseases, in particular they are not arteriosclerotic. Consequently circulatory factors are not responsible for the atrophy. Alzheimer's disease or another presenile disorder such as Jakob-Creutzfeld's disease have been excluded. None of the patients was demented. Besides these diseases do not show such a long course.

Six cases of atrophy received a series of ECTs. Whether the uncomplicated convulsive therapy might cause brain damage has been widely discussed. According to the review of Alpers (1), irreversible changes are unlikely. But mild changes may be observed after intensive treatment (2,4). Of our cases with atrophy nearly a half have not received convulsive treatment. Among the cases without atrophy there are five that have received convulsive therapy. So it seems impossible that this atrophy might have existed before the treatment. All these considerations suggest

rather a toxic effect of the drugs; at least this atrophy has been observed after prolonged therapy with the above-mentioned drugs. And the number of cases increases depending on the duration of disease or therapy, or both.

EXPERIMENTAL INVESTIGATIONS

Material and Method

Forty outbred male rats (1 year old) were divided into four groups. One group received 2.5 mg/kg of amitriptyline; the second, 2.5 mg/kg of imipramine; the third, 5 mg/kg of chlorpromazine; and the last got only saline solution. Half of each group was decapitated after 6 weeks and the rest after 12 weeks. After 24-hr fixation in 10% formalin, the brains were embedded in paraffin, and 5 μ-thick sections were cut. RNA and DNA were stained with gallocyanin-chromalum at pH 1.60. The same stain was performed after RNA extraction (10 min in 10% perchloric acid at 36°C) and DNA extraction (20 min in 10% perchloric acid at 70°C). The RNA and DNA amounts were estimated microspectrophotometrically (by means of MPV 2 of Leitz). The estimation was carried through at the level of chiasma in cortical motor neurons, i.e., first, without extraction, second, with RNA extraction, and third, with RNA and DNA extraction (20 cells in each section).

The values were computed and evaluated by the IBM Center of Ege University (Izmir). RNA values of each group and subgroup were compared. The same procedure was applied to the RNA:DNA ratio.

Results

The results are given in Tables 2 to 5. In Table 2 the distribution of RNA amounts within the groups is seen: after 6 weeks treatment with amitriptyline, the

TABLE 2. *RNA values (logarithmical)—temporal distribution*

Control	0.129 ± 0.017	0.108 ± 0.039
Amitriptyline	0.176 ± 0.051	0.139 ± 0.024
Imipramine	0.074 ± 0.036	0.057 ± 0.031
Chlorpromazine	0.102 ± 0.054	0.069 ± 0.014[a]

[a] $p < 0.01$.

TABLE 3. *RNA values (logarithmical)—groups in correlation with each other (12 weeks)*

		Little significant difference
Control	0.108 ± 0.039	
Amitriptyline	0.139 ± 0.024	1
Chlorpromazine	0.069 ± 0.014[a]	2
Imipramine	0.057 ± 0.031[a]	3

[a] $p < 0.01$.

TABLE 4. *RNA:DNA ratio—temporal distribution*

	6 Weeks	12 Weeks
Control	1.415 ± 0.308	1.353 ± 0.525
Amitriptyline	2.450 ± 0.748	2.326 ± 0.743
Imipramine	1.329 ± 0.592	0.099 ± 0.032[a]
Chlorpromazine	0.326 ± 0.129	0.220 ± 0.111[a]

[a] $p < 0.01$.

TABLE 5. *RNA:DNA ratio—groups in correlation with each other (12 weeks)*

		Little significant difference
Amitriptyline	2.326 ± 0.743[a]	1
Control	1.353 ± 0.525[a]	2
Chlorpromazine	0.220 ± 0.111[a]	3
Imipramine	0.099 ± 0.032[a]	4

[a] $p < 0.01$.

RNA amount increases. But this is temporary as after 12 weeks treatment this value approachs that of the control group, whereas the imipramine and chlorpromazine groups display a continuous decrease. This decrease seems to be more obvious with imipramine and occurs earlier. After 12 weeks treatment no significant difference can be detected between amitriptyline and the control group, whereas the values of the chlorpromazine and imipramine groups are significantly lower (Table 3).

The values of the RNA:DNA ratio represent a similar temporal distribution with some deviations (Table 4). After amitriptyline treatment, first an increase and then a decrease without significant difference may be detected. After imipramine and chlorpromazine the values fall continuously. After 12 weeks treatment all values diverge obviously (Table 5).

COMMENT

The conditions of staining, extraction, and measurement were the same in all groups. The measurements were carried through by the same person. Since the absorption of the color was measured, the possible difference in thickness of sections may be a source of mistake. The microtome was adjusted to 5μ, but the possibility still remains that the sections do not all possess the same thickness. However this factor may be ignored because an even proportion of the deviations should be expected in each group, therefore, we may assume that the values are reliable.

Consequently the RNA amount of the motor neurons has been reduced by treatment with imipramine and chlorpromazine. The RNA amount may be looked at as an indicator of the cell metabolism. Imipramine and chlorpromazine seem to inhibit this metabolism. And this evoked inhibition seems not to be temporary. It increases over time.

On the other hand, the RNA:DNA ratio may offer an indicator for the cell size. This is possible because RNA is mainly located in the cytoplasm, whereas DNA is found in a constant amount in the nucleus. The ratio between both of them therefore may be used as a measure of the cell size or cell atrophy, or both. These considerations are only valid in case there is no chromatolysis. The measured cells were free from this change. If this consideration should prove to be exact—and we are of the opinion that it is correct—then both of the drugs have influenced cell size in a negative way, i.e., they have caused atrophy of the neurons.

Can this result explain the atrophy observed in human beings? It is certainly very difficult to accept this. Two different species are in question. In addition, we have only examined one type of cell, but it supplies us with a positive hint.

SUMMARY AND CONCLUDING REMARKS

After prolonged treatment with tricyclic antidepressants, three patients under 50 years of age presented with cortical atrophy; two of them pure cortical and the last one cerebral. Out of 30 chronic schizophrenic patients, 11 showed atrophy after prolonged therapy with chlorpromazine. The criteria of selection of the patients were only age (under 50 years) and the duration of disease and treatment. All the other known causes of atrophy were excluded. Experimentally it could be proved that imipramine and chlorpromazine may influence cell metabolism and probably cell size in a negative way. Nevertheless it cannot be considered proved that the atrophy is a result of the treatment. On the other hand strong signs suggest this possibility. One should at least draw attention to this possibility.

REFERENCES

1. Alpers, B. J. (1946): The brain changes associated with electrical shock treatment: A critical review. *Digest Neurol. Psychiatr.*, 14:136–137.
2. Corsellis, J. A. N., and Meyer, A. (1954): Histological changes after uncomplicated ECT. *J. Ment. Sci.*, 100:375–383.
3. Feldman, P. E. (1957): Unusual death, associated with tranquilizer therapy. *Am. J. Psychiatry*, 113:1032–1033.
4. Ferraro, A., and Roizin, L. (1949): Cerebral morphologic changes in monkeys subjected to a large number of electrically induced convulsions (32–100). *Am. J. Psychiatry*, 106:278–284.
5. Greiner, A. C., and Nicolson, G. A. (1964): Pigment deposition in viscera associated with prolonged chlorpromazine therapy. *Can. Med. Assoc. J.*, 91:627–636.
6. Greiner, A. C., and Nicolson, G. A. (1965): New side effects in prolonged chlorpromazine therapy. *Can. Psychiatr. Assoc. J.*, 10:109–111.
7. Hollister, L. E. (1957): Unexpected asphyxial death and tranquilizing drugs. *Am. J. Psychiatry*, 114:366–367.
8. Hollister, L. E., and Kosek, J. C. (1965): Sudden death and phenothiazine derivatives. *JAMA*, 192:1035–1038.
9. Lüllmann-Rauch, R. (1974): Lipidosis-like alterations in spinal cord and cerebellar cortex of rats treated with chlorphentermine or tricyclic antidepressants. *Acta Neuropathol. (Berl.)*, 29: 237–249.
10. Reinert, R. E., and Hermann, C. G. (1960): Unexplained death during chlorpromazine therapy. *J. Nerv. Ment. Dis.*, 131:435–422.
11. Rifkin, A., Quitkin, F., and Klein D. F., (1973): Organic brain syndrome during lithium carbonate treatment. *Compr. Psychiatry*, 14:251–254.

Neurotoxicology, edited by L. Roizin, H. Shiraki,
and N. Grčević. Raven Press, New York © 1977.

Pharmacokinetics of Therapeutic and Toxic Reactions: II. Tricyclic Antidepressants

James M. Perel

Department of Psychiatry, Columbia University, College of Physicians and Surgeons; and the New York State Psychiatric Institute, New York, New York 10032

The pharmacokinetics of tricyclics, such as imipramine, are less complex than those of phenothiazines because there are fewer routes of metabolism. Following oral administration, imipramine is essentially entirely absorbed. Once in the body it is metabolized by hepatic microsomal enzymes, located in the smooth endoplasmic reticulum, via three major pathways—N-demethylation, N-oxidation, and aromatic hydroxylation (Fig. 1). These oxidations involve the participation of an electron transport chain and terminate in an oxygen transferring enzyme, cytochrome P-450. There are three principal metabolites of imipramine—desmethylimipramine, which is also an antidepressant, 2-hydroxyimipramine, and 2-hydroxydesmethylimipramine (7,18). Until recently, the 2-hydroxy metabolites were thought to be inactive, but recent data in our laboratories have shown otherwise (see below).

The N-demethylation occurs more rapidly than hydroxylation, so that repeated oral administration of imipramine at fixed intervals leads to accumulation of the drug and desmethylimipramine in the body. After some time, the drug plasma concentration reaches a constant plateau or "steady-state." The ratio of the desmethyl metabolite to parent compound in plasma was found to be 1:4. It appears that the hepatic metabolism of tricyclic antidepres-sants, such as nortriptyline, desipramine, and imipramine, are highly flow dependent, i.e., the major determinant of clearance is hepatic blood flow (8a,8b). "First pass" metabolism of tertiary tricyclic antidepressants (amitriptyline, imipramine) is mediated by N-demethylation to the active secondary metabolites which, in turn, are hydroxylated. Pathological conditions, such as cardiac disease, hepatitis, and cirrhosis, diminish the hepatic blood flow leading to slower drug metabolism and accumulation of parent compounds with subsequent toxicity (14).

Our studies (6,17) have demonstrated wide interindividual variations of as much as 12-fold, in steady-state plasma concentrations after oral administration of 3.5 mg/kg daily in three divided doses. The average plasma steady-state level for our entire sample (68 patients) was 200 ng/ml ± 137 ng/ml. Most of the observed interindividual variability is due to differences in rate of metabolism. An additional source of variability is the large volume of distribution that is a measure of extensive tissue localization (1,2,20). Twofold differences in this parameter are found to be directly related to the fraction of unbound antidepressant in plasma (19). Clinical outcome was shown to be unequivocally related to the plasma level; patients afflicted with endogenous depression (bipolar and unipolar nondelusional) have a higher rate

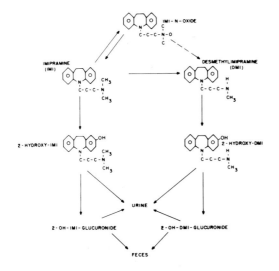

FIG. 1. Metabolic pathway of imipramine.

of response above the median plasma level of 180 ng/ml. An analysis of the relation of the plasma distribution to response indicates that with steady levels below 150, between 150 and 225, and above 225 ng/ml the respective percentage rates of recovery are 29, 64, and 93% (Fig. 2). Using a slightly different protocol, Gram and associates (9) have essentially confirmed these findings for imipramine, i.e., optimal antidepressant activity is obtained at plasma levels greater than 240 ng/ml.

Recently we have found that the 2-

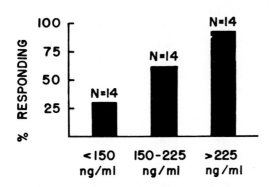

FIG. 2. Response rates for 42 patients with endogenous depression (nondelusional). The patients are divided into three equal groups by imipramine plasma level. Response rates are calculated independently for each group.

hydroxy metabolites are involved in some of the adverse cardiovascular effects observed after imipramine administration. Both 2-hydroxy imipramine and 2-hydroxy desmethylimipramine are found in myocardium and lung tissue with a binding affinity perhaps greater than for the parent drug. Cardiotoxicity studies in dogs at intravenous dosage ranges of 1 to 5 mg/kg for imipramine, desmethylimipramine, and 2-hydroxydesmethylimipramine and up to 2.5 mg/kg for 2-hydroxyimipramine show that all four compounds affect cardiac function. They significantly decrease cardiac output, left ventricular work, heart rate, and cardiac contractility while blood pressure is maintained due to a compensatory increase in peripheral vascular resistance (3,16). 2-hydroxyimipramine is exceedingly cardiotoxic and produces death in anesthetized dogs by cardiac arrest at doses above 2.5 mg/kg. Thus it appears that 2-hydroxyimipramine is the most potent and 2-hydroxy desmethylimipramine the least potent in their ability to affect cardiac function. Imipramine and desmethylimipramine were essentially similar. At present we are also studying, in patients, the effects of imipramine on conduction activity of the heart. We have found a direct relationship between plasma levels of antidepressant and conduction parameters — in 10 of 13 patients the increase in the lengthening of the QRS interval period is related to a concomitant increase in plasma level (5).

Pharmacokinetic studies have shown that imipramine persists in lungs (rabbit) for long periods of time. About 30% is in a form not readily effluxable from the lung. Analyses for the presence of unchanged imipramine and its metabolites indicate that efflux from lung exhibits two different modes of disappearance. The shorter half-life appears to be associated mainly with imipramine and its desmethylated metabolite, whereas the longer half-life is due primarily to the hydroxy metabolites (21).

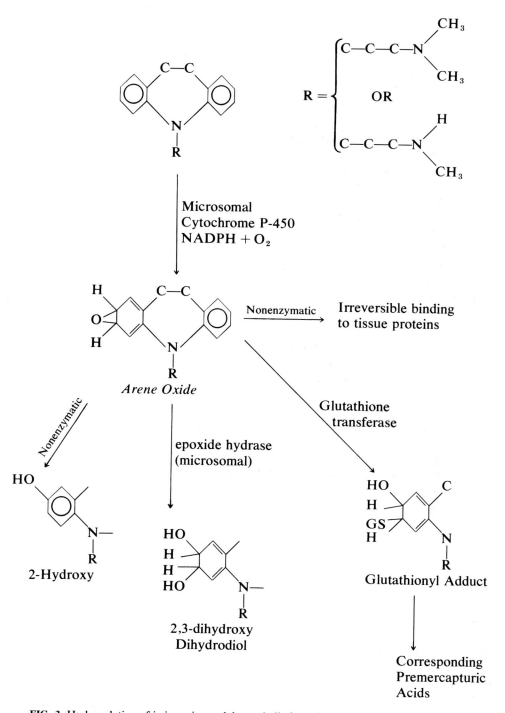

FIG. 3. Hydroxylation of imipramine and desmethylimipramine via arene oxide intermediate.

Some adverse effects reported for imipramine, such as hepatic necrosis, thrombocytopenia, and skin reactions, are probably due to irreversible binding of imipramine to tissue proteins that lead to immunochemical reactions (11,12). Evidence has been presented indicating that an epoxide intermediate is involved. The cytochrome P-450 catalyzed demethylations of imipramine do not involve epoxide intermediate formation because SH-compounds do not react with the parent compound and its N-demethyl metabolite. On the other hand, 2-hydroxylation of imipramine and of its demethylated products involves an epoxidation step leading to arene oxide formation. According to the stability of the arene oxide formed, it is converted to the corresponding phenol (2-hydroxy) or further metabolized to inert dihydrodiol compounds by epoxide hydrase or to inert premercapturic acids by reaction with glutathione or other SH-compounds (Fig. 3).

The irreversible binding of aromatic hydroxy imipramine metabolites to tissue proteins by covalent bond formation via an epoxide intermediate was demonstrated in experiments where glutathione and other cysteine derivatives diminished the binding by preferential attack on the arene epoxide, whereas *in vitro* studies with the epoxide hydrase inhibitor, trichlorpropene oxide, resulted in increased covalent binding. Irreversible protein binding of imipramine metabolites has also been shown with human liver, lung, and cardiac tissue samples.

In general, tricyclic drugs have been shown to undergo two types of epoxidation. Protriptyline, amitriptyline, nortriptyline (antidepressants), carbamazepine (anticonvulsant), and cyproheptadine (antihistaminic and antiserotonergic) undergo epoxidation at the 10,11-double bond (4,10,15). These epoxides and their hydroxy products are fairly stable and are readily detected and measured in the blood of patients receiving these agents (13,22). As previously indicated, the other tricyclics, such as imipramine, desmethylimipramine, and chlorimipramine, presumably form the less stable arene oxides (4,11,12).

In view of the toxic effects of imipramine it is interesting that serum proteins and cytoplasmic proteins of the liver irreversibly bind imipramine and/or its metabolites. The relative high drug binding of liver cytoplasmic proteins after 48 hr (11) might be due to the fact that these proteins are synthetized in the endoplasmic reticulum, where the reactive hydroxy metabolites of imipramine are formed. Most of these soluble proteins have a much longer half-life than the membrane-bound proteins. This protein-bound molecule, when present in the bloodstream, would act as a hapten so that antibodies are formed against this drug in the body during therapy.

Whether the toxicity of imipramine and other tricyclics is indeed a function of their irreversible protein bindings awaits future investigations.

ACKNOWLEDGMENT

The work reported in this chapter has been supported in part by USPHS grant no. MH-21133.

REFERENCES

1. Bickel, M. H. (1974): Binding of phenothiazines and related compounds to tissues and cell constituents. *Adv. Biochem. Psychopharmacol.*, 9:163–173.
2. Bickel, M. H., and Gigon, P. L. (1971): Intracellular binding and metabolism of imipramine and imipramine-N-oxide. *Chem. Biol. Interact.*, 3:245–246.
3. Buckley, J. P., Steenberg, M. L., Jandhyala, B. S., and Perel, J. M. (1975): Effects of imipramine, desmethylimipramine and their 2-OH metabolites on hemodynamics and myocardial contractility in dogs. *Fed. Proc.*, 34:450.
4. Frigerio, A., and Pantarotto, C. (1976): Epoxidediol pathway in the metabolism of tricyclic drugs. *J. Pharm. Pharmacol.*, 28:665–666.

5. Giardina, E. G. V., Bigger, J. T., Jr., Perel, J. M., Kantor, S. J., and Glassman, A. H. (1977): Electrocardiographic effects of imipramine at therapeutic antidepressant plasma concentrations. *Clin. Res.,* 25:454A.
6. Glassman, A. H., Perel, J. M., Shostak, M., Kantor, S. J., and Fleiss, J. L. (1977): Clinical implications of imipramine plasma levels for depressive illness. *Arch. Gen. Psychiatry,* 34:197–204.
7. Gram, L. F. (1974): Metabolism of tricyclic antidepressants. A review. *Dan. Med. Bull.,* 21:218–231.
8a. Gram, L. F., and Christiansen, J. (1975): First-pass metabolism of imipramine in man. *Clin. Pharmacol. Ther.,* 17:555–563.
8b. Gram, L. F., and Overo, F. (1975): First-pass metabolism of nortriptyline in man. *Clin. Pharmacol. Ther.,* 18:305–314.
9. Gram, L. F., Reisby, N., Ibsen, I., Nagy, A., Dencker, S. J., Bech, P., Petersen, G. O., and Christiansen, J. (1976): Plasma levels and antidepressive effect of imipramine. *Clin. Pharmacol. Ther.,* 19:318–324.
10. Hucker, H. B., Balletto, A. J., Demetriades, J., Arison, B. H., and Zacchei, A. G. (1975): Epoxide metabolites of protriptyline in rat urine. *Drug Metab. Dispos.,* 3:80–84.
11. Kappus, H. (1976): Irreversible protein binding of ^{14}C-imipramine in rats *in vivo. Arch. Toxicol. (Berl.),* 37:75–80.
12. Kappus, H., and Remmer, H. (1975): Irreversible protein binding of ^{14}C-imipramine with rat and human liver microsomes. *Biochem. Pharmacol.,* 24:1079–1084.
13. Morselli, P. L., and Frigerio, A. (1975): Metabolism and pharmacokinetics of carbamazepine. *Drug Metab. Rev.,* 4:97–113.
14. Nies, A. S., Shand, D. G., and Wilkinson, G. R. (1976): Altered hepatic blood flow and drug disposition. *Clin. Pharmacol. Ther.,* 1:135–155.
15. Pachecka, J., Salmona, M., Cantoni, L., Mussini, E., Pantarotto, C., Frigerio, A., and Belvedere, G. (1976): Activity of liver microsomal monooxygenases on some epoxide-forming tricyclic drugs. I. Kinetics *in vitro. Xenobiotica,* 6:593–598.
16. Perel, J. M., Jandhyala, B. S., Steenberg, M. L., Manian, A. A., and Buckley, J. P. (1977): Effects of imipramine, chlorimipramine and its metabolites on the hemodynamics and myocardial contractility of anesthetized dogs. *Eur. J. Pharmacol.,* 42:403–410.
17. Perel, J. M., Mendlewicz, J., Shostak, M., Kantor, S. J., and Glassman, A. H. (1976): Plasma levels of imipramine in depression. Environmental and genetic factors. *Neuropsychobiol.,* 2:193–202.
18. Perel, J. M., O'Brien, L., Black, N. B., Bellward, G. D., and Dayton, P. G. (1974): Imipramine and chlorpromazine in hepatic microsomal systems. *Adv. Biochem. Psychopharmacol.,* 9:201–212.
19. Perel, J. M., Shostak, M., Gann, E., Kantor, S. J., and Glassman, A. H. (1975): Pharmacodynamics of imipramine and clinical outcome in depressed patients. In: *Pharmacokinetics: Psychoactive Blood Levels and Clinical Outcome,* edited by L. Gottschalk and S. Merlis, pp. 229–241. Spectrum-Wiley, New York.
20. Salazar, M., Rahwan, R. G., and Patil, P. N (1976): Binding of ^{14}C-imipramine by pigmented and non-pigmented tissues. *Eur. J. Pharmacol.,* 38:233–241.
21. Wilson, A. G. E., Pickett, R. D., Hart, L. D., Eling, T. E., and Anderson, M. W. (1976): Studies on the persistence of basic amines in the rabbit lung. *Fed. Proc.,* 35:600.
22. Ziegler, V. E., Fuller, T. A., and Biggs, J. T. (1976): Nortriptyline and 10-hydroxynortriptyline plasma concentrations. *J. Pharm. Pharmacol.,* 28:849–850.

Neurotoxicology, edited by L. Roizin, H. Shiraki, and N. Grčević. Raven Press, New York © 1977.

Effects of Nortriptyline and Other Psychotropic Drugs on Neurons and Glia *In Vitro:* An Ultrastructural Study

Margaret L. Grunnet

Departments of Pathology and Neurology, University of Utah College of Medicine, Salt Lake City, Utah 84132

Numerous investigators have reported the appearance of increased numbers of dense bodies and concentrically laminated bodies (CLB) in neurons and astrocytes treated with various drugs *in vivo* and *in vitro*. Neurons *in vitro* subjected to chlorpromazine (2), LSD (6,13), chloroquine (17), and bilirubin (15) develop CLB. Similar CLB have been reported in neurons and muscles of rabbits and rats treated with chloroquine (8), in dorsal root ganglia neurons (9) and retina neurons of animals treated with tricyclic antidepressants (10) and the anorectic drug chlorphentermine (10), in lymphatic tissue of rats treated with chlorphentermine (11), and in the neurons of the substantia nigra of young hyperbilirubinemic Gunn rats (1). These CLB are similar to those found in neurons of patients with Tay–Sachs disease (16) and Chediak–Higashi disease (7).

We report here that nervous system cultures treated with the phenothiazine mesoridazine and the tricyclic antidepressant nortriptyline develop CLB and that the number and complexity of these structures appear dose- and time-related. Moreover when the drug is withdrawn from the culture media, these CLB tend to disappear.

MATERIALS AND METHODS

Explant cultures from minced newborn mouse brain were maintained on perforated cellophane tape strips, as reported elsewhere (5). After growth of explant cultures had been established for 2 weeks, nortriptyline, in concentrations of from 0.05 to 0.2 mg% for 1 to 3 weeks, or mesoridazine, in concentrations of from 0.05 to 0.2 mg% for 1 to 2 weeks, was added to the culture media. In some cases the explants were exposed to one or the other of these drugs for 1 to 2 weeks, then put back in control media for up to one week. Control cultures were run along with the experimental cultures.

At the termination of the experiment, the explant with a small portion of cellophane tape to which it was attached was fixed in 4%, cold, buffered glutaraldehyde. After several days the cultures were postfixed in osmium, dehydrated through a graded series of alcohols and toluene, and embedded in Epon. Thick sections were cut on a Porter–Blum MT-1 ultramicrotome. Thin sections were examined under an RCA EMU3H electron microscope. Control cultures not treated with any drug were run simultaneously and prepared for electron microscopic examination in the same manner.

A number of mesoridazine and nortriptyline cultures, as well as control cultures, were studied with enzyme histochemical techniques. The explants on cellophane tape were fixed in cold buffered formalin for 30 min. The Pearse methods of staining (12) for succinic acid dehydrogenase (SDH), nicotine adenine dinucleotide dehydrogenase (NADH), lactic acid dehydrogenase (LDH), and glucose 6-phosphate dehydrogenase (G6-PD) were used. Acid phosphatase staining was attempted but was not satisfactory. These cultures were examined under the light microscope and graded semiquantitatively.

In addition, random samples of cerebral cortex, caudate nucleus, and substantia nigra from three schizophrenic patients on long-term phenothiazine therapy were obtained at autopsy. These were prepared for electron microscopy and studied with an RCA EMU3H electron microscope as described above.

RESULTS

Control cultures showed only a few dense bodies and no CLB after 2 to 5 weeks *in vitro*.

Experimental Cultures

The appearance of dense bodies and simple and complex CLB was essentially the same for mesoridazine and nortriptyline. However, mesoridazine appeared to produce CLB more rapidly and at a lower dose than did nortriptyline.

Mesoridazine

At concentrations of 0.05 to 0.1 mg% for 1 to 2 weeks, a somewhat increased number of dense bodies was seen. The dense bodies were usually round or oval and densely granular with a few irregular lamellae. At concentrations of 0.2 mg% for 1 to 2 weeks, large numbers of simple and complex CLB and dense bodies could be seen as well as myelin figures. Simple CLB were made up of whorls of lamellae. Larger simple CLB had a laminated border, but toward their center lamellae appeared

to fuse and form an amorphous center of variable density. Complex CLB had several appearances. Smaller complex CLB appeared to be made up of an agglomeration of many simple CLB, some with dark, amorphous centers (Fig. 1). Dense bodies were large and often irregular in shape. Some dense bodies were fused with several CLB (Fig. 2). CLB were also fused with bodies having a finely vacuolar appearance and horizontal lamellae (Fig. 3). Round droplets of moderate density were seen alone and fused with dense bodies and CLB (Fig. 4). In many of these neurons and glia, large irregular myelin figures were present as well. These inclusions could be seen in astrocytes as well as neurons, but were fewer in number.

Nortriptyline

At concentrations of 0.05 mg% for 1 week slightly increased round dense bodies could be seen in neurons and astrocytes. At concentrations of 0.05 mg% for 1 to 2 weeks there was a moderate increase in dense bodies as well as the appearance of a few simple CLB. At a concentration of 0.2 mg% for 1 to 2 weeks increased numbers of irregular dense bodies and many simple CLB could be seen. At a concentration of 0.2 mg% for 2 to 3 weeks, many simple and complex CLB could be seen as well as large, irregular dense bodies and large, dark, irregular myelin figures.

Both simple and complex CLB in cultures treated with mesoridazine and nortriptyline were related to or even partially surrounded by rough endoplasmic reticulum. Occasionally an area of rough endoplasmic reticulum appeared to partially encircle a portion of cytoplasm, indicating the occurrence of endocytosis (Fig. 5).

Cells containing many simple and complex CLB and dense bodies often had dilated rough endoplasmic reticulum cisternae containing granular material. Mitochondria in these cells were swollen and pale and showed decreased numbers of lamellae. Dead cells with very large complex CLB could be seen.

Histochemical evaluation using techniques for SDH, NADH, LDH, and G6-PD of neurons in control cultures and cultures treated with mesoridazine and nortriptyline showed few differences. SDH was decreased from +++–++++ in control cultures to ++–+++ in cultures treated with nortriptyline and mesoridazine at a concentration of 0.2 mg% for 1 week. NADH and G6-PD were unchanged. LDH increased from ++–++++ in cultures treated with nortriptyline at a concentration of 0.2 mg% for 2 weeks. These changes may represent a decrease in oxidative metabolism.

When explants of nervous system tissue were subjected to concentrations of 0.1 to 0.2 mg% nortriptyline or mesoridazine for 1 to 2 weeks and then returned to control media for a week, the numbers of dense bodies increased. Moreover, simple and complex CLB also greatly decreased in number. Large vacuoles could be seen in some neurons and astrocytes that contained granular, membranous, and amorphous debris, suggesting intralysosomal digestion (Fig. 6). Remaining dense bodies and CLB could occasionally be seen at the periphery of cells with granular, membranous, and amorphous debris just outside the cell, suggesting that some inclusions may have been removed by a process of exocytosis.

An ultrastructural examination of thin sections of cerebral cortex, caudate nucleus, and substantia nigra from the three autopsied schizophrenic patients on long-term phenothiazine treatment was carried out. No evidence of accumulation of simple or complex CLB or dense bodies was found, although lipofuscin was present in some neurons. Melanin could be seen in neurons of the substantia nigra.

DISCUSSION

Mesoridazine and nortriptyline are amphiphilic drugs, as are other phenothiazines, tricyclic antidepressants, chlorpentermine, and bilirubin (9). These drugs may form a complex with amphiphilic phospholipids leading to impairment of phospholipid degradation and intralysosomal phospholipid accumulation (14). That CLB are lysosomal in nature has been discussed by Brosnan et al. (2), Hendelman (6), Roizin et al. (13), and others. Some studies have stated that CLB are related to and may arise from the Golgi apparatus (3,17). In the present study they appear to be often related to and formed by the rough endoplasmic reticulum. An ultrastructural study of the substantia nigra of young hyperbilirubinemic Gunn rats done in our laboratory by Batty and Millhouse in 1974 shows CLB to be within and related to rough endoplasmic reticulum also.

Simple CLB are the type of inclusion usually involved in "drug-induced lipidoses" and resemble the intraneuronal inclusions of Tay–Sachs disease (16). Complex CLB are rarely described, but some forms are illustrated in other studies, such as that in the study of lymphatic tissues of chlorphentermine-treated animals by Lüllmann-Rauch and Pietschmann (11) and in studies of neurons *in vitro* treated with LSD (6,13). Both similar and different complex CLB are shown in the ultrastructural study of the substantia nigra of young hyperbilirubinemic Gunn rats (1) and in a study of the effects of chloroquine on neurons *in vitro* (11). There is some variation in the morphology of dense and residual bodies when different drugs are used (2,6,11,13,15,17). This may indicate differences in the type of phospholipid complexed.

In the present study of the inclusions produced by the phenothiazines mesoridazine and the tricyclic antidepressant nortriptyline we found that they not only

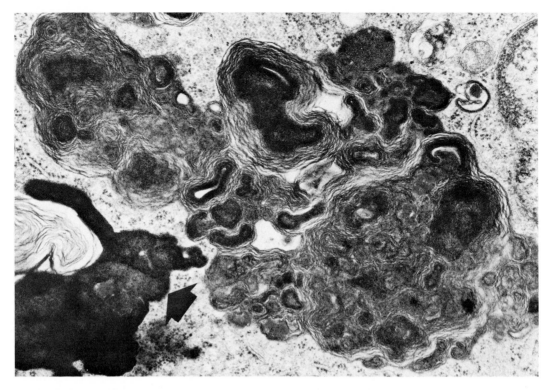

FIG. 1. Complex CLB made up of an apparent fusion of simple CLB in a neuron exposed to 0.2 mg% mesoridazine for 1 week. A dense myelin figure can be seen as well (*arrow*). ×16,000.

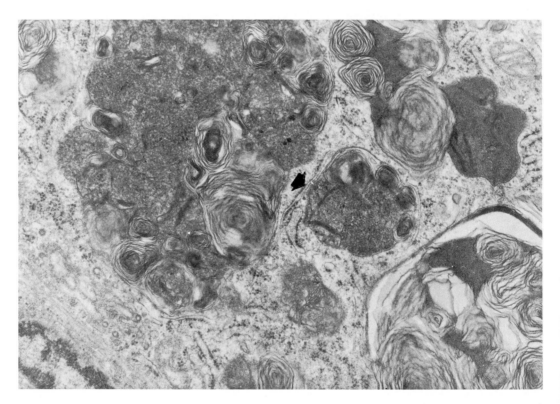

FIG. 2. Complex CLB made up of dense bodies fused with simple and small complex CLB in a neuron exposed to 0.2 mg% mesoridazine for 1 week. Note the relationship of the CLB to the rough endoplasmic reticulum (*arrows*). ×16,000.

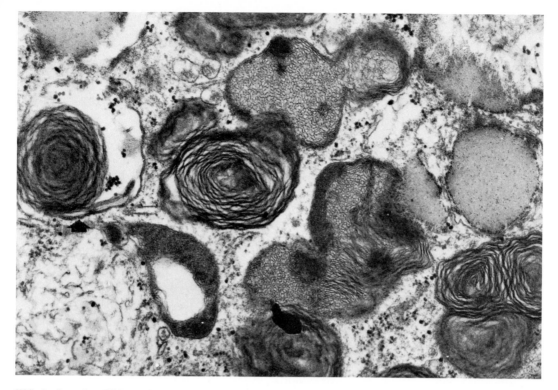

FIG. 3. Complex CLB made up of simple CLB fused with bodies having a finely vacuolar and lamellar appearance. Seen in a neuron exposed to 0.2 mg% nortriptyline for 3 weeks. Note the relationship of a simple CLB to the rough endoplasmic reticulum (*arrow*). ×16,000.

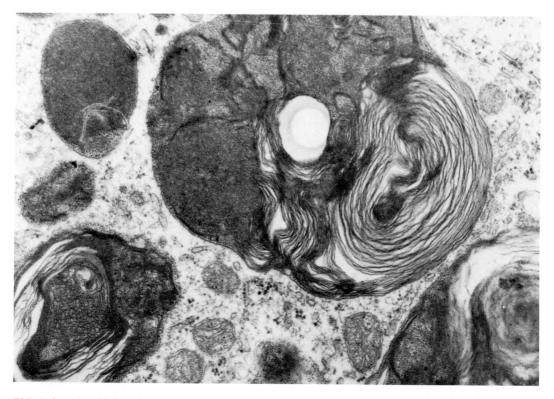

FIG. 4. Complex CLB made up of a large, irregular dense body, a round lipid droplet, and a large simple CLB in a neuron exposed to nortriptyline for 3 weeks. × 16,000.

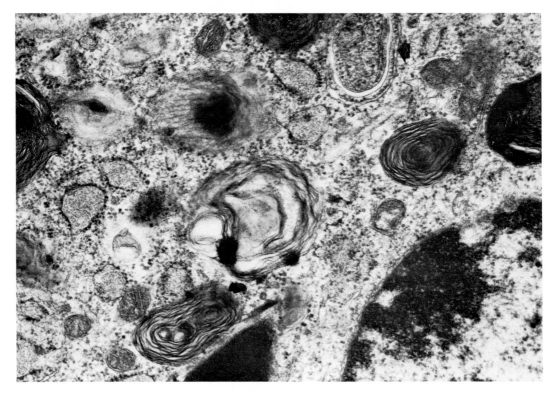

FIG. 5. Dense bodies and simple CLB in a neuron exposed to 0.2 mg% nortriptyline for 2 weeks. Note the portion of cytoplasm partially encircled by rough endoplasmic reticulum (*arrow*). ×16,000.

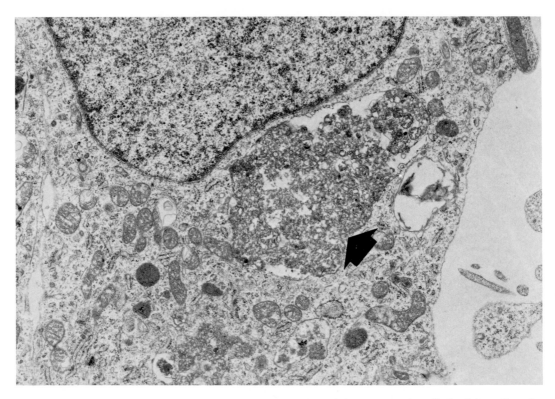

FIG. 6. Neuron exposed to 0.2 mg% mesoridazine for 2 weeks and then to control media for 5 days. Contains a large vacuole filled with granular, membranous, and amorphorous debris (*arrow*). ×16,000.

increased in number but also in complexity as the dosage of drug and time of exposure increased. The occurrence of complex CLB is probably the result of fusion of lysosomes and dense bodies, a process which has been demonstrated by Gordon et al. (4).

We have also shown that the formation of these inclusions is reversible if the drug is taken out of the media. The finding of decreased numbers of dense bodies and CLB and large vacuoles full of granular and amorphous debris suggests a process of digestion of the abnormal lipid material by hydrolytic enzymes still present in the lysosomes. The presence of these inclusions at the periphery of the cell and granular amorphous material adjacent suggests that at least *in vitro* some exocytosis may occur, although this is rare *in vivo*. It is probable that the complexed phospholipids can be metabolized but at a lower rate than uncomplexed phospholipids.

The possibility that drug-induced lipidoses may occur in patients treated with long-term phenothiazines or tricyclic antidepressants has been raised by Lüllmann-Rauch and Pietschmann (11). However, our ultrastructural study of neurons and astrocytes taken from the cerebral cortex, caudate nucleus, and substantia nigra of three autopsied schizophrenic patients on long-term phenothiazine therapy showed no CLB or dense bodies.

It is probable that a drug-induced lipidosis is reversible *in vivo* as well as *in vitro*. This is illustrated by the study of Batty and Millhouse (1) on the substantia nigra of hyperbilirubinemic Gunn rats. They found simple and complex CLB in the neurons of the substantia nigra of Gunn rats 2 to 6 weeks of age. Mature animals did not have these inclusions in their cytoplasm. Moreover, there did not appear to be a large decrease in neuronal population of the substantia nigra of mature Gunn rats.

It is apparent that accumulation of this material can be detrimental to neurons. Dead cells with very large complex CLB were seen in this study. Cells with large numbers of simple and complex CLB often showed dilated rough endoplasmic reticulum and swollen, pale mitochondria. Moreover, at drug concentrations above 0.2 mg% for 1 week, there was a slight decrease in SDH activity and an increase in LDH activity when semiquantitative histochemical techniques were used. This may well indicate a decrease in oxidative metabolism. Phenothiazines are known to uncouple oxidative phosphorylation, as is bilirubin (18).

CONCLUSIONS

In conclusion, our study of the effects of nortriptyline and mesoridazine on neurons *in vitro* has shown that these drugs promote the accumulation of simple and complex CLB and dense bodies. The number and complexity of CLB and dense bodies are related to the dosage of these drugs in the culture media and the length of exposure. Mesoridazine produced these inclusions at slightly lower doses and over shorter exposure times. The CLB in this study appeared to be related to rough endoplasmic reticulum, and in some cases autophagy could be seen. If the drugs were withdrawn from the culture media, the number of CLB and dense bodies decreased and large vacuoles containing granular and amorphous debris could be seen. This suggests that the abnormal, accumulated lipid membranes could be destroyed primarily by digestion, although there was some evidence that exocytosis could occur. The problem of such a lipidosis occurring in human patients treated with long-term phenothiazines and tricyclic antidepressants has been raised. However, we saw no evidence of accumulation of CLB or dense bodies in neurons or glia from selected areas of the cerebrums of three autopsied schizophrenics on long-term phenothiazine treatment. However, there was experimental evidence that if such a drug-induced lipidosis did occur and if there was a large accumulation of these inclusions, neurons might be damaged. It is also possible that such a drug-induced lipidosis might occur in man if some hydrolytic enzyme defect were present or if a very high dose of phenothiazines or tricyclic antidepressants were used for a long period of time.

ACKNOWLEDGMENTS

This study was supported in part by a grant from Eli Lilly and Company and by University of Utah Research Grant No. 1797.

Mesoridazine was supplied by Sandoz Pharmaceuticals and nortriptyline by Eli Lilly and Company.

Electron microscopic assistance was provided by Dee Lerdahl and Susan Carter. Histochemistry was performed by Nina Beglarian.

REFERENCES

1. Batty, H. K. and Millhouse, O. E. (1976): Ultrastructure of the Gunn rat substantia nigra I cytoplasmic changes. *Acta Neuropathol.*, 35:23–107.
2. Brosnan, C. F., Bunge, M. B., and Murray, M. R. (1970): The response of lysosome in cultured neurons to chlorpromazine. *J. Neuropathol. Exp. Neurol.*, 29:337–353.
3. Fedorko, M. E., Hirsch, J. G., and Cohn, Z. A. (1968): Autophagic vacuoles produced *in vitro.* II. Studies on the mechanism of formation of autophagic vacuoles produced by chloroquine. *J. Cell Biol.*, 38:392–402.
4. Gordon, G. B., Miller, L. R., and Bensch, K. G. (1965): Studies on the intracellular digestive process in mammalian tissue culture cells. *J. Cell Biol.*, 25:41–55.
5. Grunnet, M. L. (1973): A simple method for

maintaining neurons in vitro. *Stain Technol.*, 48:207–211.
6. Hendelman, W. J. (1972): A morphological study of the effects of LSD on neurons in culture of cerebellum. *J. Neuropathol. Exp. Neurol.*, 31:411–432.
7. Hirano, A., Zimmerman, H. M., Levine, S., and Padgett, G. A. (1971): Cytoplasmic inclusions in Chediak–Higashi and wobbler mink. An electron microscopic study of the nervous system. *J. Neuropathol. Exp. Neurol.*, 30:470–487.
8. Klinghardt, G. W. (1974): Experimentelle schädigungen von nervensystem and muskulatur durch chlorochin: Modelle verschiedenastiger speicherdystrophien. *Acta Neuropathol. (Berl.)*, 28:117–141.
9. Lüllmann-Rauch, R. (1977): Lipidosis-like alterations in dorsal root ganglion cells of rats treated with tricyclic antidepressants. *Naunyn Schmiedebergs Arch. Pharmacol. (In press.)*
10. Lüllman-Rauch, R. (1974): Retinal lesions in rats after treatment with chlorphentermine or with tricyclic antidepressants. *Virchows Arch. [Zellpathol.]*, 15:309–312.
11. Lüllmann-Rauch, R., and Pietschmann, N. (1974): Lipidosis-like cellular alterations in lymphatic tissues of chlorphentermine-treated animals. *Virchows Arch. [Zellpathol.]*, 15:295–308.
12. Pearse, A. G. E. (1972): *Histochemistry: Theoretical and Applied*, Vol. 2, pp. 922, 925, 928, 1,344. Williams & Wilkins, Baltimore.
13. Roizin, L., Schneider, J., Willson, N., Liu, J. C., and Mullen, C. (1974): Effect of prolonged LSD-25 administration upon neurons of spinal cord ganglia tissue cultures. *J. Neuropathol. Exp. Neurol.*, 33:212–226.
14. Seydel, J. K., and Wassermann, Q. (1973): NMR studies on the molecular basis of drug induced phospholipidosis. *Naunyn Schmiedebergs Arch. Pharmacol.*, 279:207–210.
15. Silberberg, D. H., and Schutta, H. S. (1967): The effects of unconjugated bilirubin and related pigments on cultures of rat cerebellum. *J. Neuropathol. Exp. Neurol.*, 26:572–583.
16. Terry, R. D., and Weiss, M. (1963): Studies in Tay-Sachs disease. II. Ultrastructure of the cerebrum, *J. Neuropathol. Exp. Neurol.*, 22:18.
17. Tischner, K. (1974): Effects of chloroquine on neurons of long term cultures of peripheral and central nervous system: A light and electron microscopic study. *Acta Neuropathol. (Berl.)*, 28:233–242.
18. Zetterstrom, R., and Ernsten, L. (1956): Bilirubin, an uncoupler of oxidative phosphorylation in isolated metochondria. *Nature*, 178:1335.

Neurotoxicology, edited by L. Roizin, H. Shiraki, and N. Grčević. Raven Press, New York © 1977.

Lithium Toxicity: A Review

†G. Michael Dempsey and Herbert L. Meltzer

Division of Internal Medicine, New York State Psychiatric Institute; and Department of Clinical Psychiatry, Columbia University College of Physicians and Surgeons, New York, New York 10032

This chapter describes the general toxicity of lithium (Li) with special reference to nervous tissue whenever possible. The focus is on human toxicity with animal research mentioned as support data.

Li has several nonmedical uses including the production of plastic and ceramics, as a dehumidifier, lithium stearate lubricants, and as a neutron-capture shielding for nuclear reactors (38). There are scattered reports of poisoning from lithium–magnesium industrial compounds in the Russian literature (36,37), but this review focuses on the medical use of Li.

MEDICAL USES

Li is well established as a therapeutic agent in psychiatry.

Cade (15) found Li to be very effective in calming excited psychotic patients. In 1954, Schou et al. (56) confirmed Li's effectiveness in treating acute mania. It is effective in preventing or reducing the severity of future manic or depressive attacks (5) and may be effective in treating ongoing depressive illnesses (42) and schizoaffective illness (25).

Sinclair (57) in 1974 reported that Li suppressed voluntary alcohol intake by rats. There have been occasional reports of the use of Li in the treatment of human alcoholism, and such applications may increase in the future.

Li has been tried in other psychiatric conditions such as schizophrenia, neuroses, epilepsy, and personality disorders and has been found to be generally ineffective (46).

In general, Li appears to be helpful in those atypical psychiatric states that have excited or overactive components to the illness.

LI TOXICITY: NONPSYCHIATRIC

In 1949, Corcoran et al. (19) and Hanlon et al. (33) presented 11 cases of Li intoxication in nonpsychiatric patients who were taking a NaCl taste substitute consisting of a 25% liquid solution of LiCl and small amounts of citric acid and potassium iodide. All these patients were suffering from severe medical illness, usually involving multiple organ systems. The average age was 44 years. The two patients who died were 70 and 66 years old, respectively, and both suffered from severe generalized arteriosclerosis manifesting itself in cardiac and central nervous system (CNS) symptoms.

The fatal episode of one patient was precipitated by her ingestion of approximately 100 mEq of Li on a hot August day. She had been using the Li salt substitute for approximately 3 months prior to this and had been on a 200-mg Na/day diet for 8 months.

---

† *Present address:* Veteran's Hospital and University of Kentucky, Lexington, Kentucky 40201.

The symptoms were quite constant in all patients. They began with tremor, muscle twitches, apathy, and difficult mentation and progressed to blurring vision, confusion, restless coma, and in two cases, death.

Objective findings were hyperactive deep tendon reflexes, muscle fasciculation, and hyperirritability to galvanic stimulation.

In 1913, Cleaveland (17) experimentally ingested 8 g of LiCl (21.9 mEq Li) in four divided doses over a 28-hr period. Slight dizziness and fullness of the head began 3 to 4 hr after the first 2-g dose. Soon after the third dose vision became blurred. After the fourth dose there was vertigo. On the third day there was severe blurred vision, vertigo, weakness, and tremors with staggering gait. The eye and ear symptoms lasted 1½ days, and weakness and tremors lasted 5 days. At no time was there abdominal pain, diarrhea, gastric irritation, or anorexia. He repeated the study "several months later" with 4 g only and noted similar but less marked symptoms. He compared the effects to cinchonism and remarked on the "entire absence" of gastrointestinal symptoms.

Earlier (1903), Good (31) had noted that cats acutely intoxicated with Li showed onset of salivation, nausea, and diarrhea within 15 min followed by death in 2 to 3 days secondary to severe diarrhea, but he did not observe striking neurological symptoms.

Good (31) did note "slight tremor in a few cases" and "stiffness and inability to use the hindquarters" in most cases. The latter symptom he attributed to gastroenteritis, but it probably represented neurological deficits.

LI TOXICITY: PSYCHIATRIC

Incidence

Allgen (1) reported on laboratory values seen in Li patients over an 11-year period in Sweden. Twenty thousand analyses in more than 1,000 patients showed only four cases in which serum Li went above 2.0 mEq/liter. The highest serum level was 3.6 mEq/liter. All four cases survived their high levels of Li. All of these patients were over 60 years old, and all were characterized by being management problems secondary to organic symptomatology with dementia. This again stresses the importance of age and organic brain disease in the etiology of Li intoxication.

CLINICAL FEATURES

Schou et al. (54) reported careful and detailed observations on eight cases of human Li toxicity accumulated over a 15-year period in Denmark (1953–1968). He stressed the slow onset, even in the single purposeful overdose case.

Premonitory symptoms of sluggishness, coarse tremor, twitching, dysarthria, anorexia, vomiting, and diarrhea occurred less than 1 week prior to diagnosis of toxicity. Symptoms during the fully developed intoxication did *not* include thirst and polyuria, and it must be assumed that when these symptoms occur in patients receiving nontoxic doses of Li they represent a specific malfunction in the renal system and not a generalized toxicity.

Renal

A moderate increase of blood urea nitrogen or creatinine, or both, occurred in seven of eight toxic patients. Those values returned to normal in all except one, in whom renal function was decreased before Li toxicity.

Two of the eight patients had autopsy or biopsy evidence of vascular sclerosis in the kidney, two of eight patients had pretoxicity elevated creatinine, and three of eight patients had evidence of urinary tract infections, i.e., five of eight patients had abnormal renal functions prior to intoxication.

Heart

Electrocardiogram stayed normal in four out of eight cases. In three of eight patients the T waves in leads 1 and 2 flattened or inverted, a common finding in patients taking nontoxic doses of Li (24). One of the three patients who died developed atrial flutter and arrhythmia with pulse deficit.

Miscellaneous

Acid-base and electrolyte imbalance problems were not encountered in these human cases although Radomski et al. (47) noted terminal renal failure with severe hyperkalemia in dogs chronically poisoned with LiCl. Many of Schou's (52) patients developed urinary tract infections, and some developed pneumonia. Respiration was occasionally irregular and usually deep. Nausea, vomiting, and diarrhea were not observed during fully developed intoxication. Li excretion, estimated by measurement of serum Li values, was approximately exponential, and half-times varied from 30 to 100 hr.

The severity of symptoms was directly proportional to serum Li level during acute phases, but the symptoms did not disappear until serum Li concentration fell to 0.1 mEq/liter or less.

All three patients who died showed bronchopneumonia and pulmonary edema at autopsy. Two of three showed old cystic changes in brain.

CNS

Schou et al. (54) noted that in dog (47) and rat (51) studies of Li toxicity there is gross damage to kidney tubules before changes are noted in myocardium or brain. In humans, however, the CNS is affected to a greater extent than heart or kidney. The clinical picture of fully developed Li intoxication is dominated by severe and protracted impairment of consciousness, and the condition has been likened to barbiturate intoxication. However, deep tendon reflexes and muscle tone are increased, findings that distinguish the condition from barbiturate intoxication. Also, the electroencephalogram (EEG) does not flatten. Asymmetrical EEG changes occur, including decrease in alpha and increase in theta and delta, the latter change sometimes as frontal paroxysms with episodes of beta and sharp waves.

EEG changes were seen in six of 12 healthy subjects given Li in a study by Reilly et al. (48). The changes were similar to those described by Schou, i.e., asymmetrical slow activity or sharp waves, or both. Four of the subjects had mild EEG abnormalities before receiving Li, and the authors concluded that "while EEG abnormalities may occur during lithium administration, they more frequently represent accentuations of previous abnormalities than they do specific drug effects upon the normal EEG." Zakowska-Dabrowska and Rybakowski (65) also found that Li accentuated preexistent EEG changes in patients and controls taking Li. They noted generalized theta and delta waves in eight of 21 subjects who had an initially normal EEG. They found no correlation between EEG changes and clinical state, outcome, or plasma Li concentration. However, they found a significantly higher erythrocyte Li concentration in subjects who had EEG abnormalities as compared to those who did not.

Schou reported several instances of transitory neurological asymmetries such as unilateral plantar reflex or lateral rotation of the head. Two cases seized, and several patients had episodic hyperextension of the arms and legs.

In no case did the poisoning leave lasting effects, but transient speech problems were seen for 8 to 17 days in some patients, one patient had abnormal movements, and another had memory problems for a few weeks before return to normal.

PERMANENT NEUROLOGICAL SEQUEL

Patients with Li intoxication either die or, more commonly, recover completely. However, von Hartitzsch et al. (62) describe two patients who were left with permanent damage to basal ganglia and cerebellar connections after Li toxicity.

One patient had residual neurological symptoms including flapping tremor of left hand, fluttering eyelids, lip pursing, and right and left arm extrapyramidal movements. She also had bilateral nystagmus and right-sided cerebellar ataxia. She was admitted to the hospital in coma after seizing and had a serum Li concentration of 5 mEq/liter. She had been taking Li for only 9 days and in that time had ingested only 363 mEq/liter (equivalent to an average of five 300-mg Li_2 CO_3 caps per day). She had also received chlorpromazine, 100 to 200 mg/day, during this same 9-day period. The other patient was medicated only with Li before her toxic episode.

She was left with a wide-based ataxia, choreiform movements of the head, tongue, and limbs, and a rhythmic tremor of the right hand.

Both of these patients seized during their toxic episodes. This is not a regular feature of Li toxicity, however Schou et al. (54) reported seizures in two out of 11 of their intoxication cases, and at New York State Psychiatric Institute we have known of one patient to seize during moderate Li intoxication. This patient had a prior history of one grand mal seizure years before. She was left without permanent neurological deficit.

Cohen and Cohen (18) reported four cases of severe permanent neurological deficits in patients who had received moderate doses of Li concurrent with relatively large doses of haloperidol.

During the acute phase of their illnesses all had fever, leukocytosis, and elevated plasma enzymes. They were left with massive deficits including stupor, dementia, and severe dyskinesias. Only one of these patients had a markedly high maximum serum Li level during the Li toxicity period. This patient had a maximum serum level of 2.45 mEq/liter. The other patients' maximum serum Li concentration levels were 1.81, 1.48, and 1.58 mEq/liter, respectively.

Verbor et al. (61) reported a single case of a 51-year-old woman who had taken chlorpromazine HCl, 50 mg t.i.d., and Li_2CO_3, 250 mg q.i.d., for 7 years without difficulties, and with good control of her recurrent mental illness. In October 1963 she became anorexic and began to lose weight. She was admitted to the hospital in a coma on 2/7/64 with a serum Li of 4.5 mEq/liter. She did not seize. By 2/14 she was much better, and serum Li was 0.1 mEq/liter. She had dysarthria and marked ataxia in late February. She was discharged in 2 months (April) and was euphoric, slightly dysarthric, and ataxic and had a tremor of the right arm. She had improved still more when seen on 5/22/64.

Thus, most of the reported cases of permanent neurological sequelae have been reported in persons who were taking phenothiazines in addition to Li.

In a recent article, Degwitz et al. (23) reported on the increased therapeutic risk of side effects when neuroleptics and Li are prescribed simultaneously for long periods of time. They noted that patients over 60 years of age were especially susceptible to side effects and recommended that the maximum Li serum level be 0.6 mEq/liter. At this level they predicted a 60 to 70% decrease in side effects.

There is very little information available concerning the structural changes induced in brain or other tissues by Li. Ellman and Gan (27) found that rats drinking 15 to 50 mm LiCl had profound depletion of the neurosecretory material in the hypophysis and swelling of the cells of the supraoptic nucleus. They interpreted these findings by postulating that Li induces an increased loss of water by the renal tubule system. Vasopressin is released, and depleted, from the storage cells in the hypothalamus in response to the lowered body water. The supraoptic nucleus cells enlarge as they synthesize larger amounts of vasopressin to replenish the depleted storage cells in the hypothalamus. These changes are not toxic *per se* but are rather an overstimulation of a normal physiological system.

MENTAL STATUS

There is very little literature concerning the effect of Li on mental status other than its obvious antimanic qualities.

Healthy volunteers taking modest doses of Li report no effect on mental status or at most a slight lassitude (53). Three subjects who took 50 mEq Li/day for 1 to 3 weeks noted passivity, a subjective sense of indifference, and a feeling of being at a distance from events. Noyes et al. (42) noted a silly giddiness in depressed patients who were being treated with heavy doses of Li. The patients were evaluated thrice weekly with modified Hamilton questionnaires, and as plasma Li concentration reached 1.5 mEq/liter level or greater many of the patients began to deny feelings of depression and give silly responses to the Hamilton.

LITHIUM DISTRIBUTION IN THE BODY

The usual form of Li used medically is Li_2CO_3 in 300-mg tablets. The type of Li salt used has little bearing on the metabolism of Li (52). LiCl is much more soluble than Li_2CO_3, but it is not used because of its propensity to cause stomach discomfort.

Orally administered Li_2CO_3 is rapidly absorbed, and serum levels peak within 2 to 4 hr (4). We have found in dogs on chronic Li administration that giving the total daily dose at one time causes the plasma concentration to peak in 2 hr to approximately three times the base-line postabsorptive level. In clinical settings the exact timing of blood sampling for determination of plasma Li concentration is not critical, just so long as the sample is taken after the 4- to 5-hr postabsorptive peak.

Li uptake into various tissues varies with time. Davenport (21) gave intraperitoneal injections of LiCl to rats and found that plasma Li peaked to 7.6 mEq/kg wet weight at 1 hr and was down to 2.0 mEq at 24 hr. Muscle Li was somewhat lower at 1 hr (3.3 mEq/kg wet weight) and slightly higher than plasma at 24 hr (2.6 mEq/kg wet weight). Li entered the brain more slowly, being only 0.7 mEq at 1 hr and increasing to 2.0 mEq/kg at 24 hr. This delayed effect of Li uptake and presumed slow release in the brain may explain the observation that the CNS symptoms of slurred speech and disorientation are invariably present for a few days after plasma levels of Li fall to insignificant levels.

LITHIUM BRAIN DISTRIBUTION

Edelfors (26) supplemented food and then assayed various regions of rat brain for Li, Na, and K. The hypothalamic area, rich in gray matter, showed the highest Li concentration, 1.10 mEq/kg wet weight tissue. This was 100% greater than some other parts of the brain, e.g., thalamus equaled 0.43 mEq/kg. Hemispherical white matter showed high Li concentration also, being 1.60 mEq/kg. Hemispherical gray matter Li concentration was 0.45 mEq/kg.

Li caused a decrease in Na content of the white matter after 3 weeks and of the hypothalamus after 5 weeks. Edelfors (26) pointed out that the Na content of the hypothalamus and white matter decreased by 7 and 16 mmol/kg, respectively, whereas the Li concentration in these areas was only about 1 mmol/kg. He concluded that a simple ion displacement mechanism cannot explain the reduction in Na content.

Li did not affect the K content in any part of the brain.

Bond et al. (14) gave rats 30 mmol LiCl/kg dry food in the diet. After 14 days plasma Li was 0.59 mmol/liter, and brain Li was 0.46 in the cerebellum and 0.63 in cortex. Plasma Mg was elevated, and brain Mg was decreased in these animals. Brain Na was also decreased. There was no change in brain water.

Cerebrospinal fluid (CSF) Li concentration has been studied in humans receiving therapeutic Li. Baker and Winokur (7) found a CSF:plasma Li concentrate ratio of 0.243 in manic patients receiving Li. This value is similar to red blood cell (RBC): plasma values.

RBC Li concentration is less than plasma concentration. The RBC:plasma ratio has been reported to vary from 0.521 (50) to 0.28.

We have found the white blood cell: plasma ratio to be of the same order, i.e., 0.31.

LITHIUM IN BONE

Birch (11) has found that Li is taken up and retained by bone in humans and rats. The growing bone of immature rats takes up more Li than does mature bone. After Li is discontinued, Li leaves the bone in two phases. The first phase lasts about 10 days, and the bone Li concentration (in rats) drops from 0.6 to 0.3 mEq/kg. Thereafter, the loss of Li is very slow.

Interestingly, human and rat bone from individuals never given Li show significant content of Li−0.16 to 0.19 mEq/kg (dry weight bone).

Birch and Jenner (9) showed that Li accumulation in bone is accompanied by a decrease in bone Ca of approximately 100 times the concentration of Li; this is further evidence indicating that Li does more than just replace other ions on a one-to-one basis.

Human tissue distribution studies are rare. Trautner et al. (60) described two autopsies of human Li fatalities. They mentioned the extreme flabbiness of all tissues and said that the Li content of heart, liver, brain, kidney, and muscles was approximately 5 mEq/kg and did not vary significantly from organ to organ.

LITHIUM EXCRETION

Li is excreted almost exclusively in urine (47,60). Thomsen and Schou (58) studied the effect of water loading and diuretics on the renal excretion of Li in six healthy adults.

He cited evidence that Li is not protein bound and therefore passes freely through glomerular membranes. Using creatinine clearance as a measure of glomerular filtration, he found that Li clearance was only about 20% of creatinine clearance (mean Li clearance = 21 ml/min).

Thus, approximately 80% of filtered Li is reabsorbed in the renal tubules, and 20% is excreted. Thomsen and Schou (58) found Li clearance and excretion fraction to be independent of serum Li concentration within the range of 0.05 to 2.0 mEq/liter. Furosemide (Lasix®), bendroflumethiazide, ethacrynic acid, mercurial diuretics, and spironolactone all failed to increase Li excretion in the urine. In contrast, sodium bicarbonate, acetazolamide (Diamox®), aminophylline, caffeine, and urea diuresis all led to significantly higher urinary Li excretion. Orally administered KCl had no effect on Li excretion. Increased Na intake only slightly increased the total amount of Li excreted, but markedly increased the filtered fraction that was excreted. Low dietary Na decreased the excretion fraction.

In 1971 Baer et al. (6) showed that Li retention occurred in response to low dietary Na or the use of thiazide diuretics.

It was suggested by Hullin et al. (35) that patients suffering from acute mania retain Li, that is, less administered Li is recovered in the urine of manics than from the urine of normal controls.

In their study 12 of 14 manic patients had a positive intake–output balance for more than 6 days after beginning the drug, whereas only two of 10 normal controls continued to retain the drug after the sixth day. Greenspan et al. (30) also found that acutely manic patients retained more Li while manic than when normothymic. During mania the apparent Li space was two to three times greater than estimated total body water, whereas during normothymia the two spaces were approximately equal. They concluded that during normothymia Li is distributed more or less throughout body water, but during mania it is sequestered intracellularly or within an extracellular compartment other than plasma. Birch's work (11) would suggest bone as a possible storage site.

DIABETES INSIPIDUS

Diabetes insipidus is an infrequent but definite side effect to the use of Li. The effect is seen only in selected patients and is not dose related in the population of patients taking Li. That is, some patients develop marked polydipsia and polyuria on modest doses of Li, whereas other patients do not develop these symptoms even at large doses. The polydipsia and polyuria cease when Li is stopped. Forrest et al. (29) found that 40% of 96 patients taking Li reported a subjective increase in thirst, and polyuria of greater than 3 liters/day was documented in 12% (11 patients).

Forrest and others (16) have found it possible to reliably and predictably induce diabetes insipidus in rats and other laboratory animals with daily administration of nontoxic doses of Li. Christensen (16) induced polyuria in rats with a 40 mmol Li/kg dry food diet such that urine volume was greater than 150 ml/24 hr and urine osmolality was less than 200 mmol/kg. Serum Li concentration was 0.5 to 0.7 mEq/liter. Oral bendroflumethiazide decreased urine osmolality beginning the first day of treatment and continuing until the drug was withdrawn. The effect was dose dependent. Chlorpropamide and carbamazepine (Tegretol®) both have selective vasopressin-like antidiuretic effect in pituitary diabetes insipidus. Neither of these agents was effective in correcting the lithium-induced polyuria. The author did not measure serum Li concentrations after diuretics were started.

Thomsen and Schou (59) fed rats a diet containing 20 mmol Li/kg dry weight of food and obtained a mean serum Li concentration of 0.36 mmol/liter. They did not measure pre-Li urine volume, therefore no data regarding polyuria were presented. However, they did find that administration of 10 mg hydrochlorothiazide/kg body weight every day caused a 35% decrease in Li clearance, from 0.18 to 0.10 ml/100 g body weight every minute. Creatinine clearance was unchanged. Concomitant with the decreased Li renal clearance, serum Li concentration increased to a mean level of 0.64 mEq/liter, nearly double the pre-thiazide level. Thus, the authors demonstrated that prolonged administration of hydrochlorothiazide leads to a fall of Li clearance and a rise of the serum Li concentration. The authors reported that there was no apparent polyuria, in contrast to Christensen (16), who found a significant polyuria. It may be that Thomsen and Schou (59) did not reach Li levels high enough to induce polyuria. Their dose was one-half of Christensen's as were the serum levels reached.

Brattleboro (rats with hereditary lack

of vasopressin) rats were also given long-term hydrochlorothiazide, but they received Li (1.0 ml of 150 mmol/liter LiCl, i.p.) only on the days when Li clearances were being determined. During administration of thiazide to Brattleboro rats, the urine flow was decreased to one-half usual values, and Li clearance was decreased 30%.

Baer et al. (6) reported a rise in serum Li in human patients who were given chlorothiazide in order to induce Na depletion. They interpreted the rise in serum Li as a secondary effect of Na depletion.

The effect of thiazide on renal Li clearance in humans has been studied by Peterson et al. (43). The subjects were nonpsychiatric patients on an internal medicine service who were suffering from edema due to various causes for which prolonged thiazide treatment was indicated. Li renal clearance was determined after giving the patients a single 600-mg (16.2 mmol) dose of Li by mouth. After the base-line Li clearance was determined, the patients received 2 months of therapy with either 25 mg/day of hydrochlorothiazide or 2.5 mg of bendrofluazide along with 3.4 g (45.7 mmol)/day of KCl. The mean Li clearance fell 24%, from 20.2 to 15.4 ml/min during thiazide treatment, but creatinine clearance did not change. Mean Na excretion increased somewhat during thiazide treatment, going to 147 mmol/min from the control value of 121 mmol/min. Interestingly, Li clearance rose when Na excretion rose (a finding also noted by Baer et al.) both with and without thiazide treatment. In addition, the authors noted that thiazide treatment reduced the Li clearance at all levels of Na excretion. They conclude that the thiazide-induced fall in Li clearance is not secondary to changes in Na excretion but rather is a direct result of thiazide treatment.

Himmelhoch et al. (34) have recently suggested that thiazides are clinically useful in the management of Li-resistant mood swings. They found that four out of seven patients who were having mood swings while taking only Li demonstrated significant mood stabilization concurrent with thiazide-induced elevation of serum Li concentration. They stress that thiazides have two effects in Li patients: (a) thiazide tends to correct Li-induced polyuria thus making it possible for patients to achieve therapeutic plasma Li concentrations once they are no longer excreting large amounts of Li and water, and (b) thiazides have a specific action on Li handling of the kidney leading to increased retention of Li and higher plasma concentrations. They suggest that renal Li clearance is decreased secondary to thiazide-induced Na loss, which in turn leads to an increased reabsorption of Na (and Li) in the proximal tubule in compensation for the Na loss. Unlike Na, however, little Li is lost at distal tubule sites, and the net result is decreased Li clearance and increased plasma Li. They postulate that thiazides might also increase the intracellular concentration of Li and cite this as an area for future research.

ADENYL CYCLASE

Much attention has been given to the possible role of adenyl cyclase inhibition by Li as the etiology of diabetes insipidus, and other observed effects of Li on hormone production and activity in the body.

Adenyl cyclase is Mg^{++} dependent, and, since Mg^{++} is susceptible to replacement by Li^1, it is an attractive hypothesis to suggest that Li affects water metabolism in the kidney by replacing Mg and thereby hindering the activation of adenyl cyclase.

This hypothesis has been studied by Forrest et al. (29) and Martinez-Maldonado

---

[1] Williams (64) calls attention to the close size relationship between Li and Mg. Both have similar ionic radii (Li = 0.60A, Mg = 0.65A) and similar ionization potentials. Li and Mg both have a preference to anions with a small radius, a high charge, or both.

Li also competes with Ca to binding sites in certain ligands.

et al. (40). Forrest et al. first studied humans who were polyuric while taking Li. Neither excessive urine volume nor low urine osmolality were significantly reduced by vasopressin or chlorpropamide (chlorpropamide is better known as Diabinese ® an oral hypoglycemic agent used in diabetes mellitus that facilitates the action of vasopressin on the distal tubule). However, chlorothiazide treatment did reduce polyuria and increase urine osmolality.

They then studied rats and found that they could make all rats polyuric at serum levels of 0.5 to 1.5 mEq/liter Li. This polyuria was resistant to vasopressin.

They then injected normal rats, Brattleboro rats (rats with hereditary lack of vasopressin), and Li-treated rats with vasopressin or dibutyryl cyclic adenosine monophosphate (cyclic AMP). Both normal and Brattleboro rats responded with lower urine volumes and higher osmolalities. However, Li-treated rats were relatively unresponsive. Urine osmolality never became greater than plasma osmolality, and urine volume was not significantly affected.

Because of the lack of effect of exogenous cyclic AMP in correcting the Li-induced diabetes insipidus in rats, Forrest concluded that Li acts, at least in part, at a site distal to adenyl cyclase-mediated production of cyclic AMP. Phosphodiesterase, for example, might be such a site.

Martinez-Maldonado et al. (40) in 1975 reached the same conclusion in a study similar to that of Forrest. They confirmed Forrest's findings that rats taking Li failed to respond to exogenous vasopressin and dibutyrl cyclic AMP.

By using phosphate and uric acid as markers of proximal tubular function and by noting that Li causes an increase in the excretion of these substances, they concluded that Li inhibits proximal tubular reabsorption.

The solubilities of various Li salts often differ from the other group I elements and tend to resemble those of Mg salts. Cotton and Wilkinson's (20) text of inorganic chemistry states that Li salts in solution generally deviate from ideal behavior to yield solutions of abnormal colligative properties such as very low vapor pressure and freezing point.

LITHIUM AND INTERMEDIARY METABOLISM

Alkali metal ions, especially K, are often required in enzyme reactions *in vivo*. They act in a structural manner rather than a catalytic manner, that is, V_{max}, the maximum velocity of a reaction, is not affected by alkali cation, but K_m, the binding strength, is strongly cation dependent (64).

In general, Li is very inefficient in replacing alkali cations in enzyme reactions and, in particular, does not compete well at K binding sites in synthetic or experimental ligands (64).

An exception, however, is Na-dependent NaK ATPase, wherein Li is more efficient than the other alkali ions in replacing Na (64).

Thus, the widespread effects of Li in mammalian tissues might be due to the replacement of relatively small amounts of physiological cations in strategic places, such as enzyme or membrane transfer activating sites.

Birch (10) suggested that Li might affect the action of Mg in Mg-dependent enzymes, such as those involved in the intermediary metabolism of sugars. The effects of Li on some of the Mg-dependent glycolytic enzymes have been studied.

The clinical observation that Li was associated with weight gain in approximately 10% of patients taking Li (55) led Mellerup and Plenge (41,44) to study the mechanism of Li-induced weight gain in rats. They found that intraperitoneal injection of LiCl caused an increase in brain and diaphragm glycogen content, a decrease in liver glycogen content, and a transient 25% rise in blood glucose followed by a return to normal or subnormal levels (41). They postulated that Li had an insulin-like effect to mediate glucose uptake into brain and muscle, and a secondary glycogenolytic action in the liver. Intracisternal injections of LiCl gave an increase in brain glycogen but had no other effects on sugar metabolism.

In a follow-up article they studied the effect of intraperitoneal Li on liver and on plasma glucagon. They found that intraperitoneal Li increased glucagon-like substance in plasma, increased liver phosphorylase-A activity in the liver, and decreased liver glycogen (44).

They postulated that Li mediated these changes by stimulating the release of glucagon from the pancreas, and in a later study demonstrated that rats treated with 600 mmol LiCl/day for 54 days gained 70% more weight than did rats injected with 600 mmol NaCl. From this data they concluded that the weight gain seen in manic-depressive patients taking Li is due to Li and not to the manic-depressive illness itself.

DeFeudis (22) showed that intraperitoneal LiCl markedly increases the uptake of glucose into the brain in mice 3 to 5 hr later. Li either decreased or did not affect the entry into the brain of D-mannose, D-fructose, D-mannitol, sucrose, or urea.

Allison et al. (2,3) demonstrated that Li given to rats caused a 30% reduction in the level of myoinositol in cerebral cortex. In a later paper, Allison (3) found that atropine and scopolamine inhibited the effect of Li on brain myoinositol. They postulated that Li is a central cholinergic agonist and that a reduction of inositol could be the result of stimulation of cholinergic synapses that in turn would affect inositol metabolism in undefined ways.

In 1962 Faust (28) reported that Li inhibited d-glucose absorption by isolated loops of rat jejunum. He postulated that Li was displacing Na from active transport sites that mediated sugar transport.

In 1965 Rosensweig et al. (49) confirmed Faust's findings and noted additionally that Li did not affect d-xylose absorption.

In 1964 Bhattacharya (8) reported that Li caused increased uptake of glucose by isolated diaphragm and epididymal fat pads of rats. He also reported that injections of Li into normal rats and rabbits produced a prolonged hypoglycemia. In rabbits the blood sugar fell steadily from 1 hr onward. In rats there was an initial increase for 1 hr, then a decrease at 3 hr. He called attention to the similarities of insulin and Li in these effects.

Gupta and Crollini (32) studied the effect of Li on RBC galactokinase, a Mg-dependent enzyme that phosphorylates galactose to galactose-1-phosphate. They could find no inhibition of the enzyme's activity by Li.

LITHIUM AND DNA

Williams (64) points out that the state of condensation of RNA and DNA are very cation-sensitive, and he speculates that Li could affect DNA and RNA conformation (and function) as much as Na does.

Birch and Goulding (12) have studied the ability of Li to replace Mg in nucleotide complexes. They found that Li does not directly substitute for Mg in adenosine diphosphate complexes, but that it does interfere with the reaction of Mg and ADP, possibly by formation of Mg–Li nucleotide complexes.

In 1962, Walwick and Main (63) found that the rate of incorporation of thymidine into DNA in a cytoplasmic system derived from rat thymus was strongly stimulated by the concentration and type of monovalent cations tested one at a time in the incubation mixture. Li had the weakest stimulatory effect; K the highest. They suggested that the ion-dependent factor in the system was the polymerase system.

In 1970 Bishop and Gill (13) found that the monovalent alkali earth cations in general and Li in particular had large inhibitory effects on DNA nuclease and DNA polymerase. The inhibition of polymerase by the relatively small alkali earth cations, Li and Na, was very similar to Mg^{++}-mediated inhibition of the polymerase. The larger alkali earth metal ions, K, Rb, and Cs, had less inhibitory effects on DNA nuclease, with Li having the strongest inhibitory effect.

The authors suggest that the alkali earth cations are essential for DNA nuclease and polymerase regulation because of their ability to balance the ionic strength of Mg in a "physiologically helpful" way.

REFERENCES

1. Allgen, L. (1969): Laboratory experience of lithium toxicity in man. *Acta Psychiatr. Scand. Suppl.,* 207:98–105.
2. Allison, J. H., and Stewart, M. A. (1971): Reduced brain inositol in lithium treated rats. *Nature* [*New Biol.*], 233:267–268.
3. Allison, J. H., and Blisner, M. E. (1976): Inhibition of the effect of lithium on brain inositol by atropine and scopolamine. *Biochem. Biophys. Res. Comm.,* 68:1332–1338.
4. Amdisen, A. (1969): Variation of serum lithium concentration during the day in relation to treatment control, absorptive side effects, and the use of slow-release tablets. *Acta Psychiatr. Scand.,* 207:55–58.
5. Baastrup, P., Poulsen, J., Schou, M., Thomsen, K., and Amidsen, A. (1970): Prophylactic lithium: Double blind discontinuation in manic-depressive and recurrent-depressive disorders. *Lancet,* 2: 326–331.
6. Baer, L., Platman, S. R., Kassir, S., and Fieve, R. (1971): Mechanisms of renal lithium handling and their relationship to mineralocorticoids: A dissociation between sodium and lithium ions. *J. Psychiatr. Res.,* 8:91–105.
7. Baker, M. A., and Winokur, G. (1966): Cerebrospinal fluid lithium in manic illness. *Br. J. Psychiatry,* 112:163–165.
8. Bhattacharya, G. (1964): Influence of lithium on glucose metabolism in rats and rabbits. *Biochim. Biophys. Acta,* 93:644–646.
9. Birch, N. J., and Jenner, F. A. (1973): The distribution of lithium and its effects on the distribution and excretion of other ions in the rat. *Br. J. Pharmacol.,* 47:586–594.
10. Birch, N. J. (1973): The role of magnesium and calcium in the pharmacology of lithium. *Biol. Psychiatry,* 7:269–272.
11. Birch, N. J. (1974): Lithium accumulation in bone after oral administration in rat and man. *Clin. Sci. Mol. Med.,* 46:409–413.
12. Birch, N. J., and Goulding, I. (1975): Lithium-

13. Bishop, C. C., and Gill, J. E. (1971): Inhibition of escherichia coli DNA polymerase by monovalent cations. *Biochim. Biophys. Acta,* 227:97–105.
14. Bond, P. A., Brooks, B. A., and Judd, A. (1975): The distribution of lithium, sodium, and magnesium in rat brain and plasma after various periods of administration of lithium in the diet. *Br. J. Pharmacol.,* 53:235–239.
15. Cade, J. F. J. (1949): Lithium salts in the treatment of psychotic excitement. *Med. J. Aust.,* 36: 349–352.
16. Christensen, S. (1976): Effect of antidiuretic drugs in rats with lithium-induced polyuria. *Acta Pharmacol. Toxicol. (Kbh.),* 38:81–89.
17. Cleaveland, S. A. (1913): A case of poisoning by lithium. *JAMA,* 60:722.
18. Cohen, W. J., and Cohen, N. H. (1974): Lithium carbonate, haloperidol, and irreversible brain damage. *JAMA,* 230 (9):1283–1287.
19. Corcoran, A. C., Taylor, R. D., and Page, I. H. (1949): Lithium poisoning from the use of salt substitutes. *JAMA,* 139:685–688.
20. Cotton, F. A., and Wilkinson, G. (1966): *Advanced Inorganic Chemistry,* 2nd ed. Wiley (Interscience), New York.
21. Davenport, V. D. (1950): Distribution of parenterally administered lithium in plasma, brain, and muscle of rats. *Am. J. Physiol.,* 163:633–641.
22. DeFeudis, F. V. (1972): Specificity of the effect of lithium injections on the entry of carbon atoms of glucose into mouse brain *in vivo. Arch. Int. Pharmacodyn.,* 197:141–146.
23. Degwitz, R., Consbruch, U., Haddenbrock, S., Neusch, B., Oehlert, W., and Umsold, R. (1976): Therapeutische risiken bei der lagzeitbehandlung mit neuroleptika und lithium. *Nervenarzt,* 47: 81–87.
24. Demers, R. G., and Heninger, G. R. (1971): Electrocardiographic T-wave changes during lithium carbonate treatment. *JAMA,* 218:381–386.
25. Dempsey, G. M., Tsuang, M. T., Struss, A., and Dvoredsky-Wortsman, A. (1975): Treatment of schizo-affective disorder. *Compr. Psychiatry,* 16:55–59.
26. Edelfors, S. (1975): Distribution of sodium, potassium and lithium in the brain of lithium-treated rats. *Acta Pharmacol. Toxicol. (Kbh.),* 37:387–392.
27. Ellman, G. L., and Gan, G. L. (1973): Lithium ion and water balance in rats. *Toxicol. Appl. Pharmacol.,* 25:617–620.
28. Faust, R. G. (1962): The effect of anoxia and lithium ions on the absorption of d-glucose by the rat jejunum *in vitro. Biochim. Biophys. Acta,* 60: 604–614.
29. Forrest, J. N., Cohen, A. D., Torretti, J., Himmelhoch, J. M., and Epstein, F. H. (1974): On the mechanism of lithium-induced diabetes insipidus

in man and rat. *J. Clin. Invest.*, 53:1115–1123.

30. Greenspan, K., Goodwin, F. K., Bunney, W. E., and Durell, J. (1968): Lithium ion retention and distribution. Patterns during acute mania and normothymia. *Arch. Gen. Psychiatry*, 19:664–673.

31. Good, C. A. (1903): An experimental study of lithium. *Am. J. Med. Sci.*, 125:273–284.

32. Gupta, J. D., and Crollini, C. (1975): Effect of lithium on magnesium-dependent enzymes. Letter, *Lancet*, 1(7900):216–217.

33. Hanlon, L. W., Romaine, M., Gilroy, F. J., and Dietrick, J. E. (1949): Lithium chloride as a substitute for sodium chloride in the diet. *JAMA*, 139:688–692.

34. Himmelhoch, J. M., Forrest, J., Neil, J. F., and Detre, T. P. (1976): Thiazide-lithium synergy in refractory mood swings. *Presented at the May 1976 Am. Psychiatr. Assoc. Meeting in Miami, Florida.*

35. Hullin, R. P., Swinscoe, J. G., McDonald, R., and Dramsfield, G. A. (1968): Metabolic balance studies on the effect of lithium salts in manic depressive psychosis. *Br. J. Psychiatry*, 114:1561–1573.

36. Il'ina, V. A., and Kochetrova, T. A. (1970): Experimental pneumosclerosis evoked by inhalation of magnesium-lithium alloy aerosols. *Gig. Tr. Prof. Zabol.*, 14:17–21.

37. Il'ina, V. A. (1970): Problems of occupational hygiene in the manufacture and working of magnesium-lithium alloys. *Gig. Sanit.*, 35:24–27.

38. Kline, N. S. (1973): A narrative account of lithium usage in psychiatry. In: *Lithium: Its Role in Psychiatric Research and Treatment*, edited by S. Gershon and B. Shopsin. Plenum Press, New York–London.

39. Kline, N. S., Wren, J. C., Cooper, T. B., Varga, E., and Canald, O. (1974): Evaluation of lithium therapy in chronic and periodic alcoholism. *Am. J. Med. Sci.*, 268:15–22.

40. Martinez-Maldonado, M., Stavroulaki-Tsapara, A., Tsaparas, N., Suki, W. N., and Ekmoyan, G. (1975): Renal effects of lithium administration in rats: Alterations in water and electrolyte metabolism and the response to vasopressin and cyclic-adenosine monophosphate during prolonged administration. *J. Lab. Clin. Med.*, 86:445–461.

41. Mellerup, E. T., Thomsen, H. G., Plenge, P., and Rafaelsen, O. J. (1970): Lithium effect on plasma glucagon, liver phosphorylase — and liver glycogen in rats. *J. Psychiatr. Res.*, 8:37–42.

42. Noyes, R., Dempsey, G. M., Blum, A., and Cavanaugh, G. L. (1974): Lithium treatment of depression. *Compr. Psychiatry*, 15:187–193.

43. Petersen, V., Hvidt, S., Thomsen, K., and Schou, M. (1974): Effect of prolonged thiazide treatment on renal lithium clearance. *Br. Med. J.*, 3:143–145.

44. Plenge, P., Mellerup, E. T., and Rafaelson, O. J. (1970): Lithium action on glycogen synthesis in rat brain, liver, and diaphragm. *J. Psychiatr. Res.*, 8:29–36.

45. Plenge, P. K., Mellerup, E. T., and Rafaelsen, O. J. (1973): Weight gain in lithium-treated rats. *Int. Pharmacopsychiatry*, 8:234–238.

46. Quitkin, F. M., Rifkin, A., and Klein, D. F. (1973): Lithum in other psychiatric disorders. In: *Lithium: Its Role in Psychiatric Research and Treatment*, edited by S. Gershon and B. Shopsin. Plenum Press, New York–London.

47. Radomski, J. L., Fuyat, H. N., Nelson, A. A., and Smith, P. K. (1950): The toxic effects, excretion and distribution of lithium chloride. *J. Pharmacol. Exp. Ther.*, 100:429–444.

48. Reilly, E., Halmi, K. A., and Noyes, R. (1973): Electroencephalographic responses to lithium. *Int. Pharmaco-psychiat.*, 8:208–213.

49. Rosensweig, N. S., Cocco, A. E., and Hendrix, T. R. (1965): A comparison of the effect of sodium and lithium on the absorption of glucose and xylose *in vivo. Biochim. Biophys. Acta*, 109:312–313.

50. Rybakowski, J., Chlopocka, M., Kapelski, Z., Hermacka, B., Szajmerman, Z., and Kasprzak, K. (1974): Red blood cell lithium index in patients with affective disorders in the course of lithium prophylaxis. *Int. Pharmaco-psychiat.*, 9:166–171.

51. Schou, M. (1958): Lithium studies: I. Toxicity. *Acta Pharmacol.*, 15:70–84.

52. Schou, M. (1973): Preparations, dosage, and control. In: *Lithium: Its Role in Psychiatric Research and Treatment*, edited by S. Gershon and B. Shopsin. Plenum Press, New York–London.

53. Schou, M., Amdisen, A., and Thomsen, K. (1968): The effect of lithium on the normal mind. In: *De Psychiatria Progrediente*, Vol. 2, edited by P. Baudis, E. Peterova, and V. Sedivec. Plenum Press, New York.

54. Schou, M., Amdisen, A., and Trap-Jensen, J. (1968): Lithium poisoning. *Am. J. Psychiatry*, 125:520–527.

55. Schou, M., Baastrup, P. C., Grof, P., Weis, P., and Angst, J. (1970): Pharmacological and clinical problems of lithium prophylaxis. *Br. J. Psychiatry*, 116:615–619.

56. Schou, M., Juel-Nielsen, N., Strömgren, E., and Volby, H. (1954): The treatment of manic psychoses by the administration of lithium salts. *J. Neurol. Neurosurg. Psychiatry*, 17:250–260.

57. Sinclair, J. D. (1974): Lithium-induced suppression of alcohol drinking by rats. *Med. Biol.*, 52:133–136.

58. Thomsen, K., and Schou, M. (1968): Renal lithium excretion in man. *Am. J. Physiol.*, 215:823–827.

59. Thomsen, K., and Schou, M. (1973): The effect of prolonged administration of hydrochlorozide on the renal lithium clearance and the urine flow of ordinary rats and rats with diabetes insipidus. *Pharmakopsychiatr.*, 6:264–269.

60. Trautner, E. M., Morris, R., Noack, C. H., and Gershon, S. (1955): The excretion and retention

of ingested lithium and its effect on the ionic balance of man. *Med. J. Aust.,* 2:280–291.

61. Verbor, J. L., Phillips, J. D., and Fife, D. G. (1965): A case of lithium intoxication. *Postgrad. Med. J.,* 41:190–192.

62. Von Hartitzsch, B., Hoenich, N. A., Leigh, R. J., Wilkinson, R., Frost, T. H., Weddel, A., and Posen, G. A. (1972): Permanent neurological sequelae despite haemodialysis for lithium intoxication. *Br. Med. J.,* 4:757–759.

63. Walwick, E. R., and Main, R. K. (1962): Monvalent cation effects on a deoxyribonucleic acid-synthesizing system. *Biochim. Biophys. Acta,* 61:876–884.

64. Williams, R. J. P. (1973): The chemistry and biochemistry of lithium. In: *Lithium: Its Role in Psychiatric Research and Treatment,* edited by S. Gershon and B. Shopsin. Plenum Press, New York–London.

65. Zakowska-Dabrowska, T., and Rybakowski, J. (1973): Lithium-induced EEG changes: Relation to lithium levels in serum and red blood cells. *Acta Psychiatr. Scand.,* 49:457–465.

Neurotoxicology, edited by L. Roizin, H. Shiraki, and N. Grčević. Raven Press, New York © 1977.

Ultrastructural Findings of the Central Nervous System in Lithium Neurotoxicology

* K. Akai, ** L. Roizin, and ** J. C. Liu

*Department of Pathology, Kyorin University School of Medicine, Mitakashi, Tokyo 181, Japan; and **Departments of Neuropathology and Neurotoxicology, New York State Psychiatric Institute, New York, New York 10032*

The beneficial effects of lithium carbonate or lithium chloride for the treatment of manic-depressive psychosis, especially mania, has been well established during recent years (5,13,15,20,24,51,54,58,71, 86,etc.).

Various degrees of adverse and toxic reactions have been observed even with therapeutic doses (2,8,12,23,32,33,35,38, 41,67,70,72,73,etc.) (ref. citation within text).

Although in most cases some of the untoward reactions, under careful clinical follow-up and serum-lithium monitoring, are readily controlled, in other instances, more severe renal (46,53,65,78,etc.), thyroid (23,37,68,84), and neurological (8,9, 25,34,38,58,59,61,74,76,79,83) disorders, and even fatalities (7,64,68,80,81) have occurred.

The mechanism of lithium toxicity (12, 17–19) is still obscure (15,20–24) and has been more recently reviewed by Dempsey and Meltzer (15).

The review of the literature on the neuropathological aspects of lithium toxicity revealed, besides our previous study of the central nervous system (CNS) in rodents (62), Srebro's report (75) on microscopic findings in the hypothalamus and Whetsell and Mire's observations (88) on the tissue cultures of dorsal root ganglia of the spinal cord.

The present study is a follow-up of our previous investigations and is concerned principally with ultrastructural observations in the CNS of nonhuman primates treated with lithium chloride.

MATERIAL AND METHODS

Six healthy male monkeys estimated to be over 7 years of age, weighing 7.0 to 11.2 kg, were used. Lithium chloride was administered by intravenous infusion in a solution containing 1 g lithium chloride in 10 ml of 5% glucose. Each animal was given different amounts according to the experimental design shown in Table 1. All animals were fed with the same standard diet.

After lithium administration all animals were under constant observation, and when marked toxicity appeared the injections were immediately discontinued. Blood samples for lithium estimations were taken at various intervals after administration. The concentration of lithium in whole blood was determined by a Beckman Model 979 atomic absorption spectrophotometer with laminar flow burner.

Two monkeys (no. 5, no. 6, Table 1) were used for recovery studies. Monkey no. 5 died 5 years after the experiment due to pneumonia, and no. 6 was sacrificed 1 year later, i.e., 6 years after completion of experiments.

Four animals were used for light micro-

TABLE 1. *Summary of experimental materials, methods, and observations*

Animal and sex	Monkey 1, male	Monkey 2, male	Monkey 3, male	Monkey 4, male	Monkey 5, male	Monkey 6, male
No. & type of injections	6 i.v.	4 i.v.	6 i.v.	9 i.v.	41 i.v.	31 i.v.
Duration of exp. (days)	14	4	11	17	70	81
Dose of LiCl/kg body wt.	200 mg	100 mg	100 mg	50 mg	50 mg	50 mg
Total amount	3,600 mg	4,000 mg	4,200 mg	3,330 mg	18,245 mg	12,400 mg
Symptomatology						
Loss of aggression	+++	+++	+++	+++	+++	+++
Increase of secretory functions (salivary, nasal, perspiratory)	+++	+++	+++	+++	++	+++
Decrease of muscle tonus and easy fatiguability	+++	+	+++	+++	++	++
Tremors	+++	0	+++	+++	++	++
Pupil reaction	Miotic	Average	Miotic	Miotic	Average	Miotic
Vomiting	Frequent	None	Frequent	None	Frequent	None
Loss of appetite	+++	+++	+++	+++	+	+
Dehydration	+++	0	+++	+++	+	0
Loss of body weight	30%	0	30%	20%	15%	0
Outcome	Sacrificed on 14th day of exp.	Died on 4th day of exp.	Died on 12th day of exp.	Sacrificed on 17th day of exp.	Died 5 years after exp.	Sacrificed 6 years after exp.

0, no remarkable changes; +, mild changes; + +, prominent changes; + + +, very pronounced changes.

scopic, histochemical, and electron microscope examinations of all organs. Immediately after death or sacrifice the animals were perfused through the left ventricle of the heart at approximately 100 mm Hg gravity. The perfusion solution was composed of 4% glutaraldehyde in 0.1 mole cacodylate buffer adjusted to pH 7.4 and adding 5 g of glucose/100 ml or with 10% buffered formalin.

After complete autospy was done, several regions of CNS, including cerebral cortex, hypothalamus, caudate nucleus, putamen, globus pallidus, thalamus, substantia nigra, dentate nucleus, pons, medulla, and spinal cord were selected. Small pieces of tissue samples were refixed in cold 4% glutaraldehyde for 90 min, rinsed with 0.1 M cacodylate buffer at pH 7.4. Dehydration was accomplished with cold grading ethanols and prophylene followed by embedding in Epon 812. The selected blocks were cut with the LKB ultratome (8800), and the sections were doubly stained with 3% uranyl acetate and lead citrate and subsequently examined with a RCA-EMU-3G electron microscope.

RESULTS

Clinical Observations

After two to four injections, all animals showed loss of appetite, decreased aggression, vomiting, hunched position, decrease of spontaneous activity, sluggishness, and frightening expressions. In the course of the experiment, the most striking changes consisted of an increase of secretory functions with salivation, discharge of mucus from the nose, and perspiration, especially on the face and hands, and, at times, edema around the mouth with reddish discoloration of the lips. Marked fatiguability, various degrees of severe hypotonicity and tremors in all extremities and neck were periodically apparent. The latter were intensified in severity by stimulation. Some monkeys also showed marked miosis. The methodology and most important findings are summarized in Table 1.

Lithium Levels in Blood

One hour before and after lithium administration, blood was drawn from the saphenous veins, and the lithium level was estimated. The concentration of lithium 1 hr after injection revealed quite constant values ranging from 2.0 to 2.22 mEq/liter. The following day, in three animals given 50 mg lithium/kg body weight once a day, levels of lithium varied from 0.07 to 1.23 mEq/liter prior to injection. Of particular interest was monkey no. 3. This animal suddenly died on the 11th day after the administration of 200 mg/kg. The postmortem blood revealed a very high concentration of lithium (8 mEq/liter). Immediately thereafter this animal was perfused with 4% glutaraldehyde to avoid postmortem changes.

Gross Pathological Findings

At autopsy, marked dehydration, pallor, and some emaciation were noted in all four lithium-treated monkeys. One monkey showed some atrophy of the thyroid and edema of the kidneys, but the others showed no remarkable changes. The rest of this report is limited to a review of the ultrastructural studies.

Ultrastructural Studies

The electron microscope observations of various regions of the CNS revealed the following outstanding findings.

The rough and smooth endoplasmic reticulum (RER and SER, respectively) showed various degrees of dilatation of RER in nerve cells and oligodendroglia (Fig. 1), particularly in the cerebral cortex (temporal and frontal lobes), hypothalamus, putamen, and medulla. The dilated cisternae of the RER presented irregular distribution and loss of ribosomes. Some membrane profiles were disorganized and disrupted.

The fine structures of the ribosomes appeared, at times, well preserved (Fig. 2A) but at other times showed various degrees of disorganization with irregular patterns of distribution and variable degrees of reduction. In some instances, such as in Fig. 2B, these changes were considered compatible with chromatolysis of the Nissl substance. In these instances, mitochondria were also severely affected, as is described in more detail in the following paragraphs.

The Golgi complex frequently showed unusual patterns of distribution. In a number of neurons in the hypothalamus, it occupied a large extension of the perikaryon, and the canaliculi assumed a multiconcentric pattern (Fig. 3A). In addition, quite often the canalicular profiles were undergoing disorganization and dissolution of the membrane structures in the neurons of various anatomotopographic regions of the brain (Fig. 3B). In these circumstances irregular distribution and pleomorphism of mitochondria or pleometabolosomes (PMS), multivesicular bodies, and lysosomes were apparent (Fig. 4A–C).

Furthermore, the PMS showed numerical variations (Fig. 5A–D) in the cellular constituents of the cerebral cortex, basal ganglia, hypothalamus, and neuropil. In addition, in several locations, they presented pronounced changes of the membranes (Fig. 5E). Still in other occasions intramitochondrial inclusions were detected (Figs. 4A and 5E).

Lysosomes and lipofuscin pigment appeared frequently associated. In these conditions they showed variations in number and pleomorphism (Fig. 6A–F). Various amounts of lipofuscin pigment were found in neurons in the basal ganglia, thalamus, and frontal and temporal lobes. Their size and shape were usually irregular but delimited by a definite membrane. Lysosomes with crystalloid inclusions were encountered in the cellular constituents of the globus pallidus (Fig. 6B and C).

Lipofuscin in various stages of metamor-

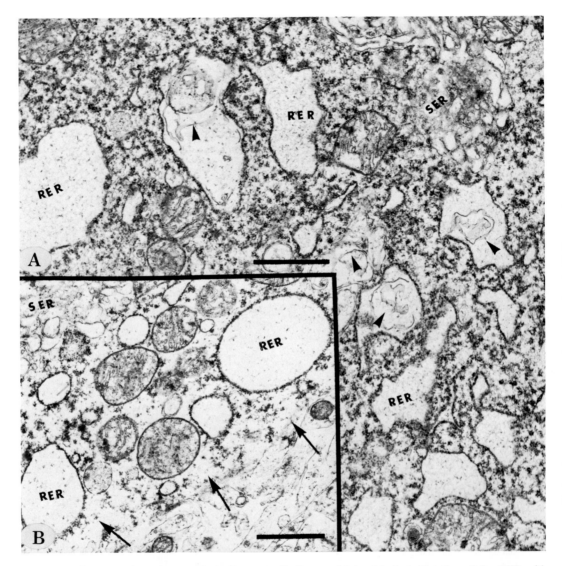

FIG. 1. Lithium-treated monkey no. 2. **A:** Putamen. **B:** Temporal lobe. Marked dilatation of the RER with irregular distribution of ribosomal fine structures and membranous changes within the cisternae of the RER (*short arrows*). Uranyl acetate and lead citrate. **A:** ×27,540; **B:** ×25,200. Scale = 1 μm. Long arrows, depletion of ribosomal fine structures.

phosis, from densely osmiophilic masses (Fig. 6A) or finger-print like (Fig. 6E and F) through particulate and granular type (Fig. 7A and B) to small vesicular (Fig. 7A and B) and multivacuolated or fenestrated features (Fig. 7C), were found in variable amounts in different cellular constituents of the CNS, but particularly in the cerebral cortex (Fig. 6E and F), thalamus (Fig. 7A and B), and cerebellum (Fig. 7C).

Many presynaptic terminals contained variable amounts of synaptic vesicles of the spherical or C (cholinergic) and dense core (monoaminergic) types. C type vesicles displayed remarkable variations in size and shape as well as dilatations and evacua-

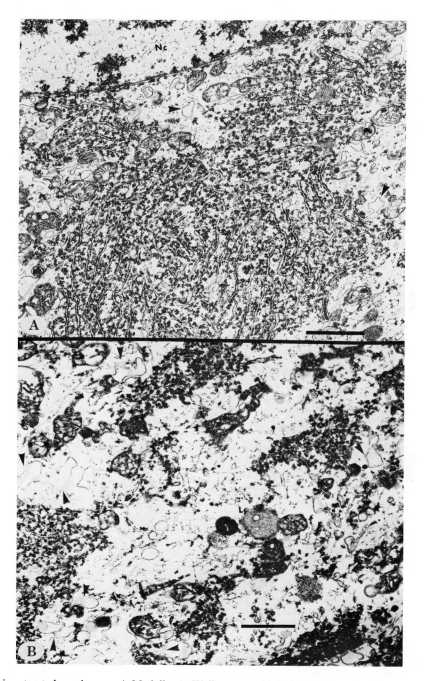

FIG. 2. Lithium-treated monkey no. 4. Medulla. **A:** Well-preserved Nissl bodies in the perikaryon. **B:** Marked disorganization of Nissl bodies with focal loss of ribosomal fine structures. Note also some membrane changes of the endoplasmic reticulum (*short arrows*) similar to those described in Fig. 1B. Uranyl acetate and lead citrate. **A:** ×28,100; **B:** ×26,200. Nc, nucleus; Lf, lipofuscin pigment.

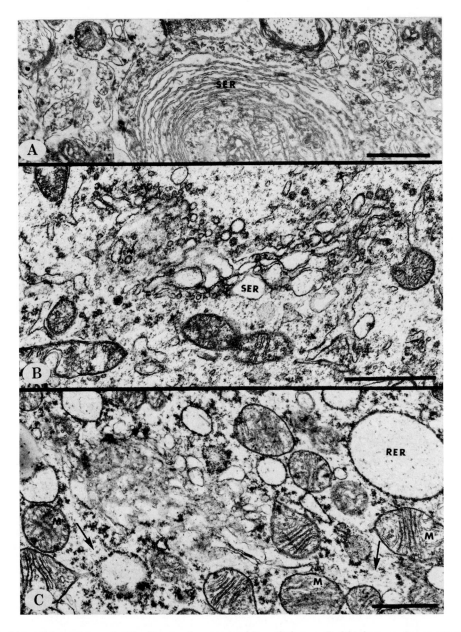

FIG. 3. Li-treated monkeys. **A:** Monkey no. 4; neuron of hypothalamus. **B:** Monkey no. 1; neuron of hypothalamus. **C:** Monkey no. 1; neuron of temporal lobe. Various degrees of fine structural changes of the Golgi complex, i.e., from some moderate proliferation to severe disorganization and disintegration of the canalicular system. Uranyl acetate and lead citrate. **A:** ×29,200; **B:** ×40,200; **C:** ×28,600. Long arrows, loss of ribosomal fine structures; M, mitochondria.

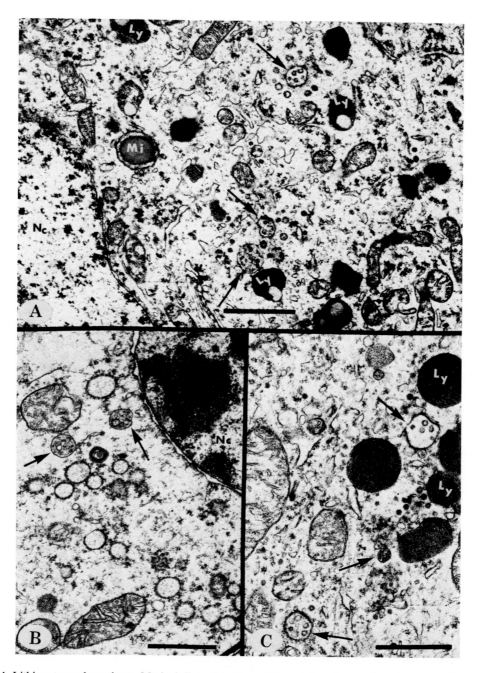

FIG. 4. Lithium-treated monkeys. Marked disorganization of the rough and smooth components of the endoplasmic reticulum, and loss of ribosomal fine structures. Note also pleomorphism of the organelles, including the presence of several multivesicular bodies (*long arrows*). **A:** Neuron of the hypothalamus, monkey no. 1. **B:** Oligodendroglia of hypothalamus, monkey no. 1. **C:** Neuron of the temporal lobe, monkey no. 2. Uranyl acetate and lead citrate. **A:** ×26,700; **B:** ×29,200; **C:** ×26,200. Ly, Lysosomes; Mi, mitochondrial inclusion.

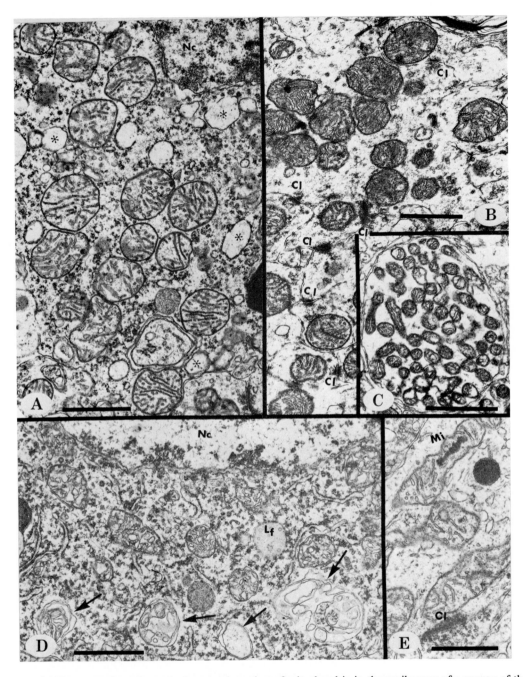

FIG. 5. Lithium-treated monkeys. **A:** Increased number of mitochondria in the perikaryon of a neuron of the caudate nucleus, monkey no. 2. **B:** In neuropil, monkey no. 2. **C:** In unmyelinated axon of the hypothalamus, monkey no. 1. **D:** Increased number and pleomorphism of mitochondria in a neuron of the temporal lobe, monkey no. 4. **E:** Note in particular abnormal membrane changes of organelles (*arrows*) and a mitochondrial inclusion (Mi; *upper corner*). Uranyl acetate and lead citrate. **A:** ×28,300; **B:** ×25,100; **D:** ×29,200; **E:** ×27,400. Cl, synaptic cleft; Lf, lipofuscin pigment; Nc, nucleus;*, RER.

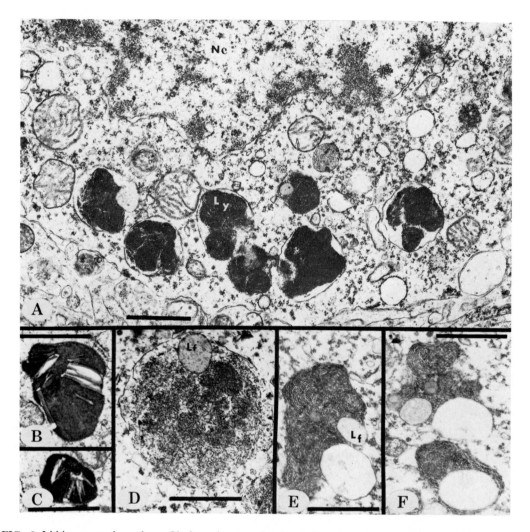

FIG. 6. Lithium-treated monkeys. Various degrees of qualitative and quantitative changes of lysosomes. **A:** Perikaryon, caudate nucleus, monkey no. 2. **B** and **C:** Lysosomes with crystalloid inclusions, globus pallidus, monkey no. 1. **D:** Cytolysosome associated with lipofuscin pigment (Lf) thalamus, monkey no. 4. **E** and **F:** Note in particular fingerprint-like features associated with lipofuscin pigment in a neuron of the temporal lobe, monkey no. 4. Uranyl acetate and lead citrate. **A:** ×25,700; **B–F:** ×29,200.

tion of their content as surmized from their translucid appearance (Fig. 8B and C). In some presynaptic terminals, accumulation of a large number of small vesicles with increased osmiophilic and incrustation-like fragmented dots or spikes along its peripheral membrane was also noted. In the basal ganglia, especially in the putamen, several unusually large presynaptic terminals (4.3 μm × 2.5 μm) revealed invaginations of the limiting membrane and a tendency to clumping or packing of the C type vesicles with many dense synaptic clefts (Fig. 8A). In many axosomatic, axodendritic, or axo-axonic types, the synaptic cleft was poorly differentiated or masked by dense osmiophilic material similar to that previously reported in acute experiments (62). At other times the synaptic cleft appeared irregular in shape with variable densities of

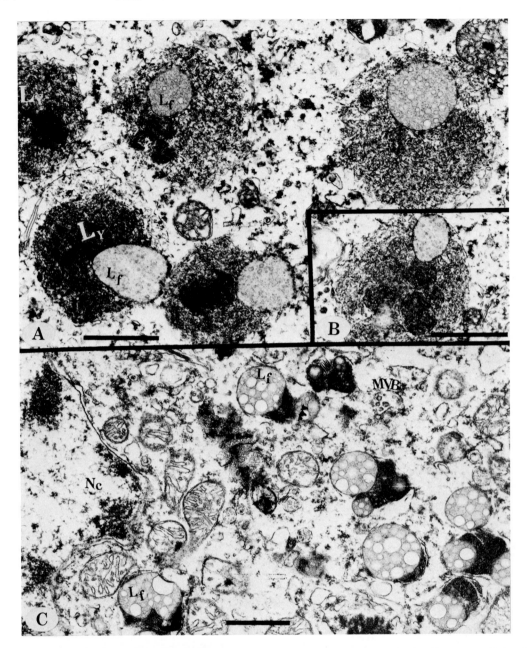

FIG. 7. Lithium-treated monkeys. **A** and **B**: Thalamus; various stages of metamorphosis of lysosomes (Ly) and lipofuscin pigment (Lf) formation, monkey no. 4. **C**: Dentate nucleus of the cerebellum. Note in particular multiple vacuoles in advanced stages of lipofuscin degradation. Uranyl acetate and lead citrate. **A–C**: ×29,200. MVB, multivesicular body; Nc, nucleus.

osmiophilic material. At times the pre- and postsynaptic membranes appeared disintegrated. In some instances dense osmiophilic material diffused to the postsynaptic region. On still other occasions partial detachment or bulging like a hump or splitting of the synaptic junction was noted at the level of the postsynaptic membrane. In

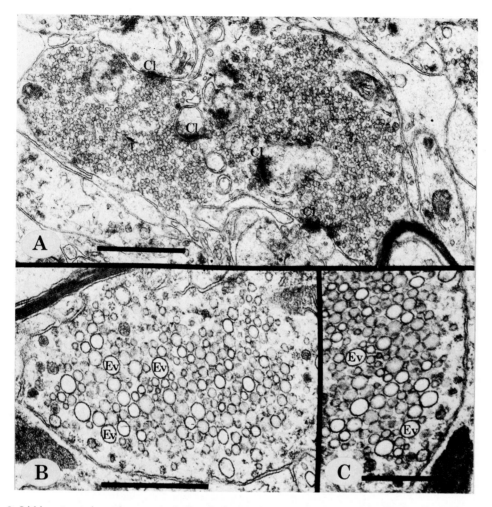

FIG. 8. Lithium-treated monkey no. 1. **A:** Lenticular nucleus; a giant synapse filled with concentrated C type vesicles and serial clefts. **B** and **C:** Hypothalamus showing, in particular, variations in size of C type synaptic vesicles, some of which appear markedly enlarged and evaculated (Ev). Uranyl acetate and lead citrate. **A:** ×29,200; **B:** ×45,100; **C:** ×26,700. Cl, synaptic cleft.

the postsynaptic region, enlarged endoplasmic reticulum and congregations of mitochondria were encountered. In several locations the spine processes were coated with dense osmiophilic material. In addition, dense core vesicles were frequently intermingled with the C type vesicles, particularly in the temporal lobe, caudate nucleus, and hypothalamus. These were presumed to be A type vesicles or neurosecretory granules (Fig. 9A–C). Along the soma or processes of the neurons of the

caudate and dentate nuclei, many small tubular, rod-shaped, or flattened vesicles were found within the presynaptic terminals (Fig. 9C). A significant number of presynaptic terminals also contained various organelles and mitochondria, some of which were undergoing degenerative changes (Fig. 9B and C).

Of particular interest was a moderate number of dense core vesicles ranging from 750 to 1,300Å in diameter. They were encountered in various processes of the neu-

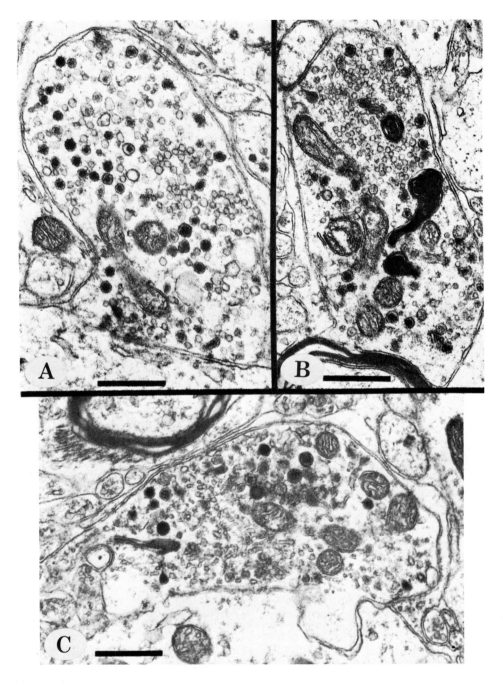

FIG. 9. Lithium-treated monkey no. 1. **A–C:** Hypothalamus, dense core synaptic vesicles showing variation in size and osmiophilia. Note also increased number of organelles, some of which are undergoing degenerative changes, especially **B** and **C.** Uranyl acetate and lead citrate. **A–C:** ×39,200.

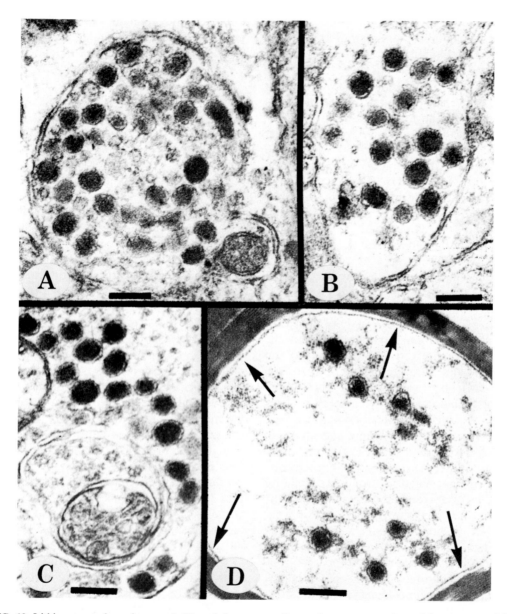

FIG. 10. Lithium-treated monkey no. 1. Hypothalamus revealing various concentrations of dense core vesicles in the neuropil (**A, B, C,** and **D**) myelinated axon containing also a significant number of dense core vesicles. Uranyl acetate and lead citrate. **A** and **B:** ×58,360; **C:** ×60,700; **D:** ×54,300. Long arrows, mesoaxon of myelinated fiber.

ropil (Fig. 10A and B) and myelinated axons (Fig. 10C) of the temporal lobe, pons, and hypothalamus.

No remarkable changes of the myelin structures were encountered. No other unusual structural abnormalities were noted except for some occasional multimembran-

ous or multiple concentric fibrillar structures randomly scattered in the neuropil.

DISCUSSION

Since Dempsey and Meltzer (15) have already reviewed the clinicopathological aspects of the adverse or toxic reaction caused by lithium administration, our discussion is limited only to ultrastructural observations of the CNS.

The most severe and diffuse ultrastructural changes were noted in the monkeys treated with the highest doses of lithium-chloride (200 mg/kg) and for the longest period of time (17 days with 50 mg/kg). The lithium level in the blood varied between 0.07 and 8 mEq/liter. This high lithium level in the blood was detected in a monkey that was treated with 200 mg/kg for a period of 11 days. In humans the highest lithium level in the tissue reported in the literature was 21.4 mEq/liter in a postmortem myocardium specimen affected by myocarditis (81).

Concerning the CNS neurohistopathological aspects of lithium toxicity, we failed to find any reference to such studies in the literature except those of Srebro (75) and Whetsell and Mire (88). In the former (75), periventricular glia and hypothalamic, and adenopituitary neurosecretory changes were observed in microscopic examinations. No other microscopic alterations of the CNS were reported nor electron microscope studies carried out. The second group of investigations concerned mature cultures of rat dorsal root ganglia of the spinal cord. Cellular responses during incubation in lithium media were examined with light and electron microscopes. In all cultures treated with lithium, most neurons developed abnormal cytoplasmic granularity with an appearance suggesting the presence of scattered cytoplasmic vacuoles. Neuronal nuclei became progressively obscured, and an increase in the size of some cells was noted. The time required for the occurrence of this response varied inversely with the concentration of lithium and directly with the concentration of Na. These neuronal changes appeared similar to those observed in cultures incubated with ouabain (strophanthin G) (87), and they were not reversible on removal of the cultures from the lithium media. The most outstanding ultrastructural changes consisted of clusters of cytoplasmic vacuoles arising in the region of the Golgi complex that appeared to replace the usual Golgi configuration.

In some of our observations qualitative PMS changes, as described and illustrated in Figs. 4 and 5, have also been noted with small lithium doses in the distal portion of the nephron and with higher doses in all portions of the nephron of rats (19).

An indirect confirmation of the effect of lithium on PMS is suggested by the experimental demonstration that brain homogenates of mice containing lithium carbonates showed activation of succinate dehydrogenase (1). It is well known that this enzyme is associated with electron transport chain linked to oxidative phosphorylation and that it is related to the function of PMS (29,30,47).

The presence of various amounts of lipofuscin pigment in different stages of degradation and abnormal lysosome metamorphosis (Figs. 6 and 7) may be the result of the combined effects of lithium ions, aging, and nutritional factors (Table 1).

A large number of synaptic terminals displayed qualitative and quantitative variations of the dense core vesicles (A type) in the basal ganglia, brainstem, and particularly the hypothalamus (Figs. 9 and 10). There is common agreement that dense core vesicles represent mainly the anatomical substrate of the catecholamines (27,28, 43,49,50,55,56,60,77) and that the integrity of their limiting membranes controls the processes of exocytosis and endocytosis (40) of these chemical transmitters (77). As a matter of fact, Figs. 8 through 10 illustrate marked variations in size or ballooning, osmiophilic density, and various degrees of thinning, blurring, disruptions, or disintegration of some limiting membranes in both postmortem as well as the sacrificed and perfused CNS specimens. In this report, it is of interest to recall the following clinical and biochemical observations.

Electrolytes as well as norepinephrine

have been implicated in mood disorders (14,15,20,63). There is indirect evidence of a relationship between mania and depression and disorders of amines, particularly norepinephrine (4,10). This is based in part on the observation that two classes of drugs that deplete the brain of norepinephrine (reserpine and alphamethyl—DOPA), acting through different mechanisms, may cause depression in some patients. The imipramine class of drugs and the monoamine oxidase inhibitors (MAOI) have been shown to benefit certain depressions. MAOI have also been found to block the breakdown pathways of norepinephrine, whereas the imipramine type of drug blocks the reuptake of norepinephrine in adrenergic tissue (1). It has been suggested that both classes of drugs increase functional norepinephrine at the receptor sites and that this effect is related to their antidepressant action. Furthermore, clinical evidence (16) suggests that mania and depression are not in all respects opposite, nor may biogenic amines and electrolytes be involved in any simple way (16). Therapeutic efficacy of lithium in mania may in part be a result of an increased reuptake of norepinephrine, with a decrease in norepinephrine available for the interaction with the receptor sites (11).

Interestingly also, lithium increases serotonin uptake into the platelets obtained from mental depressive patients (52) and increases the levels of serotonin and tryptophan in rat brain (58). Umberkoman and Joseph (82) reported significant rise in brain serotonin in mice after a 9-day treatment with lithium. However, Ho et al. (39) showed that prolonged lithium treatment produced a significant change on serotonin levels only in hypothalamus and brainstem, but no significant changes in other regions. The turnover rate of serotonin was slight but not significantly changed by lithium in the whole brain studies. Nonetheless, a significant effect was observed in regional studies. It was also noted that lithium stimulates neuro-

adrenergic cells and increases the uptake of these biogenic amines (68) or ^{3}H-norepinephrine (10) in isolated rat brain synaptosomes (3). Furthermore, chronic lithium pretreatment increases the net uptake (approximately 30%) of norepinephrine by synaptosomes from rat brain. That this effect may be due to lithium directly is consistent with the findings of relatively high concentration of lithium in synaptosomes. The mechanisms by which lithium increases the norepinephrine uptake in synaptosomes is not clear. Several possibilities may be considered. It may: (a) alter the membrane directly; (b) interact with an enzyme and/or (c) transport mechanism; (d) deplete the endogenous norepinephrine levels; (e) affect adrenergic binding site, or (f) interact with cations since they affect amine uptake (36,44,51,66, 67,69).

However, some investigators (45) observed that lithium administration decreased both the norepinephrine and 5-hydroxytryptamine content in synaptosomes, but not in mitochondria or whole brain homogenate. Lithium, according to the same authors, slightly increased the synaptosome uptake of norepinephrine in the presence of MAOI but not in that of mitochondria (45). These findings suggest that there may be a variable relationship between the tissue concentration and synthesis pathways of monoamines under both normal and lithium conditions. Furthermore, Ho and co-workers (39) concluded that the observed differences in the action of lithium on monoamines in different regions of the CNS may be related to the morphology of these "discrete areas."

Lithium treated rats also showed a marked increase in the intensity of Alcian blue staining around blood vessels, cell membranes, and nuclear membranes (85), indicating the presence of increased amounts of acid mucopolysaccharides, increased availability of carboxyl groups for dye binding, or increased dye binding due to conformational changes in the anionic polymers associated with increased hydration (6). These observations are of particular significance since it has been established (42) that the CNS mucopolysaccharides contain neuramic acid (42) and that the neuramic acid is implicated in the binding of biogenic amines (31).

CONCLUDING REMARKS

The review of the pertinent literature on lithium therapy and our experimental investigations revealed that lithium salts, like other neuropsychotropic agents (phenothiazines, antidepressants, stimulants), displayed multiple loci or targets of interaction. Adverse and toxic reactions predominantly involve the kidneys, electrolyte homeokinesis, thyroid, CNS, gastrointestinal system, and myocardium.

Ultrastructural examinations disclosed marked dilatation and fine morphological changes of the endoplasmic reticulum (both the rough and smooth components), including Golgi vesicles and vacuoles, and multivesicular bodies. These might be related to the accumulation of lithium ions and H_2O at the sodium pump sites along the Golgi membrane.

Marked numerical variations, pleomorphism, swelling, and membrane changes of mitochondria were noted in acute and subchronic experimental investigations. Significantly, Li influenced the membrane metabolism and the electron transport chain linked to oxidative phosphorylation.

Lysosomal changes were noted particularly in areas associated with lipofuscin formation. These features were noted particularly in old monkeys. Consequently, they may be the combined end result of lithium, aging, and possibly some nutritional cofactors.

Of particular interest in the CNS are the quantitative variations of the contents of the presynaptic terminals and especially synaptic vesicles. Marked concentration of the spherical or C type vesicles was observed in the temporal lobe, basal ganglia, and hypothalamus. The dense core vesicles showed marked quantitative changes in the hypothalamus and mesencephalon. In the former areas focal concentrations and variations in size and osmiophilic content of the dense core vesicles were also evident in various cellular processes of the neuropil and some myelinated axons.

The majority of multidisciplinary studies indicate that the adverse and toxic reactions of lithium salts are determined principally by the interaction of lithium salts with the physicochemical homeokinesis of the intra-extracellular electrolytes Na, K, Ca, and possibly Mg (26,57). This in turn depends also on the morphochemical integrity of the membranes of the cellular and ultracellular structures. Concerning the latter, it should be recalled that the membrane systems: (a) compartmentalize the structural organization of the organelles, which are endowed with characteristic functional and metabolic properties, (b) maintain an orderly arrangement of some of the enzyme assemblies, (c) channel the intermediary metabolites or histometabolic processes, and (d) regulate the ionic flux (active and passive transport). Consequently, the alterations of the molecular integrity of the cellular membranes of the endoplasmic reticulum (particularly of the Golgi complex) and organelles (including their subunits) may result in concomitant changes of their metabolic and functional correlates. Further elucidation of the structural and physicochemical correlates is needed.

ACKNOWLEDGMENTS

The author gratefully acknowledges the assistance and cooperation of J. C. Liu, K. M. Wu, and S. Avrin for electron microscopy procedures, V. Bystron for illustrations, W. Rivers for bibliography, and Helen Simpson for secretarial work.

REFERENCES

1. Abreu, L. A., and Abreu, R. R. (1972): Activation of brain succinate dehydrogenase by lithium. *Nature* [*New Biol.*], 236:254–255.
2. Baer, L., Glassman, A. H., and Kassir, S. (1973): Negative sodium balance in lithium carbonate toxicity. Evidence of mineral corticoid blockade. *Arch. Gen. Psychiatry*, 29:823–827.
3. Baldessarini, R. J., and Stephens, J. J. (1970): Lithium carbonate for affective disorders. *Arch. Gen. Psychiatry*, 22:72–77.
4. Bogdanaski, D. F., and Brodie, B. B. (1966): Role of sodium and potassium ions in storage of norepinephrine by sympathetic nerve endings. *Life Sci.*, 5:1563–1569.
5. Cade, J. F. J. (1949): Lithium salts in the treatment of psychotic excitement. *Med. J. Aust.*, 36:349–352.
6. Cejkova, J., and Brettschneider, I. (1969): The effect of hydration of the rabbit cornea on the histochemical demonstration of acid mucopolysaccharides. *Histochemie*, 17:327–336.
7. Chapman, A. J., and Lewis, G. (1972): Iatrogenic lithium poisoning: A case report with necropsy findings. *Oklahoma State Med. J.*, 65:491–494.
8. Cleaveland, S. A. (1913): A case of poisoning by lithium, presenting some new features. *JAMA*, 60:722.
9. Cohen, W. J., and Cohen, N. H. (1974): Lithium carbonate, haloperidol, and irreversible brain damage. *JAMA*, 230:1283–1287.
10. Colburn, R. W., Goodwin, F. K., Bunney, W. E., Jr., and Davis, J. M. (1967): Effect of lithium on the uptake of noradrenaline by synaptosomes. *Nature*, 215:1395–1397.
11. Colburn, R. W., and Maas, J. W. (1965): Adenosine triphosphate-metal norepinephrine ternary complexes and catecholamine binding. *Nature*, 208:37–41.
12. Corcoran, A. C., Taylor, R. D., and Page, I. H. (1949): Lithium poisoning from the use of salt substitutes. *JAMA*, 139:685–688.
13. Degkwitz, R., Consbruch, U., Haddenbrock, S., Neusch, B., Oehlert, W., and Unsöld, R. (1976): Therapeutische Risiken bei der Langzeitbehandlung mit Neuroleptike und Lithium. *Nervenarzt*, 47:81–87.
14. Delgado, J. M. R., and DeFeudis, F. V. (1969): Effects of lithium injections into the amygdala and hippocampus of awake monkeys. *Exp. Neurol.*, 25:255–267.
15. Dempsey, M. G., and Meltzer, M. L. (1977): Lithium toxicity: A review. In: *Neurotoxicology*, edited by L. Roizin, H. Shiraki, and N. Grčević. (*This volume.*)
16. Ebadi, M. S., Simmons, V. J., Hendrickson, M. J., and Lacy, P. S. (1974): Pharmacokinetics of lithium and its regional distribution in rat brain. *Eur. J. Pharmacol. Toxicol.*, 27:324–329.
17. Edelfors, S. (1975): Distribution of sodium, potassium and lithium in rat brain of lithium-treated rats. *Acta Pharmacol. Toxicol.*, 37:387–392.
18. Erwin, C. W., Gerber, C. J., Morrison, S. D., and James, J. F. (1973): Lithium carbonate and convulsive disorders. *Arch. Gen. Psychiatry*, 28:646–648.
19. Evan, A. P., and Ollerich, D. A. (1972): The effect of lithium carbonate on the structure of the rat kidney. *Am. J. Anat.*, 134:97–106.
20. Fieve, R. R. (1970): Clinical controversies and theoretical mode of action of lithium carbonate. *Int. Pharmacopsychiatry*, 5:107–118.
21. Foulks, J., Mudge, G. H., and Gilman, A. (1952): Renal excretion of cation in the dog during infusion of isotonic solutions of lithium chloride. *Am. J. Physiol.*, 168:642–649.
22. Francis, R. I., and Traill, M. A. (1970): Lithium distribution in the brains of two manic patients. *Lancet*, 11:523–524.
23. Franklin, L. M. (1974): Thyrotoxicosis developing during lithium treatment: Case report. *New Zealand Med. J.*, 79:782.
24. Freyhan, F. A. (1970): Lithium: Some critical considerations. *Int. Pharmacopsychiatry*, 5:77–79.
25. Gabriel, E., Karobath, M., and Lenz, G. (1976): Extrapyramidale Symptomatik bei Kombination der Lithium-Langzeittherapie mit Nortriptylin. *Nervenarzt*, 47:46–48.
26. Giacobini, E. (1969): The effect of lithium on the nerve cell. *Acta Psychiatr. Scand.* [*Suppl.*], 207:85–89.
27. Gray, E. G., and Guillery, R. W. (1966): Synaptic morphology in the normal and degenerating nervous system. *Int. Rev. Cytol.*, 19:111–182.
28. Gray, E. G. (1969): Electron microscopy of excitatory and inhibitory synapses: A brief review. In: *Mechanism of Synaptic Transmission*, edited by K. Akert, and P. G. Waser. *Prog. Brain Res.*, 31:141–155.
29. Green, D. E., and Fleischer, S. (1962): On the molecular organization of biological transducing system. In: *Horizons of Biochemistry*, edited by M. Kasha and B. Pullman, p. 381. Academic Press, New York.
30. Green, D. E., and Goldberger, R. F. (1967): *Molecular Insights Into The Living Process*, p. 222. Academic Press, London.
31. Green, J. P., Atwood, R. T., and Friedman, D. X. (1965): Studies in neuromanic acid. *Arch. Gen. Psychiatry*, 12:90–95.
32. Greenfield, I., Zuger, M., Bleak, R. M., and Bakal, S. F. (1950): Lithium chloride intoxication. *NY State J. Med.*, 50:459–460.
33. Hanlon, L. W., Romaine, M., III, Gilroy, F. J., and Deitrick, J. E. (1949): Lithium chloride as a substitute for sodium chloride in the diet, observations on its toxicity. *JAMA*, 139:688–692.
34. Hartitzsch von, B., Hoenich, N. A., and Leigh, R. J. (1972): Permanent neurological sequelae

despite hemodialysis for lithium intoxication. *Br. Med. J.*, 4:757–759.

35. Hanus, H., Bily, J., Hametova, M., and Polackova, J. (1972): Rare complications in lithium therapy: Two case reports. *Activ. Nerv. Super. (Praha.)*, 14:105.

36. Hartigan, G. P. (1963): The use of lithium salts in affective disorders. *Br. J. Psychiatry*, 159: 810–814.

37. Heltne, C. E., and Olleorich, D. A. (1973): Morphometric and electron microscopic studies of goiter induced by lithium in the rat. *Am. J. Anat.*, 136:297–304.

38. Herraro, F. A. (1973): Lithium carbonate toxicity. *JAMA*, 26:1109–1110.

39. Ho, A. K. S., Loh, H. H., Craves, F., Hitzemann, R. J., and Gersohn, S. (1970): The effect of prolonged lithium treatment on the synthesis rate and turnover of monoamines in brain regions of rats. *Eur. J. Pharmacol.*, 10:72–78.

40. Holtzman, E., Teichberg, S., Abrahams, S. J., Cittkowitz, E., Crain, S. M., and Kawai, N. (1973): Notes on synaptic vesicles and related structures, endoplasmic reticulum, lysosomes and peroxisomes in nervous tissue and the adrenal medulla. *J. Histochem. Cytochem.*, 21:349–385.

41. Hussain, M. Z., Psych, M. R., Khan, A. G., and Chaudhry, Z. A. (1973): A plastic anemia associated with lithium therapy. *Can. Med. Assoc. J.*, 108:724–728.

42. James, F., and Fotherby, J. (1963): Distribution in brain of lipid-bound sialic acid and factors affecting its concentration. *J. Neurochem.*, 10: 587–597.

43. Katz, R. I., and Kopin, I. J. (1969): Release of norepinephrine-H^3 and serotonin-H^3 evoked from brain slices by electrical-field stimulation, calcium dependency and the effects of lithum, oubain and tetrotoxin. *Biochem. Pharmacol.*, 18:1835–1839.

44. Kline, N. (1968): Lithium comes into its own. *Am. J. Psychiatry*, 125:558–560.

45. Kuriyama, K., and Speken, R. (1970): Effect of lithium on content and uptake of norepinephrine and 5-hydroxytryptamine in mouse brain synaptosomes and mitochondria. *Life Sci.*, 9: 1213–1220.

46. Lavender, S., Brown, J. N., and Berrill, W. T. (1973): Acute renal failure and lithium intoxication. *Postgrad. Med. J.*, 49:277–279.

47. Lehninger, A. L. (1965): *Bioenergetics: The Molecular Basis of Biological Energy Transformations.* Benjamin, New York.

48. Ljungberg, S., and Paalzow, L. (1969): Some pharmacological properties of lithium. *Acta Psychiatr. Scand. [Suppl.]*, 207:68–82.

49. Lund, R. D. (1972): Synaptic patterns in the superficial layers of the superior colliculus of the monkey Macaca Mulatta. *Exp. Brain Res.*, 15:194–211.

50. Lund, R. D., and Lund, J. S. (1972): Development of synaptic patterns in the superior colloiculus of the rat. *Brain Res.*, 42:1–20.

51. Maggs, R. (1963): Treatment of manic illness with lithium carbonate. *Br. J. Psychiatry*, 109: 56–65.

52. Murphy, D. L., Colburn, R. W., Davis, J. M., and Bunney, W. E. (1969): Stimulation by lithium of mono-amine uptake in human platelets. *Life Sci.*, 8:1187–1193.

53. Nielsen, T. W. (1975): Lithium effects on kidney function and ultrastructure. *Psychopharmacol. Bull.*, 11:67–68.

54. Ottosson, J. O. (1969): Introduction. *Acta Psychiatr. Scand. [Suppl.]*, 207:9–11.

55. Pappas, G. D. (1975): The fine structure of electronic synapses. In: *Golgi Centennial Symposium, Proceedings*, edited by M. Santini, pp. 339–345. Raven Press, New York.

56. Pappas, G. D., and Waxman, S. G. (1972): Synaptic fine structure—morphological correlates of the chemical and electronic transmission. In: *Structure and Function of Synapses*, edited by G. D. Pappas and D. P. Purpura, p. 1. Raven Press, New York.

57. Partridge, L. D., and Thomas, R. C. (1974): Effect of intracellular lithium on snail neurons. *Nature*, 249:578–580.

58. Perez-Cruet, J. (1971): Stimulation of serotonin synthesis by lithium. *J. Pharmacol. Exp. Ther.*, 178:325–330.

59. Peters, H. A. (1949): Lithium intoxication producing chorea athetosis with recovery. *Wis. Med. J.*, 48:1075–1076.

60. Peters, A., Palay, S. L., and Webster, de F. H. (1970): *The Fine Structure Of The Nervous System: The Cells and Their Processes*, p. 148. Harper & Row, New York.

61. Rifkin, A., Quitkin, F., and Klein, D. F. (1973): Organic brain syndrome during lithium carbonate treatment. *Compr. Psychiatry*, 14:251–254.

62. Roizin, L., Akai, K., Lawler, H. C., and Liu, J. C. (1970): Lithium neurotoxicologic effects. 1. Acute phase (preliminary observations). *Dis. Nerv. Syst.*, 31:38–44.

63. Roizin, L., Helpern, M., Baden, M., Kaufman, M., Hashimoto, S., Liu, J. C., and Eisenberg, B. (1972): Neuropathology of drugs of dependence. In: *Chemical and Biological Aspects of Drug Dependence*, edited by S. J. Mulé and H. Brill, p. 390. CRC Press, Cleveland.

64. Roberts, E. L. (1950): A case of chronic mania treated with lithium citrate and terminating fatally. *Med. J. Aust.*, 37:261–262.

65. Salomon, M. I., King, E. J., and Gallo, G. (1971): Renal functional damage during the course of lithium therapy (a case report with renal biopsy findings). *Dis. Nerv. Syst.*, 32:483–485.

66. Schou, M. (1967): Biology and pharmacology of the lithium ion. *Pharmacol. Rev.*, 9:17–58.

67. Schou, M. (1968): Lithium in psychiatric therapy and prophylaxis. *J. Psychiatr. Res.*, 6:67–95.

68. Schou, M. (1969): Lithium: Elimination rate, dosage, control, poisoning, goiter, mode of action. *Acta Psychiatr. Scand. (Suppl.)*, 207:249–254.

69. Schou, M., Amidisen, A., and Trap-Jansen, J.

(1968): Lithium poisoning. *Am. J. Psychiatry*, 125:520–527.

70. Schou, M. (1958): Lithium studies. 1. Toxicity. *Acta Pharmacol.*, 15:70–84.

71. Schou, M., Juel-Nielsen, N., Stromgnem, E., and Voldby, H. (1954): The treatment of manic psychosis by the administration of lithium salts. *J. Neurol. Neurosurg. Psychiatry*, 17:250–260.

72. Shinkey, H. S. (1970): Teratogenesis from lithium carbonate. *Ann. Intern. Med.*, 73:336–337.

73. Shopsin, B., Johnson, G., and Gershon, S. (1970): Neurotoxicity with lithium: Differential drug responsiveness. *Int. Pharmacopsychiatry*, 5:170–182.

74. Solomon, K., and Vickers, R. (1975): Dysarthria resulting from lithium carbonate, a case report. *JAMA*, 231:280.

75. Srebro, Z., and Szirmai, E. (1972): Die Periventrikulären Gliazellen und das neurosekretorische System der mit eirner Chinin-Lithium-Salicylat-Kombination Behandelten Ratten. *Acta Med. Okayama*, 26:89–97.

76. Stern, R. L. (1949): Severe lithium chloride poisoning with complete recovery. *JAMA*, 139:710–711.

77. Streit, P., Akert, K., Sandri, C., Livingston, R. B., and Moor, H. (1972): Dynamic ultrastructure of presynaptic membranes at nerve terminals in the spinal cord of rats. Anesthethized and unanesthethized preparations compared. *Brain Res.*, 48:11–26.

78. Thomsen, O. (1969): Renal lithium elimination in man and active treatment of lithium poisoning. *Acta Psychiatr. Scand. (Suppl.)*, 207:83–84.

79. Thornton, W. E., and Pray, B. J. (1975): Lithium intoxication: A report of two cases. *Can. Psychiatr. Assoc. J.*, 20:281–282.

80. Trautner, E. M., Morris, R., Noack, C. H., and Gershon, S. (1955): The excretion and retention of injested lithium and its effect on the balance of man. *Med. J. Aust.*, 2:280–291.

81. Tseng, H. L. (1971): Interstitial myocarditis probably related to lithium carbonate intoxication. *Arch. Pathol.*, 92:444–448.

82. Umberkoman, B., and Joseph, T. (1975): Effect of diphenylhydantoin and lithium on whole brain serotonin sodium and potassium in mice. *Indian J. Physiol. Pharmacol.*, 19:94–97.

83. Vinarova, E., Uhlir, O., Stika, L., and Vinar, O. (1972): Side effects of lithium administration. *Activ. Nerv. Super. (Praha)*, 14:105–107.

84. Vinarova, E., Zamrazil, V., Nemec, J., Vinar, O., and Bednar, J. (1974): Lithium treatment and thyroid function in man. *Activ. Nerv. Super. (Praha)*, 16:198–199.

85. Wagner, B. M., Cooper, T. B., and Kline, N. S. (1970): Structural basis of lithium psychopharmacology. Extracellular ground substance of rat brain. *Int. Pharmacopsychiatry*, 5:208–217.

86. Watanabe, S., and Ishino, H. (1974): Affective disorder and lithium ion. *Seishin-igaku*, 16:1028–1052.

87. Whetsell, W. O., Jr., and Bunge, R. P. (1969): Reversible alterations in the Golgi complex of cultured neurons treated with an inhibitor of active Na and K transport. *J. Cell Biol.*, 42:490–500.

88. Whetsell, W. O., Jr., and Mire, J. J. (1970): Cytoplasmic vacuole formation in cultured neurons treated with lithium ions. *Brain Res.*, 19:155–159.

Neurotoxicology, edited by L. Roizin, H. Shiraki, and N. Grčević. Raven Press, New York © 1977.

Clinical Aspects of Psychotomimetic Drugs

Herman C. B. Denber

Department of Psychiatry, University of Louisville, School of Medicine, Louisville, Kentucky 40201

The first complete description of mescaline was given by Lewin (72), while Heffter (54) made further clinical observations. Hoffman (57) described the accidental psychological effects caused by LSD, and Stoll (108) gave the first detailed clinical description. Earlier studies of both compounds, with some parallel laboratory investigations, viewed them more as a clinical curiosity until the explosion of the drug epidemic in the early 1960s in the United States.

The mass use of these drugs was foreseen by Weir Mitchell (83) and Havelock Ellis (39). Mitchell predicted, "a perilous reign for the mescal habit when this agent became attainable. The temptation to call forth again the enchanting magic of my experience, will, I am sure, be too much for some men to resist after they have set foot in the land of fairy colours where there seems to be so much charm and so little to excite horror or disgust." Mitchell also foresaw the other side of this fairyland when he said, "These shows are expensive. For two days I had a headache and for one a smart attack of gastric distress. . . . The experience however was worth one such headache and indigestion, but was not worth a second," a view shared by Havelock Ellis (39).

Although my original work was done with mescaline (30a–30c, 31a–31c) when such studies were still within the realm of experimental possibilities, at this time in history (1976), the use of psychotomimetic compounds for clinical research is fraught with much danger. Grinker (51) a decade ago was already categorical when he said that, "the drugs are indeed dangerous even when used under the best of precautions and conditions." There is little evidence for such a pessimistic view, even in 1976. However, severe restrictive regulations in most countries on the use of so-called hallucinogenic drugs, under experimental or other conditions, have more or less stopped any meaningful research in this area. It would appear that a very valuable potential tool for experimental investigation of the psychoses has been lost (82). This is unfortunate.

Some dispute a relationship between the drug-induced state and mental illness (38,94), but Behringer (11), DeShon et al. (33), Delay (28), Morselli (84), Bowers and Freedman (16), Keeler and Reifler (66), and Ludwig (75) maintain that there is a resemblance between them. Bleuler (13) was categorical in his opposition to the possible relationship, when he said, "It must be stressed that the psychopathologic picture resulting from the administration of lysergic acid diethylamide and other phantastic drugs does not correspond to the usual picture presented by schizophrenics." Furthermore, "lysergic acid diethylamide or other phantastic drugs do not induce schizophrenia."

My own observations in 350 cases[1] indi-

---

[1] Psychotic patients in remission at the Manhattan State Hospital (Research Division) studied between 1953–1960.

cate a similarity between the experimentally-induced psychotic state (mescaline) and schizophrenia. This in no way however implies identity or even equivalence, for one cannot equate any disorder to schizophrenia since its etiology is unknown.

Further clinical research would seem to be warranted and justified if we are ever to gain the maximum yield from the drug-induced model of the endogenous psychosis.

There is some agreement that the action of LSD and mescaline are similar (41,95b, 111) with perhaps variations of a pharmacological and clinical nature. Thus, for purposes of this review, and because of my own work in the field with mescaline, I will concentrate here mostly on the studies with this drug.

A great deal of the earlier interest centered on the therapeutic activity of LSD (1a,1b,3,4,29,43,48,71b,73,77,78,92,95a, 95c,95d,96,99,105,115) and mescaline (31a,45,60). Later studies after the drug pandemic were oriented more to the toxic and long-term effects.

The clinical response to mescaline and LSD has been the subject of many reports (16,30a–30c,35,46,61,68,70,77,91).

The number of subjects who have used psychotomimetic drugs[2] during the past 15 years will probably never be known although the number of chronic "acid heads" must be small (12). When studied in normals for long-term psychological effects, the results were inconclusive (80). In spite of the apparent toxicity, peyote used by the Navajo Indians in their religious ceremonies did not carry any morbidity and is regarded as "powerful and beneficial medicine" (10).

Under carefully controlled conditions, the incidence of abnormal (toxic) reactions is low (23b,79), and an important consideration in psychotomimetic drug-use

toxicity is the relevant role of the drug as well as concomitantly used drugs and a previous personality disorder (55).

Much of the illicitly available drugs contain many contaminants that may indeed be the basis of the abnormal reactions. Ungerleider et al. (113,114), Blumenfield and Glickman (15), and the Committee on Alcohol and Drug Dependence, AMA (27), have emphasized the potential dangers of these drugs, but Cohen (23b) and Cohen and Ditman (24a) gave a more balanced view of the situation indicating that with proper safeguards, LSD remained an important investigational instrument.

ABNORMAL AND TOXIC REACTIONS TO PSYCHOTOMIMETIC DRUGS

Prolonged (Psychotic) Reactions

It appears fairly clear that abnormally prolonged or psychotic reactions can occur and usually develop in those individuals with either borderline, emotionally unstable, or prepsychotic personalities (102). The drugs upset the internal biochemical–external environmental balance in individuals who have some possibly genetic defect, and the normal analytic and synthetic processes of personality functioning break down. The underlying assumptions of this review are that such functions are probably subserved through biochemical mechanisms.

Prolonged reactions were noted with mescaline (107), and two were found in this present series, which yielded rapidly to intensive treatment with chlorpromazine. Neuroleptic drugs are the best treatment, although Abramson (1a,1b) has reported that oral chlorpromazine with LSD produced an aggravation of that state. Malitz (76) found that intravenous chlorpromazine aggravated (temporarily) the mescaline-induced state in some patients producing a state of terror. He believed this to be an acute akathisia. These reactions are proba-

---

[2] For purposes of this study, LSD, mescaline, psilocybin, DMT (dimethyltriptamine), STP (diethyl, *o*-methyl amphetamine) as well as pure Δ-9-tetrahydrocannabinol (Δ-9-THC) are included.

bly the result of the patient's difficulty and inability to cope with a flood of traumatic material, which otherwise was repressed. It is highly improbable that this has a biochemical basis, at least if animal data can be extrapolated. The concentration of mescaline in rat brain at 2 hr is 0.004% of the amount injected initially (30d). This amount is incapable of producing any reaction when given as a single dose. Prolonged reactions can occur with LSD, for Fink et al. (42) reported a 2% incidence when the drug was administered to chronic psychotic patients (24a,24b,46,67,93,97). Smart and Bateman (102) analyzed the reactions to LSD and concluded that a single dose can indeed precipitate this prolonged event and the incidence from different studies was extremely variable.

Two of 350 patients in our series receiving mescaline showed a shock-like state 10 min after the 500-mg intravenous dose of the drug. They recovered rapidly without need for any specific measures. Acute panic states that require immediate termination can be observed rarely.

Flashback Phenomenon

Since the psychotomimetic drugs have almost entirely disappeared from the central nervous system (CNS) by 24 hr (30d), it is strange to observe the flashback phenomenon in about 5% of the drug users (14,46,48,90,106). Although many explanations have been offered – biochemical, neurophysiological, dissociated reaction, deconditioning (58), learned reaction, psychodynamic response – there is very little or no evidence to support any concept except perhaps the psychodynamic response. Subjects taking psychotomimetic drugs may find themselves in a similar environmental/psychological set days, weeks, or months later, setting off the same transitory train of events. This is not unlike the naloxone challenge of a detoxified and previously morphine-addicted rat which

goes into a withdrawal even though the addictive state no longer exists. One could speculate that a flashback is a partially derepressed conflict that under the stress of events similar to the LSD session attempts to repeatedly break into awareness. This is accompanied by symptoms signaling the presence of an underlying disorder, and resolution should lead to an elimination of the flashback. There is no evidence at present to support a biochemical basis.

Suicide

Mariategui and Zambrano (77) have emphasized the necessity for very close attention to depressed patients who take LSD, particularly if there is a suicidal risk. Actually, depression is a contraindication to the use of these drugs in psychotherapy or under experimental conditions, although it has been used for such cases. The exact number of patients who have attempted or completed suicide will probably never be known. Suicide can occur during psychotomimetic drug usage (48,66). Cohen (23b) related a number of anecdotal reports derived from a questionnaire to investigators of psychotomimetic drugs concerning patients who attempted or committed suicide while under the effects of LSD. One can argue that these suicides were not side effects but direct drug effects (115).

Homicide

Anxiety is one of the affects that is strongly heightened during the drug session (30b), and its intensity is usually proportional to the underlying conflict. Internalization theoretically can lead to destruction of the subject by suicide, or externalization and projection to destruction of the object that has incurred the anxiety. Thus, it should not be surprising that homicide has been reported under LSD (8,70,88). The exact underlying psychodynamic mechanisms are still unclear.

Can an analysis of events under the drug-induced homicide yield any information relevant to the many homicides taking place daily? In reviewing the few available reports it would seem that in spite of the thousands of doses of psychotomimetic drugs administered over the past 20 years, only a tiny fraction of homicides have occurred. The case histories indicate a prior unstable personality, poor impulse control (70), continued external stress that could neither be integrated nor handled appropriately, and the final defusing with LSD which placed the subject in an open indefensible position operating almost without super-ego control. It is essential to recall that the various serious psychological reactions to LSD might not in fact be due to the drug. Seriously disturbed users could very well project all of their problems on to the drug and any real acting out that possibly could have taken place in a drug-free state now is being attributed to the drug itself (49). This phenomenon is known with side effects due to psychotropic drug usage.

Data from the studies do not support the post-LSD amnesia used in defense of at least one murder case (8), for my observations indicate that the drug-induced state takes place in a clear state of consciousness. Similar observations were made for LSD by Ungerleider et al. (114) and Bromberg (17).

Organic Brain Damage

Do the psychotomimetic drugs produce organic brain damage? The evidence is unclear and poorly documented. The possibility exists, particularly if the user is exposed over long periods of time to many drugs. Cohen and Edwards (25) investigated the problem, but no definitive conclusions could be reached (23c). I have seen at least three patients, one of whom was a polydrug user, the second, of whom had a long history of heroin use with other

drugs and alcohol (he was a "tester"), and the third, with a well-defined amphetamine addiction; all had clinical evidence of organic brain damage (sensorial deficits). It is highly probable that continued use of addicting drugs in high dosages over long periods of time, particularly with the many toxic contaminants they contain, leads to CNS damage. But this still remains to be documented at the clinical level, with adequate laboratory controls and psychodiagnostic tests or through neuropathological studies.

Are There Chromosomal Effects Due to Psychotomimetic Drugs?

An analysis of this aspect of the problem reveals the introduction of sensationalism, poorly based conclusions (63), and appeals to the mass media in the science of the 1960s and early 1970s (44).

Alexander et al. (2), and Irwin and Egozcue (62) precipitated a large body of inconclusive and frustrating studies when they reported significant chromosomal abnormalities in leukocytes of LSD users compared to controls (5–7,9,18,20–22,37, 47,50,52,98,100,101,109,119).

The report by Yielding and Sterglanz (118) in which they found that LSD can bind to DNA (with all of its implications) seemed to provide some firm basis to the various reports of genetic effects. Wagner (116) further confirmed this when he found the same and suggested that "LSD may intercalate within the DNA helix in a manner similar to ethidium bromide causing changes in the configuration of the DNA." He reasoned that it would be the dissociation of the histones from chromosomal DNA that might decrease the internal stability of the DNA helix to an extent sufficient to cause breakage. This dissociation might then render the chromosomal DNA susceptible to enzymatic attack and breakage. Possible experimental errors were indicated by Smit and Borst

(103) when they could not replicate these studies and found that irradiation of DNA with ultraviolet light in the presence of LSD led to a phosphodiester bond breakage. They suggested instead that it was possibly an LSD-25-dependent photodestruction of DNA that was the basis of various reports rather than a true structural change induced by the psychotomimetic drug. Bush et al. (19) studied the binding and circular dichroism of LSD interacting with DNA. They concluded that the circular dichroism data did not favor an intercalation of LSD with DNA but rather a binding outside of the DNA helix, perhaps to the phosphate groups of DNA through an ionic mechanism.

Failure to Confirm

Many workers failed to confirm the preceding studies (26,32,34,36,40,53,59, 60,64,65,74,81,85a,104,110,117).

In spite of the enormous amount of attention paid to the effects of psychotomimetic drugs on chromosomes, no reports are available on the long-term follow-up of the psychological state of babies born of "LSD mothers" (95d). It is obviously a point of tremendous importance, for if indeed LSD or mescaline are "chromosomotoxic," one could suggest that there should be equally deleterious psychological effects. There have been no reports of this nature to date, and one cannot be certain if they are nonexistent or were simply never published.

Overview

Hoffer (56) has reviewed extensively the clinical and laboratory aspects of LSD usage. Although the entire problem was considered by a large group of investigators (1c), it is essential to separate the earlier clinical and laboratory work with the psychotomimetic drugs from those studies that appeared once the drug pandemic was

at its height. It would seem from the carefully documented studies of Behringer (11) and Kluver (69) with mescaline, and Stoll (108) as well as Rinkel et al. (89), De Shon et al. (33), Sandison (95c), Van Rhijn (115), and Leuner (71b) with LSD that these substances have specific properties that rendered them useful in studying experimentally induced aberrations of human behavior in order to make appropriate hypotheses by analogy, with regard to mental disorders. It was only with their sudden discovery by people for whom they seemed a simple solution to their seemingly insoluble personality problems, that the matter became one requiring the attention of public health authorities. The emphasis then shifted clinically from nosology, psychodynamics, and relatedness to mental illness, to the impact on youth, "the acid-head," drug-induced euphoria, the search for "inner meaning," religion, and mind expansion. Clinical toxicity was in the foreground and potential gene lethality predicted. Usage of the psychotomimetic drugs then became so restricted that many investigators simply abandoned further explorations.

One is forced to seek possible alternative explanations for this seeming wide disparity in chromosome-breaking experimental results. The scientific method should leave little room for manipulation of methods or data. Yet, the psychoanalyst could conceive of unconscious structuring of the experimental design so that the results would prove or disprove that the psychotomimetic drugs were indeed dangerous, and thus reinforce the official dictum with regard to their usage. Without any libidinal investment in the final results, it is difficult, unreasonable, and almost impossible to believe that such different findings could be obtained, so that with the same drug, one group reports chromosomal breaks and another cannot replicate these effects.

It is clear in further analyzing the data of the various papers that much of the material on the purity of LSD and dosage was unknown. Yet, the equation was made that LSD equals teratogenicity, carcinogenicity, and etc. Without doubt, one of the most serious sources of error in all of the chromosomal-break studies is an LSD of doubtful purity, with unknown contaminants, taken for ill-defined periods of time, and with an equally uncertain relationship to the gestational period. The nature of the LSD contaminants has never been reported in these studies, and they could very well be of crucial importance. In addition, most LSD users at that time, and now, take many other drugs; the polydrug abuser is the rule rather than the monodrug user.

Little is known about drug interaction phenomena (LSD–mescaline; Δ-9-THC–alcohol; etc.). Indeed Dishotsky et al. (34) concluded that when pure LSD was used, as in medically supervised treatment, 82.9% of subjects did not have any chromosomal damage. The relationship of LSD to carcinogenesis and mutagenesis was equally seen by these authors as being highly unlikely. Their conclusion seems to be the only rational and valid one in all of these studies when they state that "we believe that pure LSD ingested in moderate doses does not damage chromosomes in vivo, does not cause detectable genetic damage, and is not a teratogen or carcinogen in man"—a rational statement applicable to many nonpsychotomimetic drugs.

Obviously, not only LSD but also any pharmacological agent, including aspirin, should be used with much caution during pregnancy, especially during the first 6 weeks and particularly until 3 months have elapsed in the gestation (59). The organizer period must be passed safely, and pregnant women are best treated with less rather than more drugs.

The use of psychotomimetic drugs in clinical experimentation and for therapeutic usage is now all but extinct, and it is highly doubtful that within the present or near future their use will be permitted, except under such severe safeguards that most everyone will be discouraged. I make no mention here of the University Human Studies Committees which take up where the government leaves off. There is no question that some of the earlier work was filled with personal expectations rather than solid experimental observations. But this general review of the work throughout the world shows a theme that suggests some therapeutic activity. It is doubtful if this will ever be proved one way or the other.

It is a sad commentary on our times that one of the most promising research tools used in the quest for an etiology of mental disorder has been virtually eliminated by legislative fiat. The literature on clinical research with psychotomimetic drugs is small for the years 1970–1976, and in time will probably become smaller and then extinct. One cannot help but conclude from this review, as did Grace et al. (50) that "the social debate on the uses and abuses of LSD (and perhaps all other psychotomimetic drugs) be based on what is actually known, from rigorously controlled experiments, rather than from conjecture, insufficient sample size, isolated case histories lacking rigorous controls, and from subjective experiences."

The potential of this research area was perhaps best described by Huxley (61) when he ended his description of the *Doors of Perception* by stating, "For the man who comes back through the Door in the Wall will never be quite the same as the man who went out. He will be wiser but less cocksure, happier but less satisfied, humbler in acknowledging his ignorance, yet better equipped to understand the relationship of words to things, of systematic reasoning to the unfathomable Mystery which it tries, forever vainly, to comprehend."

It could be in this twilight of the 20th century with political power on the wane, and military and executive power in the ascendancy (86), that such insights will be considered dangerous. Psychiatry will thus have to look toward another model for study, and perhaps to consider the fearsome thought that society, in this age in which it sponsors the "right to no treatment," as well as "the right to die," does not fundamentally care to have the door to this mystery unlocked.

SUMMARY

The clinical as well as toxic responses to psychotomimetic drug usage have been described. Some general conclusions have been drawn from this work with reflections of a sociopsychological nature.

REFERENCES

1a. Abramson, H. A. (1960): A. Discussion. The nature of the psychological response to LSD. In: *The Use of LSD in Psychotherapy,* edited by H. A. Abramson, p. 129. The Josiah Macy, Jr. Foundation, New York.

1b. Abramson, H. A. (1960): B. Psychoanalytic psychotherapy with LSD. In: *The Use of LSD in Psychotherapy,* edited by H. A. Abramson, pp. 25–80. The Josiah Macy, Jr. Foundation, New York.

1c. Abramson, H. A. (editor) (1967): *The Use of LSD in Psychotherapy and Alcoholism,* pp. 1–669. Bobbs-Merrill, New York.

2. Alexander, G. J., Miles, B. E., Gold, G. M., and Alexander, R. (1967): LSD: Injection early in pregnancy produces abnormalities in offspring of rats. *Science,* 157:459–460.

3. Alnaes, R. (1964): Therapeutic application of the change in consciousness produced by psycholytica (LSD, Psilcybin, etc.) The psychedelic experience in the treatment of neurosis. *Acta Psychiatr. Scand.* (Kobenhavn), 40:397–409.

4. Arendsen-Hein, G. W. (1963): LSD in the treatment of criminal psychopaths. In: *Hallucinogenic Drugs and Their Psychotherapeutic Use,* edited by R. Crocket, R. A. Sandison, and A. Walk, pp. 101–106. Charles C Thomas, Springfield, Illinois.

5. Assemany, S., Neu, R., and Gardner, L. (1970): Deformities in a child whose mother took LSD. *Lancet,* 1:1290.

6. Auerbach, R. (1970): LSD: Teratogenicity in mice. *Science,* 170:558.

7. Auerbach, R., and Rugowski, J. A. (1967): Lysergic acid diethylamide: Effect on embryos. *Science,* 157:1325–1326.

8. Barter, J. T., and Reite, M. (1969): Crime and LSD: The insanity plea. *Am. J. Psychiatry,* 126:531–537.

9. Bender, L., and Siva-Sankar, D. (1968): Chromosome damage not found in leukocytes of children treated with LSD-25. *Science,* 159:749.

10. Bergman, R. L. (1971): Navajo Peyote use: Its apparent safety. *Am. J. Psychiatry,* 128:695–699.

11. Behringer, K. (1927): *Der Meskalinrausch,* p. 114. Springer-Verlag, Berlin and New York.

12. Blacker, K. H., Jones, R. T., Stone, G. C., and Pferrerbaum, D. (1968): LSD, STP, and marihuana. *Am. J. Psychiatry,* 125:341–351.

13. Bleuler, M. (1959): Comparison of drug-induced and endogenous psychoses in man. In: *Neuropsychopharmacology,* edited by P. B. Bradley, P. Deniker, and C. Radouco-Thomas, pp. 161–165. Elsevier, Amsterdam.

14. Blumenfield, M. (1971): Flashback phenomena in basic trainees who enter the U.S. Air Force. *Milit. Med.,* 136:39–41.

15. Blumenfield, M., and Glickman, L. (1967): Ten months experience with LSD users admitted to County Psychiatric Receiving Hospital. *NY State J. Med.,* 67:1849–1853.

16. Bowers, M. B., and Freedman, D. X. (1966): "Psychedelic" experiences in acute psychoses. *Arch. Gen. Psychiatry,* 15:240–248.

17. Bromberg, W. (1970): LSD-induced amnesia. *Am. J. Psychiatry,* 126:1182.

18. Browning, L. S. (1968): Lysergic acid diethylamide: Mutagenic effects in drosophila. *Science,* 161:1022–1025.

19. Bush, C. A., Pesce, A., Gaizutis, M., and Nair, V. (1972): Binding and circular dichroism studies on interactions of lysergic acid diethylamide with deoxyribonucleic acid. *Mol. Pharmacol.,* 8:104–109.

20. Cohen, M., Hirschhorn, K., and Frosch, W. (1967): In Vivo and In Vitro chromosomal damage induced by LSD-25. *N. Engl. J. Med.,* 277:1043–1049.

21. Cohen, M., Hirschhorn, K., Verbo, S., Frosch, W., and Groeschel, M. (1968): The effect of LSD-25 on the chromosomes of children exposed in utero. *Pediatr. Res.,* 2:486–492.

22. Cohen, M., and Mukherjee, A. B. (1968): Meiotic chromosome damage induced by LSD-25. *Nature,* 219:1072–1074.

23a. Cohen, S. (1960): Discussion. Communication processes under LSD. In: *The Use of LSD in Psychotherapy,* edited by H. A. Abramson, pp. 226–229. The Josiah Macy, Jr. Foundation, New York.

23b. Cohen, S. (1960): Lysergic acid diethylamide: Side effects and complications. *J. Nerv. Ment. Dis.,* 130:30–40.

23c. Cohen, S. (1969): The personality of the user—before and after. In: *Psychedelic Drugs,* edited by R. E. Hicks and P. J. Fink, pp. 76–82. Grune & Stratton, New York.

24a. Cohen, S., and Ditman, K. S. (1962): Complications associated with lysergic acid diethylamide (LSD-25). *JAMA*, 181:161–162.

24b. Cohen, S., and Ditman, K. S. (1963): Prolonged adverse reactions to lysergic diethylamide. *Arch. Gen. Psychiatry*, 8:475–480.

25. Cohen, S., and Edwards, A. E. (1969): Does chronic LSD user risk brain damage? *JAMA*, 204:29.

26. Corey, M. J., Andrews, J. C., McLeod, M. J., MacLean, J. R., and Wilby, W. E. (1970): Chromosome studies on patients (In Vivo) and cells (In Vitro) treated with lysergic acid diethylamide. *N. Engl. J. Med.*, 282:939–943.

27. Council on Mental Health and Committee on Alcoholism and Drug Dependence on LSD and Other Hallucinogenic Drugs. (1967): *JAMA*, 202:141–144.

28. Delay, J. (1959): Discussion for symposium. Comparison of drug-induced and endogenous psychoses in man. In: *Neuropsychopharmacology*, edited by P. B. Bradley, P. Deniker, and C. Radouco-Thomas, pp. 167–172. Elsevier, Amsterdam.

29. Delay, J., and Benda, P. (1958): L'Expérience lysergique, LSD-25. A propos de 75 observations cliniques. *L'Encephale*, 3:1–77.

30a. Denber, H. C. B. (1956): Studies on mescaline. VII: The role of anxiety in the mescaline-induced state and its influence on the therapeutic result. *J. Nerv. Ment. Dis.*, 124:74–77.

30b. Denber, H. C. B. (1958): Drug-induced states resembling naturally occurring psychoses. In: *Psychotropic Drugs*, edited by S. Garattini and V. Ghetti, pp. 27–35. Elsevier, Amsterdam.

30c. Denber, H. C. B. (1958): Studies on mescaline. VIII: Psychodynamic observations. *Am. J. Psychiatry*, 115:239–244.

30d. Denber, H. C. B. (1967): Intracellular Localization of Psychotomimetic and Psychotropic Drugs. Doctoral dissertation, Graduate School of Arts and Sciences, New York University.

31a. Denber, H. C. B., and Merlis, S. (1954): A note on some therapeutic implications of the mescaline-induced state. *Psychiatr. Q.*, 28:635–640.

31b. Denber, H. C. B., and Merlis, S. (1955): Studies on mescaline. I: Action in schizophrenic patients. *Psychiatr. Q.*, 29:421–429.

31c. Denber, H. C. B., and Merlis, S. (1955): Studies on mescaline. VI: Therapeutic aspects of the mescaline-chlorpromazine combination. *J. Nerv. Ment. Dis.*, 122:463–469.

32. DiPaolo, J. A., Givelber, H. M., and Erwin, H. (1968): Evaluation of teratogenicity of lysergic acid diethylamide. *Nature*, 220:490–491.

33. DeShon, H. J., Rinkel, M., and Solomon, H. C. (1952): Mental changes experimentally produced by LSD. *Psychiatr. Q.*, 26:33–53.

34. Dishotsky, N., Loughman, W., Mogar, R. E., and Lipscomb, W. (1971): LSD and genetic damage. *Science*, 172:431–440.

35. Ditman, K. S., Tietz, W., Prince, B., Forgy, E., and Moss, T. (1968): Harmful aspects of the LSD experience. *J. Nerv. Ment. Dis.*, 145:464–471.

36. Dorrance, D., Janiger, O., and Teplitz, R. L. (1970): In Vivo effects of illicit hallucinogens in human lymphocyte chromosomes. *JAMA*, 212: 1488–1491.

37. Egozcue, J., Irwin, S., and Maruffo, C. A. (1968): Chromosomal damage in LSD users. *JAMA*, 204:122–126.

38. Elkes, J. (1959): On the relationship of drug-induced mental changes to the schizophrenias. In: *Neuropsychopharmacology*, edited by P. B. Bradley, P. Deniker, and C. Radouco-Thomas, p. 166. Elsevier, Amsterdam.

39. Ellis, H. (1897): A note on the phenomena of mescal intoxication. *Lancet*, 1:1540–1542.

40. Fabro, S., and Sieber, S. M. (1968): Is lysergide a teratogen? *Lancet*, 1:639–640.

41. Fischer, R., Marks, P., Hill, R. M., and Rockey, M. A. (1968): Personality structure as the main determinant of drug-induced (model) psychoses. *Nature*, 218:296–298.

42. Fink, M., Simeon, J., Haque, W., and Itil, T. (1966): Prolonged adverse reactions to LSD in psychotic subjects. *Arch. Gen. Psychiatry*, 15:450–454.

43. Fordham, M. (1963): Analytic observations on patients using hallucinogenic drugs. In: *Hallucinogenic Drugs and Their Psychotherapeutic Use*, edited by R. Crocket, R. A. Sandison, and A. Walk, pp. 125–130. Charles C Thomas, Springfield, Illinois.

44. Fort, J. (1970): Social aspects of research with psychoactive drugs. In: *Hallucinogenic Drug Research: Impact on Science and Society*, edited by J. R. Gamage, and E. L. Zerkin, pp. 115–123. Stash Press, Beloit, Wisconsin.

45. Frederking, W. (1955): Intoxicant drugs (mescaline and lysergic acid diethylamide) in psychotherapy. *J. Nerv. Ment. Dis.*, 121:262–266.

46. Frosch, W. A., Robbins, E. S., and Stern, M. (1965): Untoward reactions to lysergic acid diethylamide (LSD) resulting in hospitalization. *N. Engl. J. Med.*, 273:1235–1239.

47. Geber, W. F. (1967): Congenital malformations induced by mescaline, lysergic acid diethylamide, and bromolysergic acid in the hamster. *Science*, 158:265–266.

48. Geert-Jörgenson, E., Hertz, M., Knudsen, K., and Kristensen, K. (1964): LSD-treatment experience gained within a three-year-period. *Acta Psychiatrica Scand.* (Kobenhavn), 40:373–382.

49. Glickman, L., and Blumenfield, M. (1967): Psychological determinants of "LSD reactions." *J. Nerv. Ment. Dis.*, 145:79–83.

50. Grace, D., Carlson, E. A., and Goodman, P. (1968): Drosophila melanogaster treated with LSD: Absence of mutation and chromosome breakage. *Science*, 161:694–696.

51. Grinker, R. R., Sr. (1964): Bootlegged ecstasy. *JAMA*, 187:768.

52. Grossbard, L., Rosen, D., McGilvray, E., de Capoa, A., Miller, O., and Bank, A. (1968): Acute leukemia with Ph¹-like chromosome in an LSD user. *JAMA*, 205:791–793.

53. Hecht, F., Beals, R., Lees, M. H., Jolly, H., and Roberts, P. (1968): Lysergic-acid-diethylamide and cannabis as possible teratogens in man. *Lancet*, 2:1087.

54. Heffter, A. (1898): Ueber Pellote. *Archiv für Experimentelle Pathologie und Pharmakologie,* 34:385–429.

55. Hensala, J. D., Epstein, L. J., and Blacker, K. H. (1967): LSD and psychiatric inpatients. *Arch. Gen. Psychiatry,* 16:554–559.

56. Hoffer, A. (1965): D-Lysergic acid diethylamide (LSD): A review of its present status. *Clin. Pharmacol. Ther.,* 6:183–255.

57. Hoffman, A. quoted in Stoll, Von W. A. (1947) (ref. 108).

58. Horowitz, M. J. (1969): Flashbacks: Recurrent intrusive images after the use of LSD. *Am. J. Psychiatry,* 126:565–569.

59. Houston, B. K. (1969): Review of the evidence and qualifications regarding the effects of hallucinogenic drugs on chromosomes and embryos. *Am. J. Psychiatry,* 126:251–253.

60. Hungerford, D. A., Taylor, K. M., Shagass, C., LaBadie, G. U., Balaban, M. A., and Paton, G. R. (1968): Cytogenic effects of LSD 25 therapy in man. *JAMA,* 206:2287–2291.

61. Huxley, A. (editor) (1954): *The Doors of Perception,* pp. 1–79. Harper & Brothers, New York.

62. Irwin, S., and Egozcue, J. (1967): Chromosomal abnormalities in leukocytes from LSD-25 users. *Science,* 157:313–314.

63. Jacobsen, C. B. (1968): Risk of LSD to mothers and fetuses gauged. *JAMA,* 204:28.

64. Jarvik, L. F., Yen, F., Dahlberg, C. C., Fleiss, J., Jaffe, J., Kato, T., and Moralishvili, E. (1974): Chromosome examinations after medically administered lysergic acid diethylamide and dextroamphetamine. *Dis. Nerv. Syst.,* 35:399–407.

65. Kato, T., and Jarvik, L. (1969): LSD-25 and genetic damage. *Dis. Nerv. Syst.,* 30:42–46.

66. Keeler, M. H., and Reifler, C. B. (1967): Suicide during an LSD reaction. *Am. J. Psychiatry,* 123:884–885.

67. Kleber, H. D. (1967): Prolonged adverse reactions from unsupervised use of hallucinogenic drugs. *J. Nerv. Ment. Dis.,* 144:308–319.

68. Klee, G. D., and Weintraub, W. (1959): Paranoid reactions following lysergic acid diethylamide (LSD-25). In: *Neuropsychopharmacology,* edited by P. B. Bradley, P. Deniker, and C. Radouco-Thomas, pp. 457–460. Elsevier, Amsterdam.

69. Kluver, H. (1966): *Mescal and Mechanisms of Hallucinations,* pp. 1–108, Univ. of Chicago Press, Chicago.

70. Knudsen, K. (1964): Homicide after treatment with lysergic acid diethylamide. *Acta Psychiatr. Scand.,* 40:389–395.

71a. Leuner, H. C. (1960): *Die Experimentelle Psychose,* pp. 1–237. Springer–Verlag, Berlin.

71b. Leuner, H. C. (1963): Psychotherapy with hallucinogens: A clinical report with special reference to the revival of emotional phases of childhood. In: *Hallucinogenic Drugs and Their Psychotherapeutic Use,* edited by R. Crocket, R. A. Sandison, and A. Walk, pp. 67–73. Charles C Thomas, Springfield, Illinois.

72. Lewin, L. (1888): Ueber anhalonium lewinii. *Arch für Experimentelle Pathologie und Pharmakologie,* 21:401–411.

73. Ling, T. M., and Buckman, J. (1960): The use of lysergic acid in individual psychotherapy. *Proc. R. Soc. Med.,* 53:927–929.

74. Loughman, W. D., Sargent, T. W., and Israelstam, D. M. (1967): Leukocytes of humans exposed to lysergic acid diethylamide: Lack of chromosomal damage. *Science,* 158:508–510.

75. Ludwig, A. (1970): Discussion of "relevance of chemically-induced psychoses." In: *Psychotomimetic Drugs,* edited by D. H. Efron, pp. 245. Raven Press, New York.

76. Malitz, S. (1959): Discussion. The nature of psychological response to LSD. In: *The Use of LSD in Psychotherapy,* edited by H. A. Abramson, p. 129. The Josiah Macy, Jr. Foundation, New York.

77. Mariategui, J., and Zambrano, M. (1957): Psicosindromes experimentales con los derivados del acido lisergico. *Rev. Neuro-Psychiatria* (Lima), 20:451–474.

78. Martin, J. (1963): A case of psychopathic personality with homosexuality treated by LSD. In: *Hallucinogenic Drugs and Their Psychotherapeutic Use,* edited by R. Crocket, R. A. Sandison, and A. Walk, pp. 112–115. Charles C Thomas, Springfield, Illinois.

79. McGlothlin, W. (1962): *Long-Lasting Effects of LSD on Certain Attitudes in Normals: An Experimental Proposal,* pp. 1–56. Rand Corp., Santa Monica, California.

80. McGlothlin, W., Cohen, S., and McGlothlin, M. (1967): Long lasting effects of LSD on normals. *Arch. Gen. Psychiatry,* 17:521–532.

81. McGlothlin, W., Sparkes, R. S., and Arnold, D. O. (1970): Effect of LSD on human pregnancy. *JAMA,* 212:1483–1487.

82. McKellar, P. (1957): Scientific theory and psychosis: The "model psychosis" experiment and its significance. *Int. J. Soc. Psychiatr.,* 3:170–182.

83. Mitchell, S. W. (1896): Remarks on the effects of anhalonium lewinii (the mescal button). *Br. Med. J.,* 2:1625–1629.

84. Morselli, E. (1959): Discussion for symposium. Comparison of drug-induced and endogenous psychoses in man. In: *Neuropsychopharmacology,* edited by P. B. Bradley, P. Deniker, and C. Radouco-Thomas, p. 185. Elsevier, Amsterdam.

85a. Nielsen, J., Friedrich, U., and Tsuboi, T. (1968): Chromosome abnormalities and psychotropic drugs. *Nature,* 218:488–489.

85b. King, P. and Richards, J. (1968): Accessory nuclei and annulate lamellae in hymenopteran oocytes. *Nature,* 218:488–489.

86. Nisbet, R. (1975): *Twilight of Authority,* pp. 1–287. Oxford Univ. Press, New York.

87. Ostertag, W. (1966): Koffein-und theophyllinmutagenese bei zellund leukozytenkulturen des menschen. *Mutat. Res.,* 3:249–267.

88. Reich, P., and Hepps, R. (1972): Homicide during a psychosis induced by LSD. *JAMA,* 219:869–871.

89. Rinkel, M., DeShon, H. J., Hyde, R. W., and Solomon, H. C. (1952): Experimental schizophrenia-like symptoms. *Am. J. Psychiatry,* 108:572–578.
90. Robbins, E., Frosch, W. A., and Stern, M. (1967): Further observations on untoward reactions to LSD. *Am. J. Psychiatry,* 124:393–395.
91. Ropert, M. (1957): La Mescaline en Psychiatrie Clinique et Expérimentale. Thesis, pp. 1–427. University of Paris.
92. Rosen, I. (1963): Clinical observations on aggression in the treatment of affective disorders with obsessions by the use of lysergic acid and intensive psychotherapy. In: *Hallucinogenic Drugs and Their Psychotherapeutic Use,* edited by R. Crocket, R. A. Sandison, and A. Walk, pp. 136–140. Charles C Thomas, Springfield, Illinois.
93. Rosenthal, S. H. (1964): Persistant hallucinosis following repeated administration of hallucinogenic drugs. *Lancet,* 121:238–244.
94. Roubicek, J. (1958): Similarities and differences between schizophrenia and experimental psychoses. *Rev. Czech. Med.,* 4:125–134.
95a. Sandison, R. A. (1956): The clinical uses of lysergic acid diethylamide. In: *Lysergic Acid Diethylamide and Mescaline in Experimental Psychiatry,* edited by L. Cholden, pp. 27–34. Grune & Stratton, New York.
95b. Sandison, R. A. (1959): Discussion for symposium. Comparison of drug-induced endogenous psychoses in man. In: *Neuropsychopharmacology,* edited by P. B. Bradley, P. Deniker, and C. Radouco-Thomas, pp. 176–182. Elsevier, Amsterdam.
95c. Sandison, R. A. (1960): The nature of the psychological response to LSD. In: *The Use of LSD in Psychotherapy,* edited by H. A. Abramson, pp. 81–149. The Josiah Macy, Jr. Foundation, New York.
95d. Sandison, R. A. (1963): Discussion. Hallucinogenic agents and their general application. In: *Hallucinogenic Drugs and Their Psychotherapeutic Use,* edited by R. Crocket, R. A. Sandison, and A. Walk, p. 55. Charles C Thomas, Springfield, Illinois.
96. Sandison, R. A., Spencer, A. M., and Whitelaw, J. D. A. (1954): The therapeutic value of lysergic acid diethylamide in mental illness. *J. Ment. Sci.,* 100:491–507.
97. Sarwer-Foner, G. J. (1972): Some clinical and social aspects of lysergic acid diethylamide. *Psychosomatics,* 13:309–316.
98. Sato, H., and Pergament, E. (1968): Is lysergide a teratogen? *Lancet,* 1:639–640.
99. Savage, C. (1956): The LSD psychosis as a transaction between the psychiatrist and patient. In: *Lysergic Acid Diethylamide and Mescaline in Experimental Psychiatry,* edited by L. Cholden, pp. 35–43. Grune & Stratton, New York.
100. Singh, M. P., Kalia, C. S., and Jain, H. K. (1970): Chromosomal aberrations induced in barley by LSD. *Science,* 169:491–492.
101. Skakkebaek, N. E., and Rafaelsen, O. J. (1968): LSD in mice: Abnormalities in meiotic chromosomes. *Science,* 160:1246–1248.
102. Smart, R., and Bateman, K. (1967): Unfavorable reactions to LSD: A review and analysis of available case reports. *Can. Med. J.,* 97:1214–1221.
103. Smit, E. M., and Borst, P. (1971): LSD-25 does not intercalate in DNA. *Nature,* 232:191–192.
104. Sparkes, R. S., Melnyk, J., and Bozzetti, L. P. (1968): Chromosomal effect in vivo of exposure to lysergic acid diethylamide. *Science,* 160:1343–1344.
105. Spencer, A. M. (1963): Permissive group therapy with LSD. In: *Hallucinogenic Drugs and Their Psychotherapeutic Use,* edited by R. Crocket, R. A. Sandison, and A. Walk, pp. 61–66. Charles C Thomas, Springfield, Illinois.
106. Stanton, D., and Bardoni, A. (1972): Drug flashbacks: Reported frequency in a military population. *Am. J. Psychiatry,* 129:751–761.
107. Stevenson, I., and Richards, T. W. (1960): Prolonged reactions to mescaline. A report of two cases. *Psychopharmacologia,* 1:241–250.
108. Stoll, Von W. A. (1947): Lysergsäure-diäthylamid, ein phantastikum aus mutterkorngruppe. *Schweiz. Arch. Neurol. Psychiatr.,* 60:1–45.
109. Sturelid, S., and Kihlman, B. A. (1969): Lysergic acid diethylamide and chromosome breakage. *Hereditas,* 62:259–270.
110. Tjio, J., Pahnke, W. N., and Kurland, A. A. (1969): LSD and chromosomes: A controlled experiment. *JAMA,* 210:849–856.
111. Unger, S. M. (1963): Mescaline, LSD, psilocybin, and personality change. *Psychiatry: J. Study Interpersonal Processes,* 26:111–125.
112. Ungerleider, J. T. (1970): LSD and the courts. *Am. J. Psychiatry,* 126:1179.
113. Ungerleider, J. T., Fisher, D. D., and Fuller, M. (1966): The dangers of LSD. *JAMA,* 197:389–392.
114. Ungerleider, J. T., Fisher, D. D., Goldsmith, S. R., Fuller, M., and Forgy, E. (1968): A statistical survey of adverse reactions to LSD in Los Angeles County. *Am. J. Psychiatry,* 125:352–357.
115. Van Rhijn, C. H. (1960): Discussion. Communication processes under LSD. In: *The Use of LSD in Psychotherapy,* edited by H. A. Abramson, p. 227. The Josiah Macy, Jr. Foundation, New Jersey.
116. Wagner, T. E. (1969): In Vitro interactions of LSD with purified calf thymus DNA. *Nature,* 222:1170–1172.
117. Warkany, J., and Takacs, E. (1968): Lysergic acid diethylamide (LSD): No teratogenicity in rats. *Science,* 159:731–732.
118. Yielding, K. L., and Sterglanz, H. (1968): Lysergic acid diethylamide (LSD) binding to deoxyribonucleic acid (DNA) (33203). *Proc. Soc. Biol. Med.,* 128:1096–1098.
119. Zellweger, H. (1967): Is lysergic-acid-diethylamide a teratogen? *Lancet,* 2:1066–1068.

Neurotoxicology, edited by L. Roizin, H. Shiraki, and N. Grčević. Raven Press, New York © 1977.

Hallucinogenic Compounds: Biochemical Aspects

David N. Teller

Department of Psychiatry and Behavioral Sciences, University of Louisville Medical School, Louisville, Kentucky 40201

Why hallucinogens are, why some close structural analogs are not, and why such diverse structures produce such similar psychotomimetic activity is still a puzzle (26,31,36,45,57,58). There is not enough space here to review marijuana, cocaine, amphetamines, and potential endogenous psychotomimetics that may also produce hallucinations. I will try to relate hallucinogen biochemistry and pharmacology to current ideas of dopaminergic involvement in psychotomimesis. There is some difficulty fitting data to this format, but aspects of the dopaminergic hypothesis are encompassed in current theories of schizophrenia, addiction, psychotomimesis, and parkinsonism—excessive dopamine (DA) release or disinhibition of dopaminergic neurons produces behavioral disorganization and stereotyped behavior and exacerbates the symptoms of schizophrenia. In contrast, blockade of postsynaptic receptors for DA reverses such effects. The ramifications of this are drug-induced parkinsonism and the proposal of strong DA receptor blockers for neuroleptics. Compounds that can substitute for DA and stimulate postsynaptic DA receptors can be euphorigenic (apomorphine). Moreover, large doses of L-DOPA, the precursor of DA in the treatment of DA-insufficiency (Parkinson's disease), produce transient euphoria and hallucinogenic effects. These observations fit well into support of the dopaminergic hypothesis.

LSD AND INDOLES

LSD stimulates DA-sensitive adenylate cyclase (60,72). A direct effect of D-LSD on adenylate cyclases associated with DA receptors appears not only in striatum, but also in other brain areas containing dopaminergic terminals, e.g., parts of the limbic brain that play an important role in the psychotomimetic action of D-LSD. The specific antidopaminergic action of neuroleptics that may block the LSD syndrome thus acquires special significance. LSD diminishes DA output in perfusates from the feline caudate nucleus. In the rat striatum, LSD increases the level of adenylate cyclase (13). However, the confused and psychotic states that other dopaminergic agonists (L-DOPA and amphetamine) occasionally cause in man are not identical to those produced by LSD (73). Therefore the stimulation of DA receptors probably does not explain the full psychotomimetic action of LSD, but is likely to be one of several mechanisms. Most investigators (60,72) acknowledge the possible role of serotonergic receptors and note that the general psychotomimetic effect of LSD "may be related to complex interactions of this drug with central receptors for serotonin (5-HT), dopamine, and norepinephrine, rather than a single action on one neurotransmitter system" (72). Dixon (25) suggested that β-adrenergic blockade blocks LSD-induced stereotypy.

Palmer and Burks (46) concluded that some of the central and peripheral actions of LSD and Bromo-LSD (BOL) include relatively nonspecific blockade of adrenergic receptors.

LSD was shown to be antagonized by 5-HT in the peripheral nervous system. However, centrally no tolerance appears as a result of LSD antagonism of 5-HT. For example, 18 hr after the last dose of LSD at 20 μg/kg given every day orally for 30 days, there was a 25 to 30% increase in 5-HT turnover as well as an increase in brain tryptophan and 5-HT (24). Thus, the direct psychotomimetic action of LSD, by competing with or substituting for 5-HT, although once likely, now seems incorrect, since tolerance develops very rapidly to the stereotypic behavior induced by LSD (and to its hallucinogenic activity in man), and still 5-HT responses remain. Furthermore, chlorpromazine (CPZ) blocks LSD behavioral activity but does not modify the LSD-induced increase in 5-HT (40). Moreover, Appel and Freedman (2) showed that the 5-HT effect was not proportional to the LSD level in brain.

A striking pharmacokinetic property of LSD in comparison with other hallucinogens is its short half-life in brain— 7 min (4). It may be actively transported (77). Moreover 20 to 25% of LSD is irreversibly bound *in vivo* and *in vitro* to brain synaptosomes over the range of 5×10^{-9}M to 2×10^{-5}M, binding preferentially in the protonated form (28). The binding is inhibited by hallucinogenic compounds, but not by nonhallucinogens. Prostaglandin E_1 and cyclic AMP increase LSD binding, whereas CPZ inhibits LSD binding. Mescaline at 10^{-6}M has very little effect on LSD binding, whereas *delta*-9-tetrahydrocannabinol (THC) significantly inhibits, as do 5-HT, tryptamine, and the methoxylated derivatives of tryptamine and amphetamine.

Unlike effects observed with CPZ on mescaline uptake (where a higher level of mescaline occurs), CPZ (30 μg/kg) was *not* found to alter LSD uptake (after 130 μg/kg), although the same dose of CPZ attenuated the behavioral effect (2). Similar lack of effect on LSD uptake was found with CPZ from 2 to 20 mg/kg. Yet interaction, which blocked behavioral activity, of a neuroleptic with the psychotomimetic could increase the half-life of LSD from 7 to 15 min (4). Thus, if we examine dose/response of LSD, alone, its effects outlast its presence. If a neuroleptic is given before, the situation is qualitatively inverted —half-life is increased, but the behavioral effects are blocked. Therefore, the brain concentration of the psychotomimetic is a comparator only when one drug is present.

There are two classes of LSD binding sites, one of high affinity ($K_{D1} = 9.0 \times 10^{-9}$M) and one of medium affinity ($K_{D2} = 1.2 \times 10^{-6}$M) (28). The high affinity sites are sparse in synaptosomes—6.4 pmol/g fresh brain tissue. Such sites are, however, twice as concentrated in synaptosomal membranes as in the entire synaptosome, in contrast to medium affinity sites. No significant saturability of binding of LSD to mitochondria or myelin was observed. Further, there was no significant binding of a saturable type to synaptosomes from areas other than cerebral cortex. Therefore, if the binding sites were identical to those producing effects on DA release or DA receptors, one would have expected the high affinity binding to appear primarily in striatum.

If LSD has *direct* activity on so many catecholamine systems, its half-life in brain should certainly be longer than 7 min. For example, LSD increases catecholamine cell body fluorescence in the septal region of rats (17). BOL, which does not pass the blood-brain barrier and is rapidly inactivated, did not have the same effect. These central effects of LSD last 24 hr despite the fact that the drug is totally excreted within a few hours after administration. This suggested that residual action is maintained by changes in the brain metabolism that occur within an hour after the drug is given.

We can probably also exclude 5-HT as a direct mediator of hallucinations, although LSD displaces 5-HT (1), mescaline does not. Peripherally, mescaline has some effects on 5-HT receptors, e.g., vasoconstriction (44). Furthermore, although some amino acids produce behavioral changes reminiscent of hallucinogenic agents, patients given L,5-hydroxytryptophan + the peripheral decarboxylase inhibitor MK-486 showed some improvement in the psychotic state (78). When the medication was stopped, the improvement reversed to the former, deep chronic psychosis. This is also of interest because of the acute effect of LSD in reducing the 5-HT level in the central nervous system (CNS) for which this combination of a 5-HT precursor + its peripheral metabolic blocker would seem to have the reverse effect of raising the central 5-HT levels.

Some of the diverse properties of hallucinogens in different models are results of differential toxicity. Lajtha (39) reviewed the early biochemistry of hallucinogens, the relative rate of metabolism of mescaline and its congeners in comparison with LSD, and the effects of these compounds on brain and liver enzyme activity. He also was among the first to emphasize the problems of equating even the simplest pharmacological measurement of hallucinogens in animals to humans; the LD_{50} of intravenous LSD is 60 mg/kg in mice, but in rats, it is 17 mg, and in rabbits, only 0.3 mg. Unfortunately, animal models of psychotomimetic behavior versus dose or compound are influenced not only by the choice of animal (37), but by strain, dosage schedule (61), time of day (48), and perhaps, even the local pollution level (12).

INDOLEALKYLAMINES

McIsaac et al. (41) reviewed the relationship and history of bufotenine, psilocybin, psilocin, *olioliuqhui,* substituted trypta-

mines, and beta-carbolines (harmala alkaloids). Kang et al. (35) calculated that psilocin and mescaline could assume energetic conformations similar to LSD (see also Baker et al., ref. 6). Molecular orbital calculations show that psilocin and mescaline can form structures congruent with LSD, although these are not the most stable conformers (35). The energy necessary for these structures (although it is less than is needed for hydrogen bonding) might reduce the amount of the conformer present in that shape and account for the relatively low potency of psilocybin and mescaline versus LSD.

Psilocybin is more potent than mescaline, (69) and its fate in the rat has been studied (34). The compound is remarkably stable, as are its isomers bufotenine, dimethyltryptamine, and psilocin. Oxidative deamination and oxidative demethylation of the dimethyl-aminoethyl group play only a minor role in the metabolism of psilocin. The resultant secondary and primary amines do not appear as end-products but are metabolized to 4-hydroxyindoleacetic acid (4-HIAA). After the administration of N-methyl-^{14}C-psilocin, only 4% of the substance is degraded in this manner to CO_2. Up to 25% of psilocin is excreted unaltered, but the main metabolic reactions appear to be conjugations to form hydrophilic substances. As long as 7 days after administration, derivatives of psilocin that were radioactively labeled were still appearing in the urine. In contrast to the rapid removal of mescaline from the CNS, psilocin is still found in the brain after 24 hr, and the concentration is 15.5 μg/g after only 1 min (32). Psilocin therefore enters the brain extremely rapidly (as rapidly as LSD) and is held for a longer period of time than mescaline.

MESCALINE AND PHENYLETHYLAMINES

Mescaline is the most frequently cited phenylethylamine hallucinogen and is usually the reference against which other compounds are measured (74,79). In some ways this is unfortunate, because although mescaline has an older history than LSD or amphetamines, we really do not know much about it. For instance, D-LSD at 0.13 mg/kg reduced the average bar-pressing activity by 50% (3). If this disruption is set equal to unity, then L-LSD, BOL, psilocybin, and *d*-amphetamine are approximately 1/10th as active. Mescaline is 10-fold less active than the second group, i.e., 1/100th as effective as D-LSD.

How mescaline acts as a psychotomimetic to produce hallucinations is still unknown. Early research concentrated on metabolism of the drug. Winter (76) suggested that the assumption that mescaline and LSD acted at the same central receptor (on the basis of cross-tolerance between the two drugs) was unwarranted until the mechanism could be explained. He stated that the results "don't rule out a metabolic basis nor do they confirm the possibility of a metabolic basis." Mokrasch and Stevenson (42) found no correlation between the blood or urine level of mescaline and psychological effects. They felt that the complex excretion curve for the compound's metabolites was due to the autonomic effects of mescaline on blood pressure and renal clearance function. Nieforth (45) reviewed psychotomimetic phenethylamines for the period of 1966 to early 1970, covering syntheses, identification and assay, biological implications, and structure-activity relationships. The oxidative pathway for mescaline in the brain passes through the same intermediate step as for DA, and this pathway can be blocked by disulfiram and iproniazid in the same fashion as the formation of homovanillic acid (HVA) and dihydroxyphenylacetic acid (DOPAC) from DA is blocked.

Prior to this period Denber and co-workers completed a series of clinical and biochemical investigations with mescaline. These have been reviewed elsewhere

(23,47), and by 1967 Denber completed the first subcellular distribution study of mescaline-^{14}C in rat brain (20). His work was later confirmed by Cohen and Vogel (11) and then by Seiler and Demisch (49,50); mescaline has a short half-life in brain. Similarly Korr et al. (38) indicated that the half-life of mescaline-^{14}C in mice was 55 min and noted that motility increased parallel to the increase of radioactivity in Ammon's horn; 6 hr after injection the remnants of radioactivity were concentrated in the hippocampus, while the choroid plexus was essentially free of radioactivity. Meanwhile, mescaline's effects as a motor stimulant had disappeared. Other sites of β-adrenergic receptors – Kupffer's cells, adrenal medulla, and Langerhans isles – were marked selectively after the autoradiographic experiment. In the liver, the radioactivity accumulated in bile ducts around central veins, possibly indicating an excretion route.

Thereafter, Shah (52), *apparently* independently, repeated and expanded upon the earlier work of Denber's group, using mice instead, reporting the subcellular distribution of mescaline-^{14}C in mice in a generalized way. The dose he used was about five times the human equivalent dose of 10 mg/kg, and considerable unmetabolized and unbound material was reported. Such a study suffers from the same design defects as an earlier study of Snyder and Reivich (59) on subcellular distribution of LSD in the monkey (see review by Ehrenpreis and Teller, ref. 27), where doses considerably higher than the LD_{50} were used to enable radioactive measurement. These studies confirmed what had been found earlier by Denber and colleagues – over 80% of the mescaline in the brain is unchanged in the first $1\frac{1}{2}$ hr. (20,65), and the mescaline concentration peaks within the first hr (66). Incubation of rat and mouse brain mitochondria with radioactive mescaline to determine if there was specific transport of mescaline into brain homogenates or brain mitochondria (54) confirmed our earlier results (66); no evidence of transport mechanism or highly specific binding was obtained.

Shah et al. (56) confirmed the earlier clinical and animal findings of Denber and colleagues (18–20,22,23,47) that showed that CPZ, but not haloperidol, injected prior to mescaline, effectively blocks mescaline-induced behavior. Moreover, Shah et al. also could confirm that an injection of CPZ maintains a higher level of mescaline in the CNS of mice and in other organs, whereas haloperidol did not affect the disposition of radioactive mescaline in mice. Shah and co-workers state that "the paradoxical effects of CPZ emphasize that it would be pharmacologically irrational to treat toxicity caused by a compound with a drug that prolongs its stay in the body" (56). I strongly disagree with this particular concept, because CPZ has been shown, *in effective dose,* to be one of the strongest antagonists of psychotomimetics. Furthermore, it is not the concentration in the various tissues of mescaline or LSD or amphetamine that appears important for production of the hallucinations; in the presence of effective concentrations of CPZ or other neuroleptics, the psychotomimetic levels may be raised much higher than those necessary to provoke hallucinogenic activity, yet none is observed. This apparent paradox and its implications have been discussed extensively (20,21,65,66).

In humans, haloperidol is not as effective a blocker of mescaline activity as it is a neuroleptic, in comparison with CPZ (23,47). Moreover, in mice, prior treatment with haloperidol does not disturb the distribution of mescaline, nor does it block the mescaline-induced behavioral agitation (56), which indicates that the level of mescaline in tissues treated with another drug may be misleading for assessment of hallucinogenic potential. The mescaline symptoms appeared in haloperidol-treated mice (which would seem to rule out direct

dopaminergic stimulation by mescaline, since haloperidol is a very potent DA receptor blocker), whereas in CPZ-pretreated mice, the brain and other tissues' mescaline levels rose significantly for hours, yet no symptoms appeared. Therefore, the actual concentration of mescaline in each tissue beyond a certain minimal level, as Denber and I have pointed out, may also be irrevelant to the mechanism of action.

The interaction of mescaline with phenothiazines with regard to effects on behavior, body temperature, and the level of mescaline in various mouse tissues (55,56) are similar to those Denber and I reported for rats (20,21). Speculation that the increased brain level of mescaline after treatment with neuroleptics is caused by stabilization of membranes (55) has also been extensively discussed earlier (20,65). However, this is merely speculation, because the effect of CPZ on urinary pH may modify mescaline's excretion (8,9). Further definitive studies, rather than repetition of the same experiments, are required.

In humans, the mescaline concentration peaks in plasma 2 hr after oral administration. The concentration in the cerebrospinal fluid reaches a peak at perhaps 4 to 5 hr (10). This is in marked contrast to the rapid peak appearance of radioactivity in the rat brain after intravenous administration within the first hr, but also it disappears by the fourth hr. Thus, we can see that the passage of mescaline into the brain is much slower than that of LSD and that CNS levels of mescaline are unrelated to increases in plasma. Oral mescaline has an average half-life of 6 hr in humans. One metabolite, relatively unique after this route, is the nonpsychotomimetic *N*-acetyl mescaline (43).

For man, the significance of this rapid passage out of the CNS was obscured by concern that a metabolite of mescaline was responsible for its action and by the discovery of 3,4 DMPEA (3,4-dimethoxy-phenylethylamine) in human urine. Two metabolic pathways may exist for mescaline (49) in the brain—N-acetylation and oxidative deamination to 3,4,5-trimethoxyphenylacetic acid. Both the N-acetyl mescaline and its demethylation product, N-acetyl-beta-3,4-dimethoxy, 5-hydroxyphenylethylamine, have been found in human urine. *In vivo* another breakdown product is 3,4,5-trimethoxybenzoic acid formed by microsomal enzymes rather than by mitochondrial monoamine oxidase. However, the *major* metabolic pathway of mescaline in the brain is to trimethoxyphenylacetic acid (51).

The distribution of mescaline in mouse brain correlates with that of radioactive LSD in the brain of monkeys, being primarily in the limbic system in basal ganglia. However, Seiler and Demisch (50) very strongly suggested that the metabolism of mescaline causes the hallucinogenic activity, in marked distinction to most of the pharmacological evidence indicating that in the presence of compounds that block mescaline's oxidative deamination mescaline activity is enhanced. For instance, they believe that it is due to the metabolism of mescaline that the motor activity is observed in mice 5 to 8 hr after mescaline administration, perhaps because Seiler and Demisch used a huge dose, 120 mg/kg (~8.4 g/human) or approximately 16- to 40-fold the human dose (51); whereas Denber and I believe that it is the aftereffects of the mescaline having once been present that causes secondary changes in activity. I consider that it is not the presence of the compound or its metabolism that causes the psychotomimetic activity, but rather its effects on cellular structure; when CPZ is administered before mescaline, as our group and others have shown, the level of mescaline in the CNS increases markedly, yet the behavioral effects are completely blocked. If Seiler and Demisch were correct, the mescaline in the CNS would not be metabolized any differently (because the CNS concentration of CPZ is too low to alter mescaline metabolism) than if the blocking agent had not been present at all. Therefore, we still feel that it is the effect of mescaline in passage through the CNS that produces the behavioral disorder.

Shah (53) has shown that 20 mg of SKF-525A/kg, i.p., does not affect mescaline activity in mice, although the metabolic inhibitor does enhance the blockade of mescaline by the weaker psychotropic drugs, promazine and mesoridazine. Thus, Shah has been able to experimentally demonstrate that blockade of methylation, demethylation, or hydroxylation does not affect mescaline activity.

Despite the effort expended in tracing the metabolism of mescaline and the testing of the metabolites for behavioral activity, it appears that after 5- to 20-mg/kg doses, the parent compound is the psychotomimetic. Furthermore, the mescaline analogs dimethoxy- and monomethoxyphenylethylamine are not psychotomimetic in man (29,70,71), although they may have pressor effects common to mescaline and many β-adrenergic blockers (33).

There is other evidence that mescaline may indirectly alter membrane structure; Datta and Ghosh (14–16) incubated brain slices with mescaline and isolated ribosomes, and studied their ability to incorporate amino acids. With up to 10 mg of mescaline per mg of ribosomal protein there was only slight inhibition of the incorporation of C^{14}-leucine, arginine, and phenylalanine. Polyamines (spermine or spermidine) block most of the mescaline inhibition. Goat brain cortex slices treated with mescaline at 5 to 10 mg/g also showed marked decreases in the amino acid incorporating ability by their ribosomes and a decrease in the stabilization of the slices, which released protein, RNA, acid-soluble nucleotides, and ninhydrin-positive materials. This loss of material decreased the ribosomal enzyme activity. The ribosomes, when tested with digestants such as trypsin and ribonuclease, also broke down more rapidly after being obtained from mescaline-treated cortex slices, but mescaline did not directly alter the stability of the ribosomal particles. Such alterations in the stability of ribosomes obtained from treated slices were also found after convulsant drugs (strychnine and picrotoxin). The action of mescaline on slice ribosomal RNA was due to the reduction of hydrogen bonding in the RNA species. However, the concentrations that Datta and Ghosh used were much above those expected in brain after a human equivalent dose of 10 to 20 mg/kg. For example, they used 10 μg/g of brain cortex slices, whereas the level of mescaline present in brain tissue seldom reaches 1 μg/g after 10- to 20-mg/kg doses. I have observed that synaptosomes from mescaline-treated rats are less stable than those from saline-injected controls (63), and prior treatment with CPZ before mescaline, *in vivo*, stabilizes the synaptosomes, so that they do not lose their contents, e.g., norepinephrine (NE), during sucrose gradient centrifugation (27).

How does mescaline act in the CNS? There are many possibilities other than the simple one proposed by Teller and Denber (65). Various neurons in the brainstem of decerebrate cats were examined for response to the depressant effects of mescaline (30). Those responding negatively to NE or DA are the ones that are particularly affected by mescaline. Therefore, the iontophoretic administration of mescaline may prevent synaptic depression after NE or DA, mescaline acting to antagonize the depressant effects of the two neurotransmitters. The acute effects of mescaline have been referred to as "stress" (7,18,19). Mescaline is a β blocker, and single intraperitoneal doses of mescaline (5 to 100 mg/kg) decreased significantly the resistance of male mice to histamine challenge 40 min later (75), but after 2 weeks, a development of rapid tolerance to the acute autonomic effects of mescaline was similar to that shown after LSD.

A general scheme of the neuropharmacological action of various psychotomimetics has been synthesized (73), based on the changes that occur in gross behavior, electroencephalogram (EEG), and reticular formation multiple unit activity. LSD, mescaline, and phencyclidine produce either intermittent or continuous hypersynchrony in the EEG, increase reticular formation multiple unit activity, and produce an inappropriate behavior. In man, the same agents produce changes in affect and perception. Visual perceptions are most dramatically affected (74). Mescaline and LSD are typically associated with various phenomena including distortion of body image and room shapes, but auditory hallucinations are generally absent. A second group of compounds, essentially CNS stimulants such as cocaine or amphetamine, when taken in large doses, are associated with a different syndrome. After these stimulants, a paranoid psychotic ideation is most prominent, although some hallucinations of threatening type have been noted. This second group of compounds induce stereotyped behavior and a desynchronized EEG in cats. Similar effects were observed on the EEG and arousal after L-DOPA in rabbits and cats. Amphetamine, cocaine, and L-DOPA induce common behavioral and EEG changes in cats that differ from the effects reported after certain other psychotomimetic agents (73).

Depending upon the research interest, mescaline's properties are interpreted according to the model, rather than determining whether the mescaline effects are independent and irrelevant to the model. If one studies each drug in a group, marked differences in activity stand out well — psilocybin (25 mg/kg) and amphetamine (2 mg/kg) increased ^{3}H-normetanephrine after ^{3}H-NE had been injected intracisternally (62). Mescaline (25 mg/kg) had a biphasic effect—first it increased ^{3}H-deaminated catechol metabolites, but after $1\frac{1}{2}$ to 4 hr, it markedly increased normetanephrine. Stolk et al. (62) conclude that there may be specific and peculiar mechanisms of action for each of the psychotomimetic drugs, although "an imbalance between central noradrenergic and serotonergic function remains viable" as a hypothesis dating back to 1963 (7).

A possibility to describe mescaline's activity in terms of the dopaminergic hypothesis appears remote: mescaline may release noradrenergic inhibition of dopaminergic pathways by locally depleting NE from inhibitory neurons. Mescaline does not appear to be blocked as well by "pure" DA blockers (haloperidol) as by mixed antiadrenergic-dopaminergic agents (CPZ) and is markedly enhanced by small doses of adrenergic stimulants (amphetamine). However, insufficient pharmacokinetic analyses of human brain capability to utilize Phe or Tyr *in vivo* (5) and the lack of knowledge regarding relative pool size and source of catecholamine precursors in human brain areas suggest that we lack some ability to directly extrapolate from animals to man with regard to hallucinogen biochemical pharmacology. Nonetheless, Teller and Denber noted that serum Phe in fasting humans was depleted by mescaline (64). If rapid conversion of peripheral Phe to Tyr is used to restore catecholamines, and as shown elsewhere, mescaline rapidly releases NE (27,62) and then stimulates NE uptake (10a), it could be that such apparently unrelated observations may be presumptuously organized towards a general synthesis of the hallucinogen's biochemical pharmacology. First, mescaline causes destabilization of the vesicular and presynaptic membrane, leading to rapid release of NE. Second, stimulation of NE uptake occurs to replace NE stores, coupled with increased conversion of Phe to Tyr to NE via DA. This rapid appearance of DA might be responsible for the psychotomimetic effects. The postulated utilization of Phe for DA, NE, and epinephrine synthesis may be responsible for the general fall in blood amino acids (23), particularly of Phe, observed peripherally (64). Rat plasma amino acids are also affected by hallucinogens (67,68).

As with LSD, although mescaline's activity is slower in onset, its behavioral effects outlast its presence in the brain. Unlike LSD, it does not appear to have high affinity binding sites, nor does it have much of an effect on 5-HT, and mescaline is very poorly and slowly taken up into brain, so that whole body dose comparisons with LSD or amphetamines (which are taken up very well into the CNS) are totally misleading.

SUMMARY

Within this restricted space it can be seen that although LSD-induced hallucinogenic activity can be explained via dopaminergic mechanisms, that which is induced by mescaline cannot. Further, the marked differences between LSD and mescaline or psilocybin in uptake rate into the CNS, binding affinities, effects on 5-HT, and clearance from the CNS militate against holistic comprehensive theories of hallucinogenic mechanisms. In part, these differences may be only apparent due to incomplete knowledge, and thus they suggest further comparative work. However, analyses of biochemical effects of THC, amphetamine, and potential endogenous psychotomimetic compounds also indicate discrete modes of action, variable degrees of tolerance development, and specific interactions with biorhythms or strains, in addition to those differences noted to occur between LSD and mescaline or psilocybin which were reviewed here. Therefore, despite the utility of the dopaminergic hypothesis in broad clinical areas, present knowledge of biochemical aspects of hallucinogenic compounds indicates that there may be some mechanisms of disordered thought and affect that are tangential or unrelated to dopaminergic activity.

REFERENCES

1. Alivisatos, S. G. A., Unger, F., Seth, P. K., Georgiu, D. C., and Geroulis, A. J. (1971): Subcellular localization and specificity of binding of serotonergic receptors in the CNS. A method for binding 5HT to its receptor molecule for characterization of the *in vivo* interaction. *Proc. 2nd Natl. Mtg. Am. Soc. Neurochem.*, Trans. 2:55.

2. Appel, J. B., and Freedman, D. X. (1964): Chemically-induced alterations in the behavioral effects of LSD-25. *Biochem. Pharmacol.*, 13:861–869.

3. Appel, J. B., and Freedman, D. X. (1965): The relative potencies of psychotomimetic drugs. *Life Sci.*, 4:2182–2186.

4. Axelrod, J., Brady, R. O., Witkop, B., and Evarts, E. V. (1967): The distribution and metabolism of lysergic acid diethylamide. *Ann. NY Acad. Sci.*, 66:435–444.

5. Bagchi, S. P., and Zarycki, E. P. (1975): Catecholamine formation in brain from phenylalanine and tyrosine – effects of psychotropic drugs and and other agents. *Biochem. Pharmacol.*, 24:1381–1390.

6. Baker, R. W., Chothia, C., Pauling, P., and Weber, H. P. (1972): Molecular structure of LSD. *Science*, 178:614–615.

7. Barchas, J. D., and Freedman, D. X. (1963): Brain amines: Response to physiological stress. *Biochem. Pharmacol.*, 12:1232–1235.

8. Borella, L. E., and Herr, F. (1971): Effect of ammonium chloride on the potentiation of amphetamine by psychotropic drugs in the rat. *Biochem. Pharmacol.*, 20:589–595.

9. Borella, L. E., Pinski, J., and Herr, F. (1970): Effect of chlorpromazine on the disposition and excretion of amphetamine in the rat. *Res. Commun. Chem. Pathol. Pharmacol.*, 1:667–676.

10. Charalampous, K. D., Walker, K. E., and Kinross-Wright, J. (1966): Metabolic fate of mescaline in man. *Psychopharmacologia*, 9:48–63.

10a. Chen, T. C. (1976): Effect of mescaline on the uptake of ^{3}H-L-norepinephrine in synaptosomal preparations of rat brain. *Pharmacologist*, 18:133 (Abstr. 110).

11. Cohen, I., and Vogel, W. H. (1970): An assay procedure for mescaline and its determination in rat brain, liver and plasma. *Experientia*, 26:1231–1233.

12. Conney, A. H., and Burns, J. J. (1972): Metabolic interactions among environmental chemicals and drugs. *Science*, 178:576–586.

13. Da Prada, M., Saner, A., Burkard, W. P., Bartholini, G., and Pletscher, A. (1975): Lysergic acid diethylamide: Evidence for stimulation of cerebral dopamine receptors. *Brain Res.*, 94:67–73.

14. Datta, R. K., and Ghosh, J. J. (1971): Mescaline-induced changes of brain-cortex ribosomes. *Biochem. J.*, 117:961–968.

15. Datta, R. K., and Ghosh, J. J. (1971): Mescaline-induced changes of brain-cortex ribosomes. *Biochem. J.*, 117:969–980.

16. Datta, R. K., and Ghosh, J. J. (1971): Mescaline-induced changes of brain-cortex ribosomes. Effect of mescaline on amino acid incorporating ability of ribosomes. *Brain Res.*, 33:193–203.

17. De La Torre, J. C. (1968): Effect of LSD-25 on the septal region of the rat brain. *Nature*, 219:954–955.

18. Denber, H. C. B. (1956): Studies on mescaline VII: The role of anxiety in the mescaline-induced state and its influence on the therapeutic result. *J. Nerv. Ment. Dis.*, 124:74–77.

19. Denber, H. C. B. (1959): Studies on mescaline IX: Comparative action of various drugs on the mescaline-induced state. In: *Biological Psychiatry*, edited by J. Masserman. Grune & Stratton, New York.

20. Denber, H. C. B., and Teller, D. N. (1968): Studies on mescaline XVIII: Effect of phenothiazines, amphetamine and amobarbital sodium on uptake into brain and viscera. *Agressologie*, 9:127–135.

21. Denber, H. C. B., and Teller, D. N. (1969): Studies on mescaline XX: Comparative effects of phenothiazines, amphetamine and amobarbital sodium on ^{14}C-mescaline content in rat brain after intravenous or intraperitoneal injection. *Excerpta Medical, I.C.S.*, 180:347.

22. Denber, H. C. B., and Teller, D. N. (1970): Subcellular localization of mescaline at the synapse. *Arzneim. Forsch.*, 20:903–906.

23. Denber, H. C. B., Teller, D. N., Rajotte, P., and Kauffman, D. (1962): Studies on mescaline XIII: The effect of prior administration of various psychotropic drugs on different biochemical parameters: A preliminary report. *Ann. NY Acad. Sci.*, 96:14–36.

24. Diaz, J. L., and Huttunen, M. O. (1971): Persistent increase in brain serotonin turnover after chronic administration of LSD in the rat. *Science*, 174:62–63.

25. Dixon, A. K. (1968): Evidence of catecholamine mediation in the 'aberrant' behavior induced by lysergic acid diethylamide (LSD) in the rat. *Experientia*, 24:743–747.

26. Efron, D. H. (editor) (1970): *Psychotomimetic Drugs.* Raven Press, New York.

27. Ehrenpreis, S., and Teller, D. N. (1972): Interaction of drugs of dependence with receptors. In: *Chemical and Biological Aspects of Drug Dependence*, edited by S. Mulé and H. Brill, pp. 177–217. CRC Press, Cleveland.

28. Farrow, J. T., and Van Vunakis, H. (1973): Characteristics of D-lysergic acid diethylamide binding to subcellular fractions derived from rat brain. *Biochem. Pharmacol.*, 22:1103–1113.

29. Friedhoff, A. J., and Hollister, L. E. (1966):

Comparison of the metabolism of 3,4-dimethoxy-phenylethylamine and mescaline in humans. *Biochem. Pharmacol.*, 15:269–273.

30. Gonzalez-Vegas, J. A. (1971): Antagonism of catecholamine inhibition of brain stem neurones by mescaline. *Brain Res.*, 35:264–267.

31. Harris, R. T., McIsaac, W. M., and Schuster, C. R., Jr., (editors) (1970): *Drug Dependence, Advances in Mental Science*, Vol. 2. Univ. Texas Press, Austin.

32. Hopf, A., and Eckert, H. (1969): Autoradiographic studies on the distribution of psychoactive drugs in the rat brain III. ^{14}C-psilocin. *Psychopharmacologia*, 16:201–222.

33. Iwasawa, Y., Ohashi, M., Yamamura, S., Saito, S., and Kiyomoto, A. (1975): Studies of mode of antagonism between adrenergic beta-mimetics and beta-blocking agents. *Jpn. J. Pharmacol.*, 25:525–533.

34. Kalberer, F., Kreis, W., and Rutschmann, J. (1962): The fate of psilocin in the rat. *Biochem. Pharmacol.*, 11:261–269.

35. Kang, S., Johnson, C. L., and Green, J. P. (1973): Theoretical studies on the conformations of psilocin and mescaline. *Mol. Pharmacol.*, 9:640–648.

36. Keup, W. (editor) (1969): *Origin and Mechanisms of Hallucinations*. Plenum Press, New York.

37. Koella, W. P., Beaulieu, R. F., and Bergen, J. R. (1964): Stereotyped behavior and cyclic changes in response produced by LSD in goats. *Int. J. Neuropharmacol.*, 3:397–403.

38. Korr, H., Lehr, E., Seiler, N., and Werner, G. (1969): Autoradiographische untersuchungen zur verteilung von mescalin und dessen einflusz auf de zentrale erregung bei mausen. *Psychopharmacologia*, 16:183–200.

39. Lajtha, A. (1958): The biochemistry of hallucinogens. In: *Progress in Neurobiology*, Vol. 3, edited by H. Pennes, pp. 126–151. Harper (Hoeber), New York.

40. Matin, M. A., and Vijayvargiya, R. (1967): Chlorpromazine-lysergic acid diethylamide antagonism. *J. Pharm. Pharmacol.*, 19:192–193.

41. McIsaac, W. M., Harris, R. T., and Ho, B. T. (1970): The indole hallucinogens. In: *Drug Dependence, Advances in Mental Science*, Vol. 2, edited by R. T. Harris, W. M. McIsaac, C. R. Schuster, Jr., pp. 41–54. Univ. Texas Press, Austin.

42. Mokrasch, L. C., and Stevenson, I. (1959): The metabolism of mescaline with a note on correlations between metabolism and psychological effects. *J. Nerv. Ment. Dis.*, 129:177–183.

43. Musacchio, J. M., and Goldstein, M. (1967): The metabolism of mescaline-^{14}C in rats. *Biochem. Pharmacol.*, 16:963–970.

44. Nair, X. (1974): Contractile responses of guinea pig umbilical arteries to various hallucinogenic agents. *Res. Commun. Chem. Pathol. Pharmacol.*, 9:535–542.

45. Nieforth, K. A. (1971): Psychotomimetic phenethylamines. *J. Pharmacol. Sci.*, 60:655–665.

46. Palmer, G. C., and Burks, T. F. (1971): Central and peripheral adrenergic blocking actions of LSD and BOL. *Eur. J. Pharmacol.*, 16:113–116.

47. Rajotte, P., Denber, H. C. B., and Kauffman, D. (1962): Studies on mescaline XII: Effects of prior administration of various psychotropic drugs. In: *Recent Advances in Biological Psychiatry*, Vol. 4, edited by J. Wortis, pp. 278–286. Plenum Press, New York.

48. Scheving, L. E., Vedral, D. F., and Pauly, J. E. (1968): Daily circadian rhythm in rats to D-amphetamine sulphate: Effect of binding and continuous illumination on the rhythm. *Nature*, 219:621–622.

49. Seiler, N., and Demisch, L. (1971): Oxidative metabolism of mescaline in the central nervous system – II. Oxidative deamination of mescaline and 2,3,4-trimethoxy-β-phenylethylamine by different mouse brain areas *in vitro*. *Biochem. Pharmacol.*, 20:2485–2493.

50. Seiler, N., and Demisch, L. (1974): Oxidative metabolism of mescaline in the central nervous system – III. Side chain degradation of mescaline and formation of 3,4,5-trimethoxy-benzoic acid *in vivo*. *Biochem. Pharmacol.*, 23:259–271.

51. Seiler, N., and Demisch, L. (1974): Oxidative metabolism of mescaline in the central nervous system – IV. *In vivo* metabolism of mescaline and 2,3,4-trimethoxy-β-phenylethylamine. *Biochem. Pharmacol.*, 23:273–287.

52. Shah, N. S. (1971): Subcellular distribution of 8-^{14}C-mescaline in the mouse brain and liver. *Biochem. Pharmacol.*, 20:3207–3210.

53. Shah, N. S. (1976): Influence of psychotomimetic drugs and β-diethylaminoethyl-diphenylpropyl-acetate (SKF 525-A) on mescaline-induced behavior and on tissue levels of mescaline in mice. *Biochem. Pharmacol.*, 25:591–597.

54. Shah, N. S., and Himwich, H. E. (1971): A comparative study of mescaline and 3,4-dimethoxy-phenylethylamine in isolated brain mitochondria and brain homogenates. *Brain Res.*, 34:163–170.

55. Shah, N. S., Jacobs, J. R., Jones, J. T., and Hedden, M. P. (1975): Interaction of mescaline with phenothiazines: Effect on behavior, body temperature, and tissue levels of hallucinogen in mice. *Biol. Psychiatry*, 10:561–573.

56. Shah, N. S., Shah, K. R., Lawrence, R. S., and Neeley, A. E. (1973): Effects of chlorpromazine and haloperidol on the disposition of mescaline-^{14}C in mice. *J. Pharmacol. Exp. Ther.*, 186:297–304.

57. Shulgin, A. T. (1970): Chemistry and structure-activity relationships of the psychotomimetics. In: *Psychotomimetic Drugs*, edited by D. H. Efron, pp. 21–41. Raven Press, New York.

58. Shulgin, A. T. (1975): Centrally active phenylethylamines. *Psychopharmacol. Commun.*, 1:93–98.

59. Snyder, S. H., and Reivich, M. (1966): Regional localization of lysergic acid diethylamide in monkey brain. *Nature*, 209:2093–2095.

60. Spano, P. F., Kumakura, K., Tonon, G. C., Govoni, S., and Trabucchi, M. (1975): LSD and

dopamine-sensitive adenylate-cyclase in various rat brain area. *Brain Res.*, 93:164–167.

61. Sparber, S. B. (1975): Neurochemical changes associated with schedule-controlled behavior. *Fed. Proc.*, 34:1802–1812.

62. Stolk, J. M., Barchas, J. D., Goldstein, M., Boggan, W., and Freedman, D. X. (1974): A comparison of psychotomimetic drug effects on rat brain norepinephrine metabolism. *J. Pharmacol. Exp. Ther.*, 189:42–50.

63. Teller, D. N. (1972): Scattered light measurement for molecular pharmacology. In: *Methods in Pharmacology*, vol. 2, edited by A. Schwartz and C. F. Chignell, Chapter 8, pp. 277–301. Appleton-Century-Crofts, New York.

64. Teller, D. N., and Denber, H. C. B. (1964): Studies on mescaline XV: The influence of mescaline on the free amino acid patterns of serum. *Neuropsychopharmacology*, 3:423–426.

65. Teller, D. N., and Denber, H. C. B. (1968): Defining schizophrenia with the techniques of molecular biology. *Dis. Nerv. Syst.*, 29:93–112.

66. Teller, D. N., and Denber, H. C. B. (1970): Mescaline and phenothiazine tranquilizers: Recent studies on uptake into brain, subcellular localization and effects upon membrane and protein structure. In: *Protein Metabolism of the Nervous System*, edited by A. Lajtha, Chapter 37, pp. 685–697. Plenum Press, New York.

67. Tonge, S. R., and Leonard, B. E. (1970): The effect of some hallucinogenic drugs on the amino acid precursors of brain monamines. *Life Sci.*, 9:1327–1335.

68. Tonge, S. R., and Leonard, B. E. (1971): Hallucinogens and non-hallucinogens: A comparison of the effects on 5-hydroxytryptamine and noradrenaline. *Life Sci.*, 10:161–168.

69. Uyeno, E. T. (1967): Effects of mescaline and psilocybin on dominance behavior of the rat. *Arch. Int. Pharmacodyn. Ther.*, 166:60–64.

70. Vogel, W. H. (1968): Physiological disposition and metabolism of 3,4-dimethoxy-phenylethyl-amine in the rat. *Int. J. Neuropharmacol.*, 7:373–381.

71. Vogel, W. H. (1970): Determination and physiological disposition of *p*-methoxy-phenylethylamine in the rat. *Biochem. Pharmacol.*, 19:2663–2665.

72. Von Hungen, K., Roberts, S., and Hill, D. F. (1975): Interactions between lysergic acid diethylamide and dopamine-sensitive adenylate cyclase systems in rat brain. *Brain Res.*, 94:57–66.

73. Wallach, M. B., and Gershon, S. (1971): A neuropsychopharmacological comparison of *d*-amphetamine, *l*-dopa, and cocaine. *Int. J. Neuropharmacol.*, 10:743–752.

74. Wallach, M. B., Hine, B., and Gershon, S. (1974): Cross tolerance or tachyphylaxis among various psychotomimetic agents on cats. *Eur. J. Pharmacol.*, 29:89–92.

75. Weltman, A. S., Sackler, A. M., and Johnson, L. (1970): Effect of mescaline HCl on resistance of male mice to histamine stress. *J. Pharm. Sci.*, 59:1659–1661.

76. Winter, J. C. (1971): Tolerance to a behavioral effect of lysergic acid diethylamide and cross-tolerance to mescaline in the rat: Absence of a metabolic component. *J. Pharmacol. Exp. Ther.*, 178:625–630.

77. Wright, E. M. (1972): Active transport of lysergic acid diethylamide. *Nature*, 240:53–54.

78. Wyatt, R. J., Vaughan, T., Galanter, M., Kaplan, J., and Green, R. (1972): Behavioral changes of chronic schizophrenic patients given L-5-hydroxytryptophan. *Science*, 177:1124–1126.

79. Yamamoto, T., and Ueki, S. (1975): Behavioral effects of 2,5-dimethoxy-4-methyl-amphetamine (DOM) in rats and mice. *Eur. J. Pharmacol.*, 32:156–162.

Neurotoxicology, edited by L. Roizin, H. Shiraki, and N. Grčević. Raven Press, New York © 1977.

Effects of LSD on Membranous Organelles in Cultured Neurons

Nicholas J. Willson, Leon Roizin, *Joseph F. Schneider, and Jevons C. Liu

*New York State Psychiatric Institute, New York, New York 10032; and * The New York State Research Institute for Mental Retardation, Staten Island, New York 10314*

Although considerable effort has been expended in an attempt to obtain a better understanding of how lysergic acid diethylamide-25 (LSD-25) affects neural tissues, knowledge concerning its actions, particularly the biochemic, physiologic, and structural alterations that it produces in nervous system tissues, is still limited. We do know that the drug is widely distributed in the body (2), that it crosses the blood-brain barrier, and that it probably accumulates in greater concentrations in some parts of the brain than in others (4,9).

In vivo, morphologic studies of LSD's effects on nervous system cells have been limited to light microscopic observations in animals. The results of these experiments were not very conclusive although Denber et al. (3) did find that a large (2.5 mg/100 g) dose of LSD caused nonspecific degenerative changes in cerebral cortical neurons. Similar alterations occurred in hepatic cells. A smaller dose (0.1 mg/100 g) did not produce any detectable pathology.

TISSUE CULTURE

Several light microscopic studies of LSD's effects on cultured central nervous system tissues have been carried out. Miura et al. (7) observed that LSD stimulated culture fiber outgrowth. Geiger (5) reported that time-lapse cinematography revealed changes in neuron nuclei, diminu-tion of Nissl substance, and eventually chromatolysis in cells treated with the drug.

During the last several years investigators in two different laboratories, Walter J. Hendelman (6) in Ottawa, Canada and a group at the New York State Psychiatric Institute under the supervision of Leon Roizin (8), carried out apparently simultaneous studies of the effects of LSD on cultured neural tissues. Although the two projects were not coordinated, fortuitously, Hendelman's experiments involved short-term (up to 53 hr) exposure of cultured cerebellar neurons to concentrations of LSD in the medium ranging from 1×10^{-3}M to 1×10^{-5}M, whereas Roizin's involved a more chronic, up to 19-day, exposure of spinal cord and dorsal root ganglion neurons to LSD having a concentration of 1×10^{-6}M in the medium.

Light Microscopy

In both the short- and long-term studies, light microscopic examination of living cultures revealed increased granularity in some nerve cells—a change that was related to both LSD concentration and exposure time. More specifically, in cerebellum cultures exposed to a 10^{-3}M LSD concentration, a few neurons became granular within 5 to 6 hr, and a majority eventually became granular. In contrast, neurons in cultures exposed to a 10^{-5}M concentration for periods of up to 53 hr showed no significant differences from controls. Cultures in media with intermediate concentrations showed qualitatively similar, less extensive, more delayed changes. Interestingly, in the chronic studies, increased granularity appeared in the neurons exposed to 10^{-6}M concentrations of LSD, but not until the 10th day.

Electron Microscopy

In addition to the granularity noted with the light microscope, neurons exposed to LSD showed significant ultrastructural alterations. The most striking change in the short-term experiments was an increase in the number of lysosomes and perhaps multivesicular bodies. Many lysosomes also showed morphologic changes. The most common of these was an increase in organelle size. A number of lysosomes developed structural modifications, some quite unusual. In general, these were characterized by the accumulation of differing numbers of variably configured membranous structures and amorphous material within the organelles. Hendelman felt that the appearance of some lysosomes was so distinctive that he coined the term "heterogeneous dense body" (HDB) to describe them. He classified these HDBs into four types, which he believed represented progressive stages of lysosome evolution. According to Hendelman's formulation, early stage HDBs contain vesicles and small collections of membranous material, but in later phases, membranous, then amorphous material is predominant.

Similar lysosomal changes were seen in

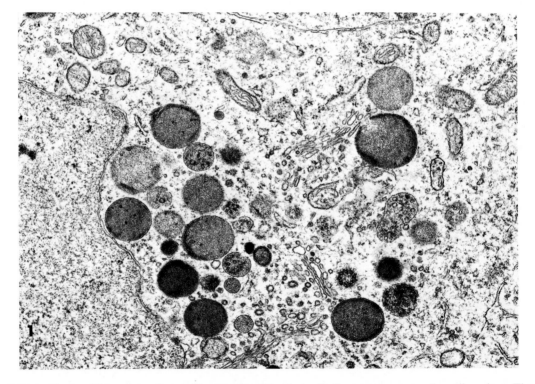

FIG. 1. Clustered lysosomes, along with several multivesicular bodies, are seen near the cell nucleus. The lysosomes differ somewhat in size and osmophilia. LSD-treated, 11 days *in vitro*. ×23,800. (From Roizin et al., ref. 8.)

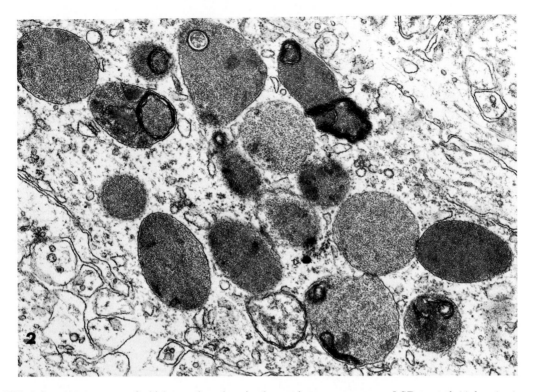

FIG. 2. Lysosomes, some of which contain rather simple membranous structures. LSD-treated, 11 days *in vitro*. ×29,500. (From Roizin et al., ref. 8.)

the chronic experiments. A segment of a neuron that contains increased numbers of somewhat pleomorphic lysosomes is seen in Fig. 1. In other neurons, clustered lysosomes containing fairly simple membranous structures were observed (Fig. 2). The development of simple membrane patterns within lysosomes seems to be an early manifestation of LSD's effects on these organelles. It should be pointed out that organelles showing similar alterations were seen in some control neurons. They were, however, much more numerous in the cultures exposed to LSD. Some lysosomes contained more complex membranous arrays, often along with amorphous material (Fig. 3). Other lysosomes (Fig. 4) were seemingly filled with the amorphous material. Hendelman believed that the accumulation of large quantities of amorphous material within the lysosomes

represented a late stage of evolution. In addition to the changes just described a few lysosomes contained variable numbers of generally loosely packed, curvilinear structures (Fig. 5). These organelles bear some resemblance to the curvilinear bodies that have been found in one form of neuro-visceral storage disease. A number of rather large, complex, membranous bodies (Fig. 6) were also encountered.

In addition to the lysosome changes seen after both acute and chronic LSD exposure, chronic exposure was marked by an increase in the number of neuronal mitochondria. In some cells this was associated with a rather marked degree of mitochondrial pleomorphism. Sometimes the mitochondria were arranged in clusters (Fig. 7). Many mitochondria had very unusual shapes, and some were gigantic. The cristae were variably configured, and the

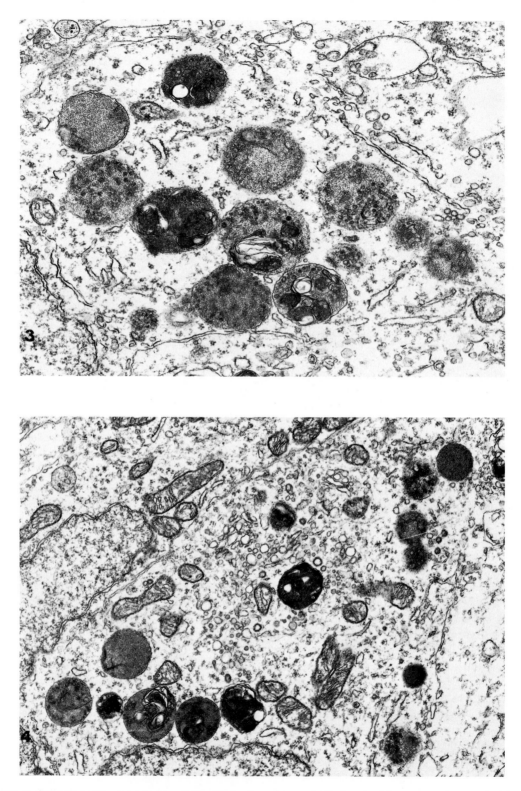

FIG. 3. Collection of lysosomes, some with membranous arrays, small clumps of dense amorphous material, or both. LSD-treated, 11 days *in vitro*. ×29,500. (From Roizin et al., ref. 8.)

FIG. 4. Lysosomes, several filled with dense amorphous material. LSD-treated, 11 days *in vitro*. ×35,400. (From Roizin et al., ref. 8.)

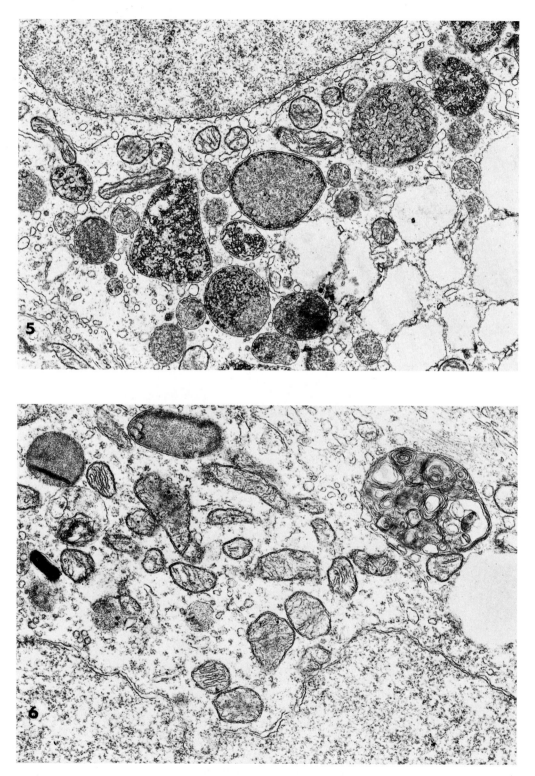

FIG. 5. Dark-staining curvilinear structures are seen in lysosomes. Dilated endoplasmic reticulum cisternae are seen at right. LSD-treated, 11 days *in vitro*. ×16,000. (From Roizin et al., ref. 8.)

FIG. 6. Aggregated organelles and a rather large, complex, membranous structure are seen near the cell nucleus. LSD-treated, 11 days *in vitro*. ×23,600. (From Roizin et al., ref. 8.)

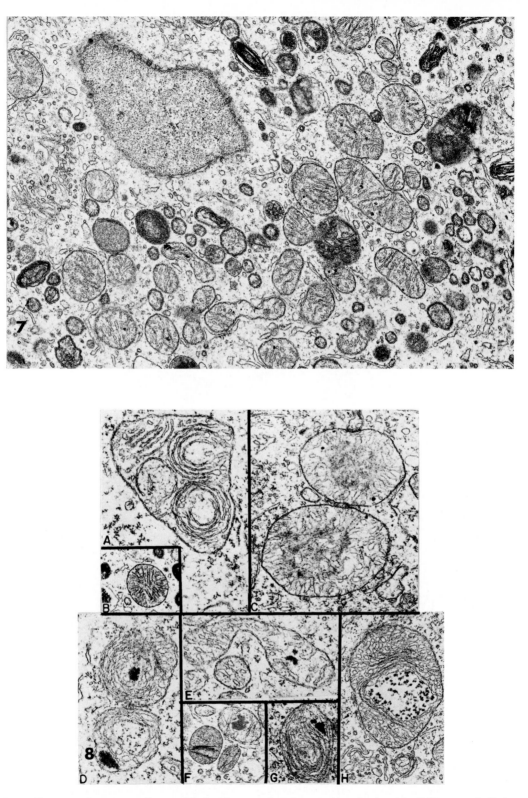

FIG. 7. Segment of neuron perikaryon filled with somewhat pleomorphic mitochondria. LSD-treated, 19 days *in vitro.* ×9,400. (From Roizin et al., ref. 8.)

FIG. 8. Pleomorphic mitochondria. LSD-treated, 19 days *in vitro.* **A:** ×21,470; **B–H:** ×15,370. (From Roizin et al., ref. 8.)

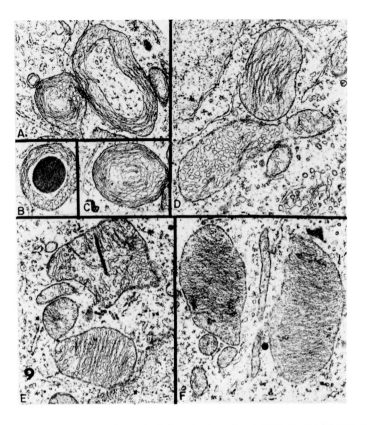

FIG. 9. Pleomorphic mitochondria. LSD-treated, 19 days *in vitro*. **A:** ×14,500; **B–C:**×20,250; **D:** ×21,000; **E–F:** ×14,500. (From Roizin et al., ref. 8.)

mitochondrial matrixes differed in density. Selected mitochondria, which illustrate these remarkable differences in external form and cristae configuration, are seen in Figs. 8 and 9. These changes were most pronounced in the older cultures.

DISCUSSION

Now what does all of this mean? Do the observed changes give any important information about the interactions of LSD and cells, and can these changes be related to LSD's clinical manifestations? It should be pointed out that there are dangers inherent in trying to correlate structural alterations in cultured rodent tissues with behavioral effects in humans. However, definite changes do occur in nerve cells exposed to LSD, and it seems important to say something about the possible, with emphasis on the word "possible," significance of these alterations. Admittedly, the changes are not necessarily specific for LSD. They do, however, represent cell modifications produced by the drug and for this reason are of importance.

In attempting to explain the actions of LSD on cells, Hendelman related the changes that occur in lysosomes to other investigators observations concerning electrophysiologic abnormalities induced by the drug. He concluded that the basic pathology was probably in cell membranes. Chronic experiments show that LSD's effect on cell organelles is more widespread than suggested by Hendelman's work. In addition to changes in lysosome morphology, long-term exposure leads to alterations in mitochondrial form. We believe that the pathologic findings in both sets of experiments support the theory that LSD produces rather widespread modifications of cell membranes. Furthermore, it seems possible that the minute blood and tissue concentrations encountered clinically (1) may produce biochemic changes in surface or synaptic membranes, or both, that are not necessarily associated with structural pathology detectable by presently available methods. If such changes do occur, perhaps they play a role in the bizarre psychic disturbances produced by LSD. How long such alterations might persist after drug withdrawal is problematic. Hendelman's work suggests that the morphologic changes are reversible, at least partially, when the cells are exposed for short periods of time. Whether structural alterations play a role in the flashbacks that some people experience is a matter for speculation, but this seems to be at least possible.

REFERENCES

1. Aghajanian, G. K., and Bing, O. H. L. (1964): Persistence of lysergic acid diethylamide in the plasma of human subjects. *Clin. Pharmacol. Ther.*, 5:611–614.
2. Axelrod, J., Brady, R. O., Witkop, B., and Evarts, E. V. (1956–57): The distribution and metabolism of lysergic acid diethylamide. *Ann. NY Acad. Sci.*, 66:435–444.
3. Denber, H. C. B., Charipper, H. A., and Roizin, L. (1964): Cytological effects of lysergic acid diethylamide (LSD-25) in rat brain and liver. *Fed. Proc.*, 23:147.
4. Diab, I. M., Freedman, D. X., and Roth, L. J. (1971): (^{3}H) Lysergic acid diethylamide: Cellular autoradiographic localization in rat brain. *Science*, 173:1022–1024.
5. Geiger, R. S. (1959): Effects of LSD-25, serotonin and sera from schizophrenic patients on adult mammalian brain cultures. *J. Neuropsychiatr.*, 1:185–199.
6. Hendelman, W. J. (1972): A morphologic study of the effects of LSD on neurons in cultures of cerebellum. *J. Neuropathol. Exp. Neurol.*, 31:411–432.
7. Miura, T., Tsujiyama, Y., Makita, K., Nakazawa, T., Sato, K., and Nakahara, M. (1957): The effect of psychotropic substances on nerve and neuroglia cells developed in tissue culture. In: *Psychotropic Drugs*, edited by S. Garattini, and V. Ghetti, pp. 478–481. Elsevier, Amsterdam.
8. Roizin, L. Schneider, J., Willson, N., Liu, J. C., and Mullen, C. (1974): Effects of prolonged LSD-25 administration upon neurons of spinal cord ganglia tissue cultures. *J. Neuropathol. Exp. Neurol.*, 33:212–225.
9. Snyder, S. H., and Reivich, M. (1966): Regional localization of lysergic acid diethylamide in monkey brain. *Nature*, 209:1093–95.

Neurotoxicology, edited by L. Roizin, H. Shiraki, and N. Grčević. Raven Press, New York © 1977.

Neuropathology of Minamata Disease in Kumamoto: Especially at the Chronic Stage

Tadao Takeuchi

Department of Pathology, Kumamoto University, School of Medicine, Kumamoto, Japan

The pathology of Minamata disease has occasionally been described in detail and has already been reviewed (6–8). The changes, however, resulting from the time dependency of prolonged and chronic cases are not known in detail yet, although a few results have been reported in Japanese (3,10,11). The neuropathology of mild cases must also be brought into focus.

MATERIAL

About 60 autopsy cases were obtained ranging from cases of severe death (12 cases) and prolonged disease (over 16 cases) to relatively mild cases of chronic occurrence in which death resulted from another illness. Although the adult (senile) cases were larger in number, because of which death did not result from poisoning itself, the autopsy cases contained five child cases and four fetal-type infants or children who had gotten intrauterine intoxication.

RESULTS

Atrophy of the Brain

The most severe atrophy of a brain affected with Minamata disease was observed in infants and children who were pre- and postnatally poisoned, whereas the brain atrophy in the adult victims, in general, was less severe.

The atrophy rate of the most severe cases observed in child victims was 55%, and the weight of the brain was reduced to less than half showing a remarkable disappearance of brain substances that resulted in formation of a spongy state in almost all of the cerebral cortices except for Ammon's horn, uncus, amygdaloid nucleus, hippocampal fusiform, and cingulate gyri. The most severe atrophy in fetal-type Minamata disease was seen in a 6-year-old child whose brain was reduced to about half, indicating a 49% atrophy rate, but there was no spongy state in the brain cortex, which was accompanied instead by considerable hypoplasia which might have reduced the brain weight.

Because, as a rule, the clinical course in acute and subacute severe cases observed in adults resulted in death within 100 days and thus the course was too short to reduce brain weight, the average atrophy rate was only 5% (−5 to 17%). This means that the nerve cells were intensely involved and disintegrated, but their loss was still smaller in number, and acute swelling and severe changes with edema remained.

The brains reduced in weight were, as a rule, seen in the cases in which a few years had passed since the onset of acute and subacute symptoms and signs. The gradual disappearance of nerve cells and dendrites effected by the poisoning had occurred then, and the reduction in weight could increase in prolonged cases in which secondary degeneration of white matter including disappearance of dendrites and nerve fibers was noticed. In those cases, particularly in the adult cases, the brain weight was reduced by about 10 to 20%. Such decrease of brain substance also resulted in the clinical symptoms of Minamata disease.

No close relationship between mercury content and atrophy rate of the brain was identified, but there was a close relationship between age and atrophy rate of the brain. The infantile and child victims more frequently had a tendency to lose brain substances including nerve cells involved than did adults.

The gyrus atrophy was widely distributed in severe cases, but it was noted in the occipital lobes, particularly in the bilateral calcarine cortex. The post- and precentral regions were also reduced often in gyri. The lateral superior gyri in both sides also atrophied occasionally.

NEUROHISTOPATHOLOGY OF MINAMATA DISEASE, PARTICULARLY FROM AUTOPSIES OF THE CHRONIC STAGE

Neuropathology of Minamata disease was characterized by disturbances of nerve cells in the cerebral and cerebellar cortices, including particular cortices of brains that were preferentially involved (Fig. 1). The cortices of whole lobes, of course, were also involved in various degrees, although there were no outstanding features in the diencephalon, brainstem, or spinal cord except for secondary degeneration and little changes of neurons.

The most intense damage could result in a macroscopic spongy state from complete loss of neurons and nerve substances of the gray matter. The next most severe disorder resulted in a microscopic spongy state in the brain cortex. The third degree of damage frequently formed a loosening of nerve tissues. The fourth degree of damage was divided further into three degrees in which the most intense change was an intense depopulation or thinning-out decrease of neurons (over 50% in number) in the brain cortex, and the second was a moderate depopulation of neurons there (30 to 50% in number) in the brain cortex, which characteristically occurred following the scattered single cell necrosis (Fig. 2).

The thinning-out loss or decrease of neurons with slight gliosis usually occurred in varying degrees according to the grade of involvement of the brain cortex, particularly observed in the second, uppermost third, and fourth layers. In chronic cases, however, a process of gradual disappearance of nerve cells could be followed. When slightly involved, the thinning-out decrease of neurons was sometimes unnoticed on microscopic observation, and it was found finally in comparison with controls (Fig. 3).

The calcarine cortex which is the center for the visual field was involved in all cases autopsied. The disturbance of nerve cells was, as a rule, much more pronounced in the anterior portions of the calcarine cortex and became less marked toward the occipital poles, although there was some rule-out of those pathological changes. In severe cases with blindness observed in children, the entire visual cortex was involved. In chronic cases that occurred after longer term contamination, however, the changes were, in general, less severe. The cortex along the depth of the calcarine fissure was predominantly involved, whereas the damage became less severe or was even absent at the crest of the convolutions, particularly in the mild chronic cases.

The varied involvements of whole layers in the calcarine area resulted in the symmetrical concentric constriction of visual fields in varying degrees. The disintegration of calcarine cortices was accompanied by varied involvements of neurons in the 18th

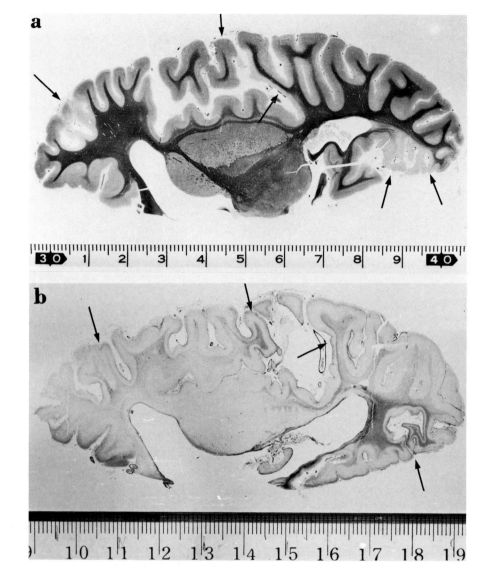

FIG. 1. **a** and **b:** Horizontal-cut sections of lateral cerebral hemisphere through calcarine regions of a severe case of prolonged Minamata disease (23 years old, female). The preferential lesions are identified by arrows. Klüver-Barrera stain **(a)** and Holzer stain **(b).**

and 19th visual association areas. These changes sometimes gave rise to abnormal ocular movements which were caught by electroophthalmography in the clinic (12). Thereby, the internal sagittal stratum, consisting of corticofugal fibers passing from the occipital lobe to the superior colliculus and the lateral geniculate body, was in-volved secondarily (Figs. 4 and 5), contrary to the relatively intact fibers of geniculo-calcarine passing in the external sagittal stratum. The fibers of the corpus callosum designated as the tapetum were also in-volved secondarily, resulting from rela-tively intense damage to neurons in the occipital cortex. There must be a disturb-

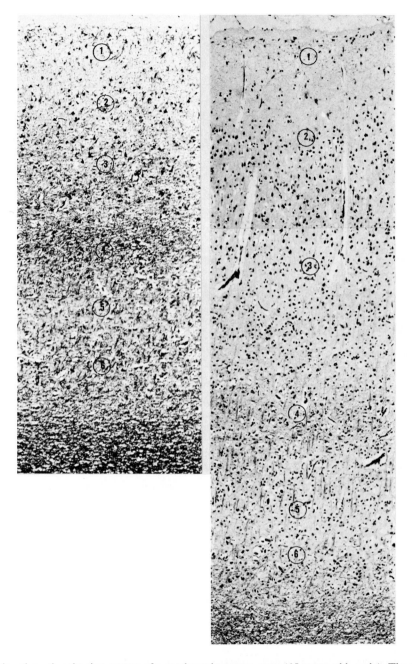

FIG. 2. Section through calcarine cortex of a moderately severe case (65 years old, male). The thinning-out decrease of neurons of over 50% is seen. Paraffin section. Klüver-Barrera stain.

FIG. 3. Section through calcarine cortex of case of minor involvement (75 years old, male). The slight thinning-out decrease of nerve cells of lower than 30% accompanied by proliferation of glial cells is revealed by Klüver-Barrera stain. Atrophic changes of nerve cells are identified.

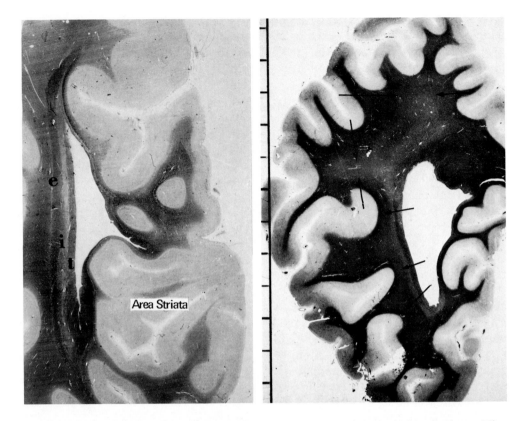

FIG. 4. Frontal-cut section near the splenium of the corpus callosum of the brain from fetal-type Minamata disease (13 years old, male). Secondary degeneration of internal sagittal stratum (I) is more intensely demonstrated, whereas the external sagittal stratum (E) is relatively well preserved. The tapetum (T) is less involved secondarily.

FIG. 5. Frontal-cut section of the brain through the splenium of the corpus callosum in chronic Minamata disease (72 years old, female). Diffuse degeneration can be recognized in the white matter in the center as well as in the internal sagittal stratum. Paraffin section. Klüver-Barrera stain. Arrows identify the internal sagittal stratum which is degenerated.

ance of binocular depth perception in methylmercury poisoning because of the cutting by this involvement of an interhemispheric link for binocular disintegration in the central vision (5,9). Indeed, the corpus callosum, particularly in the posterior parts, occasionally looked reduced macroscopically in relatively severe cases of Minamata disease.

The neurofibrillar tangles were often found in the brain cortex in prolonged and chronic cases, even when the patient was relatively young.

The changes of the other preferential cortices in the cerebrum were similar to those of the calcarine cortex, but, as a rule, were less severe. The disturbance of the precentral cortex resulted, in cases of severe involvement, in development of secondary bilateral degeneration of the pyramidal tracts in the brainstem and spinal cord. These involvements might occur mainly in the cortex along the depth of the rolandic fissure. The postcentral cortex was involved similarly.

Similar slight changes were sometimes observed in the frontal cortex of both hemispheres, particularly in the ninth area. Ammon's horn, uncus, amygdaloid nucleus, and hippocampal and cingulate gyri showed a few or no abnormalities, except for the occasional finding of ischemic nerve cells. A few or no lesions were found in the nuclei of the diencephalon or hypothalamus, except for acute severe cases.

The white matter, corresponding to the involvement of the cortex, was degeneratively reduced in prolonged cases (Fig. 5), although there were little or no changes in the acute or subacute cases. The diffuse leukodystrophy-like unstaining was often observed by the myelin-staining.

Changes of the cerebellar cortex were present in all cases examined. The granule cells were most susceptible and were affected in varying degrees, but began, as a rule, to disintegrate beneath the Purkinje cell layer of the crests of the deeper gyri in the central portions. The Purkinje cells were more resistant than granule cells, although they commonly disintegrated and then were followed by proliferation of Bergmann glial cells. Basket, climbing, and parallel fibers were also involved. There was glial proliferation of astrocytes and rod cells and occasionally of phagocytes laden with myelin debris in acute and subacute cases, but there was no such phagocytosis in chronic cases. A small number of disorganized Purkinje cells with focal thickening of their dendrites was noticed in the molecular layer of chronic cases. A fair number of torpedoes and cactus of varied types also developed in the axons of the Purkinje cells in prolonged and chronic cases. The white matter corresponding to the cerebellocortical involvements was degeneratively reduced in chronic cases, but not in the acute or subacute cases.

The above-mentioned changes predominantly involved the cortex around the depth of sulci, but were indistinct or even absent on the outer surface of each hemisphere and at the crests of folia. The topographic distribution of the changes varied from case to case. In some instances, almost all folia were widely involved, particularly in severe cases with acute and subacute occurrence, accompanied by reduced molecular layers.

However, the lesions were, in general, restricted to a circumscribed area, particularly in the deeper portion in central areas both in the neo- and paleocortices. The slight loss of granule cells under the Purkinje cell layer at the crests of gyri resulted in the "apical scar" formation, named by Takeuchi (8), after a prolonged course or in chronic cases (Fig. 6). The mildest of the chronic prolonged cases showed only the apical scar formation or a slight thinning-out decrease of granule cells in the central regions near the fourth ventricle. No abnormalities were found in the deeper white matter or dentate nuclei, except occasionally.

The basal ganglia were less severely in-

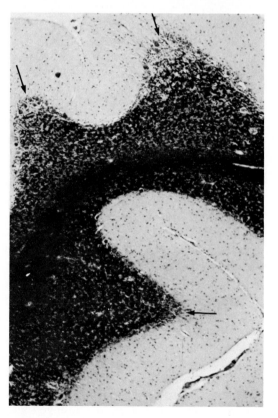

FIG. 6. Section of the cerebellar cortex obtained from a case of chronic Minamata disease. The so-called apical scar formation following mild loss of nerve cells at the crests of gyri is noted. Paraffin section. Klüver-Barrera stain. Arrows indicate the apical scar formation of lesions.

volved, except for the putamen where the cranial portion in particular was frequently disturbed. No remarkable lesions were observed in the brainstem or spinal cord, except for a secondary degeneration of the pyramidal tracts occasionally observed in severe cases with intense precentral involvement and a secondary degeneration of the posterior columnal roots, particularly of the Goll's tract, in chronic, prolonged cases. The latter degeneration was characterized by an intense involvement of posterior roots and sensory nerve fibers in which disappearance of nerve fibers with collagen increases, irregular regeneration in size, arrangement of nerve fibers with incomplete myelination, and proliferation of Schwann's cells were noticed. The disappearance of ganglion cells in spinal ganglions was also noticed, but the changes in ganglion were not so severe in chronic cases. Fewer changes were occasionally observed in cranial nerves, including the optic nerve, except for the reversible degenerations.

In general, changes in the brain became less severe in chronic cases, in which the most severe changes were restricted exclusively to the visual and visual association areas and to the pre- and postcentral areas. Slight cerebellar changes were also observed, showing only the apical scar formation of the crests of gyri and thinning-out decrease of granule cells in the central deeper portions surrounding the fourth ventricle. Nevertheless, the fine involvement of peripheral sensory spinal nerves still remained.

In the fetal-type cases that were affected in intrauterine life as well as in childhood, the neurons throughout the whole cortex of the cerebrum tended to be involved as a result of the methylmercury compound. The cortical lesions of the brain were distributed more widely and more severely in the fetal type, which had two characteristic patterns in its pathology (7,8). One was quite similar to the neuropathology common in Minamata disease mentioned above,

but cerebellar involvement with granule cell disappearance was generally less than in the child and adult cases. Another change was related to the age at fetal exposure, the time the mother had consumed the sea foods contaminated by methylmercury, and the hypoplastic changes of the brain cortex, including resting matrix cells at the ventricular wall, columnar grouping of nerve cells, abnormal cytoarchitecture of nerve cells, status marmoratus, specific thinning granular layer of the cerebellar cortex or outstanding hypoplasia of the corpus callosum, and retention of nerve cells in the cerebral medulla. These pathological changes revealed clinically the cerebral palsy in infancy. However, there were no experiences in which neuropathological changes could be identified in mild cases of children with mental deterioration that presumably had resulted from the methylmercury poisoning in the intrauterine life.

Aging with diffuse disappearance of nerve cells could stimulate onset of Minamata disease that had continued in a latent period during which no remarkable clinical symptoms and signs were identified in spite of slight neuropathological changes in the nerve system. In other words, the methylmercury poisoning could stimulate aging in the human body. The low age level of death of the residents in the Minamata area [about 50 to 52 years in Minamata as opposed to 70 to 73 years in control Japanese (4)] seemed to show this fact in practice.

BIOPSY FINDINGS OF SURAL NERVE

Sural nerve biopsy was performed and examined under both light and electron microscopes by Eto (2) and Eto et al. (3), using six chronic, prolonged cases who volunteered and two fetal-type child victims whose families volunteered.

The results obtained from these observations were characterized by an increase of incomplete myelination and amyelination

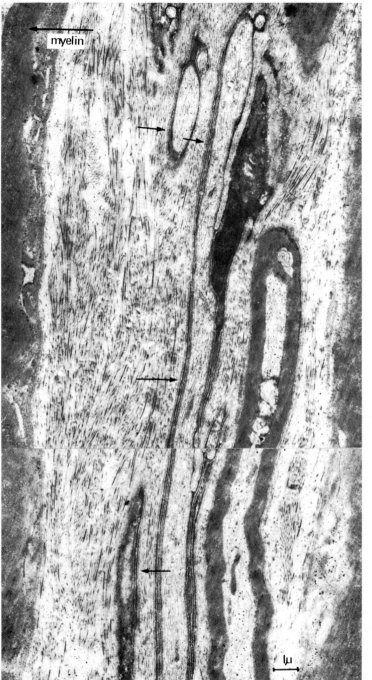

FIG. 7. Electron micrograph of longitudinal section of sural nerve biopsied from a case of chronic Minamata disease. Incomplete regeneration of myelinated nerve and regenerative small nerve fibers with lamellar processes of Schwann cell cytoplasm (*arrows*) are identified, accompanied by collagen increase. ×6,800.

of small nerve fibers and by a proliferation of Schwann's cells with collagen increase in both fetal-type and nonfetal adult cases. There may be some differences in the mechanism of myelination of nerve fibers between fetal and nonfetal Minamata dis-ease; it might mean hypoplastic and aplastic myelination of nerve fibers in the fetal-type cases, whereas it would mean incomplete regeneration of nerve fibers already destroyed in the nonfetal cases.

In the adult cases, the morphological

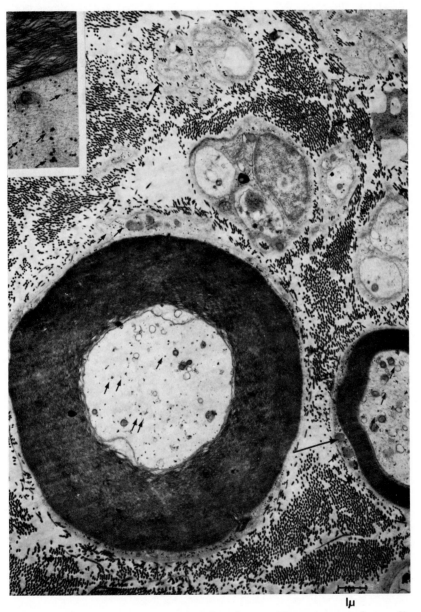

0.7cm

1μ

FIG. 8. Electron micrograph of crosscut section of sural nerve. Disarrangement of nerve fibers with increased collagen. Glycogen deposits (*small arrows*) increase in axons as well as in the cytoplasm of Schwann cells. ×7,700. Left upper corner demonstrates glycogen deposits in the axon. ×20,000. Large arrows show the regenerated fibers of the myelinated and unmyelinated fibers, which also contain glycogen deposits.

changes of the sural nerve represented an incomplete regeneration including abnormal small nerve fibers, incomplete myelination and absence of myelination (Fig. 7), abnormal regeneration with irregular branching and deformation of regenerated fibers, formation of onion bulb and regenerating unit, and a sprouting formation of small nerve fibers, whereas the sural nerve changed in repair with proliferation of Schwann's cells, irregular Schwann's cells, and fibrocyte appearance with an increase of collagen. Accordingly, the nerve fibers smaller than 5 μm in diameter increased relatively. Regressive changes were characterized by degeneration re-

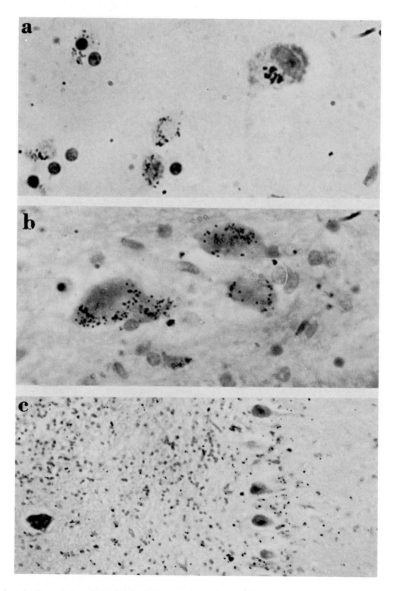

FIG. 9. Histochemical sections of the brain. Mercury is demonstrable in the body of nerve cells as well as in a microglial cell in the cerebral cortex (**a**). The ganglion cells in some nuclei of pons contain abundant silver grains as mercury deposits (**b**). Silver grains also appear in phagocytes or microglial cells and more abundantly in the Purkinje cell layer. Purkinje cells contain less granules (**c**).

TABLE 1. *Mercury content in tissues of a severely prolonged case of Minamata disease*

Tissues	Total mercury (μg/g wet weight) atom absorption method			Methyl mercury (μg/g)	
	Present chron. case 18 yrs.	Control acute 19 days[a]	Control acute 96 days[a]	Present chron. case 18 yrs.	Control acute 96 days[a]
Cerebral cortex	2.785	13.11	7.36	0.035	2.34
Cerebral medulla	1.762	13.64	—	0.043	—
Cerebellum	4.237	15.81	8.78	0.063	2.95
Liver	2.399	155.8	84.3	0.055	6.80
Kidney	5.585	147.9	62.4	0.064	9.67
Brain/liver × 100	122	8.6	9.5	86	38.8
Brain/kidney × 100	52	9.0	12.9	73	27.5

[a] Results of acute cases obtained from the formalin-fixed specimens of the autopsy performed 18 years ago.

vealing swollen myelins, wavy and whirled deformation of myelins, and destructive myelin structures released from mesoaxon into axons or whirled mesoaxon released, as well as by degeneration of axons containing dense bodies, irregular myelin structures, and glycogen deposits (Fig. 8). These regressive changes presumably resulted from the mercury storage that still occurred in Minamata areas.

In the fetal-type cases, the same findings were, as a rule, observed in varied degrees, but they were particularly characterized by aplastic and hypoplastic myelination of small nerve fibers and by an abnormal finding of small nerve fibers with outstanding whirled degeneration of myelins.

The degeneration described above was presumably caused by the methylmercury compound that was still being deposited in small amounts by consumption of contaminated fish and seafoods, because some fishermen and their families were still fishing in the Minamata Bay area, in spite of the warning described previously.

DISTRIBUTION OF MERCURY IN THE TISSUES OF MAN: LEVELS OF MERCURY IN THE HUMAN BODY

Histochemically, the mercury deposits were demonstrated in nerve cells in the brain cortices as well as in basal and stem nuclei independently from the preferential disintegration (Fig. 9 a–c). They were also demonstrated in phagocytes, rod cells, and special glial cells such as Bergmann's glia. Purkinje cells, however, tended to contain less metal particles. These findings were also demonstrated in a severe female case who died 18 years after the onset of poisoning, in spite of there being no deposits in liver cells.

Chemically, in the first outbreak of Minamata disease, the distribution of mercury in tissues of human victims who died within 100 days after the onset was found to be on an average of 46.1 ppm in kidney, 38.1 ppm in liver, and 10.7 ppm in brain, wet weight by the dithizone method. The lethal dose of mercury in the brain was calculated to be about 10 ppm, and the critical level of mercury in the brain for onset of the disease was calculated to be about 1 ppm.

Mercury contents decrease gradually from the whole body by the rule of biological half-life, which was calculated to be about 70 days in man (1). However, the half-life in the human brain, as a target organ that is easily disturbed by methylmercury, was calculated from our autopsy materials to be about 240 days. The distribution pattern in the individual organ could be changeable time-dependently (Table 1).

The average ratio of the percentage of

mercury in the brain to that in other organs amounted in acute cases to 24 in brain per liver, 22 in brain per kidney, and 2.5 in brain per hair, whereas the average ratio in chronic cases was 50 in brain to liver, 100 in brain to kidney, and 5 to 10 in brain to hair. The distribution pattern of mercury in chronic cases was different from that in acute cases. It may be very important for the pathogenesis of chronic Minamata disease that methylmercury compounds tend to remain longer in nerve tissues.

REFERENCES

1. Aberg, B., Eckman, L., Falk, R., Greitz, U., Persson, G., and Snihs, J-O. (1969): Metabolism of methyl mercury ^{203}Hg compound in man. *Arch. Environ. Health,* 19:478–484.
2. Eto, K. (1971): Pathological changes of peripheral nerve in human Minamata disease: An electron microscopic observation. *Adv. Neurol. Sci.* (Japanese ed.), 15(3):606–618.
3. Eto, K., Kojima, H., Sakai, K., Miyayama, H., Suko, S., and Takeuchi, T. (1974): Pathological study of Minamata disease 10 years after the first outbreak. Chronic occurrence and its autopsy cases. *J. Kumamoto Med. Soc.* (Japanese ed.), 48(2):162–188.
3a. Eto, K. and Takeuchi, T. (1977): Pathological changes of human sural nerves in Minamata disease (methylmercury poisoning). Light and electron microscopic studies. *Virchows Arch. B Cell Pathol.,* 23:109–128.
4. Nomura, S., Matsushita, T., Futatsuka, N., Arimatsu, T., Ueda, A., Misumi, T., Tomio, T., and Teraya, N. (1973): Progress on Minamata disease and its epidemiological study. In: *Pathological, Clinical and Epidemiological Research about Minamata Disease, 10 Years After,* Vol. I, Report of Kumamoto Univ. Study Group, T. Takeuchi, chairman. Eibun-sha, Kumamoto, Japan.
5. Okamura, R., Ito, Y., Eto, K., and Takeuchi, T. (1974): Pathology of the occipital white matter of Minamata disease (2), especially the passing route of the internal sagittal stratum in prolonged and chronic cases. *Acta Soc. Ophthalmol. Jpn.* (Japanese ed.), 78(10):1045–1058.
6. Shiraki, H., and Takeuchi, T. (1971): Minamata disease. In: *Pathology of Nervous System,* Vol. II, edited by J. Minckler, pp. 1651–1665. McGraw-Hill, New York.
7. Takeuchi, T. (1968): Pathology of Minamata disease. In: *Minamata Disease, Study Group of Kumamoto Univ.,* edited by S. Kutsuna, pp. 141–228. Shuhan Press, Kumamoto, Japan.
8. Takeuchi, T. (1972): Biological reactions and pathological changes of human beings and animals under the condition of organic mercury contamination. In: *Environmental Mercury Contamination,* edited by R. Hartung, and B. D. Dinman, pp. 247–289. Ann Arbor Scientific Publ., Ann Arbor, Michigan.
9. Takeuchi, T., Eto, K., Tsutsui, J., Okamura, R., and Mayuzumi, K. (1974): Neuropathology of medullary roots corresponding to visual cortex and associated area in Minamata disease. *Jpn. Rev. Clin. Ophthalmol.* (Japanese ed.), 68:113–117.
10. Takeuchi, T., Eto, K., Kojima, H., Otsuka, Y., Miyayama, H., Suko, S., Sakurama, N., and Iwamawa, T. (1972): Minamata disease: Pathological findings in 10 years long-term survivors. *J. Kumamoto Med. Soc.* (Japanese ed.), 46(11):666–705.
11. Takeuchi, T., Eto, K., Suko, S., Miyayama, H., Fujisaki, A., and Harada, Y. (1972): An electron microscopic study of sural nerve in prenatally acquired Minamata disease. *J. Kumamoto, Med. Soc.* (Japanese ed.), 46(11):706–719.
11a. Takeuchi, T. and Eto, K. (1977): Pathology and pathogenesis of Minamata disease. In: *Minamata Disease, Methylmercury Poisoning in Minamata and Niigata, Japan,* pp. 103–141. Kodansha Ltd. Tokyo.
12. Tsutsui, J., Fukai, S., and Nakamura, Y. (1974): Disturbance of binocular vision in Minamata disease. *Jpn. Rev. Clin. Ophthalmol.* (Japanese ed.), 68:529–531.

Neurotoxicology, edited by L. Roizin, H. Shiraki, and N. Grčević. Raven Press, New York © 1977.

Essential Neuropathology of Alkylmercury Intoxications In Humans from the Acute to the Chronic Stage With Special Reference to Experimental Whole Body Autoradiographic Study Using Labeled Mercury Compounds

H. Shiraki, and *K. Nagashima

*Department of Neuropathology, Institute of Brain Research; and *Department of Pathology, Tokyo University Medical School, Tokyo, Japan*

The scientists of the world are more or less acquainted with the epidemioclinical features of Minamata disease. In addition, several important papers on the neuropathology of Minamata disease have already been published by certain Japanese scientists (4,8–12,14–17). The present chapter deals particularly with the essential neuropathology not only of Minamata disease but also of other alkylmercury intoxications in humans from the most acute to the most chronic stage through experimental results of time-dependent whole body autoradiography in different animals using labeled alkylmercury and/or inorganic mercury compounds (13,18,19).

ESSENTIAL NEUROPATHOLOGY OF ALKYLMERCURY INTOXICATIONS IN HUMANS WITH SPECIAL REFERENCE TO TIME-DEPENDENT WHOLE BODY AUTORADIOGRAMS IN MONKEYS

Concerning central nervous system (CNS) involvements in alkylmercury intoxications including Minamata disease (Table 1), their clinical symptomatology and neuropathology indicate clearly certain topographical selectivity of foci particularly from the acute to the subacute stage as evidenced by their consistency and severity. The visual cortices of the occipital lobe were the main site of the most severe and consistent lesions in the initial stage (Fig. 6A–C), and were succeeded by cerebellar (Fig. 5A–C), pre- and postcentral, first temporal, and other cerebral cortices.

The mercury content of the monkey's brain 1 hr after the intravenous injection of ^{203}Hg ethylmercury chloride (^{203}Hg EtHgCl; 800 μg Hg/kg/100 μCi) reached its highest level in both the cerebellar (0.214 ppm) and the occipital pole (0.213 ppm; Figs. 1A and 2A). In addition, radioactivity of cerebellar cortices was more accentuated in deeper folia than in the convexity (Fig. 2A). Thus, these findings in quantity and in topographical difference of mercury indicate one reason why cerebellar cortices of deeper folia were preferentially involved in humans (Fig. 5A; Case 3 in Table 1). Radioactivity of the brain 20 hr after intraperitoneal injection of ^{203}Hg EtHgCl (800 μg Hg/kg/96 μCi), on the other hand, became moderately increased (Fig. 1C), but topographical difference of activity in each cerebral region was not

TABLE 1. *Summarized clinical features of different alkylmercury intoxications*

Case number, age, sex	Causative agent (Occupation)	Total duration of illness	Main clinical features
Minamata disease in Kumamoto intoxicated with peroral eating of contaminated seafood			
1 34, M	Methylmercury (Fisherman)	19 d	Numbness of all limbs & lips, impaired auditory acuity, spastic paraplegia, tremor of hands & upper limbs, atactic gait, slurred speech, psychomotor excitement, comatose, convulsions
2 58, F	Methylmercury (Wife of fisherman)	60 d	Numbness of fingers, impaired auditory acuity, impaired gait, rigidity of all limbs, slurred speech, comatose
3 4 yr 5 mo, F	Methylmercury (Child of fisherman)	553 d	Total blindness, spastic tetraplegia, pathological reflexes, atactic gait, slurred speech, psychomotor excitement
4 8, F	Methylmercury (Child of fisherman; two families fell ill)	993 d	Blindness, deafness, spastic tetraplegia, pathological reflexes, dysphagia, impaired coordination, atactic gait, slurred speech, nystagmus, convulsions
5 6 yr 10 mo, M	Methylmercury (Child of fisherman)	1,467 d (4 yr 7 d)	Total blindness, impaired auditory acuity, spastic tetraplegia, pathological reflexes, impaired coordination, *apallic or akinetic mutistic state at fixed stage*
Percutaneous intoxication with liniment for scabies containing methylmercury			
6 19, M	Methylmercury thioacetoamide for 5 mo (Student)	9 mo	Numbness of hands, tongue, & lower limbs, impaired visual acuity, impaired auditory acuity, unable to walk, pathological reflexes, atactic gait, ataxia of upper limbs, slurred speech, hyperhidrosis, *apallic state from intermediate to terminal stage*
Hunter-Russell's case intoxicated with pesticide dusts containing methylmercury			
7 38, M	Absorption of methylmercury phosphate or nitrite from lung and/or skin respectively for 4 mo (Worker of factory manufacturing pesticides)	15 yr	*Acute to subacute stage:* Numbness of hands, arms, lips & tongue, impaired stereognosis of hands, two-point discrimination of finger tips, concentric constriction of visual field, impaired speech, atactic gait, dysdiadochokinesia, dysmetria, nystagmus *Chronic stage:* Blindness of one eye, severe constriction of right visual field, dysphagia, impaired gait & standing, ataxia, *persistent hypertension (190/135)* *Cause of death:* Cardiac arrest & infarction
Ethylmercury intoxication with intravenous injection of LHP			
8 13, M	9,000 ml of LHP containing 0.01% of ethylmercury sodium salcylate for 29 days almost continuously (None)	Hunter-Russell's syndrome for 10 days	*Protein-losing enteropathy for 13 years:* Initiated at age of 7 mo *SMON for 6 yr & 11 mo:* Initiated at age of 7 years *Hunter-Russell's syndrome at terminal stage:* Numbness of fingers, hands & lips, itching feeling of whole body, tetraplegia, dysarthria, dyspnea, involuntary movement of hands, intention tremor, hyperhidrosis, hypersalivation, psychomotor excitement, comatose

LHP, liquid human plasmanate; SMON, subacute myeloopticoneuropathy.

clear-cut, whereas the same autoradiogram using ^{203}Hg mercury chloride (^{203}Hg HgCl; 800 μgHg/kg/96 μCi) disclosed highest activity in liver, renal cortex, urine, and intestinal walls and contents, etc. (Fig. 1D). Activity was low in different muscles and almost negative in the CNS, except for the choroid plexi (Fig. 1D). Thus, a comparison of both autoradiograms, i.e., of ethyl mercury and inorganic mercury, indicates clearly that excretion of inorganic mercury was fairly rapid, whereas that of ethylmercury was extremely retarded, since with ethylmercury activity of both intestinal contents and urine remained almost negative (Figs. 1A and C). An 8-day autoradiogram, after a single intraperitoneal injection of the same and/or almost the same amount and activity of ^{203}Hg EtHgCl, disclosed the highest activity in the CNS together with the renal cortex and salivary gland and moderate activity in intestinal contents (Fig. 1F), indicating an active migrating and/or accumulating process of mercury into the CNS. The mercury content of such monkey's brain, measured by Geiger counter, reached its highest level in the cortex of the occipital pole (1.68 ppm), whereas the homogeneous activity in either the convexity or deeper folia of cerebellar cortex indicated the lowest value (1.22 ppm; Fig. 2B).

In addition, the mercury that migrated into the cerebral parenchyma, even at this stage, consisted of over 90% ethylmercury itself (19). So, these time-dependent shifts of autoradiographic characteristics and values of mercury content correspond well with the essential neuropathology in humans in which visual cortices were more consistently and severely involved than cerebellar cortex. However, although the cerebellar autoradiogram disclosed almost the same amount of mercury in each cortical layer and/or dentate nucleus (Fig. 2B), granule cells were most susceptible, succeeded by Purkinje cells, whereas nerve cells of the dentate nucleus and Golgi

type II cells of the granular layer were highly resistent (Figs. 5B and C).

Consequently, it can be assumed that a greater accumulation of mercury comprises a necessary but not a sufficient condition for the development of nerve cell disintegration. This view also can be applied to the occipital foci, because the most severe foci were restricted to visual cortices (Fig. 6A and B), although homogeneous migration of mercury in all occipital cortices and layers was observed in the autoradiogram (Fig. 2B). Higher activity was also visualized in subthalamus and substantia nigra (Fig. 2B), compatible with that of the occipital cortices, whereas human neuropathology never developed conspicuous alterations in basal ganglia, except for putamen and/or brainstem. Thus far it seems that the determining factors for the development of foci are a time-dependent shift of different mercury contents in each region and the different susceptibility of each cellular element for alkylmercury compounds.

EXISTENCE OF HEMODYNAMIC CIRCULATORY DISTURBANCE ASSOCIATED WITH THE MORPHOPATHOGENESIS OF ALKYLMERCURY INTOXICATIONS

The existence of a circulatory disturbance of hemodynamic origin should seriously be considered in understanding the morphopathogenesis of the disease. Supporting neuropathology for this aspect can be summarized as follows. In the most acute case of only 10 days' duration and intoxication from intravenous injection of ethylmercury compound (cast 8 in Table 1), typical ischemic nerve cells with a few neuronophagia and activated rod cells were exceedingly widespread not only in the different cortical layers but also in the subcortical gray matter (Fig. 10A). In other acute and subacute cases (case 1 in Table 1), similar ischemic nerve cells were pre-

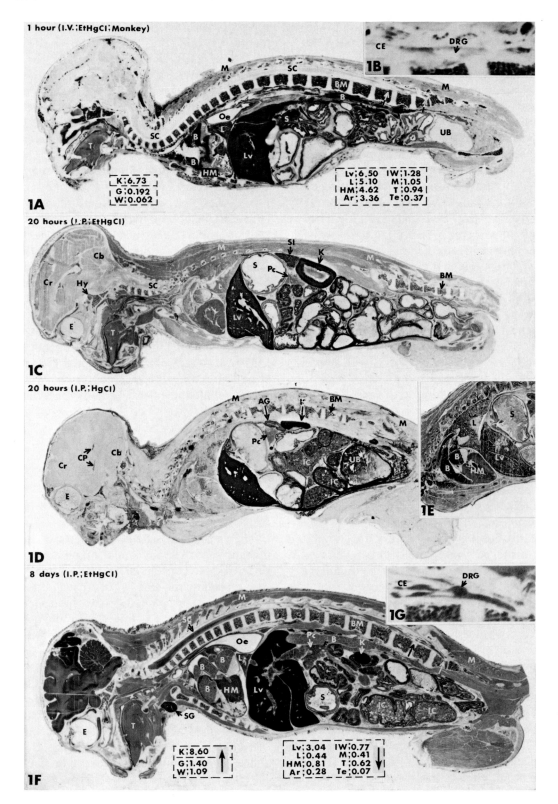

dominant in the second and upper third cortical layers and from the convexity to the depth of the sulci (Fig. 7A and B). In subchronic and chronic cases, therefore, cortical deterioration and resulting atrophy with calcified nerve cells (Fig. 6D) were pronounced in the same regions but were inconspicuous or even absent at the convexity (Fig. 6C). Disintegration of the cerebellar granular layer, coarse spongy tissue disruption, and migrated edema fluids began to develop just beneath the Purkinje cell layer (Fig. 5B).

Considering these features, one can postulate the existence of impaired hemodynamic circulation and/or occurrence of cerebral edema particularly at the acute and the subacute stage. Consequently, in an understanding of the morphopathogenesis of alkylmercury intoxications, another factor—circulatory disturbance of a hemodynamic origin—should be added to the above-mentioned two factors.

CEREBROVASCULAR SCLEROSES IN ALKYLMERCURY INTOXICATIONS IN HUMANS AND AUTORADIOGRAPHIC FINDINGS IN MONKEYS

Whether these circulatory disturbances are associated with cardiac arrest or are of a cerebral focal nature, such as functional vasospasm, is unknown. Actually, radio-activity of heart muscles 1 hr after administration of ^{203}Hg EtHgCl was high (4.62 ppm), but it became low 8 days later (0.81 ppm). The absolute value of 8-day heart muscles, however, was still the highest among those of other muscles (Fig. 1F). The aorta and large-calibered arterial walls adjacent to the heart in each 20-hour (Fig. 4A and B) and 8-day autoradiogram (Fig. 1F) also demonstrated high activity, whereas activity of the large-calibered veins in the same region was absent or minimal, except for slight activity of the intimal layer (Figs. 4A and B). Thus, the higher activity of the arterial vessel walls suggests migration of mercury into their muscle layers.

The 20-hr autoradiogram of ^{203}Hg HgCl, on the other hand, disclosed almost negative activity not only in heart muscle but also in other muscles (Figs. 1D and E). The following findings were interesting: in the case of ^{203}Hg HgCl, radioactivity was present in plasma but far less conspicuous in corpuscles (Fig. 1D and E), whereas in the case of ^{203}Hg EtHgCl, the activity was present in corpuscles but almost negative in plasma (Figs. 1F, 4A and B). These observations correspond well with the following data in rats (19): administered alkylmercury compounds bonded almost instantly with erythrocytes particularly in their stroma-free hemolysates, and further research on the fate of ethylmercury in

FIG. 1. Time-dependent whole body autoradiograms of monkeys after administration of labeled mercury compounds. **A:** One hour after intravenous injection of ^{203}Hg ethylmercury chloride (^{203}Hg EtHgCl; 800 μg Hg/kg/100 μCi). ×0.59. **B:** Magnified area indicated by arrows in **A.** ×2.5. **C:** Twenty hours after intraperitoneal injection of ^{203}Hg EtHgCl (800 μg Hg/kg/96 μCi). ×0.45. **D:** Twenty hours after intraperitoneal injection of ^{203}Hg HgCl (800 μg Hg/kg/96 μCi). ×0.35. **E:** Frozen-dried section of the chest and adjacent areas corresponding to **D.** ×0.35. **F:** Eight days after intraperitoneal injection of ^{203}Hg EtHgCl (800 μg Hg/100 μCi). ×0.56. **G:** Magnified area indicated by arrows in **F.** ×2.2. Values in parentheses in **A** and **F** are amounts of Hg (μg Hg/g wet tissue) measured by Geiger counter. AG, adrenal gland; Ar, artery; B, blood corpuscle; BM, bone marrow; Bo, bronchus; Cb, cerebellum; CC, corpus callosum; CE, cauda equina; CN, caudate nucleus; CP, choroid plexus; Cr, cerebrum; CSC, cervical cord; DRG, dorsal root ganglion; E, eyeball; Fr, frontal; G, gray matter; GP, globus pallidus; HM, heart muscle; Hy, hypophysis; IC, intestinal content; Ir, iris; IW, intestinal wall; K, kidney; L, lung; Lv, liver; M, muscle; MB, midbrain; NM, neck muscle; Oc, occipital; Oe, esophagus; OM, ocular muscle; ON, olivary nucleus; P, plasma; Pa, parietal; Pc, pancreas; Po, pons; Pt, putamen; R, retina; S, stomach; Sb, subthalamus; SC, spinal cord; SG, salivary gland; SN, substantia nigra; T, tongue; Te, testis; Th, thalamus; TrN; trigeminal nerve root; UB, urinary bladder; W, white matter; ↑, increase; ↓, decrease.

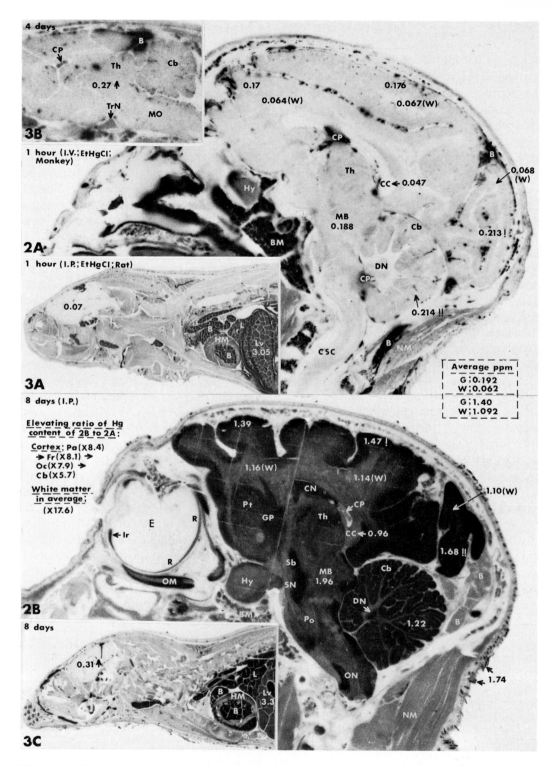

FIG. 2. Magnified autoradiograms of the brain and adjacent areas in Fig. 1. **A:** From Fig. 1A. ×1.8. **B:** From Fig. 1F. ×1.8. Values in and outside parentheses are the amounts of Hg (μg Hg/g wet tissue) measured by Geiger counter.

FIG. 3. Time-dependent autoradiograms of rats after intraperitoneal injection of [203]Hg EtHgCl (950 μg Hg/kg/ 100 μCi). **A:** One hour. ×0.8. **B:** Four days. ×2.4. **C:** Eight days. ×0.8. Values in and outside parentheses are the amounts of Hg (μg Hg/g wet tissue) measured by Geiger counter. For abbreviations, see Fig. 1.

erythrocytes revealed that ethylmercury residue accumulated inside of red corpuscles and combined with sulphatide (SH) groups of cystein residues of hemoglobulin molecules forming a mercaptide linkage.

These autoradiographic findings could have a certain significance in understanding the morphopathogenesis of cerebrovascular scleroses in both infantile and younger patients of alkylmercury intoxications. Such cases are summarized as follows. In all three infantile cases of Minamata disease, of which case 5 showed the most severe spongy or cystic cortical disruption (Fig. 8D), cerebrovascular sclerosis, as shown by concentric proliferation of intimal layers (Fig. 8E), thrombus formation, and/ or fibrohyalinous thickening mainly of the meningeal arteries, was always present (cases 3, 4, and 5). A 19-year-old male, who suffered from scabies, was treated with percutaneous inoculations of methylmercury compound for 5 months (case 6 in Table 1). During the total course of 9 months, psychic impairments became prominent, and he finally expired in an akinetic mutistic state. A conspicuous spongy cavitation similar to Fig. 8D was exceedingly widespread not only in the visual cortices but also in other cortical regions (Fig. 8A). In addition, conspicuous cerebrovascular scleroses, shown by concentric proliferation of intimal layers (Fig. 8B), fatty infiltration in the degenerated deeper layer (Fig. 8C), thrombus formation, etc., was widespread in the different-calibered meningeal arteries. In this regard, the case (2) of a 38-year-old male intoxicated with methylmercury compounds at the age of 23 years is important (case 7 in Table 1), because, after an acute illness and during a long-standing 15-year course, he developed hypertension (190/135) and finally expired of cardiac arrest and pulmonary infarctions. Postmortem, slight but similar vascular scleroses and advanced thrombus formation of the basilar vein were shown (8–10). In addition, old heart muscle scars from cornal scleroses as well as deteriorated renal cortices by ischemic process at the acute stage were found.

To summarize the findings, these cerebrovascular scleroses belong in an abnormal range and could have been caused by alkylmercury compounds, because the age of disease onset in all patients actually fell into the range of infants and younger adults and no other particular agents besides alkylmercury compounds were noticeable there.

Wakatsuki et al. (20) identified a conspicuous increase of total cholesterol of both sera and blood sugar in rabbits intoxicated with ethylmercury compounds. Actually, the time-dependent autoradiograms in the monkeys clearly showed a gradual increase of the radioactivity of ^{203}Hg EtHgCl in the pancreas and renal cortex (Fig. 1C and F). In addition, Langhans' islets, renal cortices, and heart muscles were frequently involved at the chronic stage of Minamata disease (7,16). Therefore, concerning the morphopathogenesis of cerebrovascular alterations in chronic cases of alkylmercury intoxications, one should consider the possibility that not only direct migration of mercury into the vascular system but also certain general metabolic errors directly or indirectly caused by such intoxications are responsible for the development of vascular scleroses of the whole body including the cerebrovascular system, which can play a significant role in more widespread damage of the CNS and a gradual progression of its severity during a protracted stage.

RETARDED EXCRETION OF ALKYLMERCURY COMPOUNDS FROM THE CNS IN HUMANS

The total mercury content in three brains of Minamata disease at the chronic stage, i.e., of 1.6 to 4.0 years' duration (cases 3, 4, and 5 in Table 1), ranged from 1.3 to 5.3 ppm (Figs. 5A, 6A, and 8D). These values

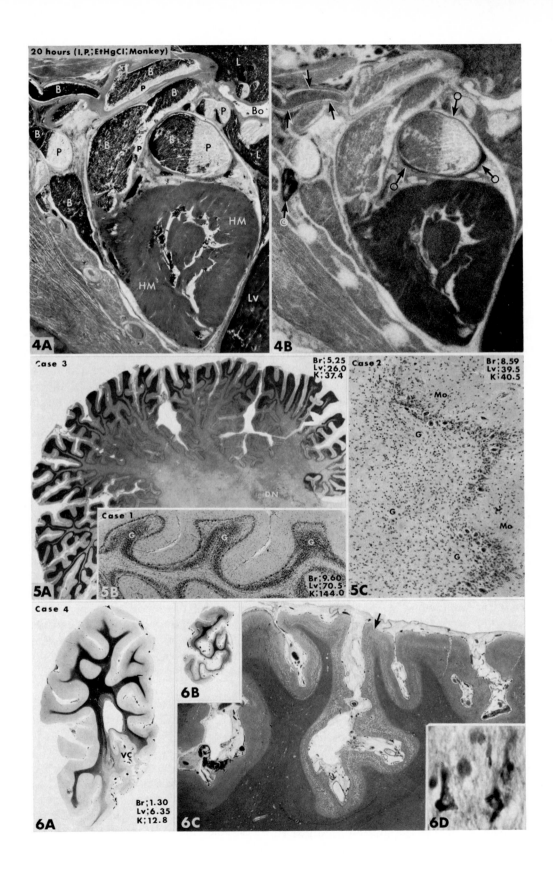

20 hours (I.P.;EtHgCl;Monkey)

4A

4B

Case 3
Br;5.25
Lv;26.0
K;37.4

5A

Case 1
G   G   G
Br;9.60
Lv;70.5
K;144.0

5B

Case 2
Br;8.59
Lv;39.5
K;40.5
Mo.
G
G   G
G   Mo

5C

Case 4

VC

Br;1.30
Lv;6.35
K;12.8

6A

6B

6C

6D

clearly exceeded controls, i.e., 0.0 to 0.05 ppm. In this regard, the case of a 23-year-old female in whom Minamata disease began at 5 years and 7 months of age and who survived for 18 subsequent years is worth referring to (1). Postmortem, the severity and topographical selectivity of the CNS foci coincided well with those of other cases of the disease. Significantly enough the total mercury content ranged from 0.4 ppm in liver, to 5.9 ppm in kidney, and *4.7* ppm in brain. It is particularly noteworthy that, even though she was hospitalized during almost the total clinical course of 18 years and was thought to have had no particular chance of taking contaminated seafood with methylmercury, the mercury content in her brain still remained at a high level. One, therefore, can postulate, concerning the determining factors for the morphopathogenesis of CNS involvement in alkylmercury intoxications, that another important factor—exceedingly retarded excretion of mercury from the CNS—should be considered.

"CACTUS-LIKE" OR "STELLATE BODY" IN CEREBELLAR MOLECULAR LAYER IN ALKYLMERCURY INTOXICATIONS AT THE CHRONIC STAGE

In the example of Minamata disease of 18 years' duration, there were multiple "cactus-like" or "stellate bodies" in the cerebellar molecular layer. Hunter and Russell (2) have already identified numerous similar bodies in an above-mentioned case

of 15 years' duration. These bodies were localized mainly in the molecular layer and less conspicuously in the Purkinje cell layer of cerebellar cortices, the granular layer of which was disintegrated severely (Fig. 9A). They consisted of focal swellings of axonal structures and radially proliferated thick- or thin-calibered dendritic processes connected with the axonal structures which were of an apical dendritic nature from Purkinje cells (Fig. 9B). These bodies were also surrounded tightly by numerous, exceedingly tiny, granular- or fibrillary-shaped structures only faintly stained with various preparations (Fig. 9B). In any case, it can be assumed that these bodies, suggesting a hypertrophic or proliferative disease process, indicate a certain regenerative phenomena of remaining Purkinje cells. In addition, in the chronic cases of alkylmercury intoxications examined, these bodies were only encountered in the two cases mentioned above, and thus, it may be that the time required for their development is very long, i.e., over 15 years.

PERIPHERAL NERVE INVOLVEMENTS IN ALKYLMERCURY INTOXICATION AT THE MOST ACUTE STAGE

Several important questions still remain open in regard to the consistency, severity, topography, and characteristics of the essential neuropathology of peripheral nerve lesions in alkylmercury intoxications. In this respect, the following case (case 8 in Table 1) is worth referring to.

←

FIG. 4. Magnified autoradiogram of the heart and adjacent areas in Fig. 1C. **A:** Frozen-dried section. ×1.7. **B:** Autoradiogram corresponding to **A.** ×1.7. Intense radioactivity of the muscle layer of aorta (*arrows with zeros*) and tangential-cut arterial vessel wall (*arrow with double zeros*), and slight radioactivity of the intimal layer of a large vein (*arrows*). For abbreviations, see Fig. 1.

FIG. 5. Cerebellar lesions in Minamata disease. **A:** *Case 3* in Table 1; sagittal-cut hemisphere. ×3.3. **B:** *Case 1* in Table 1; magnified deeper folia. ×28.0. **C:** *Case 2* in Table 1; magnified cortex. ×86. Values in **A–C** are total amounts of mercury in brain, liver, and kidney. Thionine stain. Br, brain; DN, dentate nucleus; G, granular layer; K, kidney; Lv, liver; Mo, molecular layer.

FIG. 6. Visual cortical lesions in Minamata disease; *case 4* in Table 1. **A:** Frontal-cut occipital lobe. ×1.0. **B:** Occipital pole. ×1.0. **C:** Magnified visual area in **A.** ×5.2. **D:** Magnified third cortical layer at convexity (*arrow* in **C**). ×570. **A** and **B,** Woelcke myelin method; **C** and **D,** H. & E. stain. VC, visual cortical.

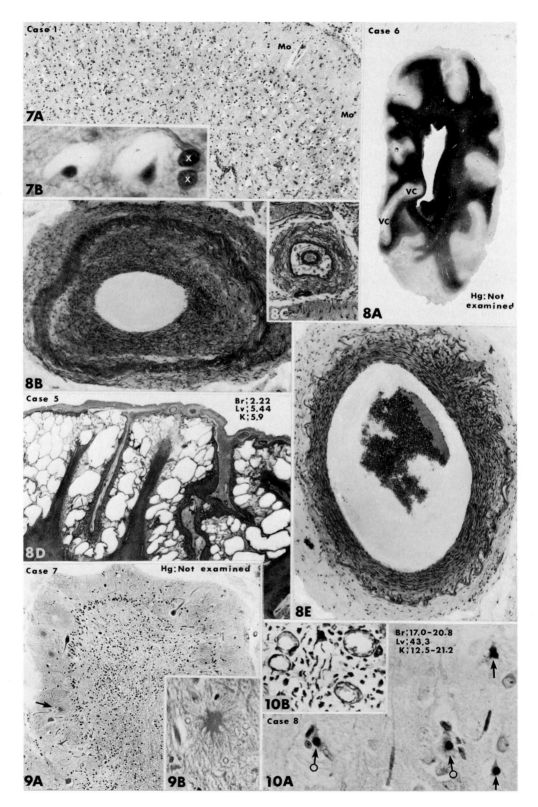

A 13-year-old boy, who suffered from protein-losing enteropathy since the age of 7 months, subsequently developed subacute myeloopticoneuropathy at the age of 7 years, and because of severe emaciation, he finally was given intravenous injections totaling 9,000 ml of "liquid human plasmanate" almost continuously for 1 month. Unfortunately, this "liquid" contained 0.01% of ethylmercury sodium thiosalcylate as an antiseptic, and thus, he developed Hunter-Russell's syndrome and died after 10 days. As has already been mentioned, ischemic degenerated nerve cells were exceedingly widespread in different cerebral cortices, basal ganglia, and brainstem (Fig. 10A). The dorsal root ganglia either at the cervical or the thoracolumbosacral level developed conspicuous alterations, such as severely disintegrated ganglion cells, multiple neuronophagia, ischemic or homogeneously degenerated neurons with vacuolar formation in their cytoplasms (Fig. 11A and B), and focal swelling, vacuolation, fragmentation, and tortuosity of the axons of nerve fiber bundles (Fig. 11A and C). Axonal alterations were also predominant in the posterior nerve rootlets including the cauda equina, whereas the anterior nerve rootlets were entirely free from lesions. Thus, these findings indicate a preferential, selective involvement of sensory peripheral nerve fibers with ethylmercury compound, and thus they correspond well with observations that experi-mentally induced methylmercury also selectively damaged posterior nerve rootlets of rats (5). This general rule can also be applied to the tract degeneration of the spinal cord and brainstem of the present example, since the posterior tract of the spinal cord (Fig. 10B), sensory trigeminal tract in the pons, etc., were degenerated in a similar way, whereas the corticospinal tract from the brainstem to the spinal cord was only minimally involved. Sciatic and femoral nerves were also similarily disintegrated.

A 1-hr autoradiogram with ^{203}Hg EtHgCl disclosed low and/or negative radioactivity of the cauda equina and adjacent dorsal root ganglia (Fig. 1A and B), whereas higher activity became manifest in both areas in an 8-day autoradiogram (Fig. 1F and G). In any case, it is true that a fairly large amount of ethylmercury compound could migrate into the dorsal root ganglia and tract, cauda equina, and spinal nerve rootlets during a protracted stage.

In the present example, it also is emphasized that the spheroid bodies, which suggested abnormal focal swelling of boutons because of the extreme difficulty of spatially identifying them adjacent to axonal structures, were widespread in subcortical gray matter, such as thalamus, subthalamus, globus pallidus, reticular zone of substantia nigra, vestibular nucleus, olivary nucleus (Fig. 11D), anterior horn and Goll's nucleus of the spinal cord, etc.

FIG. 7. Visual cortical lesion at convexity in Minamata disease; *case 1* in Table 1. **A:** Superficial layers. ×89. **B:** Magnified upper third layer in **A.** Hypertrophic astrocytes with coarse fiber formation (*crosses*). ×970. **A** and **B,** H. & E. stain. Mo, molecular layer.

FIG. 8. Percutaneous methylmercury intoxication; *case 6* in Table 1. **A:** Frontal-cut occipital lobe. ×1.7. **B:** Meningeal artery in the deteriorated frontoparietal gyri. ×97. **C:** Similar to one in **B.** ×82. Minamata disease; *Case 5* in Table 1. **D:** Parietal cortex. ×4.0. **E:** Meningeal artery in the deteriorated occipital cortex. ×86. **A,** Woelcke myelin method; **B** and **E,** H. & E. stain; **C,** van Gieson-elastica stain; **D,** Holzer method. Br, brain; K, kidney; Lv, liver; VC visual cortex.

FIG. 9. Cerebellar lesions in Hunter-Russell's case; *case 7* in Table 1. **A:** Magnified cortex. ×86. **B:** Magnified area indicated by arrow in **A.** ×437. **A** and **B,** H. & E. stain.

FIG. 10. Intravenous ethylmercury intoxication; *case 8* in Table 1. **A:** Magnified third layer of the visual cortex. Ischemic nerve cell (*arrows*), neuronophagia (*arrows with zeros*), and activated rod cells. ×570. **B:** Magnified Goll's tract at the caudal medulla oblongata. ×476. **A,** Luxol fast blue with cresylviolet stain; **B,** Bodian method. Br, brain; K, kidney; Lv, liver.

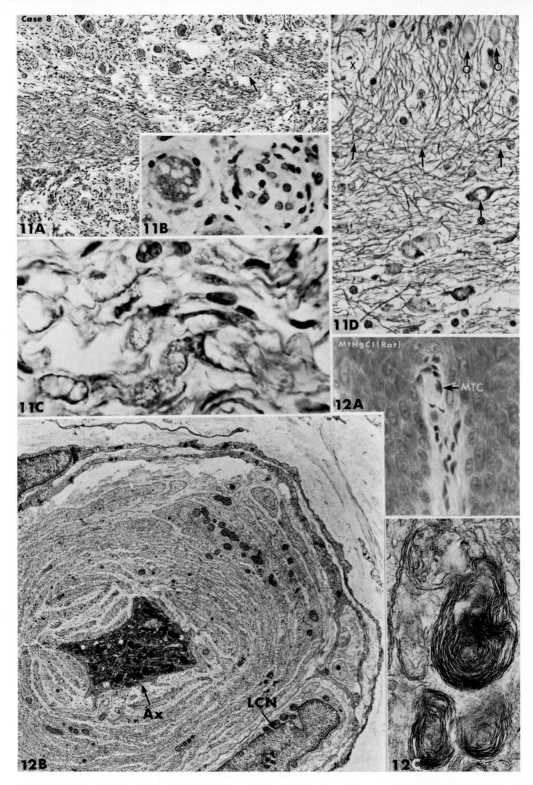

FIG. 11. Intravenous ethylmercury intoxication; *case 8* in Table 1. **A:** Dorsal root ganglion at the level of third lumbar cord. One example of multiple ganglion cells with neuronophagia (*arrow*). ×100. **B:** Two magnified degenerated ganglion cells in **A.** ×513. **C:** Magnified nerve fiber bundle in **A.** ×900. **D:** Magnified olivary nucleus. Arrows indicate the border area of the nucleus (*upper part*) to the adjacent white matter (*lower part*). One example of multiple spheroid bodies in the white matter (*arrow with double zeros*), two spheroid bodies in the nucleus (*arrow with single zero*), and degenerated nerve cell (*cross*). ×476. **A, C,** and **D,** Bodian method; **B,** Luxol fast blue with cresylviolet stain.

FIG. 12. Experimental methylmercury (MtHgCl) intoxication in rat. **A:** Magnified dermal papilla of the toe pad. **B:** Magnified Meissner's type corpuscle in **A. C:** Magnified terminal axon in **B. A,** H. & E. stain. **B** and **C,** electron microscope from fresh tissue. MTC, Meissner's type corpuscle; Ax, terminal axon; LCN, lamellar cell nucleus.

Another remarkable alteration similar to spheroid bodies is "grumose degeneration" of the cerebellar dentate nucleus at the earliest stage, the details of which are discussed in another chapter listed in this volume (Chapter 5 by H. Shiraki, A. Okumura, and S. Oyanagi, *this volume*).

Summarizing these findings, it can be assumed that one of the most conspicuous and earliest alterations of the CNS gray matter in the present example preferentially occurs in terminals and/or preterminals of centrifugal axons but not in mother nerve cells themselves.

ALTERATIONS OF CUTANEOUS SENSORY RECEPTOR IN AN EXPERIMENTAL MODEL WITH METHYLMERCURY COMPOUND

A question can arise whether a similar process can happen at the most distal endings of sensory nerve fibers projecting to skin, tendon, muscle, etc.

Four-week rats after delivery when administered peroral 20 ppm of methylmercury chloride per day developed, as a rule, certain neurological signs and symptoms (6). Dorsal root ganglia at the lumbar level corresponding to sensory innervation of the toe pad were almost normal or involved only slightly either ganglion cells or nerve fibers. The posterior nerve rootlet was severely disintegrated, however. At the level of light microscopic observations on cutaneous sensory receptors, Meissner's type corpuscles in the dermal papillae of toe pad, no particular alterations seemed to develop (Fig. 12A). Electron microscopic examination, however, disclosed clearly that although lamellar and/or capsule cells appeared normal, terminal axons of "ellipsoid" or "discoid" form were selectively affected and visualized darkly and contained degenerated mitochondria and/or electron-dense, concentrically structured, oval-shaped multiple bodies (Fig. 12B and

C), and they were never visible in control animals, detailed studies of which have recently been obtained by Ide (3). The same but less conspicuous alterations of terminal axons were also identified in preterminal axons. Although some segmental alteration was, at times here and there, visible in nerve fibers connecting cutaneous sensory receptors to dorsal root ganglia, the main site of alteration was more or less confined to these cutaneous sensory receptors and their adjacent preterminal axons, suggesting a preferential occurrence of the disease process at the most distal endings of sensory peripheral nerves.

CONCLUSION

For a sufficient understanding of the neuropathology of alkylmercury intoxications, therefore, a series of human autopsy cases is needed from the most acute to the most chronic stage with a variety of routes of administration with different alkylmercury compounds. In addition, the general pathology of the disease, particularly that of the cardiovascular system, should be associated closely with neuropathology.

In experimental models intoxicated with alkylmercury compounds, however, it is emphasized that one must be cautious in a selection of species of experimental animals, because the time-dependent whole body autoradiograms in rats never disclosed a pattern similar to that of monkeys. For example, it is true that 1-hr to 8-day autoradiograms in rats disclosed a gradual increase of radioactivity in the CNS but never demonstrated precisely a clear-cut topographical difference of radioactivity in each cerebral region, as seen in monkeys, except for a greater radioactivity of the trigeminal nerve rootlet in the protracted stage (Fig. 3A–C). In addition, radioactivity of the CNS in rats remained at a very low level through all stages in contrast to that of monkeys (Fig. 3A–C).

ACKNOWLEDGMENTS

The author gratefully acknowledges the generous cooperation of Dr. T. Takeuchi, Professor of Pathology, Kumamoto University Medical School, Kumamoto; Dr. H. Mii, Instructor of Psychiatry, Okayama University Medical School, Okayama; and Dr. D. S. Russell, London.

REFERENCES

1. Eto, K., Katsuragi, Sh., and Takeuchi, T. (1976): An autopsy case of childhood Minamata disease. A long term survival case after an acute occurrence. *Adv. Neurol. Sci.,* 20:444–457.
2. Hunter, D., and Russell, D. S. (1954): Focal cerebral and cerebellar atrophy in a human subject due to organic mercury compounds. *J. Neurol. Neurosurg. Psychiatry,* 17:235–241.
3. Ide, Ch. (1976): The fine structure of the digital corpuscle of the mouse toe pad, with special reference to nerve fiber. (*In preparation.*)
4. Ikuta, F., Makifuchi, T., Ohama, E., Koga, M., Yamamura, Y., and Oyake, Y. (1974): Morphological alterations in the autopsy cases of chronic mercury intoxication with minimal doses. *Adv. Neurol. Sci.,* 18:861–881.
5. Miyakawa, T., Deshimaru, M., Sumiyoshi, Sh., Teraoka, A., Udo, N., Hattori, E., and Tatetsu, S. (1970): Experimental organic mercury poisoning. Pathological changes in peripheral nerves. *Acta Neuropathol. (Berl.),* 15:45–55.
6. Nagashima, K., and Ohi, G. (1976): Early alterations of digital corpuscles of toe pad of rats intoxicated with methylmercury compound. Pathologic and electron microscopic observations. (*In preparation.*)
7. Shigenaga, K., Sato, K., and Takeuchi, T. (1974): Pathological changes of pancreatic islets in Minamata disease. *J. Kumamoto Med. Soc.,* 48:189–198.
8. Shiraki, H. (1967): Aging and senile phenomena of central nervous system from neuropathological viewpoint. *Adv. Neurol. Sci.,* 11:607–625.
9. Shiraki, H. (1969): The necessity of long-term follow-up study on organic mercury intoxication from neuropathological viewpoint. *Adv. Neurol. Sci.,* 13:113–120.
10. Shiraki, H. (1973): Mercury pollution in Japan. *Res. Environ. Disruption toward Interdisciplinary Cooperation,* 2:1–27.
11. Shiraki, H. (1975): The neuropathology of alkylmercury intoxication in humans with especial reference to cerebellar involvement. In a comparison with whole body autoradiographic studies in experimental animals. In: *Studies on the Health Effects of Alkylmercury in Japan,* edited by T. Tsubaki, pp. 71–128. Environment Agency, Japan.
12. Shiraki, H., and Takeuchi, T. (1971): Minamata disease. In: *Pathology of Central Nervous System,* Vol. 2, edited by J. Minckler, pp. 1651–1665. McGraw-Hill, New York.
13. Takahashi, T., Kimura, T., Sato, Y., Shiraki, H., and Ukita, T. (1971): Time-dependent distribution of ^{203}Hg-mercury compounds in rat and monkey studied by whole body autoradiography. *Eisei-gaku,* 17:93–107.
14. Takeuchi, T., Morikawa, N., Matsumoto, H., and Shiraishi, Y. (1962): A pathological study of Minamata disease in Japan. *Acta Neuropathol. (Berl.),* 2:40–57.
15. Takeuchi, T. (1972): Biological reactions and pathological changes in human beings and animals caused by organic mercury contamination. In: *Environmental Mercury Contamination,* pp. 247–289. Ann Arbor Science, Ann Arbor, Michigan.
16. Takeuchi, T., Eto, K., Kojima, H., Otsuka, Y., Miyayama, H., Suko, Sh., Sakai, K., Sakurama, N., Iwamasa, T., and Matsumoto, H. (1972): Minamata disease. Pathological findings in 10 years long term survivors. *J. Kumamoto Med. Soc.,* 46:666–705.
17. Takeuchi, T., and Eto, K. (1974): Pathogenesis of chronic Minamata disease (chronic methylmercury poisoning). *Adv. Neurol. Sci.,* 18:845–860.
18. Ukita, T., Takeda, Y., Takahashi, M., Yoshikawa, M., Sato, Y., and Shiraki, H. (1970): Distribution of ^{203}Hg-mercury compounds in monkeys studied by whole body autoradiography. *Proc. 1st Symp. Drug Metabolism and Action, November 14 to 15 in Chiba,* pp. 32–42. Pharmaceutical Society of Japan, Tokyo.
19. Ukita, T. (1971): Experimental follow-up study of mercury intoxications. I. Behaviors of mercury compounds in body of mamalians. *Kagaku,* 41:557–568.
20. Wakatsuki, T. (1967): Inapparent intoxication with especial reference to pesticides of organic mercurial origin. *Psychiatr. Neurol. Jpn.,* 69:1004–1006.

Neurotoxicology, edited by L. Roizin, H. Shiraki, and N. Grčević. Raven Press, New York © 1977.

Neuropathology of Methylmercury Intoxication in Niigata and Chronic Effect in Monkeys

Takeshi Sato and Fusahiro Ikuta

Department of Neuropathology, Brain Research Institute, Niigata University, Niigata City, Japan 951

In Japan great epidemics of methylmercury intoxication occurred in Minamata Bay in 1953 and in Niigata in 1960 (15,16). As of 1975, 627 cases had been officially documented in Niigata, and 32 patients had died.

It has been shown that methylmercury produces neuronal degeneration with astroglial proliferation in the cerebral cortex, most often in the calcarine cortex and in the granular layer of the cerebellum (4,8,13). In addition, myelin fragmentations are present in the peripheral nerves (6,14).

Several reports (4,8,13) mentioned that there were no remarkable changes in the optic nerves and lateral geniculate nuclei in Minamata disease. However, severe neuronal degeneration is present in monkeys (2,12) as well as in the bipolar cells in the retina of rat after methylmercury intoxication (11). To investigate this abnormality of the lateral geniculate nucleus, we examined two autopsy cases with acute course and monkeys after methylmercury intoxication. In addition, the abnormalities seen previously with light microscope in the nerve cells of monkeys (10) were examined in more detail with the electron microscope to define the toxic level of methylmercury in relation to the development of nerve cell damages.

REPORTS OF CASES

Case 1. A 19-year-old man developed progressive paresthesia in his fingers and speech disturbance on February 10, 1965. Subsequently he had finger tremor, difficulty in walking, hearing loss, rigidity, mutism, and dementia.

Neurological examination revealed increased muscle tonus and positive Babinski's sign. Spinal fluid was normal. The patient deteriorated steadily and died 40 days after the onset of his illness.

The main neuropathological findings on the cerebral cortex, cerebellum, and peripheral nerves were previously reported by Oyake et al. (8). They also described remarkable degeneration of nerve cells with astroglial proliferation predominantly in the calcarine, parietal, and temporal cortices.

Further neuropathological examination revealed similar neuronal changes with astroglial proliferation in the lateral geniculate nucleus (Fig. 2B). There was some involvement of neurons of the claustrum, putamen, globus pallidus, thalamus, dentate nucleus of the cerebellum, and to a lesser degree the substantia nigra. In addition to the atrophy of neurons, central chromatolysis or loss of Nissl's granules was seen in some cranial nerve nuclei in the brainstem, such as the nucleus of spinal tract of the trigeminal nerve, the vestibular nucleus, the vagal nucleus, and the cuneate nucleus as well as the dorsal nucleus in the spinal cord, and to a lesser degree the oculomotor nucleus.

There was myelin fragmentation and axonal changes in the optic chiasma and proximal end of the optic nerve associated with perivascular lymphocytic infiltration (Fig. 3). Determination of mercury showed 10.76 μg/g in the occipital cortex. (K. Hirota, *unpublished data*).

Case 2. Four weeks prior to admission, a 28-year-old man noted progressive paresthesia in the distal part of upper and lower extremities as well as perioral region. He was admitted to Niigata University Hospital because of sensory disturbance, hearing loss, ataxic gait, and visual and mental disturbance on March 27, 1965. Neurological examination revealed moderate dementia, nystagmus, visual and speech disturbance, hyperreflexia, cerebellar ataxia, finger tremor, and rigidity of his extremities. Retrobulbar neuritis was suspected by ophthalmoscopic examination. Subsequently he had an opistotonic convulsion. He received D-penicillamine, but his condition deteriorated. He died 2 months after admission.

Neuropathological findings of the cerebral cortex and cerebellum were very similar to those of case 1. Neuronal disintegration and loss with astroglial proliferation were present in the lateral geniculate nucleus, lenticular nucleus, thalamus, substantia nigra, and dentate nucleus of the cerebellum. Central chromatolysis was seen in the remaining neurons in various nuclei of brainstem and in dorsal nuclei of the spinal cord. There were several glial nodules in the inferior colliculi. In the posterior root ganglia and Gasserian ganglion severe degeneration of ganglion cells was accompanied by capsular cell proliferation. Peripheral nerves showed destruction of the myelin sheath and loss of axons. Mercury in his hair was determined to be 239.6 ppm, and in the occipital lobe, 14.4 μg/g (K. Matsukawa, *unpublished data*).

EXPERIMENTAL STUDIES IN MONKEYS

Materials and Methods

Animals

Cynomolgus monkeys (*Macaca irus*) of both sexes weighing between 1.0 and 2.0 kg were used.

Methods of Administration

Monkey pellets containing 0.1 and 0.01 mg methylmercury chloride (as Hg) were prepared by the methods of Ikeda's report (5). Methylmercury chloride was put into an egg at a rate of 50 mg per egg in a homogenizer, stirred for about 10 min, placed overnight at 4°C, and then freeze dried. The dried egg prepared in this procedure did not have the bad smell of methylmercury. It was mixed into ordinary diet for monkeys and then pelleted by evaporation. Each pellet contained 0.1 or 0.01 mg of mercury. The gas chromatographic analysis of the methylmercury concentration in the pellet showed that the reduction of mercury was 1 to 2% during the procedure. The monkeys were given orally the designated amount of pellet daily. Dose and duration of methylmercury chloride varied in each animal and are summarized in Table 1.

TABLE 1. *Methylmercury intoxication in monkeys*

						Mercury concentration (μg/g)			
No	Body weight	Dose of Hg mg/kg/day	Total Hg mg/kg	Days	(*Days of Hg administration)	Whole Blood μg/ml	Fur	Liver	Brain (occipital cortex)
1	1.03	0.21	12.8	62	(51* + 11)	3.42	248.0	27.91	30.00
2	1.55	0.04	3.7	87	(64* + 23)	1.24	2.7	11.41	5.60
3	1.55	0.02	3.6	166	(107* + 59)	0.50	63.0	2.41	1.69
4	1.02	0.03	8.7	327	(132* + 195)	0.46	61.9	3.83	1.49
5	1.96	0.02	1.1	56	(45* + 11)				
6	1.39	0.01	1.1	92	(36* + 56)				

Determination of Mercury

During the long-term experiments, methylmercury concentration in whole blood and fur were determined by gas chromatography using Shimazu GC-5A (ECD).

Autopsy

Monkeys were anesthetized with an intraperitoneal sodium pentobarbital injection. For light microscopy, the hemisphere was fixed in 10% formalin. Small specimens from various locations of coronal sections of the other side of the hemisphere were fixed in 3% glutaraldehyde, postfixed in 1% osmium tetroxide, and then embedded in Epon-araldite. Thin sections were stained with uranyl acetate and lead citrate and examined by Hitachi 11B electron microscope. For mercury assay, tissue specimens were kept at −20°C.

RESULTS

Clinical Symptoms

Monkey no. 1 developed the first symptoms 57 days after the administration of mercury (total 11.45 mg/kg) (Table 1). The monkey became clumsy in grasping raisin rewards and showed loss of activity and gross tremor of the trunk. By 62 days of administration (total 12.8 mg/kg), the monkey developed weakness of grasping, unsteady and ataxic gait, and anorexia. Subsequently, fine tremor and periodic myoclonic seizures occurred in his upper and lower extremities. Visual and hearing impairments were detected through sluggish response to light and sounds. The symptoms progressed, and the monkey developed occasionally generalized tonic and clonic seizures. An electroencephalography revealed paroxysmal bursts of polyspikes or spike-and-wave

complexes during seizure attacks. The monkey was sacrificed by anesthesia after a postexposure observation period of 21 days.

None of the other monkeys (no. 2–6) showed any evidence of symptoms. Monkey no. 5, given a total of 1.1 mg/kg, died of a common cold after an exposure period of 55 days.

Determination of Mercury

Table 1 showed the maximum mercury concentration in whole blood, fur, liver, and brain. Monkey no. 1 had clinical symptoms of 3.42 μg/ml of mercury in the blood, 248.0 ppm in the fur, and 30.0 μg/g in the occipital lobe on the 62nd day after administration.

In monkeys no. 3 and 4, mercury concentration in fur and blood was almost constant during the period of administration (Fig. 1). Monkey no. 3 showed 0.42 ± 0.069 μg/ml of mercury on the average in the whole blood and 50.0 ± 6.9 ppm in the fur. In monkey no. 4, 0.34 ± 0.072 μg/ml of mercury in the whole blood and 45.8 ± 6.4 ppm in the fur were determined.

Neuropathological Findings

In monkey no. 1, macroscopic examination of the brain demonstrated marked atrophy of the calcarine cortex (Fig. 4). The histopathological findings were severe neuronal changes with astroglial proliferation predominantly in the occipital, parietal, and temporal lobes, and in the lateral geniculate nucleus (Figs. 2 and 3) which were very similar to those observed in Minamata disease. The most severe damage was seen in the calcarine and insular cortices associated with spongy degeneration (Fig. 6). The neuronal changes were characterized by pyknosis or karyolysis with ultimate cytolysis. There was some involvement of neurons of the claustrum, putamen, globus pallidus, thalamus, and lateral geniculate

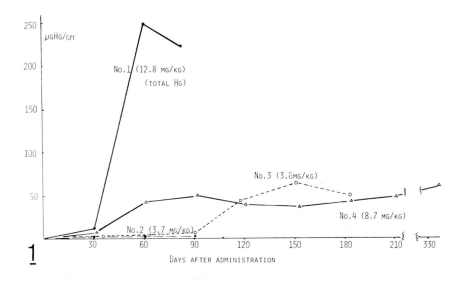

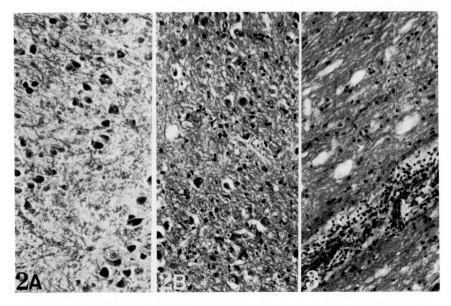

FIG. 1. Concentration of methylmercury in fur.
FIG. 2. A: Normal lateral geniculate nucleus. Kluver-Barrera. ×150.
FIG. 2. B: Case 1. Neuronal degeneration with astroglial proliferation in lateral geniculate nucleus. H. & E. × 150.
FIG. 3. Case 1. Nerve fiber degeneration with perivascular lymphocytic infiltration in optic nerve. H. & E. ×150.

nuclei (Fig. 8). Focal myelin destruction and axonal changes were revealed in the optic nerves (Fig. 9).

There was occasional mild atrophy of Purkinje cells in the cerebellum, but the number of nerve cells in the granular layer appeared normal. Moderate degeneration of nerve cells could be found occasionally in the dentate nuclei, cranial nerve nuclei in the brainstem, inferior olivary nuclei, and

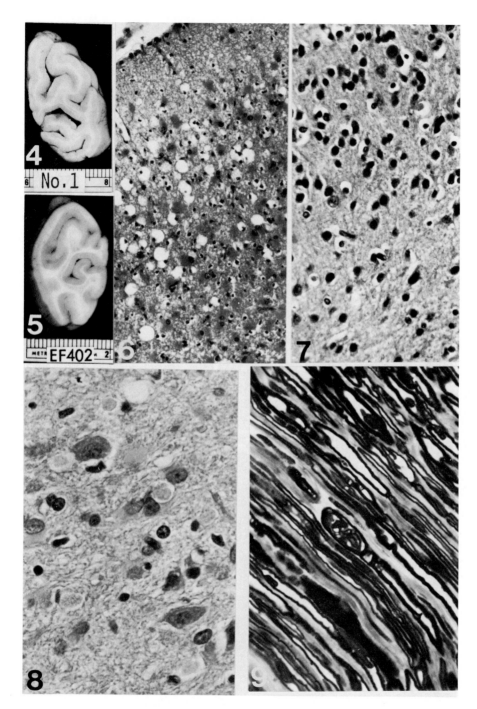

FIG. 4. Monkey no. 1. Marked atrophy of calcarine cortex.

FIG. 5. Monkey no. 4. Normal appearance of calcarine cortex.

FIG. 6. Monkey no. 1. Calcarine cortex. Severe disintegration of nerve cells and proliferation of astroglia with status spongiosus. H. & E. ×150.

FIG. 7. Monkey no. 4. Deep layer of calcarine cortex. Slight atrophy of nerve cells. H. & E. ×300.

FIG. 8. Monkey no. 1. Degeneration of neurons with astroglial proliferation in lateral geniculate nucleus. ×600.

FIG. 9. Monkey no. 1. Degeneration of myelin in optic nerve. Toluidin blue. × 600.

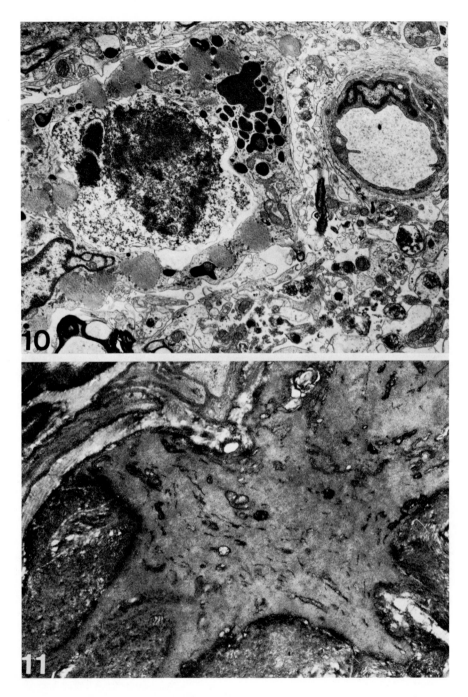

FIG. 10. Monkey no. 1. Deep layer of calcarine cortex. Cytolysis of nerve cell surrounded by a macrophage. ×8,000.

FIG. 11. Monkey no. 1. Sural nerve. Degeneration of myelin sheath and markedly increased number of neurofilaments in axon. ×12,000.

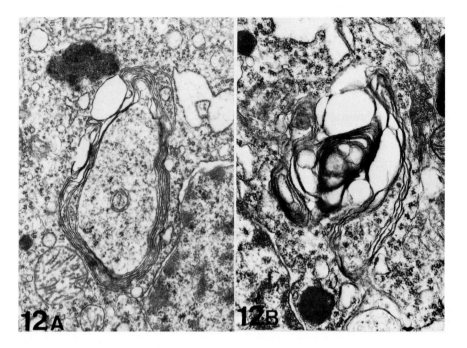

FIG. 12. Monkey no. 4. A part of nerve cell in calcarine cortex. **A:** Multimembranous structure. ×13,000. **B:** Myelin-like membranous structure. ×20,000.

dorsal nuclei in the spinal cord as well as in some dorsal root ganglion neurons.

Electron microscopic observations revealed remarkable degeneration of nerve cells in the cerebral cortex, especially in the calcarine cortex. Loss of mitochondria and endoplasmic reticulum as well as breakdown of the nuclear membrane in the nerve cells were seen. These necrotic nerve cells were surrounded by astrocytes or macrophages (Fig. 10). Similar degeneration of neurons and nerve fibers was seen in the lateral geniculate nuclei. There was occasional Wallerian degeneration of the myelinated nerve fibers in the granular layer of the cerebellum. There was a moderate increase in the number of neurofilaments of the axon and destruction of the myelin sheaths in the sural nerves (Fig. 11).

Monkeys no. 2 and 3 did not develop any clinical or histopathological abnormality.

In monkey no. 4, histopathologically, the nerve cells in the deep layer of the calcarine cortex appeared slightly atrophic (Figs. 5 and 7.) However, during this stage electron microscopic observation of the nerve cells revealed the presence of many myelin-like membranous structures in the perikarya. Cisternae of Golgi apparatus appeared to encircle a portion of the cytoplasm. The wall of these structures had increased in electron density and changed into myelin-like membranous structures (Fig. 12). Focal degeneration of myelinated nerve fibers was seen in the sural nerves resembling that found in monkey no. 1.

COMMENT

The clinical symptoms and histopathological findings in monkeys with methylmercury intoxication are very similar to those of human beings. Therefore, the experimental model in monkeys may be useful to ascertain the correlation between the amount of methylmercury accumulation and the histopathological changes in the central nervous system. Previous pathological reports by many investigators had emphasized that the preferential damage of the calcarine cortex is related to the clinical symptom of constriction of the visual fields.

Visual acuity impairment and optic atrophy were reported in patients in the Iraqi epidemics (9), whereas few patients with reduced visual acuity were reported in the Japanese epidemics. Since improvement in visual acuity has been remarkable in most of the patients in Iraq, the optic nerve involvement might have been of reversible nature, as suggested by Rustam and Hamdi (9).

In monkeys, chromatolysis of neurons with glial cell proliferation in the lateral geniculate nuclei was reported by Berlin et al. (2) and Shaw et al. (12). In addition, changes of the optic nerve were present in our monkey no. 1.

Our previous study (11) on the retina of rats after methylmercury intoxication had demonstrated swelling of synaptic terminals of bipolar cells with loss of synaptic vesicles.

Several reports on autopsy cases described that there were no remarkable changes in the optic nerves and lateral geniculate nuclei. However, the present study indicates that there is obvious involvement of the neuron in the lateral geniculate nuclei in two cases with Minamata disease as well as change of the optic nerve in case 1. Therefore, a further careful study is necessary to ascertain change of the optic nerve and lateral geniculate nuclei in patients in Japanese epidemics.

Early ultrastructural changes in the cortical neurons, seen in monkey no. 4 without clinical symptom, were swellings of the rough endoplasmic reticulum and Golgi apparatus. Then, cisternae of Golgi apparatus appeared to be encircling a portion of the cytoplasm and forming multi-lamellar structures.

The formation of myelin-like membranous structures in neurons after methylmercury intoxication is not an uncommon event in the degeneration of cytoplasm such as ischemic nerve cell changes (7). The increased electron density of the membrane of these structures suggests that biochemical components of the wall may be changed after methylmercury intoxication.

Ikeda et al. (5) investigated whether daily doses of 0.3 and 0.1 mg/kg of methylmercury chloride were definitely neurotoxic to monkeys. In our study, toxic doses of mercury in monkey no. 1 appear very similar to those of Ikeda's experiments. Monkey no. 4, administered 0.03 mg/kg daily for 327 days, did not show any detectable clinical signs. However, during this stage electron microscopic study revealed definite changes of the neuron in the calcarine cortex.

Clinically inapparent damage to the central nervous system has been demonstrated in a squirrel monkey with a maximum blood Hg level of 1.2 μg/g by Grant (3). The biological half-time for total Hg in the monkey has been reported as 49 $\pm$ 2.8 days in blood and 134 $\pm$ 2.7 days in the whole body by Berlin et al. (1). Our findings demonstrated that methylmercury in smaller doses of 0.03 mg/kg for long-term administration produces ultrastructural damage to the central nervous system.

SUMMARY

1. In addition to previous neuropathological reports on Minamata disease, further examination on two autopsy cases in Niigata revealed neuronal changes with astroglial proliferation in the lateral geniculate nuclei, basal ganglia, and brainstem.

2. Six cynomolgus monkeys were administered per os 0.01 to 0.21 mg/kg daily for 62 to 327 days. A monkey administered 0.21 mg/kg daily for 62 days (total 12.8 mg/kg) developed clinical symptoms re-

sembling those of Minamata disease in human beings. The pathological changes in the central nervous system including the lateral geniculate nuclei and optic nerves were very similar to those of acute human cases.

3. A monkey that received low doses of mercury, 0.03 mg/kg daily for 327 days (total 8.7 mg/kg), did not show any detectable clinical signs. However, electron microscopic study revealed definite changes in the calcarine cortex of the monkey, characterized by loss of ribosome, multilamellar proliferations of the membrane of endoplasmic reticulum, and formation of myelin-like structures in the perikaryon.

ACKNOWLEDGMENT

This investigation was supported in part by grants from the Japan Ministry of Environmental Health, the Ministry of Education, and Tokyo Metropolitan Bureau of Hygiene.

REFERENCES

1. Berlin, M., Carlson, J., and Norseth, T. (1975): Dose-dependence of methylmercury metabolism. *Arch. Environ. Health,* 30:307–313.
2. Berlin, M., Grant, C. A., Hellberg, J., Hellström, J., and Schütz, A. (1975): Neurotoxicity of methylmercury in squirrel monkeys. *Arch. Environ. Health,* 30:340–348.
3. Grant, C. A. (1971): Pathology of experimental methylmercury intoxication: Some problems of exposure and response. In: *Mercury, Mercurials and Mercaptans,* edited by Morton W. Miller and Thomas W. Clarkson, pp. 294–312. Charles C Thomas, Springfield, Illinois.
4. Hunter, D., Bomford, R. R., and Russell, D. S. (1940): Poisoning by methyl mercury compounds. *Q. J. Med.,* 9:193–213.
5. Ikeda, Y., Tobe, M., Kobayashi, K., Suzuki, S.,

Kawasaki, Y., and Yonemaru, H. (1973): Long-term toxicity study of methylmercuric chloride in monkeys. *Toxicology,* 1:361–375.
6. Ikuta, F., Makifuchi, T., Ohama, E., Koga, M., Yamamura, Y., Oyake, Y., Saito, H., Kanno, S., and Kitamura, S. (1974): Morphological alterations in the autopsy cases of chronic organic mercury intoxication with minimal doses. *Adv. Neurol. Sci.* (Japanese ed.), 18(5):861–881.
7. Little, J. R., Kerr, F. W. L., and Sundt, T. M., Jr. (1974): The role of lysosomes in production of ischemic nerve cell changes. *Arch. Neurol.,* 30:448–455.
8. Oyake, Y., Tanaka, M., Kubo, H., and Chichibu, M. (1966): Neuropathological studies on organic mercury intoxication, with special reference to distribution of mercury granules. *Adv. Neurol. Sci.* (Japanese ed.), 10(4):744–750.
9. Rustam, H., and Hamdi, T. (1974): Methyl mercury poisoning in Iraq. A neurological study. *Brain,* 97:499–510.
10. Sato, T., Niina, K., and Sahashi, K. (1974): An electron microscopic study on the retina of rats after methylmercury intoxication. *Brain Nerve* (Japanese ed.), 26(5):614–615.
11. Sato, T., Makifuchi, T., Ikuta, F., Masuhara, T., and Nakamura, Y. (1976): Long-term studies on the neurotoxicity of small amount of methylmercury in monkeys. *Igaku no Ayumi* (Japanese ed.), 97(4):175–176.
12. Shaw, C., Mottet, N. K., Body, R. L., and Luschei, E. S. (1975): Variability of neuropathologic lesions in experimental methylmercurial encephalopathy in primates. *Am. J. Pathol.,* 80(3):451–470.
13. Takeuchi, T., Morikawa, N., Matsumoto, H., and Shiraishi, Y. (1962): A pathological study of Minamata disease in Japan. *Acta Neuropathol.* (*Berl.*). 2:40–57.
14. Takeuchi, T., Etoh, K., Kojima, H., Otsuka, Y., Miyayama, H., Suko, S., Sakai, K., Sakurama, N., Iwamasa, T., and Matsumoto, H. (1972): Minamata disease: Pathological findings in 10 years long term survivors. *Kumamoto Med. J.,* 46(11):666–705.
15. Tokuomi, H. (1960): Minamata disease: Clinical observation and pathologic physiology. *Psychiatr. Neurol. Jpn.,* 62(13):1816–1850.
16. Tsubaki, T., Sato, T., Shirakawa, K., Kanbayashi, K., and Hirota, K. (1968): Epidemiological study of mercury poisoning in the Agano River area. *Saigai Igaku* (Japanese ed.), 11(14):1383–1389.

Neurotoxicology, edited by L. Roizin, H. Shiraki, and N. Grčević. Raven Press, New York © 1977.

Chemotoxic Blood-Brain Barrier Damage with Special Regard to Some Mercurial Effects

Oskar Steinwall

Department of Neurology, University of Göteborg, Sahlgren Hospital, 413 45 Göteborg, Sweden

The present chapter is an abstract of a number of studies stretching over a long period of time and bearing more on certain pathophysiological aspects of the blood-brain barrier (BBB) than on mercurial intoxication in general.

In the late 1950s a variety of chemicals were investigated in our laboratory with regard to their potency to damage the BBB when briefly perfused through one hemisphere in rabbits under control· of concentration *in loco* and application time. Special interest was directed toward agents known to block the transport apparatus in the tubules of the kidney because it was hypothesized that principally related bidirectional transports took part in the function of the BBB (8,9).

EXPERIMENTAL PROCEDURE

The experimental procedure implies in principal injection of the noxious agent via one internal carotid artery in rabbits with a pressure adjusted to expel the blood only from the ipsilateral hemisphere during the application period (30 sec). Afterward, the hemisphere is supplied via the circle of Willis with blood, to which indicators of barrier dysfunctions are added (for details, see ref. 9).

BBB-DAMAGING AGENTS

Examples of BBB-damaging agents are presented in Table 1. The approximate minimal molar concentration inducing BBB

TABLE 1. *Examples of chemicals damaging the blood-brain barrier*

Heavy metals		
$Hg^{++}:10^{-5}$	$Ag^+: 5 \times 10^{-5}$	$Au^{+++}:10^{-4}$
$Cu^{++}:10^{-4}$	$Pb^{++}: \quad 10^{-3}$	
"Specific" sulfhydryl-blocking agents		
p-Chloro-mercuri-benzoate		5×10^{-6}
N-ethyl-maleimide		10^{-4}
o-Iodoso-bensoate		10^{-3}
Iodo-acetate		10^{-3}
Various metabolic inhibitors		
(affecting, i.e., renal tubular transport)		
2,4-Dinitrophenol		5×10^{-3}
Fluoride		2×10^{-3}
Malonate		2×10^{-2}
Azide		10^{-1}

Approximate minimum concentration inducing extravasation of acid dyes in the brain after brief intracarotid injection (about 30 sec). See text for experimental method.

damage, here defined as a barely visible extravasation of trypan blue, shows that certain heavy metals, and particularly mercuric ions, are highly injurious to the barrier. Organic mercurials, e.g., methyl mercuric ions, showed comparable damaging potency. The dose-dependent degree of BBB injury was clearly demonstrable. A solution of 1 mM $HgCl_2$ caused massive trypan blue staining, extravasation of red cells, and macroscopical edema in the perfused hemisphere. Under similar conditions the staining was moderately strong at 0.1 mM and barely visible at 0.01 mM. The detoxifying effect of equimolar binding to dimercaprol (BAL) was obvious, rendering 1 mM $HgCl_2$ innocuous as regards trypan blue extravasation.

Some aspects of mercurial BBB damage, derived from studies with the unilateral-exposure technique, are now reviewed.

MERCURIAL EFFECTS OF BBB TRANSPORT MECHANISMS

At the time when these studies were initiated, a BBB damage was still commonly thought of in terms of merely abnormal permeability with leakage of plasma solutes. Today, the BBB concept has emerged to comprise also a variety of directed biological transport mechanisms, many serving to supply the brain with essential nutrients, others perhaps removing polar metabolites, like conjugated organic acids (cf. the hypothesis of analogies with the renal tubules).

In order to reveal a presumed inhibitory effect of mercuric ions on specific carrier-mediated blood-brain *uptake* of nutrients, the leakage component should preferably be minimized. Using very low $HgCl_2$ concentrations for the unilateral perfusion, it was possible to achieve a convincing *decrease* in the brain uptake of various nutrient tracers concomitant with a slight or invisible extravasation of conventional

BBB-damage indicators like acid dyes. With radioassay of a labeled compound (counting or autoradiography, or both), such decreased uptake was evidenced not only for metabolized nutrients like glucose, leucine, and selenomethionine but also for tracers like methyl-0-glucose and cycloleucine, which are known to share the respective biological transport of their analogs without being further metabolized (3,10,11,13). Under the conditions employed, the mercurial thus seemed to affect primarily the actual transport mechanisms.

This was supported by recent studies on ^{3}H-leucine uptake and further incorporation in different cell fractions after unilateral mercurial BBB damage (3). Unfractionated material and fractions enriched in neurons, glia, and somewhat contaminated capillaries prepared according to Blomstrand and Hamberger (1) were determined with regard to protein-incorporated radioactivity. The main results are given in Table 2. Both unfractionated material and the different cell fractions showed similarly decreased incorporation in the perfused hemisphere, fairly proportional to the overall decrease in tracer uptake. Slice incubation studies from brains, similarly damaged *in vivo*, showed no corresponding differences between perfused and control hemisphere (Table 3). These and similar short-term

TABLE 2. *Effect of unilateral Hg^{++} perfusion on uptake and incorporation of ^{3}H-leucine (bilateral carotid perfusion) into trichloracetic acid (TCA)-soluble and TCA-insoluble material from unfractionated material and into TCA-precipitable material from cell-enriched fractions*

Unfractionated		
TCA-soluble	54%	±7
TCA-precipitable	34%	±3
Neuronal fraction	42%	±6
Glial cell fraction	46%	±6
Capillary fraction	49%	±8

Value for Hg^{++}-exposed side expressed as percent of the corresponding value for the contralateral side. Mean of six experiments.

TABLE 3. *Incorporation of ^{3}H-leucine into TCA-precipitable material during brain slice incubation*

Unfractionated material	93%	±7
Neuronal fraction	86%	±9
Glial cell fraction	98%	±9
Capillary fraction	103%	

Value for the Hg^{++}-exposed side expressed as percent of the corresponding value for the contralateral side. Mean of 15 experiments.

studies seem to indicate that an early and probably essential neurotoxic effect of mercuric ions is transport inhibition and thereby starvation of cells dependent on the specifically transported nutrients.

SITE OF ACTION

Theoretically, one would expect that the mercuric ions, after brief application in very dilute solutions and according to their strong tissue affinity, should be captured mostly in the "blood-brain interphase," i.e., primarily in the endothelium, reaching brain tissue proper first when a damaged barrier permits the passage of recirculating ions, now bound to plasma proteins by about 99%. This idea has experimental support of a different type.

1. In studies with EEG recording (6), we found that a weak unilateral mercurial BBB damage could exist for up to 1 hr without neuronal damage as reflected in EEG asymmetry. Increased permeability could meantime be discovered by transient unilateral spikes after intravenous penicillin administration.

2. Catecholamines, intravenously injected after corresponding BBB damage, invaded only the barrier-damaged hemisphere, whereupon they showed a normal pattern of active uptake in axons and nerve terminals as observed with fluorescence microscopic technique (5).

3. In a recent study BBB damage was induced with ^{203}HgCl$_2$ and fluorecein sodium given as an indicator of abnormal permeability (2). The experiments were of 10 min duration. Radioactivity was assayed in neuronal-, glial-, and capillary-enriched fractions. The activity was practically wholly recovered in protein-bound form. The capillary fractions, although contaminated with cells with much lower activity, showed by far the highest activity; the glial fractions contained about half as much; and the neurons came down to very low values—in three of the nine brains practically zero (Table 4). In contrast, there was no significant difference in distribution between the cell fractions when normal brain slices were incubated in ^{203}Hg-containing medium (30 min, 37°C).

Thus, both theoretical considerations and experimental findings suggest that, under these conditions, the barrier-damaging mercuric ions primarily affect the endothelium and possibly also adjacent glial elements that may be involved in

TABLE 4. *Distribution of BBB-damaging ^{203}Hg^{++} in different cell-enriched fractions*

	Exposed hemisphere	Nonexposed hemisphere
Unfractionated	4,624 cpm/mg ± 410 (= 100%)	1,221 cpm ± 230 (= 100%)
Neuronal fraction	37%	46%
Glial fraction	138%	182%
Capillary fraction	241%	267%

Activity of ^{203}Hg in unfractionated tissue is given as mean cpm/mg protein. The values from differential cell-enriched fractions are expressed in percent of the unfractionated brain value for each hemisphere.

BBB functional activity. Whether impairment of the BBB actually constitutes a significant pathogenic factor in clinical mercuric intoxication remains to be proved. Experimental studies with systemic poisoning (4,7,12) have as yet not conclusively elucidated this question.

REFERENCES

1. Blomstrand, C., and Hamberger, A. (1970): Amino acid incorporation in vitro in proteins of neuronal and glial cell enriched fractions. *J. Neurochem.*, 17:1187–1195.
2. Blomstrand, C., and Steinwall, O.: Distribution of [203]Hg in different structural elements after acute damage to the blood-brain barrier by [203]Hg-mercuric chloride. (*To be published.*)
3. Blomstrand, C., and Steinwall, O.: Leucine incorporation in different brain cell fractions after damage to the blood-brain barrier by mercuric ions. (*To be published.*)
4. Carmichael, N., Cavanagh, J. B., and Rodda, R. A. (1975): Some effects of methyl mercury salts on the rabbit nervous system. *Acta Neuropathol. (Berl.)*, 32:115–125.
5. Flodmark, S., Hamberger, A., Hamberger, B., and Steinwall, O. (1969): Concurrent registration of EEG responses, catecholamine uptake and trypan blue staining in chemical blood-brain barrier damage. *Acta Neuropathol. (Berl.),* 12:16–22.
6. Flodmark, S., and Steinwall, O. (1963): Differentiated effects on certain blood-brain barrier phenomena and on the EEG produced by means of intracarotidally applied mercuric dichloride. *Acta Physiol. Scand.,* 57:446–453.
7. Joó, F. (1971): Increased production of coated vesicles in the brain capillaries during enhanced permeability of the blood-brain barrier. *Br. J. Exp. Pathol.,* 52:646–649.
8. Steinwall, O. (1961): Transport mechanisms in certain blood-brain barrier phenomena—a hypothesis. *Acta Psychiatr. Neurol. Scand. [Suppl. 150]*, 36:314–318.
9. Steinwall, O. (1967): Transport inhibition phenomena in unilateral chemical injury of blood-brain barrier. *Prog. Brain Res.,* 29:357–364.
10. Steinwall, O. (1969): Brain uptake of Se75-selenomethionine after damage to blood-brain barrier by mercuric ions. *Acta Neurol. Scand.,* 45:362–368.
11. Steinwall, O., and Klatzo, I. (1966): Selective vulnerability of the blood-brain barrier in chemically induced lesions. *J. Neuropathol. Exp. Neurol.,* 25:542–559.
12. Steinwall, O., and Olsson, Y. (1969): Impairment of the blood-brain barrier in mercury poisoning. *Acta Neurol. Scand.,* 45:351–361.
13. Steinwall, O., and Snyder, S. H. (1969): Brain uptake of C14-cycloleucine after damage to blood-brain barrier by mercuric ions. *Acta Neurol. Scand.,* 45:369–375.

Neurotoxicology, edited by L. Roizin, H. Shiraki, and N. Grčević. Raven Press, New York © 1977.

Modification of the Neurotoxic Effects of Methyl Mercury by Selenium

*,†Louis W. Chang, *,‡Alden W. Dudley, Jr., *,‡Mary A. Dudley, **Howard E. Ganther, and ***Milton L. Sunde

Departments of *Pathology, **Nutritional and ***Poultry Sciences, University of Wisconsin, Madison, Wisconsin 53706

Unusually high levels of selenium were reported in the organs of animals and patients who died from Minamata disease (41,42). Recently, Koeman et al. (29) also noted a definitive correlation between the accumulation of selenium and that of mercury in the liver of seals and dolphins.

Increasing evidence indicates that selenium, like sulfur, has a high affinity for certain heavy metals such as cadmium and mercury. In general, the interaction between the metal and selenium in animals leads to decreased biological activities and toxicity of both the metal and selenium. Although the neurotoxic effects of methyl mercury are well documented (2–8, 37,40), the protective potential of selenium against the toxicity of mercury is relatively unknown. However, since its discovery, the effectiveness of selenium as a protective agent against methyl mercury toxicity has attracted increasing attention.

The interaction of mercury and selenium resulting in the decreased toxicity of both has been reported by numerous investigators (19,21–23,25,27,28,32–39). Such observations were successfully obtained in both acute and chronic studies, with both inorganic and organic mercury, and with either inorganic or organic forms of selenium. Only in rare cases has an adverse interaction been reported (26,35).

Although the interaction of mercury with selenium metabolism was noted over 30 years ago (24), the effectiveness of selenium against acute inorganic mercury intoxication was not appreciated until 1967 (34). The efficacy of dietary selenium (0.5 ppm) against chronic toxicity of methyl mercury was first reported by Ganther et al. in 1972 (19) who showed that growth and survival rates were much improved in rats fed both methyl mercury and selenium as compared to those fed methyl mercury alone. Similar findings were subsequently reported by Stillings et al. (38) and Potter and Matrone (36) in 1974. Many other studies, however, have employed rather high, nonnutritional levels of selenium (as sodium selenite), typically 5 ppm or more. At such levels selenium itself may be toxic, and in such cases protection against selenium toxicity by mercury has been observed (25). Therefore, a combination of mercury and selenium may be administered to animals at levels which would be toxic when each element was given alone, but which become less toxic when given together. In short, an antagonistic rather than a synergistic effect in toxicity can be observed.

---

† Present address: National Center for Toxicological Research, Jefferson, Arkansas 72709; ‡ Department of Pathology, University of South Alabama, Mobile, Alabama 36688.

MODIFICATION OF MERCURY TOXICITY BY SELENIUM: AN EXPERIMENTAL MODEL

Effects of Selenium on the Survival of Mercury-Intoxicated Animals

We have investigated the protective effects of both sodium selenite and naturally occurring selenium. in fish against the toxic effects of methyl mercury.

Cats were fed with diets containing 3.0 ppm methyl mercury and different levels of selenium (added as sodium selenite) ranging from 0.5 to 1.0 ppm. It was found that, although all the cats were exposed to similar amounts of mercury, the animals that were on a higher selenium (1.0 ppm) diet all outlived the animals that were on a lower selenium (0.5 ppm) diet.

Similar results were obtained with rats that were injected with 2.0 ppm methyl mercury. The selenium-treated (1.0 ppm) rats all demonstrated a better growth pattern than the untreated animals. Moreover, no significant neurological disturbances were observed in the selenium-treated rats at the time when all the untreated animals became symptomatic of mercury intoxication.

Of greater environmental significance is the ability of naturally occurring selenium, at levels of the same order of magnitude as the nutritional requirement for this essential element, to reduce the toxicity of methyl mercury. An experiment was performed to investigate the effectiveness of naturally occurring dietary selenium against methyl mercury toxicity. The low selenium (0.15 ppm) food source was fresh water pike and the moderate (0.5 ppm) was tuna.

The cats were divided into several groups. There were control animals on basal fish diets without added mercury or on commercial fish-flavored cat food. There also were animals on tuna or pike diets containing either 1.5 ppm or 3.0

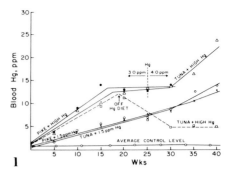

FIG. 1. Mercury levels in the blood of cats on pike and tuna diets containing various amounts of methyl mercury. No significant difference in the blood mercury was found between animals on pike and tuna diets of similar mercury content.

ppm methyl mercury. Because of the difference in the selenium content in the tuna and pike, the mercury/selenium ratio in the tuna diet was much lower than that in the corresponding pike diet.

The levels of mercury and selenium in the blood were monitored once a month. No difference in the blood mercury was observed between the tuna- and the pike-fed animals (Fig. 1). It was interesting to note that the blood selenium level was generally lower in the animals fed with higher concentrations of methyl mercury. Tissue analysis showed similar mercury contents within most organs of the tuna- and pike-fed cats (Fig. 2). However, because of the difference of selenium content in the diets, the uptake of selenium by the animals on tuna diet was much

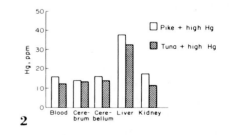

FIG. 2. Average mercury concentrations in cat tissues at time of death up to 30th week of experiment. No significant difference was observed between the tuna- or pike-fed animals.

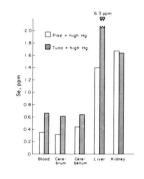

3

FIG. 3. Average selenium concentrations in cat tissues at time of death up to 30th week of experiment. Much higher selenium content was found in the tuna-fed animals.

higher (Fig. 3), resulting in a much lower mercury/selenium ratio in the tissues of these animals (Fig. 4).

Despite similar concentrations of mercury in the pike- and tuna-fed animals, approximately 12% of the animals on high mercury–pike diets displayed neurological symptoms of methyl mercury intoxication (truncal ataxia with a drunken gait; seizures; changes in personality such as aggression, apprehension, or stupor; abnormal EEG; and progression in frequency and severity of seizures to death in status epilepticus) by the 10th week of the experiment, whereas no neurological disturbances were observed in the corresponding tuna-fed animals at this time (Fig. 5). By the 30th week, 100% of the animals on the high mercury–pike diet

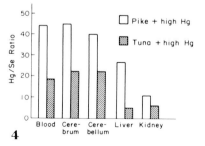

4

FIG. 4. Average mercury/selenium ratios in cat tissues at time of death up to 30th week of experiment. Significantly higher mercury/selenium ratio was observed in the pike-fed animals.

were dead, whereas about 40% of the animals in the high mercury–tuna group were still alive (Fig. 5). The animals in the low mercury groups survived longer than the high mercury groups. Once again, the animals on the tuna diet outlived those on the pike diet. It appears, therefore, that the selenium in the tuna diet offered some protection against mercury toxicity.

Effects of Selenium on the Neuropathology of Mercury-Intoxicated Animals

Ample evidence has been provided, both by other investigators and by our own laboratory, to show that selenium prolongs the survival of mercury-intoxicated animals. However, the question concerning the effects of selenium on the tissue reactions of the animals has yet to be answered. In other words, morphology correlates or anatomical substrates and the defense mechanism must be defined.

Parallel studies of the neuropathology in the cerebellum of rats subjected to methyl mercury intoxication with or without selenium treatment were performed. All animals were sacrificed at the same time when the nonselenium-treated animals became symptomatic from mercury toxicity. Tissue samples from the cerebellum were obtained from the animals and examined under a "double blind" system. It was found that, although there were severe degenerative changes in the cerebellum of mercury-intoxicated animals (Fig. 6), the brains of the selenium-treated animals appeared to be well protected from mercury toxicity at this time (Fig. 7).

Despite the initial protection against methyl mercury toxicity by selenium, the selenium-exposed animals also died at a later time. When tissues from these animals were examined, it was found that the end stage pathology was very similar to that of mercury toxicity, showing areas of cerebellar degeneration with loss of granule

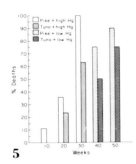

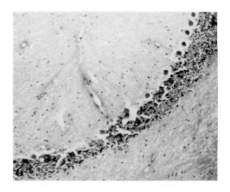

FIG. 5. Modification of methyl mercury toxicity by dietary selenium measured by the survival rate of cats on pike or tuna diets. Higher percentage of the animals on the tuna diet outlived those on pike diets containing similar amounts of mercury.

FIG. 6. Cerebellum of a rat injected with 2.0 ppm methyl mercury/day for 20 days. Thinning and degenerative changes of the granule cells were observed. H.&E. × 200.

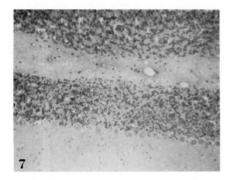

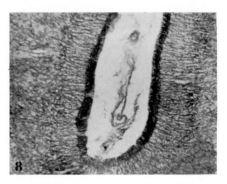

FIG. 7. Cerebellum of a rat injected with 2.0 ppm methyl mercury and 1.0 ppm sodium selenite/day for 20 days. Significant morphological protection was observed. H.&E. ×200.

FIG. 8. Cerebellum of a cat fed on tuna diet containing 3.0 to 4.0 ppm methyl mercury for 30 weeks. Animal died from methyl mercury intoxication. The end stage pathology is similar to that found in animals on pike diet. Besides loss of granule cells, there is a proliferation of Bergmann's glial fibers. Holzer's. ×400.

cells and extensive proliferation of Bergmann's glial fibers (Fig. 8). With electron microscopy, however, it was revealed that the degenerative pattern of the cerebellar granule cells was noticeably more severe and widespread in the nonselenium-exposed animals than in the selenium-treated ones (Fig. 9). Moreover, it was noted that an increase in accumulation of lysosomes and dilatation of the rough endoplasmic reticulum (Fig. 10) was present in the Purkinje neurons of the low selenium animals (e.g., cats on mercury–pike diet). Such changes of the Purkinje neurons, however, were not readily found in the animals exposed to high selenium diet as well as mercury (e.g., cats on mercury–tuna diet). Therefore, it may be concluded that selenium, although it may not offer a total or permanent protection of the animals from methyl mercury intoxication, definitely reduces and modifies the organic mercury toxicity.

DISCUSSION AND CONCLUSION

The mutual antagonism of mercury and selenium is one of the strongest and most general examples of interaction in the trace

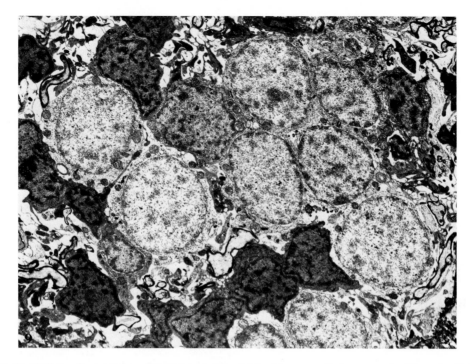

FIG. 9. Cerebellum of a cat fed on pike diet containing 3.0 to 4.0 ppm methyl mercury for 20 weeks. Extensive degeneration of the granule cells, which became shrunken and electron dense, was observed. Degenerative pattern of the cerebellum of the tuna-fed animals, however, appeared to be less extensive. ×3,500.

element field. The interaction of mercury and selenium resulting in the decreased toxicity of mercury and/or selenium has been observed on both acute and chronic studies, with either inorganic mercury or methyl mercury salts, and with both inorganic and organic forms of selenium (19,21–23,25–28, 32–39).

The mechanism of selenium in the reduction of mercury toxicity is rather complicated. It is apparent that the effect varies with the relative amounts of mercury and selenium given to the animal (22). However, when methyl mercury is given at a toxic dose (31,36,38), it seems that selenium does not reduce the accumulation of mercury in the animals. It is known that inorganic salts of selenium are rapidly reduced in animal tissues to various selenides that bind metals, such as selenotrisulfides (—S—Se—S—), selenopersulfides (—S—SeH), hydrogen selenide (H_2Se), or other low-molecular-weight metabolites, as well as the analogous selenoprotein derivatives (14–16,18,20). Such complexing, in fact, usually results in increased retention of the metal with selenium in the animal and decreased elimination via excretory pathways, milk, or offspring (12,17,30,38). The distribution of the metal and selenium within the tissues and tissue components may also be altered (1,10–12,17,30). Recent studies by Stoewsand et al. (39) and H.E. Ganther and M.L. Sunde (*unpublished observation*) indicate that brains of quail fed with methyl mercury and sodium selenite can accumulate extremely high levels of methyl mercury (as high as 40 to 50 ppm) without any occurrence of neurological symptoms or mortality. It appears, therefore, that the protective effect of selenium can be exerted within the tissue without decreasing the amount of the toxic metal in that tissue. Although it was found that the selenium levels in the nervous system are also

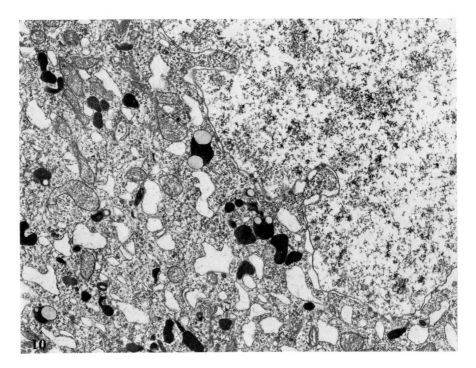

FIG. 10. Cerebellum of a cat fed on pike diet containing 3.0 to 4.0 ppm methyl mercury for 20 weeks. Dilatation of the endoplasmic reticulum and accumulation of lysosomes were observed in the Purkinje neurons. Such Purkinje changes were not readily found in the tuna-fed animals. ×12,500.

elevated [to levels of 4 to 5 ppm (28)], these levels of selenium are far below the amount equivalent to a 1:1 equimolar complex, thus selenium is not simply chelating the bulk of the brain mercury.

It has been claimed that selenium induces the "C–Hg cleavage enzyme" (13), and the possibility exists that selenium may permit greater breakdown of methyl mercury to less toxic forms. However, there is little evidence that such a mechanism is of much significance when toxic levels of methyl mercury are given (9,22). Moreover, Stoewsand (39) has demonstrated that the mercury in the brains of selenium-treated animals was still in the form of methyl mercury rather than a less toxic breakdown product. Furthermore selenium is found to be highly protective against the toxicity of inorganic mercury (mercuric mercury) *per se* (34,36). It is clear that selenium does not exert its

protective or detoxification effect by demethylation.

A recent study by Welsh (43) indicated that the mercury isolated from selenium-treated animals (selenium-complexed mercury) is much less toxic than the same amount of selenium-free mercury. Chen et al. (11) reported that after pretreatment with selenium the mercury in the soluble fraction of the cell, a major subcellular mercury-binding component, was markedly diverted from low-molecular-weight proteins to large-molecular-weight ones. With all the present information on hand, it may be postulated that the interaction of selenium and mercury for detoxification may not be a direct 1:1 molar ratio, but rather each selenium molecule may induce the formation of a large protein complex that in turn binds to multiple molecules of mercury. In such a way a high level of mercury could be "arrested" or "inactivated" by a much lesser amount of selenium. The mechanism proposed here merely represents our postulation. The precise mechanism of selenium in the modification of mercury toxicity is still unclear. Further investigation in this area is needed.

Our study with cats not only indicates that dietary selenium is effective in the reduction of methyl mercury toxicity, but also suggests that the mercury/selenium ratio in food or animal tissues, particularly the brain, may be a more accurate reference index than the mercury level alone in relation to mercury toxicity. Moreover, since many marine organisms tend to accumulate selenium with mercury in an approximately 1:1 ratio, it becomes important to be aware of the fact that mercury in marine fish may have a less toxic potential than mercury in fish from polluted fresh water containing a similar amount of mercury.

ACKNOWLEDGMENTS

Research is partially supported by National Marine Fisheries Service, NOAA, Contract No. 4–36755 and by the Food Research Institute of the University of Wisconsin, Madison, Wisconsin.

REFERENCES

1. Burk, R. F., Foster, K. A., Greenfield, P. M., and Kiker, K. W. (1947): Binding of simultaneously administered inorganic selenium and mercury to a rat plasma protein. *Proc. Soc. Exp. Biol. Med.*, 145:782–785.
2. Chang, L. W. (1977): Neurotoxic effects of mercury intoxication—a review. *Environ. Res.* (*Submitted for publication.*)
3. Chang, L. W., Desnoyers, P. A., and Hartmann, H. A. (1972): Quantitative cytochemical studies of RNA in experimental mercury poisoning. I. Changes in RNA content. *J. Neuropathol. Exp. Neurol.*, 31:389–501.
4. Chang, L. W., Desnoyers, P. A., and Hartmann, H. A. (1973): Quantitative cytochemical study of RNA in experimental mercury poisoning. II. Changes in base composition and ratios. *Acta Neuropathol. (Berl.),* 23:77–83.
5. Chang, L. W., and Hartmann, H. A. (1972): Electron microscopic histochemical study on the localization and distribution of mercury in the nervous system after mercury intoxication. *Exp. Neurol.*, 35:122–137.
6. Chang, L. W., and Hartmann, H. A. (1972): Ultrastructural studies of the nervous system after mercury intoxication. I. Pathological changes in the nerve cell bodies. *Acta Neuropathol. (Berl.),* 20:122–138.
7. Chang, L. W., and Hartmann, H. A. (1972): Ultrastructural studies of the nervous system after mercury intoxication. II. Pathological changes in the nerve fibers. *Acta Neuropathol. (Berl.),* 20:316–334.
8. Chang, L. W., and Hartmann, H. A. (1972): Blood-brain barrier dysfunction in experimental mercury intoxication. *Acta Neuropathol. (Berl.),* 21:179–184.
9. Chen, R. W., Ganther, H. E., and Hoekstra, W. G. (1973): Studies on the binding of methyl mercury by thioneine. *Biochem. Biophys. Res. Commun.*, 51:383–390.
10. Chen, R. W., Wagner, P. A., Hoekstra, W. G., and Ganther, H. E. (1974): Affinity labeling studies with [109]Cd in cadmium-induced testicular injury in rats. *J. Reprod. Fertil.*, 38:293–306.
11. Chen, R. W., Whanger, P. D., and Fang, S. C. (1974): Diversion of mercury binding in rat tissues by selenium. A possible mechanism of protection. *Pharmacol. Res. Commun.*, 6:571.
12. Eybl, V., Sykora, T., and Merth, F. (1969): Einfluss von Natriumselenit, Natriumtellurit and Natrium-sulfit auf Retention und Verteilung von Quecksilber bei maüsen. *Arch. Toxikol.*, 25:296–305.
13. Fang, S. C. (1974): Induction of C–Hg cleavage enzymes in rat liver by dietary selenite. *Res. Commun. Chem. Pathol. Pharmacol.*, 9:579–582.
14. Ganther, H. E. (1966): Enzyme synthesis of dimethyl selenide from sodium selenite in mouse liver extracts. *Biochemistry*, 5:1089–1098.
15. Ganther, H. E. (1968): Selenotrisulfides: Formation by the reaction of thiols with selenious acid. *Biochemistry*, 7:2898–2905.
16. Ganther, H. E. (1971): Reduction of the selenotrisulfide derivative of glutathione to a persulfide analog by glutathione reductase. *Biochemistry*, 10:4089–4098.
17. Ganther, H. E., and Baumann, C. A. (1962): Selenium metabolism. I. Effects of diet, arsenic, and cadmium. *J. Nutr.*, 77:210–216.
18. Ganther, H. E., and Corcoran, C. (1969): Selenotrisulfides. II. Cross-linking of reduced pancreatic ribonuclease with selenium. *Biochemistry*, 8:2557–2563.
19. Ganther, H. E., Goudie, C., Sunde, M. L., Kopecky, M. J., Wagner, P., Oh, S.-H., and Hoekstra, W. G. (1972): Selenium: Relation to decreased toxicity of methyl mercury added to

diets containing tuna. *Science,* 175:1122–1124.

20. Ganther, H. E., and Hsieh, H. (1974): Mechanisms for the conversion of selenite to selenides in mammalian tissues. In: *Trace Element Metabolism in Animals,* Vol. 2, edited by W. G. Hoekstra, J. W. Suttie, H. E. Ganther, and W. Mertz, pp. 338–353. Univ. Park Press, Baltimore.

21. Ganther, H. E., and Sunde, M. L. (1974): Effect of tuna fish and selenium on the toxicity of methyl mercury – a progress report. *J. Food Sci.,* 39:1–5.

22. Ganther, H. E., Wagner, P. A., Sunde, M. L., and Hoekstra, W. G. (1973): Protective effects of selenium against heavy metal toxicities. In: *Trace Substances in Environmental Health,* Vol. 6, edited by D. D. Hemphill, pp. 247–252. Univ. of Missouri Press, Columbia.

23. Groth, D. H., Vignati, L., Lowry, L., Mackay, G., and Stokinger, H. E. (1973): Mutual antagonistic and synergistic effects of inorganic selenium and mercury salts in chronic experiments. In: *Trace Substances in Environmental Health,* Vol. 6, edited by D. D. Hemphill, pp. 187–189. Univ. of Missouri Press, Columbia.

24. Gusberg, S. B., Zamecnik, P., and Aub, J. C. (1941): The distribution of injected organic diselenides in tissues of tumor-bearing animals. *J. Pharmacol. Exp. Ther.,* 71:239–245.

25. Hill, C. H. (1974): Reversal of selenium toxicity in chicks by mercury, copper, and cadmium. *J. Nutr.,* 104:593–598.

26. Huckabel, J. W., and Griffith, N. A. (1974): Toxicity of mercury and selenium to the eggs of carp (cyprinus carpio). *Trans. Am. Fisheries Soc.,* 103:822–824.

27. Iwata, H., Okamoto, H., and Ohsawa, Y. (1973): Effects of selenium on methyl mercury poisoning. *Res. Commun. Chem. Pathol. Pharmacol.,* 5:673–680.

28. Johnson, S. L., and Pond, W. G. (1974): Inorganic vs. organic Hg toxicity in growing rats: Protection by dietary Se but not Zn. *Nutr. Rep. Int.,* 9:135–147.

29. Koeman, J. H., Reeters, W. H. M., Kondstaal-Hol, C. H. M., Tjioe, P. S., and De Goeij, J. J. M. (1973): Mercury selenium correlations in marine animals. *Nature,* 245:385–386.

30. Moffitt, A. E., and Clary, J. J. (1974): Selenite induced binding of inorganic mercury in blood and other tissues in the rat. *Res. Commun. Chem. Pathol. Pharmacol.,* 7:593–603.

31. Ohi, G., Nishigaki, S., Seki, H., Tamura, Y., Maki, T., Maeda, H., Ochiai, S., Yamada, H., Shimamura, Y., and Yagyu, H. (1975): Interaction of dietary methyl mercury and selenium on accumulation and retention of these substances in rat organs. *Toxicol. Appl. Pharmacol.,* 32:527–533.

32. Parizek, J., Benes, I., Ostadalova, I., Babicky, A., Benes, J., and Lener, J. (1969): Metabolic interrelations of trace elements. The effect of some inorganic and organic compounds of selenium on the metabolism of cadmium and mercury in the rat. *Physiol. Bohemoslov.,* 18:95–103.

33. Parizek, J., Kalonskova, J., Babicky, A., Benes, J., and Pavlik, L. (1974): Interaction of selenium with mercury, cadmium, and other toxic metals. In: *Trace Element Metabolism in Animals,* Vol. 2, edited by W. G. Hoekstra, J. W. Suttie, H. E. Ganther, and W. Mertz, pp. 119–131. Univ. Park Press, Baltimore.

34. Parizek, J., and Ostadalova, I. (1967): The protective effect of small amounts of selenite in sublimate intoxication. *Experientia,* 23:142–143.

35. Parizek, J., Ostadalova, I., Kalouskova, J., Babicky, A., and Benes, J. (1971): The detoxifying effects of selenium. Interrelations between compounds of selenium and certain metals. In: *Newer Trace Elements in Nutrition,* edited by W. Mertz, and W. E. Cornatzer, pp. 85–122. Dekker, New York.

36. Potter, S., and Matrone, G. (1974): Effect of selenium on methyl mercury poisoning. *Res. Commun. Chem. Pathol. Pharmacol.,* 5:673–680.

37. Shiraki, H., and Takeuchi, T. (1971): Minamata disease. In: *Pathology of the Nervous System,* edited by J. Minckler, pp. 1651–1665. McGraw-Hill, New York.

38. Stillings, B. R., Lagally, H., Bauersfeld, P., and Soares, J. (1974): Effects of cystine, selenium and fish protein on the toxicity and metabolism of methyl mercury in rats. *Toxicol. Appl. Pharmacol.,* 30:243–254.

39. Stoewsand, G. S., Bache, C. A., and Lisk, D. J. (1974): Dietary selenium protection of methyl mercury intoxication of Japanese quail. *Bull. Environ. Contam. Toxicol.,* 11:152–156.

40. Takeuchi, T., and Shiraishi, Y. (1962): A pathological study of Minamata disease in Japan. *Acta Neuropathol. (Berl.),* 2:40–57.

41. Ueda, K. (1960): Experimental studies on selenium poisoning. *J. Kumamoto Med. Soc.,* 34 (Suppl. 1):141–155.

42. Uzioka, T. (1960): Analytical studies on methyl mercury in the animal organs and foodstuff. *J. Kumamoto Med. Soc.,* 34 (Suppl. 2):383–399.

43. Welsh, S. O. (1972): Physiological Effect of Methyl Mercury – Toxicity Interaction of Methyl Mercury with Selenium, Telliumum and Vit. E Ph.D. Thesis, University of Maryland.

Neurotoxicology, edited by L. Roizin, H. Shiraki, and N. Grčević. Raven Press, New York © 1977.

Metabolic Mechanisms of Neurotoxicity Caused by Mercury

J. B. Cavanagh

M.R.C. Research Group in Applied Neurobiology, Institute of Neurology, London WC1N 3AR, England 3AR, England

Methyl mercury poisoning in the rat principally causes selective damage to primary sensory neurons and to granule cells in the cerebellum (7). In the rabbit, in addition, it also causes loss of cerebellar stellate and basket cells, loss of small stellate cells from the cerebral cortex, and loss of granule cells from the dentate fascia of the hippocampus as well as from the islands of Calleja (3). Similar selectivity is found in the nervous system of other species (6,8,16). The question as to why the largest nerve cells of the nervous system (primary sensory cells) on the one hand and the smaller cells of the central nervous system (CNS) on the other should be selected for destruction on the entry of mercury into the system is an intriguing one that demands an answer.

There is evidence (1,11,13) that the capillary bed of sensory ganglia is permeable to plasma constituents owing to the presence of fenestrations between endothelial cells. Evans blue – albumin and horseradish peroxidase (HRP) readily enter, and within 2 min of intravenous injection HRP can be found within the extracellular spaces and even between satellite cells and lying against the surfaces of the neurons. It is apparent, therefore, that anything in the plasma readily reaches primary sensory neurons in greater quantity and sooner than it reaches CNS neurons which are sheltered behind the blood-brain barrier. It is doubtful, therefore, whether any other explanation is necessary for the far greater sensitivity of primary sensory cells to high circulating amounts of mercury.

The special sensitivity of small cells in the CNS certainly explains very adequately the pattern of damage found in the cerebral cortex in man (8), particularly the marked concentration of damage to the visual cortex, where the highest concentration of stellate neurons is found (14). A similar distribution of cortical lesions was found by Takeuchi et al. (16). In the damaged cerebellum often only the largest cells, namely the Purkinje cells, tend to survive, whereas most of the granule cells and the small cells of the molecular layer are destroyed. The same pattern is seen in the cat (16) and in the rabbit (3).

The reason for this latter selectivity is not obvious. Carmichael et al. (3) found no unequivocal evidence of increased vascular permeability to Evans blue–albumin or to [131I]albumin after the doses of methyl mercury used in these experiments, so that another explanation must be sought.

PERSONAL INVESTIGATIONS AND DISCUSSION

Two possible explanations spring to mind for this phenomenon. It is possible that the

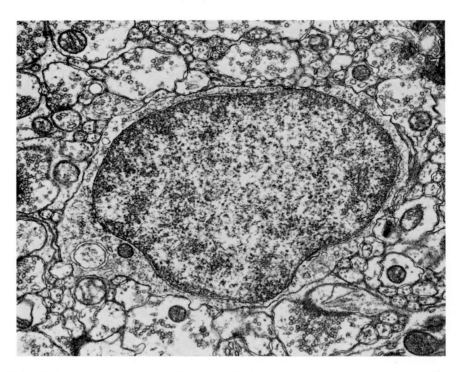

FIG. 1. Molecular layer of cerebellum of rabbit after 3 daily doses of methyl mercury acetate (7.5 mg/kg per day). Note the very narrow rim of perinuclear cytoplasm and the disappearance of ribosomes and endoplasmic reticulum. There are many dying stellate cells in the vicinity. Adjacent nerve terminals are normal. ×26,000. (Courtesy of Dr. Jean M. Jacobs.)

larger surface-to-volume ratio of small neurons might result in these cells absorbing more mercury than larger neurons from the extracellular space in relation to the size of the cell. This suggestion must assume an equal distribution of mercury in the extracellular space and an equal availability for entry of neuron surface in all cell types. It is, however, very unlikely that either of these premises is correct. The second suggested explanation is connected with the fact that small neurons have a smaller total quantity of ribosomes than large neurons (Fig. 1). If, as seems likely from our earlier study (9), cell death occurs when a certain proportion of the cell's content of ribosomes is damaged by mercury, then clearly large cells must be able to tolerate a much larger amount of mercury than small cells. In any region of the brain where mercury enters, there-

fore, small cells are more likely to be irreversibly damaged. Nerve cells seem to be able to tolerate a certain amount of loss of ribosomes which can be made good by normal replacement mechanisms, provided that the damage is not overwhelming. In general, therefore, the larger the cell the less likely it is to be overwhelmed.

The earlier demonstration that protein synthesis in the rat was inhibited by methyl mercury (4,18) and the ultrastructural finding that ribosomal damage is a very early feature of the toxic effects in neurons (9) (Fig. 2) both imply that the degeneration of the axon is a secondary consequence of these two basic changes. Moreover, it occurs independently of degeneration of the cell body and follows these two crucial changes by several days. The more recent finding in the rat that following dosing with mercuric chloride exactly the same ultra-

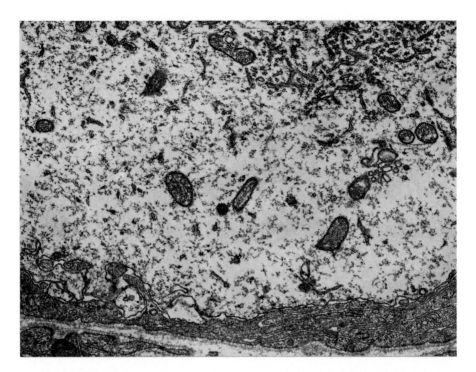

FIG. 2. Spinal root ganglion cell of rabbit 24 hr after 2 daily oral doses of methyl mercury acetate (7.5 mg/kg per day). Note loss of polyribosomes and rough endoplasmic reticulum from the periphery of the cell. Mitochondria and a few strands of smooth endoplasmic reticulum only remain. Satellite cells appear normal. × 17,500. (Courtesy of Dr. Jean M. Jacobs.)

structural features may be seen as with methyl mercury, although of lesser severity and without observable cell death, may be of particular relevance to the mechanism of intoxication by methyl-mercury (10) (Fig. 3). The earlier observation of Enders and Noetzel (5) that chronic feeding of mercuric chloride to rats leads to damage to cerebellar granule cells shows that inorganic mercury can behave similarly to methyl mercury in another way. Furthermore, the recent finding of Carmichael (2) that significant depression of protein synthesis also occurs in rats fed mercuric chloride daily for 14 days with either 1 or 2 mg/kg gives further support for the similarity of the effects of the two forms of mercury. Axon degeneration may also sometimes occasionally be found after daily dosing with 1 mg/kg, but it is uncommon and occurs only after several weeks of

dosing (10), so that mercuric chloride at this dose level is not causing a significant amount of irreversible change.

Chemical analysis of the tissues for mercury in methyl mercury poisoning by several workers has shown that methyl mercury accumulates in the brain. Dosing with inorganic mercury also leads to mercury entering the brain, but it does so less readily and does not persist for so long. It is possible that some degree of methylation of inorganic mercury might occur, and that this might account for the identity of the morphological changes, but analyses by L. Magoś found no support for this possibility. However, inorganic mercury as well as methyl mercury occur in the brain in methyl mercury-fed animals,[15] although whether by demethylation *in situ* or by the entry of inorganic mercury ions demethylated elsewhere, such as in the kidney,

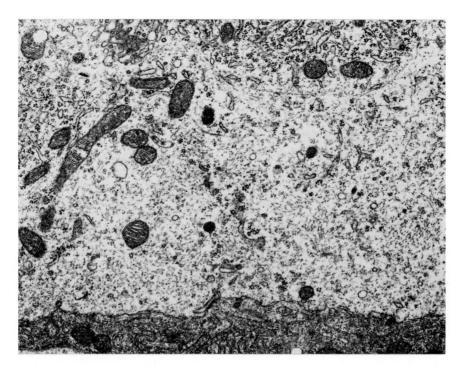

FIG. 3. Spinal root ganglion cell of rat after 14 daily oral doses of mercuric chloride (1.0 mg/kg per day). Note virtually the same changes as with methyl mercury in Fig. 2. A few polysomes and strands of smooth endoplasmic reticulum remain. Mitochondria appear normal. Satellite cells appear normal. ×17,500. (Courtesy of Dr. Jean M. Jacobs.)

is unknown. Indeed, about 3.0% mercury in the brain may be in the inorganic form (12). It is, perhaps, significant that the mercury content of brains of animals fed daily 1 mg/kg for 70 days is only 0.5 to 0.25 times the *inorganic* mercury content of brains from animals fed 7.5 mg/kg methyl mercury for eight daily doses and that the severity of the cell changes are only slightly less in the former than in the latter animals.

Although mercuric chloride (LD_{50} for rats, 37 mg/kg) is about as generally toxic as methyl mercury (LD_{50} for rats, 30 to 40 mg/kg) for the animal as a whole, methyl mercury has the greater *neurotoxicity,* which may well be correlated with its greater lipid solubility. One result of this property is its greater ease of entry into the cell and its greater capacity to dissolve in membranes with which the nervous system is particularly well endowed. Since both inorganic and organic mercury bind to -SH groups and other ligands, it may well be irrelevant for toxicity which form enters the cell provided there is a certain minimal quantity present. The fact that divalent inorganic mercury ions form more stable complexes with other radicles than do monovalent alkyl mercury ions (17) would seem very relevant to the intimate mechanism of the metabolic lesion. It is probable, however, that most of the mercury within the cell accumulates in the lipid of various membranes, and this is more likely to occur with the methyl form than with the less lipid soluble inorganic form. The essential quality of methyl mercury neurotoxicity may well, therefore, reside in its lipid solubility rather than in any other property.

SUMMARY

The lesions in the nerve cell in both methyl and inorganic mercury have been briefly discussed, and their similarity at the ultrastructural level have been emphasized. The intracellular lesion seems to begin in the ribosome with both forms of poisoning, and this correlates in both with a reduction in the tissues' capacity to synthesize proteins. At lower doses, this results in axon degeneration only, whereas with higher doses cell death occurs.

The special sensitivity of primary sensory ganglion cells to methyl mercury poisoning may be ascribed to the presence of fenestrated vessels in sensory ganglia readily allowing the penetration of mercury from the plasma into the tissue, since these cells are not protected by a blood-nerve barrier. The particular distribution of lesions in the CNS is ascribed to the tendency of the mercury compounds selectively to damage small nerve cells, hence the damage to the cerebellum and to the visual cortex. This tendency probably is a result of the relatively small ribosomal content of these cells and thus their inability to tolerate the disorganization of these organelles by mercury.

Attention is drawn to the presence of free divalent mercury in the brains of methyl mercury-fed animals, and to the greater lipid solubility of alkyl as opposed to inorganic mercury salts. The latter property would enable alkyl mercury more readily to enter the cell, and it is probable that divalent mercury would be more chemically active inside the cell than monovalent alkyl mercury.

ACKNOWLEDGMENTS

My thanks are due to my colleagues Jean M. Jacobs, Ph.D., and Neil Carmichael, B.Sc., for their achievements in helping to unravel some of the details of this problem.

REFERENCES

1. Anzil, A. P., Blinzinger, K., and Herrlinger, H. (1976): Fenestrated blood capillaries in rat craniospinal sensory ganglia. *Cell Tissue Res.,* 1:563–567.
2. Carmichael, N. (1976): *Unpublished data.*
3. Carmichael, N., Cavanagh, J. B., and Rodda, R. A. (1975): Some effects of methyl mercury salts on the rabbit nervous system. *Acta Neuropathol. (Berl.),* 32:115–125.
4. Cavanagh, J. B., and Chen, F. C.-K. (1971): Amino acid incorporation in protein during the "silent phase" before organo-mercury and p-bromophenylacetylurea neuropathy in the rat. *Acta Neuropathol. (Berl.),* 19:216–224.
5. Enders, A., and Noetzel, H. (1955): Spezifische veranderungen im kleinhirn bei chronischer oraler vergiftung mit sublimat. *Arch. Exptl. Pathol. Pharmacol.,* 225:345–351.
6. Grant, C. A. (1973): Pathology of experimental methyl mercury intoxication: Some problems of exposure and response. In: *Mercury, Mercurials and Mercaptans,* edited by M. W. Miller and T. W. Clarkson, Ch. 17, pp. 294–310. Charles C Thomas, Springfield, Ill.
7. Hunter, D., Bomford, R. R., and Russell, D. S. (1940): Poisoning by methyl mercury compounds. *Q. J. Med.,* 9:193–213.
8. Hunter, D., and Russell, D. S. (1954): Focal cerebral and cerebellar atrophy in a human subject due to organic mercury compounds. *J. Neurol. Neurosurg. Psychiatry,* 17:235–241.
9. Jacobs, J. M., Carmichael, N., and Cavanagh, J. B. (1975): Ultrastructural changes in the dorsal root and trigeminal ganglia or rats poisoned with methyl mercury. *Neuropathol. Appl. Neurobiol.,* 1:1–19.
10. Jacobs, J. M., Cavanagh, J. B., and Carmichael, N. (1975): The effect of chronic dosing with mercuric chloride on dorsal root trigeminal ganglia of rats. *Neuropathol. Appl. Neurobiol.,* 3:321–337.
11. Jacobs, J. M., Macfarlane, R. M., and Cavanagh, J. B. (1977): Vascular leakage in the dorsal root ganglia of the rat, studied with horse-radish peroxidase. *J. Neurol. Sci. (In press.)*
12. Magoś, L., and Butler, W. H. (1972): Cumulative effect of methyl mercury dicyandiamide given orally to rats. *Fd. Cosmet. Toxicol.,* 10:513–517.
13. Olsson, Y. (1968): Topographical differences in the vascular permeability of the peripheral nervous system. *Acta Neuropathol. (Berl.),* 10:26–33.
14. Ranson, S. W., and Clark, S. L. (1953): *The Anatomy of the Nervous System.* Saunders, Philadelphia and London.
15. Syverson, T. L. M. (1974): Biotransformation of

Hg-203 labeled methyl mercuric chloride in rat brain measured by specific determination of Hg2+. *Acta Pharmacol. Toxicol. (Kbh.)*, 35:277–283.

16. Takeuchi, T., Morikawa, N., Matsumoto, H., and Shiraishi, Y. (1962): A pathological study of Minamata disease in Japan. *Acta Neuropathol. (Berl.)*, 2:40–57.

17. Webb, J. L. (1966): *Enzymes and Metabolic Inhibitors*, Vol. 2, pp. 768–886. Academic Press, New York.

18. Yoshino, Y., Mozai, T., and Nakao, K. (1966): Biochemical changes in the brain in rats poisoned with an alkylmercury compound, with special reference to the inhibition of protein synthesis in brain cortex slices. *J. Neurochem.*, 13:1223–1230.

Neurotoxicology, edited by L. Roizin, H. Shiraki, and N. Grčević. Raven Press, New York © 1977.

Subcellular Mechanisms in Lead Toxicity: Significance in Childhood Encephalopathy, Neurological Sequelae, and Late Dementias

†Werner J. Niklowitz

Indiana University Medical Center, Division of Neuropathology, Indianapolis, Indiana 46202

LEAD AND MAN

The human race is burdened by an increasing load of environmental contaminants, affecting not just health and behavior, but finally survival of the species itself.

Among these chemicals, lead (Pb) is one of the most hazardous to living matter. In mammals the main target is the central nervous system (CNS), particularly in the young; but the adult population is by no means spared. Pb is widely used in increasing and almost indiscriminate quantities, so that higher Pb levels in blood and teeth of children and adults (1,3,27,49,50) should not surprise us. The number of deaths directly attributable to Pb exposure has declined in children during the last decades, what with earlier diagnosis, with more effective therapy (7,9), and with other factors, such as improvement of diet and hygiene. However, this decline should not blind us to the danger of chronic low dose Pb ingestion or, as it has been aptly referred to, the "silent epidemic" (42).

Acute as well as chronic plumbism has been recognized since antiquity (16), and what a vast literature exists! However, little yet is known about the cellular site and subcellular mechanisms of Pb toxicity.

† Present address: 4252 Glenhaven Road, Cincinnati, Ohio 45238.

Above all, what we know of long-term intake of seemingly insignificant or "safe" doses of Pb (subclinical Pb poisoning) is pitiful.

Occupational Pb intoxication takes place by the respiratory route; absorption is more rapid and complete than by any other route (18,25,39). Smoking makes available 0.8 μg per cigarette (39). Apart from occupational or accidental exposure, the entire population suffers from increased Pb intake, since Pb is present in food, water, and air (for review see ref. 55). The daily uptake of Pb through the GI tract, lung, and skin is between 200 and 500 μg. Some 10% of this is retained. Alcohol accelerates the absorption of Pb (54,54a). Absorbed Pb is distributed everywhere. Cerebral uptake occurs at any level of blood Pb (19), and there appears to be no threshold to protect the brain against absorption and storage of Pb.

MATERIALS AND METHODS

Experimental

Our studies in the last decade on experimental Pb intoxication yield some limited answers. Matched sets of young adult (postsuckling) rabbits were used in a multidisciplinary approach including light and electron microscopy, assays of enzymes, and analysis of trace metals (atomic absorption spectrophotometry). Acute Pb poisoning was produced by a single dose injection of tetraethyllead (TEL, 100 mg/kg, i.p.) (35). There is evidence that the toxic component of organo-Pb compounds is the Pb itself; TEL merely provides a means of faster passage across the blood-brain barrier (BBB). The final structural changes in the CNS after inorganic Pb poisoning (31) or organo-Pb exposure (32) are neuropathologically identical.

Human Cases

Humans with occupational or accidental exposure to Pb who revealed neurological symptoms and/or neuropathological changes of the Alzheimer's type were also studied (31).

RESULTS AND DISCUSSION

Although metal shifts are known to be early indicators of response to toxic agents (51) and occur during the course of human brain diseases such as schizophrenia, epilepsy, and Wilson's disease (41), the interaction and/or interference of toxic metals, especially of Pb, with essential trace metals in the brain is still an unexplored field. The interaction of Pb with the cations K, Na, Ca, and Mg has been preferentially studied in the blood (38,57). However, no data are available concerning the effects of Pb on essential trace metals of the brain such as Fe, Cu, and Zn.

A preliminary report indicates a proportional interference of Pb with Fe, Cu, and Zn in several rabbit brain areas after TEL poisoning (33). Subsequent trace metal studies, however, reveal specific shifts of trace metals (Cu, Fe, Zn) in several analyzed brain areas (cortex, hippocampus, cerebellum, thalamus, putamen-pallidum, caudate nucleus) after TEL poisoning of rabbits during the course of the year (34, 37). Whereas Cu and Zn levels are fairly

constant in control animals, with a slight peak during the fall, normal Fe levels exhibit considerable seasonal fluctuation, different for cortical (cortex, hippocampus, cerebellum) and subcortical tissues (thalamus, putamen-pallidum, caudate nucleus). The Pb levels of control animals vary from 1 (cortex) to 6 nmoles (thalamus), expressed per gram dry weight.

After TEL intoxication Pb levels in all brain tissues examined are about 200 nmoles. Cu levels are now increased, particularly through fall, winter, and spring. Zn levels are always depressed. The Fe levels in winter are the same (cortical areas) or somewhat less (subcortical areas) than in controls. However, during the course of the year, the Fe levels are now almost constant, although different for each brain area, and no longer season dependent. During the hottest month of the year, July, the Fe values of the cortical areas are higher and in subcortical brain tissues lower than normal (34,37).

It is this shift of essential trace metals in brain tissues after Pb poisoning that led to the development of the current concept of Pb toxicity (Model 1976) concerning the basic mechanisms and the primary site of cell injury.

The following terms are defined: extracellular compartment – vascular as well as extracellular tissue space; cell membrane – nerve and glial cell wall, also cell walls of erythrocytes and endothelial cells (as part of the BBB); cell – erythrocytes, endothelial cells, as well as neurons and glial cells.

The hypothesis is developed in stages (compare Fig. 1):

1. *Exposure to Pb leads to increased tissue Cu levels.*

The differential shifts of the trace metals Cu, Fe, and Zn in cortical (cortex, hippocampus, cerebellum) and subcortical brain tissues (thalamus, putamen-pallidum, caudate nucleus) consequent to Pb exposure have been discussed previously. All

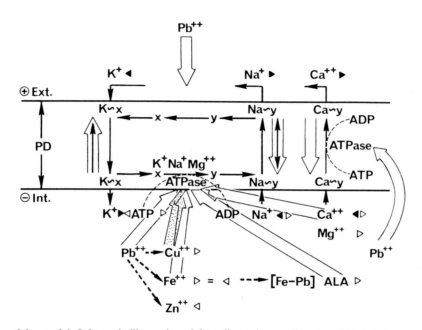

FIG. 1. Pb toxicity model. Schematic illustration of the cell membrane, direction of Na^+–K^+ pump activated as well as passive ion movement across the cell membrane, and degree of ion accumulation in normal conditions (▲) and after Pb exposure (△). ADP, adenosine diphosphate; ALA, δ-aminolaevulinic acid; ATP, adenosine triphosphate; Ext., external surface with positive charge (+); Int., internal surface with negative charge (−); PD, potential difference; x and y, carrier compounds.

investigated brain areas exhibit a significant increase of tissue Cu levels; this elevation of tissue Cu is regarded as primary in Pb poisoning. (The significance of Fe and Zn shifts are discussed later.)

Pb effects the Cu homeostasis in some way. It has been shown that Pb exposure in man (48) as well as in experimental animals (52) leads to a significant decrease of blood ceruloplasmin levels. Ceruloplasmin functions as a carrier for Cu and therefore is involved in the homeostatic control of tissue Cu levels in mammals (46). Similar observations concerning Cu balance impairment are made in Wilson's disease (58,59).

It is interesting to observe that the elevation of tissue Cu levels can be due to exposure to other agents, such as sodium diethyldithiocarbamate in brain tissue (23), morphine in the spinal cord (24), and ozone in lung tissue (51). Additionally, there is at least the suspicion that the therapeutic effectiveness of chelators in childhood lead encephalopathy (7,9) and in cases with an amyotrophic lateral sclerosis syndrome following Pb exposure (2,5) primarily relate to removal of Cu, as in Wilson's disease (56).

2. Pb-induced elevated tissue Cu inhibits cell membrane adenosine triphosphatase.

Although Cu is a vital part of a number of metalloenzymes (10) and therefore is an essential trace element, an excess of tissue Cu is toxic. Cu, like most other heavy metals, inhibits the catalytic activity of many enzymes (13), more specifically microsomal and membrane adenosine triphosphatase (ATPase) (11,12,22,53), depending on the level sometimes irreversibly.

The interference of Pb with microsomal and membrane ATPase is well documented (for review see ref. 6). For intracellular Pb, this can be expected. However, if the Pb appears in the extracellular compartment, it is likely that its effect is mediated through the now-demonstrated increase of tissue Cu that consequently inhibits the membrane ATPase; this is the thrust of our hypothesis. Reactions of heavy metals within the membrane are relatively rapid and reversible, whereas those occurring within the cell show a lag time and are sometimes irreversible or very slowly reversible (43).

3. *The inhibition of cell membrane ATPase results in breakdown of cell membrane properties.*

Increased intracellular Cu and its inhibitory action on the cell membrane ATPase interferes with the normal function of the cell membrane by impairment of the Na^+-K^+ pump. The Na^+-K^+ pump maintains the integrity of the cell by regulation of the ion transport across the membrane in both directions and preserves a sufficient intracellular ion balance. One widely accepted model for the Na^+-K^+ pump assumes that carrier compounds (in Fig. 1, x and y) or more likely ATPase itself is involved in such a carrier mechanism, as illustrated in Fig. 1. A partial impairment of the cell membrane, as documented by hydropic change in nerve and glial cells, or a total impairment, as in pyknotic and shrunken nerve cells after Pb poisoning (35), however, demonstrates morphologically a differential breakdown of the osmotic properties of the cell membrane. Whereas hydropic altered nerve cells maintain their integrity, despite an apparently higher uptake of Na^+ and subsequent swelling, pyknotic and shrunken nerve cells collapse completely. In any case, Ca, Na, Mg, and now also Pb enter the cell via diffusion and some of these intracellularly accumulating elements and other substances such as δ-aminolaevulinic acid (ALA), in addition to Cu, are able to interfere with ATPase (see Fig. 1). The extreme cerebral edema in acute lead encephalopathy is evidence of poor cellular ion handling. The breakdown of the cell membrane properties is also attested

to by the findings that tissue Zn and alkaline phosphatase, a Zn requiring enzyme, are diminished (34,36), more so in brain areas with cell pyknosis and shrinkage (cerebellum, 35).

4. *Interaction of tissue Fe with Pb.*

We have demonstrated a seasonal fluctuation of brain tissue Fe levels in untreated control animals; this fluctuation differs in cortical and subcortical brain areas (34). Pb-treated animals, however, reveal constant Fe levels, evidence of Pb interference. It is observed that Pb in Pb-poisoned cattle is bound to ferric hydroxide in liver, spleen, and kidney (44). *In vitro* investigations confirm the property of Fe compounds to absorb Pb (14). Raised Fe levels in erythrocytes, brain, and liver after Pb poisoning could have been caused by its ability to bind Pb and by subsequent storage.

Although the classic hypochromic anemia of chronic Pb intoxication reflects interference of heme synthesis, there is also a direct effect on tissue availability of Fe.

The current hypothesis points to the basic mechanisms and the primary cellular site of Pb toxicity, with (1) elevated tissue Cu levels inhibiting (2) cell membrane ATPase that (3) results in the breakdown of the cell membrane properties (Na^+-K^+ pump) and (4) leads to intracellular impairments, as summarized in Fig. 1. This model of Pb toxicity, furthermore, not only explains the breakdown of the BBB, but also offers some insight in unsolved problems concerning childhood lead encephalopathy, neurological sequelae, and late dementias.

LEAD ENCEPHALOPATHY WITH ITS NEUROLOGICAL SEQUELAE AND LATE DEMENTIAS

Lead encephalopathy is almost exclusively seen in children, often those with prior pica, typically in the summer.

Pica, that mysterious perversion of appetite, has been linked to iron deficiency and can be treated as such (29). Since (a)

Fe is bound by Pb in tissues and (b) Pb can itself produce a hypochromic anemia, subclinical Pb intoxication could well be a causative and/or additional factor in pica. Observe that pica is not seasonal (60). It typically occurs in other (iron) deficiency states, such as pregnancy.

Fe levels are normally much lower in small children; near-adult levels are not reached until age 7 to 9 (47). It is therefore small children that suffer most from excessive Pb intake, with less Fe available for Pb binding. Fe losses through perspiration are well known; the hot humid summer months see therefore the highest incidence of lead encephalopathy and death (4).

Outright lead encephalopathy or undetected subclinical cases (identified by epidemiological case finding) can be followed by various degrees of sequelae, such as mental retardation, memory and learning disabilities, and hyperactivity. These cases could represent a defect situation, but could also reflect irreversible membrane damage. Such children are quite vulnerable to further Pb exposure, with the chance of severe brain damage close to 100% (4,8).

Recently, a third and most disturbing group of cases with late (middle to late adulthood) sequelae has been identified. Cases with presenile dementia, neuropathologically quite similar to Alzheimer's disease (neurofibrillary tangles, granulovacuolar changes, argyrophilic plaques) have been reported (21,31) (Fig. 2). This is in keeping with experimental findings (32) (Figs. 3 and 4). Then cases of amyotrophic lateral sclerosis (ALS) of patients exposed to Pb are known (40). Some of the Alzheimer's changes have been seen in many other conditions, such as ALS, kuru, dementia pugilistica, postencephalitic parkinsonism, the Guam parkinson-dementia complex, Pick's disease, Creutzfeldt-Jakob disease, subacute sclerosing panencephalitis (30), Down's syndrome, vascular malformations, and doubtless others.

Our knowledge concerning the effects of chronic and low level exposure of Pb on the adult population and its involvement in human diseases is woefully deficient. Particularly in Alzheimer's disease the implications are unsettling. On microincineration, increased quantities of Fe and Ca are found in nerve cells with neurofibrillary changes, in oligodendroglia cells, and in capillaries. Goodman (20) suggested that Alzheimer's disease may be a disturbance in cerebral Fe metabolism.

It is obvious that in acute as well as in chronic cases of severe Pb poisoning only minor or nonspecific lesions are ever uncovered, although the activity of hydrolytic enzymes such as acid phosphatase is increased in cortical brain tissues with preferentially hydropic-changed pyramidal cells (36). Therefore, these findings are highly indicative that intracellular Pb interferes with hydrolytic enzymes and that such affected nerve cells undergo epigenetic mutations or transformations with resulting neurofibrillary changes, as documented in experimental Pb-poisoned animals and human cases with accidental or occupational exposure to Pb (21,31,32).

It is fashionable to declare diseases for which the causative agents as well as the pathogenesis are still unknown as being of viral origin, such as cancer, multiple sclerosis, diabetes, dementias, and others. However, clinical and basic research concerning these matters should also consider and evaluate other, somewhat neglected, factors, particularly the impact of our changing environment on human health.

In this context it is suggestive that there exists already a theoretical link between Pb exposure and kuru, the classic example of a progressive degenerative disease of the CNS of slow virus etiology (15). It is known that the soil of New Guinea (and Guam) is high in Pb, and that the blood–Pb level of its population is high as well (17). It is therefore not surprising that the brains in such cases exhibit high Pb levels (28). Furthermore, it has been suggested that the widespread astrocytosis, which is similar to cases with Pb poisoning, reveals

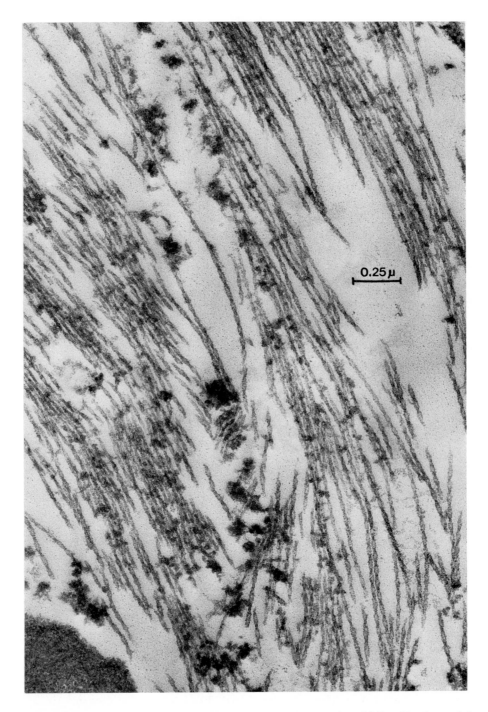

FIG. 2. Neurofibrillary tangle of a human case with Alzheimer's changes after childhood lead encephalopathy. Twisted tubules. ×50,000.

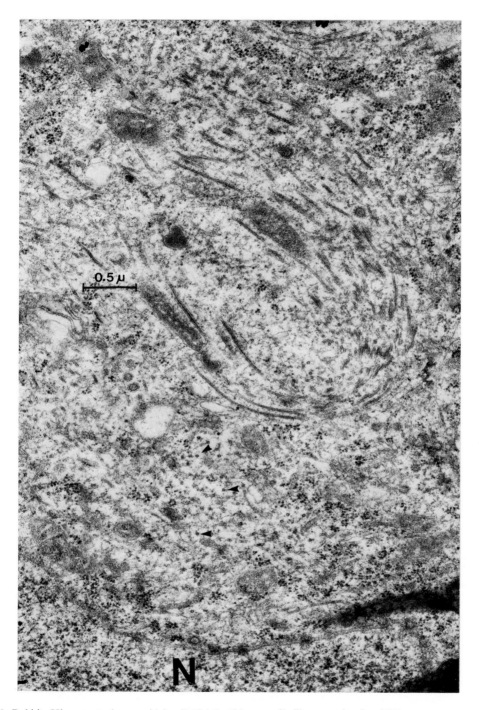

FIG. 3. Rabbit. Hippocampal pyramidal cell (CA3) with neurofibrillary tangle after TEL exposure. ×27,000. N, nucleus.

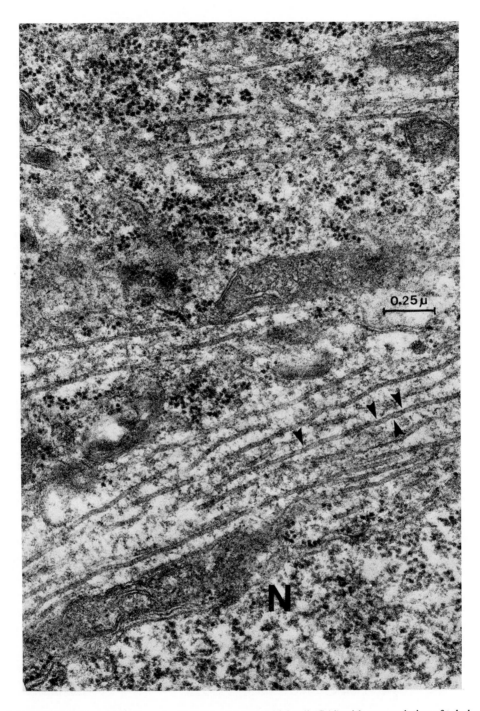

FIG. 4. Rabbit. Higher magnification of a hippocampal pyramidal cell (CA1) with accumulation of tubules after TEL exposure. Arrows indicate twists. ×52,000. N, nucleus.

the operation of a toxic substance. Cases with similar pathology, as described in other parts of the world (26,45), support our theoretical assumption. Even if there is a transmissible agent, one has to consider all the other intrinsic and extrinsic factors.

In conclusion and with support of our model of Pb toxicity we wish to advance the hypothesis that Pb and other toxic metals (Hg, Cr, Ni, Cd) could be causative or additional causative factors in certain neurological disorders, specifically in late onset of dementias.

ACKNOWLEDGMENT

These investigations were supported by USPHS Research grants ES 00900 and ES 01171.

I thank Dr. Jans Muller for encouragement and help.

REFERENCES

1. Baloh, R. W. (1973): The effect of chronic increased lead absorption on the nervous system: A review article. *Bull. Los Angeles Neurol. Soc.*, 38:91–99.
2. Boothby, J. A., deJesus, P. V., and Rowland, L. P. (1974): Reversible forms of motor neuron disease. *Arch. Neurol.*, 31:18–23.
3. Browder, A. A., Joselow, M. M., and Louria, D. B. (1973): The problem of lead poisoning. *Medicine (Baltimore)*, 52:121–139.
4. Byers, R. K. (1959): Lead poisoning. *Pediatrics*, 23:585–603.
5. Campbell, A. M. G., Williams, E. R., and Barltrop, D. (1970): Motor neuron disease and exposure to lead. *J. Neurol. Neurosurg. Psychiatry*, 33:877–885.
6. Campbell, I. R., and Mergard, E. G. (1972): *Biological Aspects of Lead: An Annotated Bibliography.* Publication No. AP-104, U.S. Environmental Protection Agency.
7. Chisolm, J. J., Jr. (1968): The use of chelating agents in the treatment of acute and chronic lead intoxication in childhood. *J. Pediatrics*, 73:1–38.
8. Chisolm, J. J., Jr., and Harrison, H. E. (1956): The exposure of children to lead. *Pediatrics*, 18:943–957.
9. Coffin, R., Philips, J. L., Staples, W. I., and Spector, S. (1966): Treatment of lead encephalopathy in children. *J. Pediatr.*, 69:198–206.
10. Davies, I. J. T. (1972): *The Clinical Significance*

of the Essential Biological Metals. Charles C Thomas, Springfield, Illinois.
11. Donaldson, J., St.-Pierre, T., Minnich, J., and Barbeau, A. (1971): Seizures in rats associated with divalent cations inhibition of Na^+–K^+–ATPase. *Can. J. Biochem.*, 49:1217–1224.
12. Epstein, P. S., and McIlwain, H. (1966): Action of cupric salts on isolated cerebral tissue. *Proc. R. Soc. Lond. [Biol.]*, 166:295–302.
13. Evans, G. W. (1973): Copper homeostasis in the mammalian system. *Physiol. Rev.*, 53:535–570.
14. Gadde, R. R., and Laitinen, H. A. (1973): Study of the sorption of lead by hydrous ferric oxide. *Environ. Lett.*, 5:223–235.
15. Gajdusek, D. C., and Gibbs, C. J., Jr. (1975): Slow virus infection of the nervous system and the laboratories of slow, latent, and temperate virus infection. In: *The Nervous System, Vol. 2: The Clinical Neurosciences*, edited by D. B. Tower, pp. 113–135. Raven Press, New York.
16. Gilfillan, S. C. (1965): Lead poisoning and the fall of Rome. *J. Occup. Med.*, 7:53–60.
17. Goldwater, L. J., and Hoever, A. W. (1967): An international study of "normal" levels of lead in blood and urine. *Arch. Environ. Health*, 15:60–63.
18. Goldsmith, J. R., and Hester, A. C. (1969): Lead intake from food and from the atmosphere. *Science*, 159:1000.
19. Goldstein, G. W., Asbury, A. K., and Diamond, I. (1974): Pathogenesis of lead encephalopathy. *Arch. Neurol.*, 31:382–389.
20. Goodman, L. (1953): Alzheimer's disease. A clinico-pathologic analysis of twenty-three cases with a theory on pathogenesis. *J. Nerv. Ment. Dis.*, 117:97–130.
21. Hess, K., and Straub, P. W. (1974): Chronische Bleivergiftung. *Praxis*, 63:177–183.
22. Hexum, T. D. (1974): Studies on the reaction catalyzed by transport (Na,K) adenosine triphosphatase. I. Effects of divalent metals. *Biochem. Pharmacol.*, 23:3441–3447.
23. Iwata, H., Watanabe, K., Miichi, H., and Matsui, Y. (1970): Accumulation of copper in the central nervous system on prolonged administration of sodium diethyldithiocarbamate to rats. *Pharmacol. Res. Commun.*, 2:213–220.
24. Iwata, H., Watanabe, K., and Matsui, Y. (1971): Change of copper concentrations in the central nervous system after morphine treatment and effect of copper on morphine analgesia in rats. *Pharmacol. Res. Commun.*, 3:147–153.
25. Kehoe, R. A. (1961): The metabolism of lead in man in health and disease. I. The normal metabolism of lead. *J. Roy. Inst. Public Health*, 24:81–97.
26. Krücke, W., Beck, E., and Gräfin Vitzthum, H. (1973): Creutzfeld-Jakob disease. Some unusual morphological features reminescent of kuru. *Z. Neurol.*, 206:1–24.
27. Lin-Fu, J. S. (1973): Vulnerability of children to lead exposure and toxicity. *N. Engl. J. Med.*, 289:1229–1233 and 1289–1293.
28. Lowenthal, A. (1970): The metals of the human

nervous system. In: *Neuropathology: Methods and Diagnosis,* edited by C. G. Tadeschi. Little, Brown, Boston.

29. McDonald, R., and Marshall, S. R. (1964): The value of iron therapy in pica. *Pediatrics,* 34:558–562.

30. Mandybur, T. I., Nagpaul, A., Pappas, Z., and Niklowitz, W. J. (1977): Alzheimer neurofibrillary change in subacute sclerosing panencephalitis. *Ann. Neurol.,* 1:103–107.

31. Niklowitz, W. J., and Mandybur, T. I. (1975): Neurofibrillary changes following childhood lead encephalopathy. *J. Neuropathol. Exp. Neurol.,* 34:445–455.

32. Niklowitz, W. J. (1975): Neurofibrillary changes after acute experimental lead poisoning. *Neurology (Minneap.),* 25:927–934.

33. Niklowitz, W. J., and Yeager, D. W. (1973): Interference of Pb with essential brain tissue Cu, Fe, and Zn as main determinant in experimental tetraethyllead encephalopathy. *Life Sci.,* 13:897–905.

34. Niklowitz, W. J. (1977): Seasonal behavior of essential trace metals of various brain areas in comparison to trace metal shifts after lead poisoning. (*In preparation.*)

35. Niklowitz, W. J. (1974): Ultrastructural effects of acute tetraethyllead poisoning on nerve cells of the rabbit brain. *Environ. Res.,* 8:17–36.

36. Niklowitz, W. J., and Murthy, R. C. (1976): Lead induced changes of alkaline and acid phosphatase activity. I. *In vivo* effects of acute tetraethyllead poisoning in subcellular fractions of specific brain areas. *Arch. Environ. Health.* (*Submitted for Publication.*)

37. Niklowitz, W. J. (1975): Lead: The perspectives of childhood encephalopathy, persistent neurological sequelae, and Alzheimer's disease. *Neurosci. Abstr.,* 1:1081.

38. Passow, H., Rothstein, A., and Clarkson, T. W. (1961): The general pharmacology of the heavy metals. *Pharmacol. Rev.,* 13:185–224.

39. Patterson, C. C. (1965): Contaminated and natural environments of man. *Arch. Environ. Health,* 11:344–360.

40. Petkau, A., Swatzky, A., Hillier, C. R., and Hoogstraten, J. (1974): Lead content of neuromuscular tissues in amyotrophic lateral sclerosis; case report and other considerations. *Br. J. Ind. Med.,* 31:275–287.

41. Pfeiffer, C. C. (1975): *Mental and Elemental Nutrients.* Keats Publ., New Canaan, Connecticut.

42. Rothschild, E. O. (1970): Lead poisoning—the silent epidemic. *N. Engl. J. Med.,* 283:704–705.

43. Rothstein, A. (1959): Cell membrane as site of action of heavy metals. *Fed. Proc.,* 18:1026–1035.

44. Rüssel, H. A. (1970): Über die Bindung von Blei an eisenoxidhaltige Stoffe in Leber, Niere und Milz vergifteter Rinder. *Bull. Environ. Contam. Toxicol.,* 5:115–124.

45. Schaltenbrand, G., Trostdorf, E., Orthner, H., and Henn, R. (1968): Kuruähnliche sclerosierende Panencephalo-myelitis in Europa. *Dtsch. Z. Nervenheilkunde,* 193:158–194.

46. Scheinberg, I. H. (1966): Ceruloplasmin. A review. In: *The Biochemistry of Copper,* edited by J. Peisach, P. Aisen, and W. E. Blumberg. Academic Press, New York.

47. Schicha, H., Kasparek, K., Feinendegen, L. E., Siller, V., and Klein, H. J. (1971): Eisen-Konzentrationen in verschiedenen Abschnitten des menschlichen Gehirns und ihre Beziehungen zum Lebensalter. *Beitr. Pathol.,* 142:268–274.

48. Soliman, M. H. M., El-Sadik, Y. E., El-Kashlan, K. M., and El-Waseef, A. (1970): Biochemical studies of Egyptian workers exposed to lead. *Arch. Environ. Health,* 21:529–532.

49. Stack, M. V., Burkitt, A. J., and Nickless, G. (1975): Lead in children's teeth. *Nature,* 255:169.

50. Shapiro, I. M., Mitchell, G., Davidson, I., and Katz, S. H. (1975): The lead content of teeth. *Arch. Environ. Health,* 30:483–486.

51. Stokinger, H. E., Dixon, J. R., and Keenan, R. G. (1966): Metal shifts as early indicators of response to toxic agents. *15th Int. Congr. Occupational Health, Vienna,* pp. 43–44. Verlag der Wiener Medizinischen Akademie, Vienna.

52. Stowe, H. D., Goyer, R. A., Krigman, M. M., and Cates, M. (1973): Experimental oral lead toxicity in young dogs. *Arch. Pathol.,* 95:106–116.

53. Ting-Beall, H. P., Clark, D. A., Suelter, C. H., and Wells, W. W. (1973): Studies on the interaction of chick brain microsomal (Na$^+$ + K$^+$)-ATP-ase with copper. *Biochim. Biophys. Acta,* 291:229–236.

54. Valyi-Nagy, T., Kelentei, B., and Kocsar, L. (1954): II. The influence of alcohol ingestion upon lead poisoning. *Acad. Sci. Hung.,* 5:537–542.

54a. Valyi-Nagy, T., Kelentei, B., and Kocsar, L. (1954): III. Effect of alcohol in acute lead poisoning. *Acad. Sci. Hung.,* 5:543–547.

55. Waldron, H. A., and Stöfen, D. (1974): *Subclinical Lead Poisoning.* Academic Press, London.

56. Walshe, J. M. (1966): Wilson's disease. A review. In: *The Biochemistry of Copper,* edited by J. Peisach, P. Aisen, and W. E. Blumberg, pp. 475–498. Academic Press, New York.

57. White, J. M., and Selhi, H. S. (1975): Lead and the red cell. *Br. J. Haematol.,* 30:133–138.

58. Williams, A. O. (1965): Studies on copper, ceruloplasmin, and cirrhosis in relation to Wilson's disease. *Br. J. Exp. Pathol.,* 46:504–568.

59. Williams, A. O. (1967): Studies on azide, ceruloplasmin and copper in relation to Wilson's disease. *Br. J. Exp. Pathol.,* 48:180–187.

60. Williams, H., Kaplan, E., Couchman, C. E., and Sayers, R. R. (1952): Lead poisoning in young children. *Public Health Rep.,* 67:230–236.

Neurotoxicology, edited by L. Roizin, H. Shiraki, and N. Grčević. Raven Press, New York © 1977.

An Appraisal of Rodent Models of Lead Encephalopathy

Martin R. Krigman, Paul Mushak, and Thomas W. Bouldin

Department of Pathology, University of North Carolina School of Medicine, Chapel Hill, North Carolina 27514

The involvement of the nervous system in lead poisoning is well known. Encephalopathy with seizures and coma is one of the most striking and serious complications of lead poisoning. Despite the interest in and number of studies on lead poisoning over the last century, we still have much to learn about the encephalopathic effects of lead. Experimental studies are limited by available paradigms, insofar as most experiments involve protracted periods of lead exposure and yield variable results.

Pentschew and Garro (1) in 1966 recognized these deficiencies of existing models of lead encephalopathy and concluded that young animals should be treated. This strategy was based on the assumption that the immature or developing nervous system is more sensitive to toxins than the adult nervous system. Intoxication of suckling Long-Evans rats produced an encephalopathy in almost all of the pups from every litter treated.

Pregnant rats must be available. Immediately after parturation, they are placed on a lead-supplemented diet (4% lead carbonate); presumably, the suckling rats are intoxicated via their mothers' milk. The effects are almost immediate — the intoxicated pups are obviously smaller than controls within the first week of life, opening of the eyes is retarded by about a day, about 21 days of life most of the pups show evidence of urinary incontinence,

and suddenly at about 25 to 26 days the intoxicated pups develop hindlimb paralysis. The last feature usually heralds death within 24 hr. Many animals, at 24 to 28 days, exhibit seizure-like activity at this time. Macroscopically, the central nervous system of these 25- to 26-day-old animals shows petechial cerebral hemorrhages and gross cerebellar and spinal cord hemorrhages. Microscopically, there are small blood vessel changes, multiple hemorrhages, and parenchymal edema, particularly in the cerebellum. Endothelial cell hypertrophy and increased capillary cellularity constitute the principal vascular changes. The original study utilized the Long-Evans strain, but, essentially the same findings are noted with other strains.

The Pentschew and Garro model is somewhat deceptive. The significant exposure to lead is not from the mother's milk, but from the lead-enriched food. The milk from lead-exposed nursing dams contains about 50 μg of lead per g of milk(1), whereas the mothers' lead-supplemented diet (4% lead carbonate) contains about 27,000 μg of lead per g of food. When the pups open their eyes at about 2 weeks of age and begin to explore the cage, they invariably enter the mother's food dish. Contamination at this time means a new level of exposure. Michaelson and Sauerhoff (2) have clearly demonstrated that if the pups do not have access to the food,

TABLE 1. *Lead dose response – survival*

Age, days	Pb dose, μg/g body wt daily								
	100	200	300	400	750	1,000	1,500	2,500	3,000
5							±	D	D
10					±	D	D		
15					D				
20				D					
25									
30	S	S	±						

Pups dosed at day 2 of life, and daily thereafter. D, all dead by this time; ±, about half survive; S, all survive lead effects.

they do not develop the encephalopathy, even with continued exposure to the lead-containing milk.

In order to minimize the uncertainties of the lead exposure, we initiated feeding the suckling pups a defineable daily lead dose by gastric gavage (μg Pb/g body weight daily). A total of 12 different doses of lead ranging from 10 to 3,000 μg Ph/g body weight daily was investigated. Litters were started on the second day of life and dosed 6 out of 7 days until death or the 30th day of life. Predictable survival (Table 1) was limited to doses of 300 μg or less. Weight gain studies (Table 2) with carefully controlled litters revealed no effect with doses up to 50 μg over the first 30 days of life compared to sodium acetate-treated controls. However, the intubation procedure does affect weight gain when the intubated animals are compared to naive or nonintubated controls at 30 days of life. Cerebral, cerebellar, and spinal cord hemorrhages and edema regularly develop with lead doses greater than 400 μg. Moreover, the higher the dose, the earlier the appearance of the hemorrhages. Animals under 5 days of age with hemorrhages (2,500 μg dose) generally show more prominent cerebral than cerebellar hemorrhages, whereas at the lower doses, the converse is true. In an attempt to define whether all ages were equally vulnerable, we started litters on a daily dose of 2,500 μg. These litters were first started at eight

different ages, ranging from the second through the 60th day of life. Only the rats first exposed to lead at age 20 days or younger developed the hemorrhages and edema. The vulnerability of the animals 20 days or younger was age-dose related; the older the animal when first exposed to lead, the higher the dose (greater than 400 μg) required to produce hemorrhages and edema. The cerebral vascular damage is obviously age and dose related and may in part be related to the absorption of lead, such that there may be a critical blood level. As the rat pups mature, they absorb less lead and the blood lead concentrations drop. From our studies, we found with the 2,500-μg dose, the blood lead concentrations of rats older than 20 days were still above levels (1,000 to 2,000 μg Pb/dl of whole blood) that would yield hemorrhages and edema in younger animals. In addition, suckling pups first given a 1,000-μg dose at

TABLE 2. *Lead dose response – weight gain**

Age, days	Pb dose, μg/g body wt daily					
	10	25	50	100	200	300
5						D
10						D
15					D	D
20					D	D
25					D	D
30	NC	NC	NC	D	D	D

Pups dosed at day 2 of life, and daily thereafter. NC, no change; D, drop in weight gain.

5 days of life and treated bidaily thereafter, develop brain hemorrhages, but survive. However, when sacrificed at 20 days of age or older (after at least seven doses), the pups have no acute hemorrhages or edema. The only changes noted are a discolored cerebellum and microscopic evidence of resolving edema and hemorrhage with a concommittant astrocytosis accentuated about the capillaries. Even in these animals that survive in the face of regular dosing, blood lead concentrations are higher (greater than 1,000 μg Pb/dl of whole blood) than levels associated with the acute vasculopathy. These results suggest that as the newborn rat gets older, the cerebral capillaries mature or differentiate in the face of a high lead dose and are consequently resistant to the lead. The actual mechanisms by which endothelial cells cope with the lead are still to be defined. Related to the mechanism for handling the lead is the pathogenesis of the acute vascular (endothelial) damage. Intrinsic to this question is whether the lead enters the capillary. Thomas et al. (3) demonstrated by autoradiography that lead does enter the capillary. We (4) have also demonstrated lead in capillaries isolated from both acutely and chronically exposed pups. Interestingly, the capillaries from the chronically exposed rats with a resolving encephalopathy contained as much lead as those obtained from the acutely intoxicated pups.

The vulnerability of capillaries in the developing nervous system is not unique to the rat. Hirano and Kochen (*this volume*), in a series of studies, have clearly demonstrated the sensitivity of the chicken endothelium to lead. Lorenzo (A. V. Lorenzo, *personal communication*) has noted the same changes in newborn rabbits and also that it was limited to the first weeks of life. Rosenblum and Johnson (5) noted changes in the mouse brain that could be the result of endothelial damage from lead. Press (6), utilizing a rat model with a

defineable lead dosage, demonstrated that development of the brain capillary network was perturbed by the lead damage. How universal the sensitivity of the cerebral capillaries is and what forms it may take are not clear at this time.

The Pentschew and Garro suckling rat model has been an important contribution to our understanding of the nervous system's vulnerability in lead poisoning. However, it is not the only model of lead encephalopathy. Prior to the Pentschew and Garro report, all attempts at producing lead encephalopathy were based on adult animals, but encephalopathy was sometimes noted. These earlier experiments are reviewed by Weller (7), and in this paper, he also presents a guinea pig model of lead encephalopathy. This guinea pig model has received little attention, possibly because it utilizes animals with a mature nervous system, and the neuropathologic changes are minimal.

This guinea pig model was thoroughly studied by Weller, and we have had no problem reproducing his results (8). The animals are given a single dose of lead daily, 155 μg of lead carbonate. The animals rapidly lose weight and after four or five successive doses, they develop clonic seizures. Brain lead is significant at this time. Many animals die during the seizures. Six or more doses are invariably fatal. We have not explored the dose range but have noted that age is not a factor. Animals found dead or dying with seizures have edematous and congested brains. However, those sacrificed after four or more doses show no appreciable structural alterations. Ultrastructural analysis, including tracer studies with horse radish peroxidase, revealed no discernible capillary changes nor blood-brain barrier dysfunction, even in animals that had seizures.

The pathogenesis of lead encephalopathy is obviously different in these two rat models. In the neonatal rat, vasculopathy is a prominent feature, whereas in the guinea pig, despite the encephalopathy, pathologic features are minimal. The vascular findings in the suckling rat have been utilized to support the thesis that the encephalopathic effects of lead are the consequence of a vasculopathy. Although there are morphologic correlates for such a conclusion, particularly in human cases of lead encephalopathy (9,10), a direct effect of lead on neuronal function cannot be dismissed. Lead certainly enters the nervous system, and the brain concentration may be quite high in clinical and experimental cases of lead poisoning with encephalopathy. Although experimental studies indicate two apparently different mechanisms in the genesis of lead encephalopathy, they are not necessarily mutually exclusive. One or both mechanisms may be instrumental in the development of the encephalopathy, depending on the species, age, and nature of the lead exposure. This is particularly true considering that the vasculopathy of lead is dependant on the dose, the apparent state of vascular development, and that it may be reversible despite a continued burden.

SUMMARY

Two forms of models of lead encephalopathy are considered. In the rat, the encephalopathy is limited to the neonatal period and is characterized by an acute cerebral vasculopathy with hemorrhages and edema. The generation of the vasculopathy is both age and dose dependant. In the guinea pig, the encephalopathy is independant of age. After four or five daily doses of lead, guinea pigs have seizures that are often fatal. Vascular changes are not discernible, and blood-brain barrier function is intact.

Both models are highly reproducible and obviously different models of lead encephalopathy. However, they clearly demonstrate the mechanism by which lead may be toxic to the central nervous system.

ACKNOWLEDGMENT

This report was supported by grant no. ES 01104 from the National Institutes of Health.

REFERENCES

1. Pentschew, A., and Garro, F. (1966): Lead encephalo-myelopathy of the suckling rat and its implications of the porphyrinopathic nervous diseases. *Acta Neuropathol. (Berl.)*, 6:266–278.
2. Michaelson, I. A., and Sauerhauff, M. W. (1974): An improved model of lead-induced brain dysfunction in the suckling rat. *Toxicol. Appl. Pharmacol.*, 28:88–96.
3. Thomas, J. A., Dallenbach, F. D., and Thomas, M. (1973): The distribution of radioactive lead (210 Pb) in the cerebellum of developing rats. *J. Pathol.*, 109:45–50.
4. Krigman, M. R., Mushak, P., Hayward, J. C., Toews, A. D., and Morell, P. (1977): Acute lead encephalopathy in the suckling rats: A study of isolated capillaries. *Am. J. Pathol.*, 86:40a.
5. Rosenblum, W. I., and Johnson, M. G. (1968): Neuropathologic changes produced in suckling mice by adding lead to the maternal diet. *Arch. Pathol.*, 85:640–648.
6. Press, M. (1977): Lead encephalopathy in neonatal Long-Evans rats:Morphologic studies. *J. Neuropathol. Exp. Neurol.*, 36:169–193.
7. Weller, C. V. (1927): Tolerance in respect to the meningocerebral manifestations of acute and subacute lead poisoning. *Arch. Intern. Med.*, 39:45–59.
8. Bouldin, T. W., and Krigman, M. R. (1975): Acute lead encephalopathy in the guinea pig. *Acta Neuropathol. (Berl.)*, 33:185–190.
9. Pentschew, A. (1965): Morphology and morphogenesis of lead encephalopathy. *Acta Neuropathol.*, 5:133–160.
10. Popoff, N., Weinberg, S., and Feigin, I. (1963): Pathologic observations in lead encephalopathy. *Neurology (Minneap.)*, 13:101–112.

Neurotoxicology, edited by L. Roizin, H. Shiraki, and N. Grčević. Raven Press, New York © 1977.

Relationship of Blood and Brain Lead Levels to Morphologic Changes in Lead-Induced Chick Embryo Encephalopathy. I. Morphologic Studies

Asao Hirano and *Joseph A. Kochen

*Departments of Pathology and *Pediatrics, Montefiore Hospital and Medical Center, Bronx, New York, 10467, and The Albert Einstein College of Medicine, Bronx, New York 10467*

Lead is an environmental pollutant the effects of which in the human have been well known for many years (9,29). In children, one of its major effects is encephalopathy (1,2,17,18,21,25). A number of experimental studies in the young, developing animal have been performed (5,8, 11–13,15,16,19,22,26–28), but the mechanism of the action of lead on the central nervous system of the young child is, however, poorly understood.

We have chosen the chick embryo as an experimental model for the study of the mode of action of lead on the central nervous system (4,10,14). The lack of a uterine environment and the accessibility of the embryo to precisely controlled doses of lead salts makes this animal model a convenient tool.

PERSONAL INVESTIGATIONS

When 75- to 100-μg doses of lead acetate trihydrate are injected into the yolk sacs 4 days after incubation, many embryos die. A substantial number of the survivors, however, develop a progressively enlarging hydrocephalic cyst (Fig. 1).

Our study began with an anatomic investigation of this hydrocephalic cyst. Most often it was found in the occipital area, but occasionally in other areas as well. The

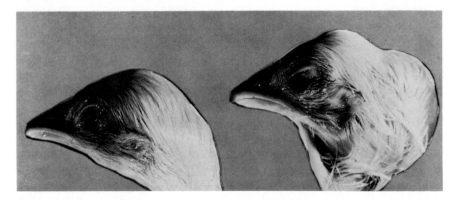

FIG. 1. Eighteen-day-old normal (*left*) and lead-treated (*right*) chick embryos. The treated animal shows a distinct cyst in the occipital area. (From Hirano and Kochen, ref. 10, © 1973 U.S. Canadian Division of the International Academy of Pathology.)

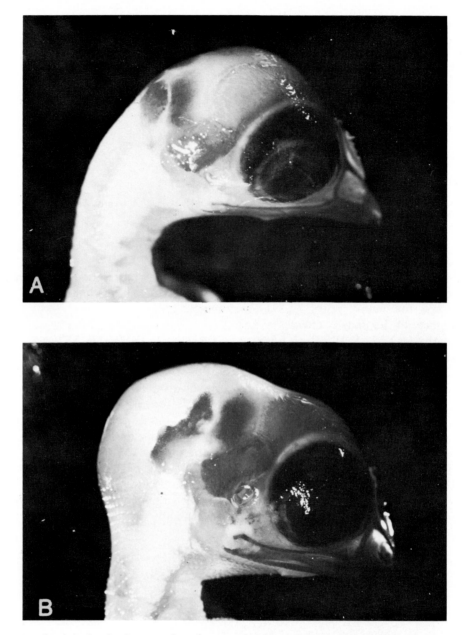

FIG. 2A: An alizarin red-stained preparation of a normal eighteen-day-old chick embryo. B: An alizarin red-stained preparation of a lead-treated eighteen-day-old chick embryo showing a cyst in the occipital area.

extent of the lesion could be seen most effectively after staining the occipital bones with alizarin red (3) (Figs. 2A and B). Instead of the normally closed suture line, the occipital bones were separated to a varying extent, depending on the size of the cyst (Figs. 3A and B).

When examined microscopically, the cysts were found to contain a clear fluid that occasionally contained hemorrhagic

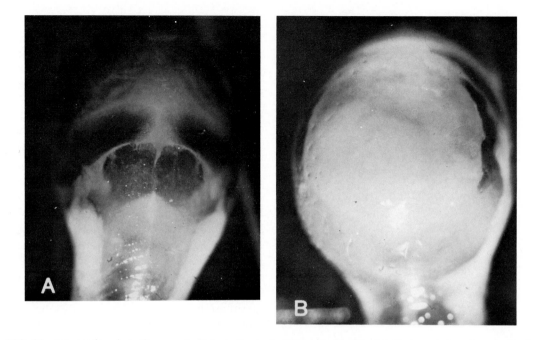

FIG. 3A: A posterior view of a normal chick similar to that illustrated in Fig. 2A. **B:** A posterior view of a lead-treated chick similar to that illustrated in Fig. 2B. Wide separation of the occipital bones is evident.

material. The cysts were expansions of the fourth ventricle that extended from the floor of the ventricle to the subcutaneous tissue over the head (Fig. 4). The walls of the cyst consisted of the edges of the interrupted layers of the brain, leptomeninges, skull, and subcutaneous tissue (Fig. 5).

In order to understand the formation of the cysts, we examined lead-intoxicated embryos at stages prior to the appearance of the hydrocephalic cyst. The major finding was that of hemorrhage into the central nervous system within 48 hr after injection of lead (Figs. 6A and B). The degree of central nervous system bleeding varied a great deal, but sometimes was so massive that the extraembryonic vessels appeared devoid of blood. Microscopic examination revealed that the hemorrhages were confined to the central nervous system. In those animals that survived, the hemorrhage gradually subsided and by the 10th day the ventricles began to expand to form the hydrocephalic cyst.

There seems to be a definite correlation between the hemorrhage and hydrocephalic cyst formation (Fig. 7), however, the precise mechanism relating the two events is not clear. Presumably the hemorrhage and

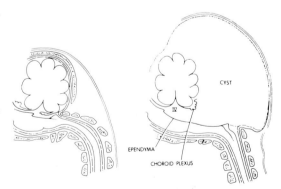

FIG. 4. Diagram of the anatomy of the posterior fossa in the normal (*left*) and lead-treated (*right*) eighteen-day-old chick embryo. In the treated animal there is a large cyst-like expansion communicating with the fourth ventricle. (From Hirano and Kochen, ref. 10, © 1973 U.S. Canadian Division of the International Academy of Pathology.)

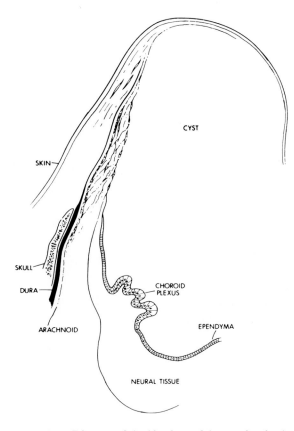

SKIN

SKULL

DURA

ARACHNOID

CYST

CHOROID
PLEXUS

EPENDYMA

NEURAL TISSUE

FIG. 5. Diagram of the histology of the cyst in a lead-treated chick. (From Hirano and Kochen, ref. 10, © 1973 U.S. Canadian Division of the International Academy of Pathology.)

subsequent hemolysis as well as destruction of neuronal tissue leads to an increase of osmotic pressure that results in cyst formation. The possible destruction of the arachnoid granulation—the site of cerebrospinal fluid absorption—may also lead to increased fluid accumulation. We cannot overlook the possibility of some obstruction of the cerebrospinal fluid pathways. The means by which the lead induces the hemorrhage and the reason for its restriction to the central nervous system are obscure. That the lead itself is responsible for these changes is suggested by the fact that ethylenediaminetetraacetic acid prevents the lead effects but only if administered within 8 hr of the lead treatment. It

should also be noted that the period during which lead is effective in producing hemorrhage, i.e., day 4 to day 10, corresponds to a period during which blood vessel development in the central nervous system parenchyma is very active (6,7,20). On day 4 the endothelial cells are poorly differentiated clusters with little or no intercellular specialization. By day 10 blood vessels are well developed, and tight junctions are present between adjacent endothelial cells. It is at that point that the blood-brain barrier becomes established (6). We have studied the developing blood vessels in both lead-treated and control chicks (23,24). No qualitative differences were detected between the two groups. However, certain features such as endothelial attenuation, mitochondrial alterations, accumulation of dense bodies, pinocytotic vesicles, and surface infoldings all seemed increased in the lead-treated chicks.

CONCLUSIONS

It is clear that lead intoxication, at least in the chick embryo, can lead to changes resembling meningoencephalocele in the human. This suggests the possibility that some of the changes generally ascribed to congenital deformation may in fact be related to environmental lead pollution.

ACKNOWLEDGMENTS

The authors wish to thank Dr. H. M. Dembitzer for his helpful suggestions and advice, and Yigal Greener and Ernestine Middleton for their technical assistance. We are also grateful to Dr. Leopold G. Koss for his help in the preparation of this manuscript.

This investigation received financial support from the United Cerebral Palsy Research and Education Foundation, Inc., and The National Foundation–March of Dimes.

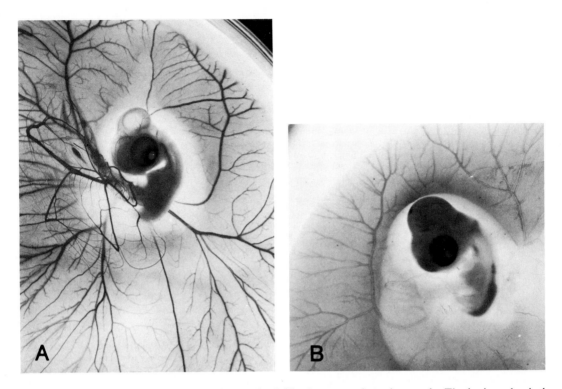

FIG. 6A: A normal six-day-old chick embryo. Blood fills the extraembryonic vessels. The brain and spinal cord appear relatively clear. **B:** A lead-treated six-day-old chick embryo. The extraembryonic vessels are collapsed, and the blood seems to fill the brain and spinal cord.

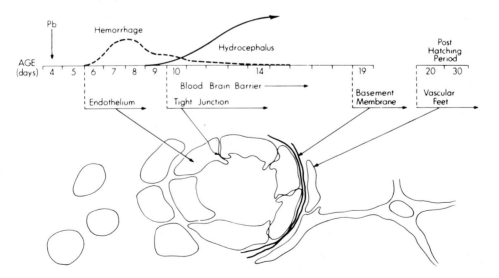

FIG. 7. A diagram of the temporal relationship between the effects of lead treatment and blood vessel development in the chick brain. (From Hirano and Kochen, ref. 10, © 1973 U.S. Canadian Division of the International Academy of Pathology.)

REFERENCES

1. Akelaitis, A. J. (1941): Lead encephalopathy in children and adults: A clinicopathological study. *J. Nerv. Ment. Dis.*, 93:313–332.
2. Blackman, S. S., Jr. (1930): The lesions of lead encephalitis in children. *Bull. Johns Hopkins Hosp.*, 61:1–61.
3. Burdi, A. R. (1965): Toluidine blue-alizarin red S staining of cartilage and bone in whole mount skeletons *in vitro*. *Stain Technol.*, 40:45–48.
4. Butt, E. M., Pearson, H. E., and Simonsen, D. G. (1952): Production of meningoceles and cranioschisis in chick embryos with lead nitrate. *Proc. Soc. Exp. Biol. Med.*, 79:247–249.
5. Clasen, R. A., Hartman, J. F., Starr, A. J., Coogan, P. S., Pandolfi, S., Laing, I., Becker, R., and Hass, G. M. (1974): Electron microscopic and chemical studies of the vascular changes and edema of lead encephalopathy. *Am. J. Pathol.*, 74:215–234.
6. Delorme, P., Gayet, J., and Grignon, G. (1970): Ultrastructural study on transcapillary exchanges in the developing telencephalon of the chicken. *Brain Res.*, 22:269–283.
7. Delorme, P. (1972): Différenciation ultrastructurale des jonctions intercellulaires de l'endothélium des capillaires télencéphaliques chez l'embryon de poulet. *Z. Zellforsch. Mikrosk. Anat.*, 133:571–582.
8. Goldstein, G. W., Arsbury, A. K., and Diamond, I. (1974): Pathogenesis of lead encephalopathy. Uptake of lead and reaction of brain capillaries. *Arch. Neurol.*, 31:382–389.
9. Goyer, R. A., and Rhyne, B. (1973): Pathological effects of lead. In: *International Review of Experimental Pathology*, Vol. 12, edited by G. W. Richter and M. A. Epstein, pp. 1–77. Academic Press, New York.
10. Hirano, A., and Kochen, J. A. (1973): Neurotoxic effects of lead in the chick embryo. Morphologic studies. *Lab. Invest.*, 29:659–668.
11. Hirano, A., and Kochen, J. A. (1975): Some effects of intracerebral lead implantation in the rat. *Acta Neuropathol. (Berl.)*, 33:307–315.
12. Hirano, A., and Kochen, J. A. (1976): Further observations on the effects of lead implantation in rat brains. *Acta Neuropathol. (Berl.)*, 34:87–93.
13. Hirano, A., and Kochen, J. A. (1976): Experimental lead encephalopathy. In: *Progress in Neuropathology*, Vol. 3, edited by H. M. Zimmerman, pp. 319–342. Grune & Stratton, New York.
14. Karnofsky, D. A., and Ridgway, L. P. (1952): Producing of injury to the central nervous system of the chick embryo by lead salts. *J. Pharmacol. Exp. Ther.*, 104:176–186.
15. Krigman, M. R., Druss, M. J., Traylor, T. D., Wilson, M. H., Newell, L. R., and Hogan, E. L. (1974): Lead encephalopathy in the developing rat: Effect upon myelination. *J. Neuropathol. Exp. Neurol.*, 33:58–73.
16. Lampert, P. W., Garro, F., and Pentschew, A. (1967): Lead encephalopathy in suckling rats. In: *Symposium on Brain Edema*, edited by I. Klatzo and F. Seitelberger, pp. 207–222. Springer Publ., New York.
17. Okazaki, H., Aronson, S. M., DiMaio, D. J., and Olvera, J. E. (1963): Acute lead encephalopathy of childhood. Histologic and chemical studies with particular reference to angiopathic aspects. *Trans. Am. Neurol. Assoc.*, 88:248–250.
18. Pentschew, A. (1958): Intoxikationen. In: *Handbuch der Speziellen Pathologische Anatomie und Histologie, Vol. 13, Part 2*, edited by W. Scholz, pp. 1929–2502. Springer-Verlag, Berlin, Göttingen, Heidelberg.
19. Pentschew, A., and Garro, F. (1966): Lead encephalopathy of the suckling rat and its implications on the porphyrinopathic nervous diseases. With special reference to the permeability disorders of the nervous system's capillaries. *Acta Neuropathol. (Berl.)*, 6:266–278.
20. Peterson, R. G. (1968): Vascularization and basement membranes of the chick brain in light microscopy. *Anat. Rec.*, 161:37–44.
21. Popoff, N., Weinberg, S., and Feigin, I. (1963): Pathologic observations in lead encephalopathy: With special reference to the vascular changes. *Neurology (Minneap.)*, 13:101–112.
22. Rosenblum, W. I., and Johnson, M. G. (1968): Neuropathologic changes produced in suckling mice by adding lead to the maternal diet. *Arch. Pathol.*, 85:640–648.
23. Roy, S., Hirano, A., Kochen, J. A., and Zimmerman, H. M. (1974): The fine structure of cerebral blood vessels in chick embryo. *Acta Neuropathol. (Berl.)*, 30:277–285.
24. Roy, S., Hirano, A., Kochen, J. A., and Zimmerman, H. M. (1974): Ultrastructure of cerebral vessels in chick embryo in lead intoxication. *Acta Neuropathol. (Berl.)*, 30:287–294.
25. Smith, J. F., McLaurin, R. L., Nichols, J. B., and Asbury, A. (1960): Studies in cerebral edema and cerebral swelling. I. The changes in lead encephalopathy in children compared with those in alkyltin poisoning in animals. *Brain*, 83:411–424.
26. Thomas, J. A., Dallenbach, F. D., and Thomas, I. M. (1971): Considerations on the development of experimental lead encephalopathy. *Virchows Arch. Abt. A. [Pathol. Anat.]*, 352:61–74.
27. Thomas, J. A., Dallenbach, F. D., and Thomas, M. (1973): Distribution of radioactive lead (210 Pb) in the cerebellum of developing rats. *J. Pathol.*, 109:45–50.
28. Thomas, J. A., and Thomas, I. M. (1974): The pathogenesis of lead encephalopathy. *Indian J. Med. Res.*, 62:36–41.
29. Waldron, H. A., and Stöfen, D. (1974): *Subclinical Lead Poisoning*. Academic Press, New York.

Neurotoxicology, edited by L. Roizin, H. Shiraki, and N. Grčević. Raven Press, New York © 1977.

Relationship of Blood and Brain Lead Levels to Morphologic Changes in Lead-Induced Chick Embryo Encephalopathy. II. Biochemical Studies

*Joseph A. Kochen, *Yigal Greener, and **Asao Hirano

*Departments of *Pediatrics and **Pathology, Montefiore Hospital and Medical Center, Bronx, New York; and The Albert Einstein College of Medicine, Bronx, New York 10467*

Lead intoxication in early childhood can result in a severe hemorrhagic and edematous encephalopathy (4,7). Despite the well-documented association between high blood lead levels and the encephalopathic effects of lead, little is known about the relationship between red blood cell lead, plasma lead, and the entry of lead into the central nervous system (CNS). The purpose of this study was to explore this relationship in the chick embryo with lead encephalopathy.

Lead encephalopathy in the chick embryo is characterized by vascular endothelial cell injury, CNS hemorrhage, and encephalocele formation. Exposure of 4-day embryos to lead at a time when primitive CNS blood vessel formation begins results within 48 hr in electron microscopic evidence of vascular endothelial cell injury and focal extravasation of red cells. In most severely affected embryos, this progresses to massive CNS hemorrhage and death. In the remaining embryos bleeding subsides by day 12, when mature microvessels with tight endothelial junctions have replaced much of the more primitive microvasculature. In the surviving embryos, this is followed by expansion of the ventricles and subarachnoid space and by encephalocele formation (see Chapter 31, Hirano and

Kochen, *this volume,* and refs. 2,3,5, and 6).

PERSONAL INVESTIGATIONS

The primary objective was to determine the extent to which extravasation of lead-containing red cells and diffusion of plasma lead contribute to the accumulation of lead in the brain. For the purpose of the present study, two doses of lead were selected for injection into the yolk sacs of 4-day chick embryos. The injection of 75 μg lead acetate trihydrate resulted by day 18 in only a 2% incidence of encephaloceles, whereas 100 μg resulted in 35% incidence of encephaloceles.

The use of ^{59}Fe permitted quantitation of the extent of red cell sequestration in the brain. The radio-iron was injected in tracer doses into the yolk sac on day 4 simultaneously with the administration of lead. The ^{59}Fe was incorporated during erythropoiesis and served as a convenient red cell marker. The administration of lead did not result in a significant change in the uptake of radio-iron by red cells. In contradistinction, the injection of lead resulted in a marked increase in the localization of ^{59}Fe in the brain. Exposure to 75 μg lead acetate resulted in a twofold increase and 100 μg in a fourfold increase in brain ^{59}Fe uptake. This corresponded to an increase in red cell volume from 18.4 μl/g brain in the controls to 38.2 μl at the lower dose of lead and 69.5 μl at the higher dose.

The volume of red cells in the nonlead-treated control group represented the extent of trapping of red cells in the brain vasculature at the time the embryos were killed by exsanguination. Exposure to toxic levels of lead clearly resulted in substantially increased retention of red cells in the brain. This increased trapping of red cells was consistent with morphologic finding of focal hemorrhages and quantitatively reflected the extent of red cell extravasation due to lead-induced microvascular injury.

The use of ^{210}Pb tracer facilitated the measurement of lead uptake by blood and brain. The radiolead was injected with and without nonradioactive lead acetate on day 4. The administration of 75 and 100 μg lead acetate resulted in a decreased uptake of radioactive lead by red cells, reflecting the dilutional effect of the nonradioactive lead. Despite its dilutional effect, 75 μg lead acetate resulted in a twofold increase and 100 μg in an eightfold increase in ^{210}Pb uptake by brain.

Blood lead levels did not differ significantly at the 75- and 100-μg doses. However, at the higher dose of lead there was a marked increase in the accumulation of lead in brain. At the 75-μg dose the brain lead level was 2.14 μg/g dry weight of brain and at the 100-μg dose this increased to 7.48 μg lead/g. This increase in brain lead correlated well with the increased CNS hemorrhage and encephalocele formation seen at the higher dose of lead.

Based on volume of red cells trapped in the brain, red cell lead level, and concentration of lead in the brain, it was possible to calculate the proportion of brain lead attributable to the presence of red cells. Following the administration of a tracer dose of lead in the absence of nonradioactive lead, 60% of the brain lead uptake

was attributable to the presence of red cells trapped in the vasculature. At 75- and 100-μg lead acetate doses, the proportion of brain lead attributable to red cells was reduced to 18 and 16%, respectively. However, when expressed in absolute terms, the increase in dose from 75 to 100 μg resulted in an increase in the red cell fraction of brain lead from 0.37 to 1.13 μg lead/g dry weight of brain. This threefold increase in brain lead attributable to trapped red cells corresponded to the increased extravasation of red cells at the higher dose of lead.

The remaining and larger fractions of brain lead, 1.13 μg/g at the 75 μg-dose and 6.35 μg/g at the 100-μg dose, were not attributable to red cells and presumably reflected the diffusion of plasma lead across the lead-damaged brain microvasculature.

The linear correlation coefficient between the red cell and non-red cell fractions of brain lead was 0.830 ($p < 0.001$) at 75 μg and 0.884 ($p < 0.001$) at 100 μg lead acetate. This strong and highly significant correlation suggests that the extravasation of red cells and the diffusion of plasma lead may have occurred by a common mechanism, namely, lead-induced capillary injury.

CONCLUSIONS

In conclusion, our studies have shown that chick embryo encephalopathy is associated with morphologic and functional evidence of injury to CNS microvessels. This microvascular injury results in CNS hemorrhage and is presumably responsible for the ensuing encephalocele formation. As in the case of the immature rat model (1), the amount of lead entering into the brain and the severity of the microvascular injury are related to the extent of lead exposure. The movement of lead into the brain occurs in the form of both extravasated lead-containing red cells and plasma lead that has diffused across damaged vascular endothelium. Although the metabolic consequences of increased lead deposition in the CNS are unknown, it appears likely that lead-induced microvascular injury is an important factor in the pathogenesis of lead encephalopathy.

ACKNOWLEDGMENT

This investigation received financial support from The United Cerebral Palsy Research and Educational Foundation and The National Foundation–March of Dimes.

REFERENCES

1. Goldstein, G. W., Asbury, A. K., and Diamond, I. (1974): Pathogenesis of lead encephalopathy. Uptake of lead and reaction of brain capillaries. *Arch. Neurol.,* 31:382–389.
2. Hirano, A., and Kochen, J. A. (1973): Neurotoxic effects of lead in the chick embryo. Morphologic studies. *Lab. Invest.,* 29:659–668.
3. Hirano, A., and Kochen, J. A. (1977): Experimental lead encephalopathy. In: *Progress in Neuropathology,* Vol. 3, edited by H. M. Zimmerman. Grune & Stratton, New York.
4. Lin-Fu, J. S. (1973): Vulnerability of children to lead exposure and toxicity. *N. Engl. J. Med.,* 289:1229–1233.
5. Roy, S., Hirano, A., Kochen, J. A., and Zimmerman, H. M. (1974): The fine structure of cerebral blood vessels in chick embryo. *Acta Neuropathol. (Berl.),* 30:287–294.
6. Roy, S., Hirano, A., Kochen, J. A., and Zimmerman, H. M. (1974): Ultrastructure of cerebral vessels in chick embryo in lead intoxication. *Acta Neuropathol. (Berl.),* 30:287–294.
7. Waldron, H. A., and Stofen, D. (1974): *Subclinical Lead Poisoning.* Academic Press, New York.

Neurotoxicology, edited by L. Roizin, H. Shiraki, and N. Grčević. Raven Press, New York © 1977.

Neurotoxicity of Aluminum

H. M. Wisniewski, *J. K. Korthals, †L. M. Kopeloff, *R. Ferszt, **J. C. Chusid, and *R. D. Terry

*NYS Institute for Basic Research in Mental Retardation, Staten Island, New York 10314; *Albert Einstein College of Medicine, Bronx, New York, 10461; **St. Vincent's Hospital and Medical Center of New York, New York, New York 10011; †NYS Psychiatric Institute, New York, New York 10032*

Neuroscientists for the first time became interested in aluminum in 1942 when Kopeloff and associates (8,9,12) found that in monkeys after direct application of the metal to the cortex, this atom produces a chronic state of convulsive reactivity with recurrent seizures that simulate epilepsy in man. Aluminum for the second time drew the attention of brain researchers in 1965 when Klatzo, Terry, and I (7,13,16) reported that aluminum induces neurofibrillary degeneration in rabbits.

As we all know, one of the most common and devastating diseases, presenile and senile dementia, is characterized by the presence of neurons with neurofibrillary changes. So when we found that aluminum is the cause of neurofibrillary degeneration, we thought that we had an experimental model of Alzheimer's disease and had possibly found one of the agents responsible for these changes. Ultrastructural studies of the affected neurons from aluminum-treated animals and from humans with presenile and senile dementia showed differences between the species regarding the individual elements forming the neurofibrillary tangle. In aluminum-treated rabbits the tangles are made of 100-Å filaments, ultrastructurally similar to the normal neurofilaments, whereas in Alzheimer's disease they are made of paired helical filaments each about 120 Å in diameter. These filaments are helically wound with periodic twists about 800 Å apart (14,15).

Since that time it was found that several other compounds, such as colchicine and other spindle inhibitors, induce neurofibrillary degeneration. Like aluminum, all these compounds cause the accumulation of 100 Å filaments and not the paired helical filaments found in the majority of human diseases. So aluminum appeared to be an interesting atom in neurofibrillary pathology, but its relevance to Alzheimer's disease remained uncertain.

Some new observations, however, again drew our attention to aluminum with regard to a possibly important role in the pathogenesis of Alzheimer's changes in presenile and senile dementia. The Canadian group of investigators led by Crapper (4) found that in brain specimens from patients with Alzheimer's disease there is an increased concentration of aluminum in areas showing neurofibrillary degeneration. Their behavioral studies of cats with aluminum encephalopathy also showed an alteration in short-term retention and associative learning as measured by delayed task response (2,3). At this point we must recall that aluminum does not induce neurofibrillary changes in all species. The animals that do respond to aluminum treatment with neurofibrillary changes are rabbits, cats,

313

and dogs. In mice and rats aluminum only produces epilepsy. As mentioned, it has been known since 1942 that application of aluminum to the rhesus monkey cortex induces epilepsy. We recently examined seven monkeys with 15-year clinical histories of epilepsy after intracortical injections of 0.5 to 1.0 cc of aluminum paste. At the site of injection we found a glial scar with some debris of aluminum paste. However, none of the neurons around the area where aluminum was injected showed evidence of neurofibrillary changes. We also injected up to 1.5 ml of 1% $AlCl_3$ into the subarachnoid space of another five monkeys. These animals, 10 to 15 days after the aluminum injection, showed weakness of all extremities and severe ataxia. However, both light and electron microscopic studies of the central nervous system revealed only some degeneration of the Purkinje cells and tri-ethyl-tin-like changes in the white matter. The latter observation is of great interest in the light of recent reports that in patients undergoing dialysis, there was dementia, increased levels of aluminum in the blood, and vacuolar degeneration in the brain (1). In the literature there are only two reports of well-documented human cases of aluminum encephalopathy. The first was a 49-year-old man who had worked for $13\frac{1}{2}$ years in an aluminum powder factory and died following a 10-month period of progressive mental deterioration, complete aphasia, and focal and general epileptic seizures. Postmortem examination of his brain showed 17 times the normal concentration of aluminum. However, there is no information whether neurofibrillary changes were present, nor are other histologic changes documented (11). The second case was a 37-year-old alcoholic who died after a 10-year course of mental and motor deterioration with palatal myoclonus. His brain had numerous concretions in the white matter with high concentrations of

aluminum. Again the cortex, by implication, was normal (10).

These data indicate that in both humans and animals epilepsy is the constant feature of aluminum encephalopathy. In presenile and senile dementia, epileptic seizures are not common. Therefore it is doubtful whether aluminum is responsible for alterations in neuronal fibrous protein in age-associated dementias. However, since recent data indicate (5,6) that the human paired helical filament tangles are made of protein similar if not identical to the normal 100-Å filaments, we can not exclude the possibility that in some species aluminum may produce paired helical filaments instead of the 100-Å filaments found to date.

REFERENCES

1. Alfrey, A. C., LeGendre, G. R., and Haehny, W. D. (1976): The dialysis encephalopathy syndrome: Possible aluminum intoxication. *N. Engl. J. Med.,* 294:184–188.
2. Crapper, D. R., and Dalton, A. J. (1973): Alterations in short term retention, conditioned avoidance response acquisition and motivation following aluminum induced neurofibrillary degeneration. *Physiol. Behav.,* 10:925–933.
3. Crapper, D. R., and Dalton, A. J. (1973): Aluminum induced neurofibrillary degeneration, brain electrical activity and alterations in acquisition and retention. *Physiol. Behav.,* 10:935–945.
4. Crapper, D. R., Krishnan, S. S., and Dalton, A. J. (1973): Brain aluminum distribution in Alzheimer's disease and experimental neurofibrillary degeneration. *Science,* 180:511–513.
5. Iqbal, K., Wisniewski, H. M., Grundke-Iqbal, I., Korthals, J. K., and Terry, R. D. (1975): Chemical pathology of neurofibrils, neurofibrillary tangles of Alzheimer's presenile-senile dementia. *J. Histochem. Cytochem.,* 23:563–569.
6. Iqbal, K., Wisniewski, H. M., Shelanski, M. L., Brostoff, S., Liwnicz, B. H., and Terry, R. D. (1974): Protein changes in senile dementia. *Brain Res.,* 77:337–343.
7. Klatzo, I., Wisniewski, H., and Streicher, E. (1965): Experimental production of neurofibrillary degeneration. I. Light microscopic observations. *J. Neuropathol. Exp. Neurol.,* 24:187–199.
8. Kopeloff, L. M., Barrera, S. E., and Kopeloff, N. (1942): Recurrent convulsive seizures in animals produced by immunologic and chemical means. *Am. J. Psychiatry,* 98:881–902.

9. Kopeloff, N., Kopeloff, L. M., and Pacella, B. L. (1947): The experimental production of epilepsy in animals. In: *Epilepsy,* edited by P. H. Hoch and R. P. Knight, pp. 163–180. Grune & Stratton, New York.

10. Lapresle, J., Duckett, S., Galle, P., and Cartier, L. (1975): Documents cliniques, anatomiques et biophysiques dans une encephalopathie avec presence de depots d'aluminum. *Soc. Biologie (Comptes Rendus),* 169:282–290.

11. McLaughlin, A. I. G., Kazantzis, G., King, E., Teare, D., Porter, R. J., and Owen, R. (1962): Pulmonary fibrosis and encephalopathy associated with the inhalation of aluminum dust. *Br. J. Ind. Med.,* 19:253–263.

12. Pacella, B. L., Kopeloff, N., Barrera, S. E., and Kopeloff, L. M. (1944): Experimental production of focal epilepsy. *Arch. Neurol. Psychiatry,* 52:183–186.

13. Terry, R. D., and Pena, C. (1965): Experimental production of neurofibrillary degeneration. II. Electron microscopy, phosphatase histochemistry and electron probe analysis. *J. Neuropathol. Exp. Neurol.,* 24:200.

14. Wisniewski, H. M., Narang, H. K., and Terry, R. D. (1976): Neurofibrillary tangles of paired helical filaments. *J. Neurol. Sci.,* 27:173–181.

15. Wisniewski, H., Terry, R. D., and Hirano, A. (1970): Neurofibrillary pathology. *J. Neuropathol. Exp. Neurol.,* 29:163–176.

16. Wisniewski, H., Terry, R. D., Pena, C., Streicher, E., and Klatzo, I. (1965): Experimental production of neurofibrillary degeneration. *J. Neuropathol. Exp. Neurol.,* 24:139.

ADDENDUM

Our recent studies [J. R. McDermott, K. Iqbal, and H. M. Wisniewski, *Lancet* (*in press*)] of AL content in 274 brain samples from 9 mentally normal and 10 patients with clinical diagnosis of senile dementia confirmed by histopathologic studies failed to show any significant differences in aluminum concentration between normal and demented patients, either overall or in the regions rich in neurofibrillary tangles. In the material studied 23% of senile dementia samples showed elevated aluminum concentration, however the same was true in 22% of the non-demented age matched control samples. This suggests that high aluminum levels are an age-associated phenomenon, unrelated to dementia.

Crapper et al. at the workshop-conference on Alzheimer's disease, senile dementia and related disorders (National Institutes of Health, Bethesda, Maryland, June 6–9, 1977) reported that human neurons taken from aborted fetuses and exposed to aluminum, develop neurofibrillary tangles made of 100 Å filaments and not of the Alzheimer's paired hellical filaments.

Neurotoxicology, edited by L. Roizin, H. Shiraki, and N. Grčević. Raven Press, New York © 1977.

Effect of Triethyltin on the Developing Brain of the Mouse

Itaru Watanabe

Veterans Administration Hospital, Kansas City, Missouri 64128, and the Departments of Pathology and Oncology, University of Kansas College of Medical Science and Hospital, Kansas City, Kansas 66103

Acute triethyltin (TET) encephalopathy is characterized morphologically by a transient edema of the central nervous system caused by extensive intramyelinic vacuolation (1,2,11,13,15,19). The edema is restricted within the myelin sheath and is not accompanied by enlargement of the extracellular space (12,16,27,29). The edema fluid consists of water containing high levels of sodium and chloride, but, except for one report (11), no blood proteins have been detected (2,3,12,19,21,24). In spite of the marked alteration in the myelin sheath, the myelin composition of the intoxicated brain is normal (7). The edema is not associated with any morphologic changes of the blood vessels (2,15,26,29). Vital stains with Trypan blue have yielded negative results (2,3,23). The blood-brain barrier has remained impermeable to ^{131}I-labeled albumin (3). The edema can be prevented, but only partially, by steroid administration (23,25).

The mechanism of the myelinotoxicity of TET still remains to be elucidated. Direct effects to the myelin sheath have been observed after intracerebral TET implantation (10) and after TET administration into the spinal cord culture (9). Purified rat brain myelin binds triethyltin (18). Action by TET metabolites can also be considered when the encephalopathy is produced through systemic routes. Biochemically,

and also histochemically, TET inhibits oxidative phosphorylation and ATPase activities in the mitochondria (4,5,20,22,28). It has further been found that TET inhibits glucose oxidation by rat brain cortex slices (6,17). Mitochondrial damage by TET has also been observed in the culture study (9). In addition to mitochondrial injury, it has been considered that TET may alter permeability of the cell membrane, particularly that of the myelin lamellae (29,30).

In TET encephalopathy, neurons and glial cells show only minor changes when intramyelinic edema has fully developed. Torack et al. (29) observed, however, that immediately after a single injection of TET the development of the myelin vacuoles is preceded by axonal and astrocytic edema. Peripheral myelin is less sensitive to TET (24), but extensive myelin splitting has been produced by Graham and Gonatas (8).

PERSONAL INVESTIGATIONS

In order to know the effects of TET on the central myelination, four experiments have been undertaken to observe morphologic changes occurring in the cerebral white matter of the developing mice at the stage of active myelin production. For this study, suckling mice, Charles River outbred, aged 5 to 20 days were treated with a single intraperitoneal injection of 0.1% bis-triethyltin sulfate (Organische Chemische Institute, Utrecht, The Netherlands) in physiologic saline. The intoxicated animals were sacrificed by decapitation, and the corpus callosum and the adjacent areas were fixed by immersion with a solution containing glutaraldehyde (1%), paraformaldehyde (1%), and sucrose (3%) in 0.1 M phosphate buffer. The Epon-embedded tissue was examined with light and electron microscope.

Severity of TET Encephalopathy and Morphologic Changes

Fifty-five suckling mice aged 5, 10, 15, and 20 days and 15 mature ones aged 40 days received TET according to the schedule shown in Table 1. With a dose of 10 mg/kg body weight (BW), all the developing mice died within 24 hr, whereas the 40-day-old animals survived more than 2 weeks. With 7.5 mg/kg BW, 10-day-old mice survived only 3 days; 15-day-old ones lived up to 6 days; whereas none of the 20- and 40-day-old animals died. With 5 mg/kg BW, all the mice recovered from intoxications spontaneously. Thus, the younger mice were more sensitive to TET than the mature.

TABLE 1. *Severity of TET encephalopathy and mortality*

Age of mice when dose given (days)	Time of death at dose of TET (mg/kg BW)			
	2.5	5.0	7.5	10.0
5				< 24 hr[a]
10	nil	nil	day 3[b]	< 24 hr[a]
15		nil	days 5 & 6[c]	< 24 hr[a]
20		nil	nil	< 24 hr[a]
40		nil	nil	nil

A group consists of five mice; one each was sacrificed at days 1, 2, 3, 7, and 14. Nil, no spontaneous death occurred in the group.
[a] All five mice died within 24 hr.
[b] All three nonsacrificed mice died spontaneously on day 3.
[c] Spontaneous death of one mouse each on day 5 and 6.

In the above schedule, the intoxicated mice were sacrificed at days 1, 2, 3, 7, and 14. Regardless of age and dose, intramyelinic vacuolation was present at 24 hr (Figs. 1 and 5). The vacuoles were increased in number and size by the third day, measuring up to 20 μm in diameter (Fig. 2). The vacuolation occurred mostly in the thick fibers, consisting of an axon larger than 1 μm in diameter and a myelin sheath possessing more than five major dense lines (Fig. 3). The small myelinated fibers were only minimally affected. At day 4, intramyelinic vacuoles were markedly reduced in number and size. Many vacuoles were now surrounded by a thin tag of oligodendroglial cytoplasm which contained abundant microtubules (Fig. 4); this suggests a participation of oligodendroglia in reorganization of the myelin sheath. At days 7 and 14, a large majority of the myelin sheaths were normal in structure, arrangement, and distribution. There were only a few myelinic vacuoles present.

In the animals administered high doses of TET, there were severe axonal and glial changes, which were absent in those that received low doses (Fig. 5). Namely, both myelinated and unmyelinated axons were edematously swollen, and their microtubules and filaments were disrupted (Fig. 7). In the oligodendroglias, there was a marked intracytoplasmic vesicle formation, but rough endoplasmic reticulum and mitochondria appeared intact (Fig. 6). Astrocytes were also edematously swollen. In spite of severe axonal edema, the neuronal perikarya in the adjacent gray matter appeared intact.

Remote Effect

In order to observe a remote effect on myelination of a single TET administration, 15-day-old mice received 5 mg/kg BW TET and were sacrificed 1, 2, 3, 4, and 5 weeks later. When compared with the control brains, there was no appreciable evidence of hypomyelination.

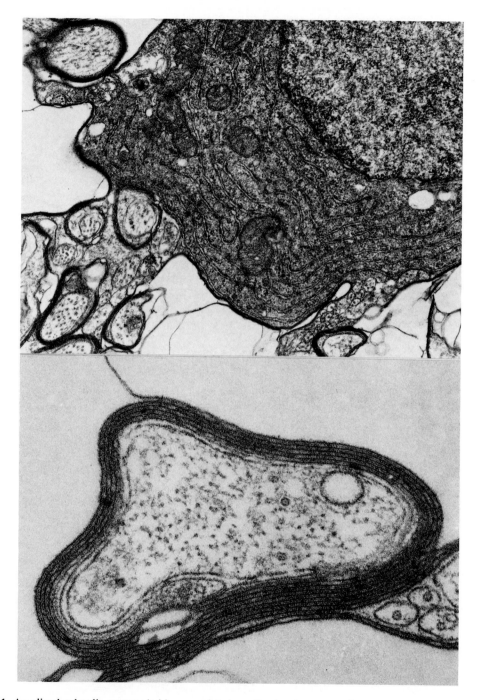

FIG. 1. An oligodendroglia surrounded by vacuolated myelin sheaths appears intact except for a few vesicles. 15-day-old mouse, 24 hr after TET (7.5 mg/kg BW). ×19,000.
FIG. 2. Intramyelinic vacuolation due to splitting of myelin sheath at the intraperiod line. 15-day-old mouse, 72 hr after TET (7.5 mg/kg BW). ×83,000.

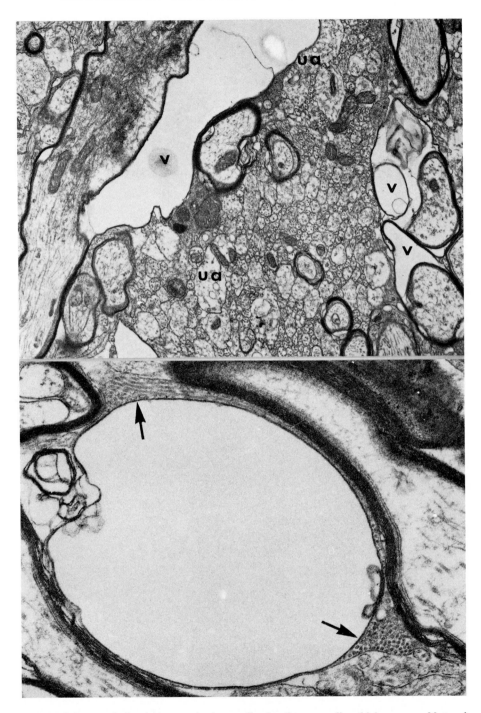

FIG. 3. Intramyelinic vacuolation (v) occurs in the myelin sheath surrounding thicker axons. Note edematous swelling of some unmyelinated axons (ua). 15-day-old mouse, 24 hr after TET (7.5 mg/kg BW). ×12,000.
FIG. 4. A myelinic vacuole surrounded by a thin cytoplasmic tag of oligodendrocyte (*arrows*). 20-day-old mouse, 4 days after TET (5 mg/kg BW). ×29,000.

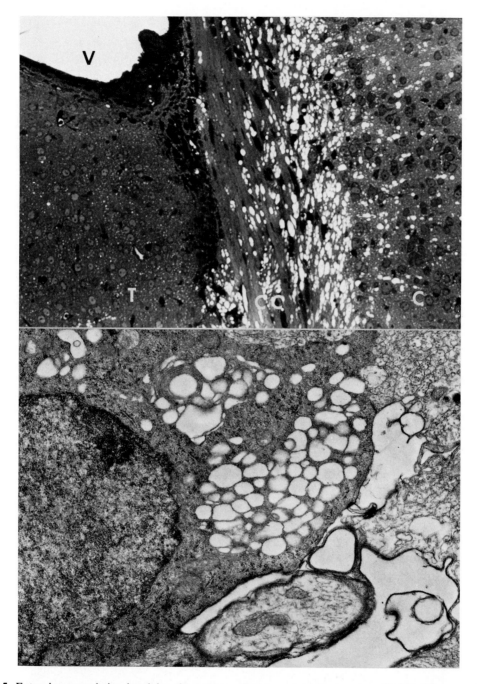

FIG. 5. Extensive vacuolation involving the corpus callosum and cerebral cortex. 10-day-old mouse, 24 hr after TET (7.5 mg/kg BW). C, cerebral cortex; CC, corpus callosum; T, thalamus; V, lateral ventricle. ×170.
FIG. 6. Intracytoplasmic vesicle formation in an oligodendrocyte. 10-day-old mouse, 24 hr after TET (7.5 mg/kg BW). ×15,000.

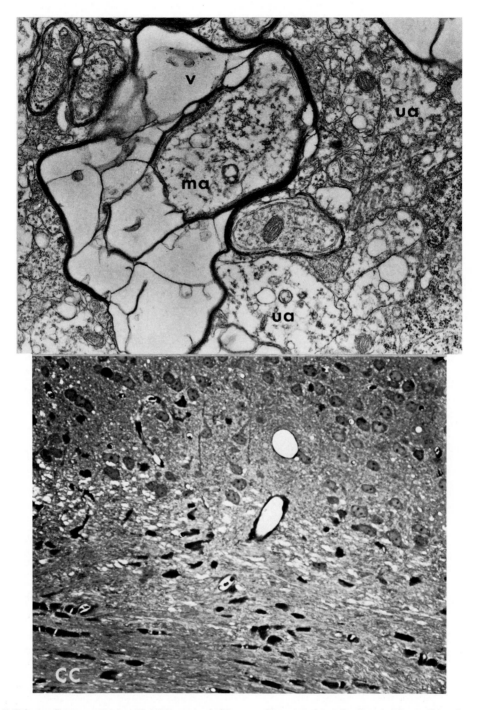

FIG. 7. Edema of an axon (ma), which is surrounded by a multiloculated myelin sheath. Unmyelinated neuronal branches (ua) are also edematously swollen. 10-day-old mouse, 48 hr after TET (7.5 mg/kg BW). v, intramyelinic vacuole. ×23,000.
FIG. 8. Vacuolation of the deeper cortex of the cerebrum. 19-day-old mouse, 6 hr after TET (5 mg/kg BW). CC, corpus callosum. ×230.

Cumulative Effect

In order to observe whether repeated TET administration produces any cumulative effects on myelination, TET (3 mg/kg BW) was given every 4 days from the 13th day of life. Two mice were sacrificed 3 days after each injection. The last four mice received 10 injections and were sacrificed at days 40 and 51 (3 and 14 days, respectively, after the last injection). Although there was a myelinic vacuolation in all the brains, no recognizable evidence of hypomyelination could be observed.

Initial Changes in Axons and Astroglia Which Precede Myelinic Vacuolation

Nineteen-day-old mice that had received TET (5 mg/kg BW) developed, within a half-hour, a lethargic condition that lasted 6 hr. These mice were sacrificed at 3, 6, 9, 12, 24, and 48 hr. At 3 hr, there was a moderate astrocytic edema at the deeper cortex adjacent to the corpus callosum (Fig. 9). Six hours after the TET injection, edematous swelling of both myelinated and unmyelinated axons became obvious (Figs. 8 and 10). At 9 hr, the astrocytic edema had almost subsided, whereas the axonal edema predominated. Twenty-four hours after TET administration, the intramyelinic vacuolation was outstanding, whereas the edema of the unmyelinated fibers had disappeared. Throughout this time period, no significant changes were observed in the neuronal perikarya, oligodendroglias, and myelinated axis cylinders. Vital stain with Evans blue was negative at all stages of this experiment, indicating unaltered permeability of the blood vessels to the serum protein (14).

Increased Vascular Permeability to Quinacrine

Quinacrine hydrochloride (3 mg/kg BW) was injected intravenously at the various stages of the TET encephalopathy, and the mice were then sacrificed 30 min later. Frozen sections of the brains were examined for the autofluorescence of the compound as a clue of increased permeability of the blood vessels. In the control animals, fluorescence was observed only in the choroid plexus, but not in the brain parenchyma. In the brain of the experimental animals, the autofluorescence started to be seen in the gray matter at 2 hr; became marked both in the gray and white matter at 4 hr; faint at 6 hr; and negative at 24 hr. Thus, marked penetration of quinacrine occurred in a very short period of time immediately after TET injection.

CONCLUSION

1. TET caused intramyelinic vacuolation in the growing mouse brain in the same manner as in the mature brain. It occurred, however, predominantly in the thick myelin sheaths surrounding large axons.

2. With a lethal dose, there was severe edema in astrocytes and neuronal branches, vacuolation of oligodendroglial cytoplasm, and fragmentation of myelin membranes in the vacuoles.

3. At a sublethal dose, long-term studies indicate that TET did not appreciably prevent the myelin production of oligodendroglia.

4. Immediately after intraperitoneal administration, TET affected deeper cortex first, as manifested by astrocytic edema, followed by edematous swelling of myelinated and unmyelinated axons including axonal terminals, and, finally, myelin splitting and vacuolation.

5. TET did not produce increased permeability of blood vessels to Evans blue in the stage of active myelinization, as it did not in the adult brain. Vascular permeability to quinacrine, as tested in the mature mice, was abnormally increased immediately after TET injection.

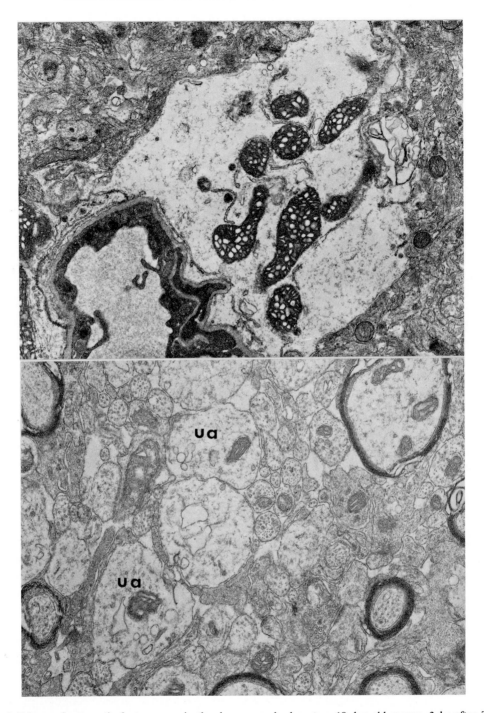

FIG. 9. Edema of astrocytic foot process in the deeper cerebral cortex. 19-day-old mouse, 3 hr after TET (5 mg/kg BW). ×15,000.
FIG. 10. Edema of unmyelinated (ua) and myelinated axons. 19-day-old mouse, 6 hr after TET (5 mg/kg BW). ×21,000.

ACKNOWLEDGMENT

This work was supported by the Medical Research Service of the Veterans Administration.

REFERENCES

1. Adachi, M., and Aronson, S. M. (1967): Studies on spongy degeneration of the central nervous system (Van Bogaert–Bertrand type). In: *Inborn Disorders of Sphingolipid Metabolism, Proc. IIIrd Int. Symp. Cerebral Sphingolipidosis,* edited by S. M. Aronson and B. W. Volk, pp. 129–148. Pergamon Press, Oxford.
2. Aleu, F. P., Katzman, R., and Terry, R. D. (1963): Fine structure and electrolyte analyses of cerebral edema induced by alkyltin intoxication. *J. Neuropathol. Exp. Neurol.,* 22:403–413.
3. Bakay, L. (1965): Morphological and chemical studies in cerebral edema: Triethyltin induced edema. *J. Neurol. Sci.,* 2:52–67.
4. Brody, T. M., and Moore, K. E. (1962): Biochemical aspects of triethyltin toxicity. *Fed. Proc.,* 21:1103–1106.
5. Cremer, J. E. (1962): The action of triethyltin, triethyl lead, ethyl mercury and other inhibitors on the metabolism of brain and kidney slices in vitro using substrates labeled with C^{14}. *J. Neurochem.,* 9:284–298.
6. Cremer, J. E. (1970): Selective inhibition of glucose oxidation by triethyltin in rat brain in vivo. *Biochem. J.,* 119:95–102.
7. Eto, Y., Suzuki, K., and Suzuki, K. (1971): Lipid composition of rat brain myelin in triethyltin-induced edema. *J. Lipid Res.,* 12:570–579.
8. Graham, D. I., and Gonatas, N. K. (1973): Triethyltin sulfate-induced splitting of peripheral myelin in rats. *Lab. Invest.,* 29:628–632.
9. Graham, D. I., Kim, S. U., Gonatas, N. K., and Guyotte, L. (1975): The neurotoxic effects of triethyltin sulfate on myelinating cultures of mouse spinal cord. *J. Neuropathol. Exp. Neurol.,* 34:401–412.
10. Hirano, A., Zimmerman, H. M., and Levine, S. (1968): Intramyelinic and extracellular spaces in triethyltin intoxication. *J. Neuropathol. Exp. Neurol.,* 27:571–580.
11. Kalsbeck, J. E., and Cummings, J. N. (1963): Experimental edema in the rat and cat brain. *J. Neuropathol. Exp. Neurol.,* 22:237–247.
12. Katzman, R., Aleu, F. P., and Wilson, C. (1963): Further observations on triethyltin edema. *Arch. Neurol. (Chic.),* 9:178–187.
13. Kolkman, W., and Ule, G. (1967): Tin poisoning edema. In: *Brain Edema,* edited by I. Klatzo and F. Seitelberger, pp. 530–535. Springer-Verlag, New York.
14. Lee, J. C. (1971): Evolution in the concept of the blood-brain barrier phenomenon. In: *Progress*
15. Lee, J. C., and Bakay, L. (1965): Ultrastructural changes in the edematous central nervous system. I. Triethyltin edema. *Arch. Neurol.,* 13:48–57.
16. Lee, J. C., and Bakay, L. (1967): Electron microscopic studies on experimental brain edema. In: *Brain Edema,* edited by I. Klatzo and F. Seitelberger, pp. 590–597. Springer-Verlag, New York.
17. Lock, E. A. (1976): The action of triethyltin on the respiration of rat brain cortex slices. *J. Neurochem.,* 26:887–892.
18. Lock, E. A., and Aldridge, W. N. (1975): The binding of triethyltin to rat brain myelin. *J. Neurochem.,* 25:871–876.
19. Magee, P. N., Stoner, H. B., and Barnes, J. M. (1957): The experimental production of edema in the central nervous system of the rat by triethyltin compounds. *J. Pathol. Bact.,* 73:102–124.
20. Moore, K. E., and Brody, T. M. (1961): The effect of triethyltin on mitochondrial swelling. *Biochem. Pharmacol.,* 6:134–142.
21. Reed, D. J., Woodbury, D. M., and Holtzer, R. L. (1964): Brain edema, electrolytes and extracellular space. Effect of triethyltin on brain and skeletal muscle. *Arch. Neurol. (Chic.),* 10:604–616.
22. Rose, M. S., and Aldridge, W. N. (1972): Oxidative phosphorylation: The effect of anions on the inhibition of triethyltin of various mitochondrial functions, and the relationship between this inhibition and binding of triethyltin. *Biochem. J.,* 127:51–59.
23. Scheinberg, L. C., Herzog, I., and Taylor, S. M. (1969): Cerebral edema in brain tumors: Ultrastructural and biochemical studies. *Ann. NY Acad. Sci.,* 159:509–532.
24. Scheinberg, L. D., Taylor, J. M., Herzog, I., and Mandell, S. (1966): Optical and peripheral nerve response to triethyltin intoxication in the rabbit: Biochemical and ultrastructural studies. *J. Neuropathol. Exp. Neurol.,* 25:202–213.
25. Siegel, B. A., Studer, R. K., and Potchen, E. J. (1972): Effect of dexamethasone on triethyltin-induced brain edema and the early edema in cerebral ischemia. In: *Steroids and Brain Edema,* edited by H. J. Reulen and K. Schürann, pp. 113–121. Springer-Verlag, New York.
26. Smith, J. F., McLaurin, R. L., Nichols, J. B., and Asbury, A. (1960): Studies in cerebral edema and cerebral swelling. I. The changes in lead encephalopathy in children compared with those in alkyltin poisoning in animals. *Brain,* 83:411–424.
27. Streicher, E. (1962): The thiocyanate space of rat brain in experimental cerebral edema. *J. Neuropathol. Exp. Neurol.,* 21:437–441.
28. Torack, R. M. (1965): The relationship between adenosine triphosphatase activity and triethyltin toxicity in the production of cerebral edema of the rat. *Am. J. Pathol.,* 46:245–262.
29. Torack, R. M., Gordon, J., and Prokop, J. (1970):

Pathobiology of acute triethyltin intoxication. In: *International Review of Neurobiology,* Vol. 12, edited by C. C. Pfeiffer and J. R. Smythes, pp. 45–86. Academic Press, New York.

30. Webster, H. DeF., Ulsamer, A. G., and O'Con-nell, M. F. (1974): Hexachlorophene induced myelin lesions in the developing nervous system of Xenopus Tadpoles: Morphological and biochemical observations. *J. Neuropathol. Exp. Neurol.,* 33:144–163.

Neurotoxicology, edited by L. Roizin, H. Shiraki, and N. Grčević. Raven Press, New York © 1977.

Neuropathology of Subacute Myeloopticoneuro-pathy in Humans with Special Reference to Experimental Whole Body Autoradiographic Studies Using Labeled Quinoform Compounds

H. Shiraki

Department of Neuropathology, Institute of Brain Research, Tokyo University Medical School, Tokyo, Japan

Subacute myeloopticoneuropathy (SMON), which is characterized by subacute onset of the illness and almost systemic combined degeneration of long tracts of the spinal cord with polyneuropathy and optic nerve involvement, has been observed sporadically since late 1950 in Japan as a myelitic illness preceded by abdominal pain or diarrhea prior to the onset of neurological impairments. In 1963, a sharp increase in sporadic cases and some regional and/or hospital-centered outbreaks developed, followed by the sudden disappearance of the disease in 1971 continuing until present.

The authentic neuropathology of SMON was described for the first time by Shiraki and Oda (15) and Matsuyama et al. (7) and was supplemented again by Shiraki (17) and others (11). The tentative conclusion at that time, when the causative agent of the disease was still unknown, was as follows: SMON could belong to a subgroup of endemic diseases that is characterized by degeneration of long tracts of the spinal cord combined with polyneuropathy and is associated with complex nutritional deficiency or toxic interference of tissue metabolism (15).

In the present chapter, the briefly summarized clinicoepidemiology and etiology of SMON as well as its essential neuropathology at different stages at which quinoform (Qf) was medicated without exception (18,20,21), are described and discussed in relation to the time-dependent shift of whole body autoradiographic findings in monkeys and mice using labeled Qf compounds (20).

CLINICOEPIDEMIOLOGY AND ETIOLOGY OF SMON

Clinical Features (Reviewed by Kono, ref. 4)

In SMON initiating acutely or subacutely, as a rule, ascending paresthesia or dysesthesia developed preceded by bouts of abdominal pain and/or diarrhea, which either had been a chronic complaint for months or years or preceded onset of neurological impairments by only days or weeks. Exceptionally, the neurological manifestations occurred without prior abdominal discomforts. Without exception, the initial symptoms and signs consisted of paresthesias and/or dysesthesias in the lower extremities, particularly in their distal portions, and these symptoms distressed patients for many years even after the other impairments subsided;

weakness of the legs was found in 74%, but complete paraplegia was encountered only in 12%, indicating a more benign prognosis for motor disturbances than for sensory impairments. Diminution in visual acuity, predominantly of a central scotoma type, often developed, with total blindness in 3% and blurred vision in 19%. Exacerbations and remissions were often observed, and, thus, there is no doubt that these cases were at first considered to be neuromyelitis optica. Subsequently, it was discovered that the exacerbations of SMON were not infrequently associated with the development of "green tongue."

Green Tongue, Green Urine, and Green Feces (4)

In 1970, Takasu et al. (22) noticed greenish-colored fur on some SMON patients' tongues. In May of the same year, Igata et al. (1) found two patients excreting greenish urine or greenish feces, or both. Subsequently, it was discovered that the green pigment appearing in urine and feces was the *iron (III) chelate of Qf(5-chloro-6-ido-8-hydroxyquinoline)*, and the urine also contained crystals of nonconjugated Qf in a large amount (25). Later, the presence of Qf in the green fur of tongue was confirmed by gas chromatography (2).

Epidemiology of SMON Associated with Medication of Qf (4)

The SMON Research Commission (SRC), which was organized in 1969, conducted a large scale retrospective study to find out how many SMON patients had actually been medicated with Qf 6 months before or any time after the development of neurological impairment. The overall results were as follows: 632 of 742 cases (85.2%) had been medicated with Qf; 110 (14.8%) had not been or it was unclear. In the newspaper on August 7, 1970, Tsubaki presented the Qf hypothesis of SMON onset based on his observation that a common characteristic of SMON was hospital- or doctor-centered outbreak, or both. Judging from his and other similar observations, the SRC strongly urged the Japanese Government to ban the sale of Qf. In September 8, 1970, the Japanese Government made the decision to stop the sale of Qf compounds.

The SRC, on the other hand, took action to collect information on new SMON cases in a prospective orientation. As a result, it was discovered that there were 371 new patients in 1970, whereas from September 8, 1970 to January 31, 1971, the number dropped sharply to only 19. Such a dramatic drop in new monthly cases of SMON could be considered far beyond a natural decrease and was ascribed to the banning of the sale of Qf. From then until the present, i.e., June, 1976, the outbreak of new SMON patients has been almost nil (13,14). Thus far this is the most beautiful epidemiological result, strongly supporting the Qf theory of SMON onset.

Miscellaneous Clinicoepidemiology (4)

From 1967 to the end of February, 1972, SMON patients totaled 9,131 (confirmed cases 5,570, suspected cases 3,361). The prevalence and annual incidence rates of patients were higher in the middle west and/or southern prefectures of Japan, but they were more or less widespread throughout all the territories of Japan. The prevalence and incidence rates of SMON by age and sex were impressive because infants and children were affected extremely rarely, whereas the peaks of both curves occurred at the age of 60 to 69 in either sex, and the rates for females averaged twice as high as those for male. About 50% of SMON patients could return to the family and social life within 1 to 2 years with some sequelae left behind, whereas 10 to 15% were completely unable to take care themselves. SMON occurred often in hospitalized patients with other chronic illnesses, such as malignant neoplasm, chronic hepatitis, tuberculosis, diabetes, etc., as well as with preceding surgical operations to abdominal viscera (Table 1). Deaths were, as a rule, ascribed to different complications such as decubiti, cystitis, or other intercurrent infections, but it is also true that SMON *per se* could cause death, particularly at the acute and subacute stage.

Summary

From the epidemioclinicoetiological viewpoints mentioned above, it, therefore, can be concluded that there is overwhelming evidence implicating the significant role of Qf medication in the outbreak of SMON in a great majority of SMON patients. In addition, this conclusion is strongly supported by findings that experimental neuropathology, particularly in mongrel and beagle dogs and cats medicated with Qf either by the increasing-daily-dose method or the fixed-dose method, almost exactly reconstructed the neuropathology of human SMON, in both main characteristics and topography of foci (23,24).

NEUROPATHOLOGY OF SMON IN HUMANS AND TIME-DEPENDENT AUTORADIOGRAMS IN ANIMALS

The essential clinical features and medication of Qf in the SMON cases presented here are summarized in Table 1. Actually, the total number of autopsy cases listed in different laboratories in Japan up to 1976 was approximately 150.

Dorsal Root Ganglia

Ganglia cells were severely disrupted by vacuoles at the acute stage (Fig. 15A, Case 2), whereas at the next stage, nerve cell disintegration with advanced neurono-

phagia became predominant (Fig. 15B, C, and E, Case 8), and the tangle formation of a glomerular appearance with different-calibered axons prevailed at places of disintegrated and/or degenerated ganglion cells, suggesting a regenerating process of axons (Fig. 15D). In addition, the disintegration of nerve fibers in each nerve fiber bundle became clear-cut (Fig. 15C). It is emphasized that the deterioration of these ganglia was far more severe at the thoracolumbosacral level than at the cervical (Fig. 15B and C); this corresponds well with clinical features in which sensory impairments are dominant in the lower body half of SMON patients.

The radioactivity of root ganglia in monkeys even 5 min after intravenous injection of ^{14}C-Qf (20 mg Qf/kg/40 μCi) disclosed a greater accumulation of Qf at the lumbosacral level than at the cervical (Fig. 4A and B), and this became more accentuated 20 min later (Fig. 4C–E). Thus far these findings in quantity and in topographical difference of Qf show one of the reasons why root ganglia at the lumbosacral level are preferentially involved in humans.

Spinal Nerve Rootlets and Pre- and Postganglionic Tracts

Alterations of spinal nerve rootlets, which consisted of more severely disrupted axons rather than deteriorated myelin sheaths predominantly at the acute stage (Fig. 10A–C, Cases 1 and 2), were pronounced particularly in the posterior at the sacrolumbothoracic level, less conspicuous in the anterior, and most predominant in the cauda equina through all stages (Fig. 10A–D, Cases 1, 2, and 6).

Even 5 min after the intravenous injection of ^{131}I-Qf in the monkey (10 mg Qf/kg/66.5 μCi) as well as 20 min after that of ^{14}C-Qf, both lumbosacral spinal nerve rootlets and cauda equina disclosed a higher radioactivity and exceeded that of

TABLE 1. *Summary of clinical features and Q f administration in SMON*

Case number Age (years) Sex	Previous illness (Surgical operation)	Total duration of illness (A, B, and C)	Main clinical features and Qf administration (→ Shift)
Acute stage			
1 70 M	Diabetes mellitus, hypertension, arteriosclerosis (Gastric carcinoma)	A: 25 days B: 13 days C: 12 days	Epigastric pain, diarrhea → *Qf, 42 g for 14 days* → impaired vision, paraplegia → paralysis of upper limbs → total blindness → hypesthesia & dysesthesia below L_1 → shock-like syndrome → tetraplegia → semicomatose → bulbar paresis
2 76 F	Hypertension, pyelitis (Polyposis of colon, postoperative peritonitis & pancytopenia)	A: 30 days B: 12 days C: 18 days	Abdominal pain, diarrhea → *Qf, 37.5 g for 25 days* → blurred vision → weakness of lower limbs → hypesthesia of lower limbs → somnolent, weakness of upper limbs ? → intestinal bleeding, broncheal atelectasis
Subacute stage			
3 42 M	Hypertension, anemia, nephritis (Peritoneal dialysis for 1 month)	A: 3 months B: 5 days C: 55 days	Diarrhea → *Q f, 10.5 g for 7 days* → *Qf, 24.5 g for 23 days* → "shivering" feeling of lower legs → ascended to lumbar region, abdomen, & upper limbs → oliguria → *Qf, 27.5 g for 11 days* → pain sensation, paralysis, impaired vision → bleeding → uremia
4 26 F	None (None)	A: 3 months & 2 weeks B: 10 days C: 56 days	Abdominal pain → *Qf, 108.5 g for 58 days* → inability to walk & stand, hypesthesia & paresthesia of lower limbs → tetraplegia → blurred vision → paresthesia below umbelicus → blindness → dysphagia, dysarthria → respiratory paralysis
5 46 F	Nephritis, pyelitis, hepatitis, herniation, & ileus (Elongated sigma & operated)	A: 4 months & 10 days B: 22 days C: 125 days	Abdominal pain → *Qf, 76.5 g for 51 days* → shivering feeling below lower abdomen, weakness of lower limbs → impaired sensations to mamillary line → shivering feeling & weakness of fingers → "green tongue," hypesthesia of upper limbs, paraplegia, dysarthria → *Qf, 58 g for 29 days* → *pronounced amnesia* → impaired vision → meteorism, dysphagia → stuporous → coma, anuria, ascites
Chronic stage			
6 81 F	Hypertension, venous thrombus (None)	A: ? (No description of abdominal discomfort) B: 8 months & 15 days C: 2 years & 3 months	*Qf, 514 g for 275 days* → epigastric distress, weakness of lower limbs, pathological reflexes → *Qf, 156 g for 78 days* → weakness of lower limbs → weakness of upper limbs, slurred speech, paralytic ileus → dyspnea → tracheotomy → broncheal atelectasis due to spontaneous removement of tracheal canule

TABLE 1. (*continued*)

Case number Age (years) Sex	Previous illness (Surgical operation)	Total duration of illness (A, B, and C)	Main clinical features and Qf administration (→ Shift)
7 37 F	Schizophrenia treated with neuroleptics, nephritis (Mesenterium cyst of intestine)	A: 2 years & 9 months B: Over 8 days C: 2 years & 8 months	Diarrhea → *Qf, 45 g for 15 days* → shivering feeling of lower limbs → impaired gait → *Qf, 123 g for 41 days* → impaired vision → inability to walk, weakness of upper limbs, shivering feeling of finger tips → pathological reflexes, hypesthesia, & dysesthesia below C_4, optic atrophy → capable of walking with great difficulty → uremia
8 40 F	Heavy drinker, unbalanced diet (Gastrectomy to duodenal ulcer, reoperated to adhesion)	A: 6 years & 6 months B: ? (Unknown history of Qf administration before admission) C: 3 years & 6 months	Watery diarrhea → *possible administration of Qf* → reoperated → hypesthesia, pain, & dysesthesia of legs → 5x admissions; hypesthesia, dysesthesia, & weakness of legs, persistent diarrhea, anemia, edema, hepatic impairments, occasional fits of impaired consciousness, & abnormal behavior; *Qf, 222.5 g for 11 months* → *green tongue, urine, & stool* → clouded consciousness → oliguria, petechiae

*A, From onset of abdominal pain and/or diarrhea to death; B, from administration of Qf to onset of neurological impairments; C, From onset of neurological impairments to death.

the spinal cord parenchyma (Figs. 1A and B and 4F). It also is noted that demyelination and resulting collagenosis were, as a rule, more pronounced in the preganglionic tract than in the postganglionic, particularly at the cervical cord level (Fig. 12C and D, Case 6). Actually, the 20-min autoradiogram disclosed higher activity in the preganglionic tract at the cervical level, whereas the activity of the ganglion itself remained exceedingly low (Fig. 4C).

Extravertebral Peripheral Nerves and Vagus Nerve Rootlets

Foci of peripheral nerves were discontinuous and/or focal, and their severity differed in each nerve fiber and bundle (Fig. 11A, Case 6). The neurogenic muscular atrophy of lower limbs developed focally even at the acute stage. In an interpretation of clinical features in which impaired sensations of SMON patients, as a rule, began at the most distal part of lower limbs and then ascended to the umbilical level, the following 20-min autoradiogram in the dog after intravenous injection of ^{14}C-Qf (20 mg Qf/kg/40 μCi) could be significant: the activity of crosscut extravertebral peripheral nerves at the coccygeal cord level was higher and more symmetrically bilateral in the distal portion than in the proximal (Fig. 3A and B). Such a clear-cut difference of the radioactivity in each nerve, however, was not identified in the monkey (Fig. 4E).

Intravenously injected ^{14}C-Qf (30 mg Qf/kg/60 μCi) in mice migrated very rapidly into the central nervous system, (CNS), i.e., 30 sec (Fig. 2A), but was excreted from there very quickly and still remained in the trigeminal nerve root and brainstem 7 min later (Fig. 2B). The radioactivity of peripheral nerves of the lower body, on the other hand, became ac-

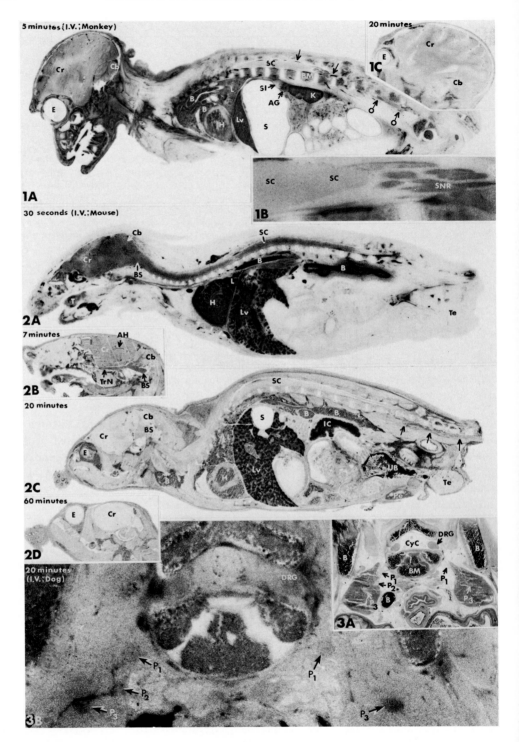

centuated 20 min later (Fig. 2C), and the activity of the CNS became almost negative 1 hr later (Fig. 2D).

Among alterations of the vegetative nervous system, in which similar but mild changes to those of the dorsal root ganglia and tracts were encountered in the sympathetic and parasympathetic ganglia and tracts but were assumed to be of an abnormal range, it is emphasized that the vagus nerve rootlets at the level of medulla oblongata were involved in a majority of cases, particularly from the acute to the subacute stage (Fig. 11B), and, thus, comprise one of the causes of SMON death at these stages. In a 5-min autoradiogram of the monkey, it is noted that the vagus nerve rootlets developed a higher activity (Fig. 7C). However, although an even higher activity was observed in dorsal vagus nuclei (Fig. 7C), disintegration of nerve cells never occurred in human SMON, indicating a different susceptibility of each cellular element for Qf.

Spinal Cord

Changes of the spinal cord at the acute stage that consisted of more severely disrupted axons rather than deteriorated myelin sheaths as seen in peripheral nerves (Figs. 12A and B, Cases 3 and 4) were bilaterally widespread in almost the entire area of the posterior tract at the lumbar level, gradually shifting to Goll's tract of the thoracic cord (Fig. 12A), and were most pronounced and restricted to Goll's tract of the upper cervical cord. In long-standing cases, the demyelination, gliosis, and mobilization of fat granule cells became more clear-cut (Fig. 12C–F, Case 6). Involvements of both the lateral and/or anterior corticospinal tract similar to those of the posterior tract, on the other hand, were consistently found but milder than those of the posterior tract. They, as a rule, began to be pronounced from the middle thoracic cord and became more distinct at the lumbar level (Fig. 12C–F). In all cases, nerve cells of the entire gray matter at all cord levels were only minimally involved, whereas cytoplasmic axonal alteration of nerve cells as well as spheroid bodies were frequently encountered, particularly in the anterior horn of the lumbosacral cord (Fig. 13A and B, Cases 2 and 3).

In short, the foci of two long tracts of

←——————

Fig. 1. Time-dependent autoradiograms of monkeys after intravenous injection (i.v.) of ^{131}I-Qf (10 mg Qf/kg/66.5 μCi). **A:** Five minutes. Moderate radioactivity of the ischiadic nerve (*arrows with zeros*). ×0.56. **B:** Magnified area indicated by *arrows* in **A**. ×3.3. **C:** Twenty minutes. ×0.67. *Abbreviations:* AG, adrenal gland; AH, Ammon's horn; Am, amygdaloid nucleus; B, blood corpuscle; BM, bone marrow; BP, brachial plexus; BS, brain stem; Cb, cerebellum; CbC, cerebellar cortex; CbW, cerebellar white matter; CC, corpus callosum; CE, cauda equina; Ch, choroid; CN, caudate nucleus, CP, choroid plexus; Cr, cerebrum; CyC, coccygeal cord; DG, dentate gyrus; Di, disc; DRG, dorsal root ganglion; DVN, dorsal vagus nucleus; E, eyeball; F, fat tissue; GP, globus pallidus; H, heart; H_1, H_2 & H_3, each region of Sommer's sector of Ammon's horn; Hy, hypophysis; IC, intestinal content; K, kidney; L, lung; LC, lumbar cord; LGB, lateral geniculate body; Lv, liver; MCC, middle cervical cord; MO, medulla oblongata; Oe, oesophagus; OM, ocular muscle; ON, optic nerve; Ov, olivary nucleus; P_1, proximal peripheral nerve; P_2, distal peripheral nerve; P_3, more distal peripheral nerve than P_2; PB, pontine basis; Pc, pancreas; Pe, penis; PF, prefrontal lobe; Po, pons; PoT, postganglionic tract; PrT, preganglionic tract; PT, posterior tract; Pt, putamen; R, retina; RC, renal cortex; Sb, subiculum; SC, spinal cord; SG, sympathetic ganglion; Sl, spleen; SN, substantia nigra; SNR, spinal nerve root; T, tongue; Te, testis; Th, thalamus; Tr, trachea; TrN, trigeminal nerve root; UB, urinary bladder; Un, uncus; USC, upper sacral cord; VNR, vagus nerve root.
FIG. 2. Time-dependent autoradiograms of mice after i.v. of ^{14}C-Qf (30 mg Qf/kg/60 μCi). **A:** Thirty seconds. ×1.8. **B:** Seven minutes. ×1.8. **C:** Twenty minutes. Intense radioactivity of the peripheral nerves of lower body (*arrows*). ×1.8. **D:** 60 minutes. ×1.8. For abbreviations, see Fig. 1.
FIG. 3. Autoradiogram of dog 20 min after i.v. of ^{14}C-Qf (20 mg Qf/kg/40 μCi) in crosscut section. **A:** Frozen-dried section of the coccygeal cord and adjacent areas. ×1.5. **B:** Magnified autoradiogram corresponding to **A**. ×4.0. For abbreviations, see Fig. 1.

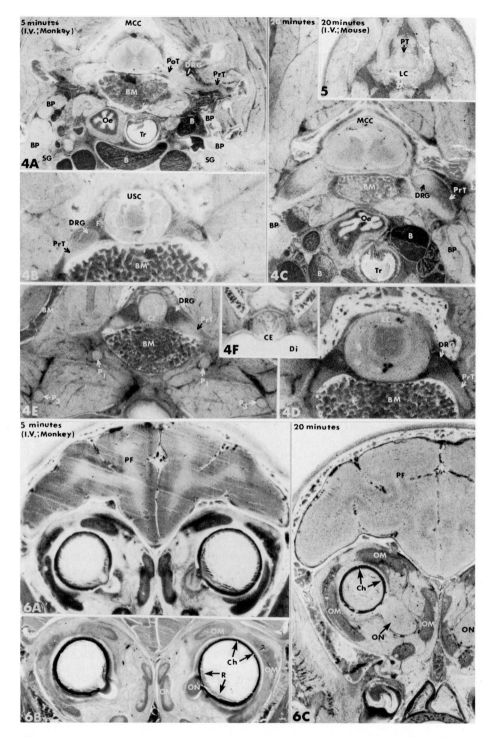

FIG. 4. Time-dependent autoradiograms of monkeys after i.v. of ^{14}C-Qf (20 mg Qf/kg/40 μCi) in crosscut sections. **A:** Five minutes. Middle cervical cord level. ×2.0. **B:** Five minutes. Upper sacral cord level. ×4.1. **C:** Twenty minutes. Middle cervical cord level. ×3.0. **D:** Twenty minutes. Lumbar cord level. ×4.0. **E:** Twenty minutes. Cauda equina level. ×2.8. **F:** Twenty minutes. More caudal part of cauda equina level than **E.** ×2.5. For abbreviations, see Fig. 1.

FIG. 5. Autoradiogram of lumbar cord and adjacent areas of mouse 20 min after i.v. of ^{14}C-Qf (30 mg Qf/kg/60 μCi) in crosscut section. ×3.0. For abbreviations, see Fig. 1.

FIG. 6. Time-dependent autoradiograms of brain and adjacent areas of monkeys after i.v. of ^{14}C-Qf (20 mg Qf/ kg/40 μCi) in crosscut sections. **A:** Five minutes. Eyeballs and prefrontal lobes. ×2.2. **B:** Frozen-dried section corresponding to **A.** ×2.2. **C:** Twenty minutes. ×2.5. For abbreviations, see Fig. 1.

the spinal cord, i.e., sensory and motor pathways corresponding to an innervation of lower part of the body, were continuously and symmetrically bilateral in all cases, resulting in systemic degenerative features, particularly in distal portions of these long tracts. The short tract of the spinal cord, corresponding to an innervation of the upper part of the body, on the other hand, was absent or less frequently and less severely affected.

Autoradiograms in monkeys and dogs, however, never disclosed a positive relationship between the severity of foci in humans and a time-dependent shift of a regionally greater accumulation of Qf as seen in the dorsal root ganglia and peripheral nerves. Both 5- and 20-min autoradiograms showed a high activity in the spinal gray matter rather than in its white matter, whereas a greater accumulation of Qf either in the posterior or in Goll's tract never occurred (Figs. 3B and 4A–D). In mice, on the other hand, the 5-min radioactivity of spinal gray matter began to decrease 20 min later, whereas that of the spinal white matter, in which the activity of the posterior tract was slightly predominant, increased 20 min later (Fig. 5).

Optic Nerve and Retina

According to clinical symptomatology, optic nerves were not infrequently disintegrated. Confluent, widespread demyelination occurred in almost the entire length and/or circumscribed areas of bilateral optic nerves, chiasm, and tracts (Fig. 16A and D, Case 7). In addition, the distal most part of the optic tract closely adjacent to the lateral geniculate body, the nerve cells of which were well preserved, was most severely disintegrated, again suggesting a preferential involvement of the distal portion of optic nerves (Fig. 16E). Ganglion cells of the inner ganglion cell layer of the retina, particularly in the papillomacular region, were selectively disintegrated, indicating a positive relationship between impaired visual acuity of a central scotoma's type and the characteristic topography of foci (Fig. 16B and C). In chronic cases (Case 7), disintegration of the optic nerve was predominant in the ventral part of its proximal portion, while gradually shifting to the central part of its more distal portion, suggesting preferential involvement of papillomacular nerve fibers, presumably of a secondary degenerative nature originating from severely disintegrated retinal ganglion cells of the papillomacular region (Fig. 16A).

The 5-min autoradiogram indicated clearly a high activity in the retina and a slight to moderate one in the optic nerves, whereas the retinal activity conspicuously decreased 20 min later (Fig. 6A–C). It also is noted that the highest activity was observed in the choroid of both autoradiograms (Fig. 6A–C). However, although there was almost the same amount of Qf in all regions and layers of retina, the papillomacular region and inner ganglion cells were almost preferentially involved in human SMON. In addition, there were no remarkable changes of the choroid in humans even when its radioactivity remained highest. Consequently, it can be assumed that a greater accumulation of Qf in both retina and choroid is one of the necessary conditions for the development of retinal deterioration but never a satisfactory condition. However, the 20-min autoradiogram, in which the activity of the central portion of the optic tract was greater than its marginal area (Fig. 7D), could correspond with the human neuropathology of SMON in which a cystic cavity formation occurred in its central part but its marginal area was spared (Fig. 16D).

Olivary Nucleus, Cerebellum, and Brainstem

Multiple, coalescent, conspicuous vacuoles occasionally occurred in cytoplasms of nerve cells of the olivary nucleus

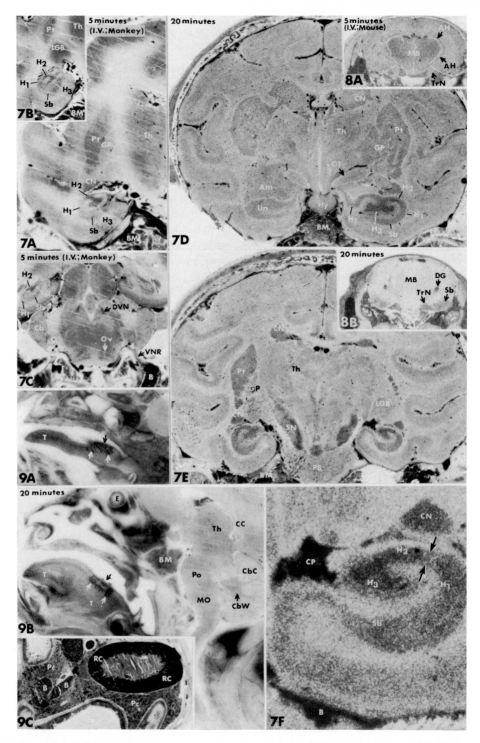

FIG. 7. Time-dependent autoradiograms of brain and adjacent areas of monkeys after i.v. of ^{14}C-Qf (20 mg Qf/kg/40 μCi) in crosscut sections. A: Five minutes. Striatum and hippocampus. ×2.0. B: Five minutes. Lateral geniculate body and hippocampus. ×1.9. C: Five minutes. Medulla oblongata and hippocampus. ×1.8. D: Twenty minutes. Through the amygdaloid nucleus. ×2.5. E: Twenty minutes. Through the substantia nigra. ×2.0. F: Magnified hippocampus in E. Arrows indicate the border area of H_2 to H_1. ×8.0. For abbreviations, see Fig. 1.

FIG. 8. Time-dependent autoradiograms of brain and adjacent areas of mice after i.v. of ^{14}C-Qf (30 mg Qf/kg/60 μCi) in crosscut sections. A: Five minutes. ×3.0. B: Twenty minutes. ×3.0. For abbreviations, see Fig. 1.

FIG 9. A & B: Time-dependent autoradiograms of tongue and adjacent areas of monkeys after i.v. of ^{131}I-Qf (10 mg Qf/kg/66.5 μCi) in sagittal-cut sections. A: Five minutes. ×1.2. B: Twenty minutes. ×1.2. C: Autoradiogram of kidney and pancreas of monkey 5 min after i.v. of ^{14}C-Qf (20 mg Qf/kg/40 μCi) in crosscut section. ×1.6. For abbreviations, see Fig. 1.

from the acute to the subacute stage, and a severe disintegration of nerve cells and intense gliosis finally developed (Fig. 17A and B, Cases 4 and 6). In these cases, a torpedo formation of the Purkinje cells was firmly combined with (Fig. 18, Case 4). The intracytoplasmic axonal alteration of large-typed pyramidal cells was occasionally disseminated in the tegmentum from the medulla to the pons as seen in the spinal cord anterior horn (Fig. 14, Case 6).

Ammon's Horn, Cerebral and Cerebellar White Matter, Globus Pallidus, and Substantia Nigra

SMON comprises essentially a neurological disorder. The following exceptional case with severe amnesia, however, is worth referring to in relation to time-dependent autoradiographic findings (ref. 20, Case 5). SMON with green tongue developed in a 46-year-old female. One month prior to death, she experienced a pronounced amnesia that persisted until death. Convulsive seizures, however, were never observed during the total clinical course. The postmortem examination indicated clearly the neuropathology of typical and most severe SMON as well as bilateral, severe, and advanced deterioration of Sommer's sector of Ammon's horn, i.e., most severe in the H_1 and subiculum (Fig. 19B), severe in the H_3, and moderate in the H_2 (Fig. 19A). Kaeser and Scollo-Lavizzari (3) have reported several clinical cases of SMON with retrograde anmesia of either reversible or irreversible character. For example, a 24-year-old male was suffering from diarrhea and following the medication of 30 tablets of iodochlorhydroxquin (Entero-vioform®), he became incoherent, semicomatose, and developed hallucinations that were succeeded by retrograde anmesia and a transient abnormal electroencephalogram (EEG). Therefore, the amnesia based on the bilateral Ammon's horn involvement in the present Japanese SMON case was not coincidental.

In 5-min autoradiograms in the monkey, the cerebral cortices and subcortical gray matter developed a higher activity, whereas only minimal activity was seen in the white matter, except for the occipital and cerebellar white matter (Figs. 1A, 6A, and 7A). Among cerebral cortices, the Sommer's sector of Ammon's horn disclosed a higher activity than that of the adjacent hippocampal cortex (Fig. 7A–C). This selective high activity of Ammon's horn became more accentuated in the 20-min autoradiogram, even when the activity of other cerebral cortices conspicuously decrease and that of the white matter increased (Figs. 1C and 7D, and E). It was the same in the time-dependent autoradiograms in mice (Fig. 8A and B). Among the medullary radioactivity, those of both occipital and cerebellum still disclosed a high activity (Fig. 9B). Actually, a moderate astrocytosis was not infrequently visualized in the white matter of both regions of human SMON.

A careful observation of the radioactivity of Ammon's horn in the 20-min autoradiogram demonstrated the highest activity in the H_3 and H_2 area that was succeeded by an activity not as high in the H_1 and subiculum (Figs. 7E and F). This characteristic distribution of different radioactivity in each area may correspond with the different amounts of zinc in these same regions demonstrated histochemically in the following findings: (a) particularly in the subcortical white matter of these regions in the guinea pig, i.e., most intense in the end plate, H_3 and H_2 area, and minimal or absent in the H_1 and subiculum (Fig. 20A and B); (b) particularly in cortices of the same regions in the cat, i.e., intense in the H_3 and H_2 area and slight to moderate in the H_1 and subiculum (Fig. 20C); and (c) in both animals, zinc-positive tiny granules are visible around nerve

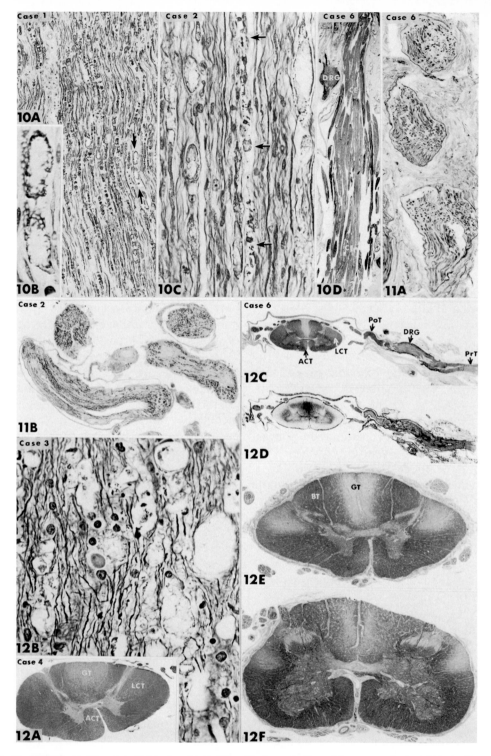

FIG. 10. SMON. **A:** Case 1 in Table 1. ×84. **B:** Magnified area indicated by arrows in **A.** ×513. **C:** Case 2 in Table 1. Fragmented single axon (*arrows*). ×440. **D:** Case 6 in Table 1. Cauda equina. ×2.5. (**A, B, & D;** Luxol fast blue with cresylviolet. **C,** Bodian.) ACT, anterior corticospinal tract; BT, Burdach's tract; CE, cauda equina; Ch, choroid; DRG, dorsal root ganglion; FD, fascia dentata; GT, Goll's tract; H_I, H_2 & H_3, each region of Sommer's sector of Ammon's horn; HK, hyperkeratosis; LCT, lateral corticospinal tract; LGB, lateral geniculate body; OT, optic tract; Pa, papilla; PoT, postganglionic tract; PrT, preganglionic tract; R, retina; RN, renal cortex; SN, substantia nigra; TC, tuber cinereum.

FIG. 11. SMON. **A:** Case 6 in Table 1. Sciatic nerve. ×87. **B:** Case 2 in Table 1. Vagus nerve rootlets at the level of medulla oblongata. ×96. (**A & B,** Luxol fast blue with cresylviolet.) For abbreviations, see Fig. 10.

FIG. 12. SMON. **A:** Case 4 in Table 1. Third thoracic cord. ×5.8. **B:** Case 3 in Table 1. Magnified longitudinal-cut lateral corticospinal tract of the lower thoracic cord. ×460. **C:** Case 6 in Table 1. Seventh cervical cord. **D:** Same section as in **C. E:** Tenth thoracic cord. **F:** Second lumbar cord. (**A, C, E, & F;** Luxol fast blue with cresylviolet. **B,** Bodian. **D,** Holzer.) For abbreviations, see Fig. 10.

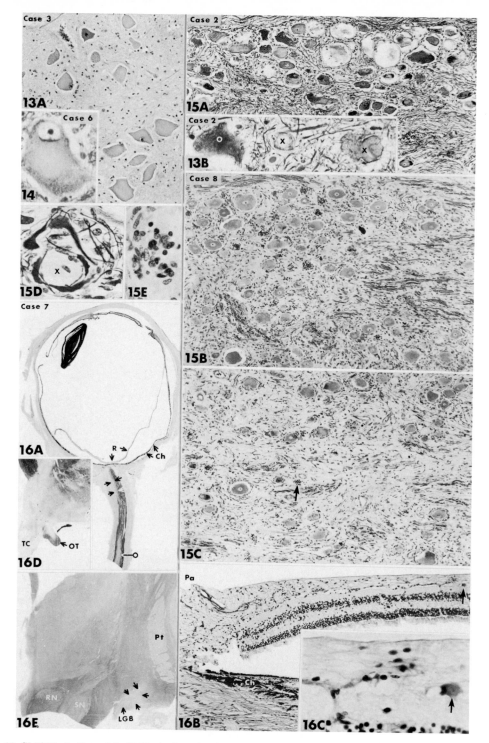

FIG. 13. SMON. **A:** Case 3 in Table 1. Anterior horn of the sacral cord. H. & E. ×100. **B:** Case 2 in Table 1. Anterior horn of the fifth lumbar cord. Two spheroid bodies (*crosses*) and nerve cell (*zero*). Bodian. ×460.
FIG. 14. SMON. Case 6 in Table 1. Large pyramidal cell in the tegmentum of medulla oblongata. Luxol fast blue with cresylviolet. ×476.
FIG. 15. SMON. **A:** Case 2 in Table 1. Cauda equina level. ×105. **B:** Case 8 in Table 1. Dorsal root ganglion. Cervical level. ×96. **C:** Lumbar level. ×96. **D:** Magnified disintegrated ganglion cell (*cross*) in **C.** ×476. **E:** Magnified neuronophagic ganglion cell (*arrow in* **C**). ×476. (**A & D,** Bodian. **B,C,** & **E;** Luxol fast blue with cresylviolet.)
FIG. 16. SMON. Case 7 in Table 1. Ocular bulb and optic nerve. **A:** Restricted demyelination (*arrows*) and central one (*arrow and zero*) of the optic nerve. ×2.3. **B:** Retina adjacent to the papilla (*R with arrows in* **A**). Remaining single nerve cell (*arrow*). **C:** Magnified degenerated nerve cell (*arrow*) in **B.** ×440. **D:** Optic tract at the level of tuber cinereum. ×2.0. **E:** Optic tract (*arrows*) adjacent to the lateral geniculate body. ×1.5. (**A,** Woelcke myelin. **B–E,** Luxol fast blue with cresylviolet.) For abbreviations, see Fig. 10.

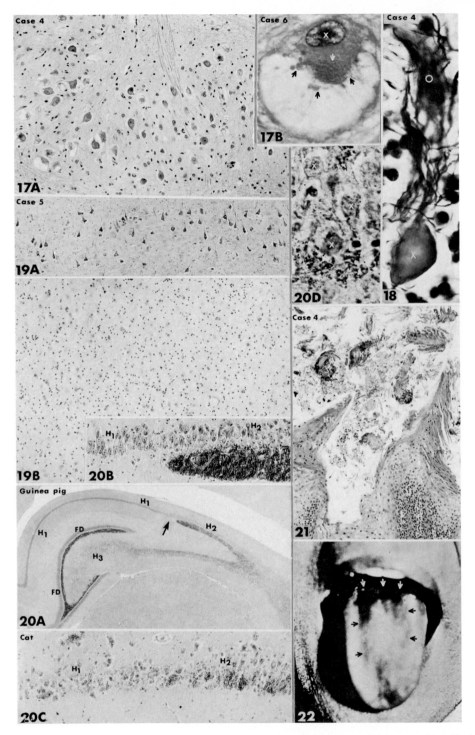

FIG. 17. SMON. A: Case 4 in Table 1. Olivary nucleus. H. & E. ×120. B: Case 6 in Table 1. Magnified nerve cell of the olivary nucleus. Eccentric nucleus (*cross*) and aggregated small eosinphilic granules (*arrows*). H. & E. ×950.

FIG. 18. SMON. Case 4 in Table 1. Purkinje cell layer. Degenerated Purkinje cell (*zero*) and torpedo (*cross*). Bodian. ×570.

FIG. 19. SMON. Case 5 in Table 1. Sommer's sector of the Ammon's horn. A: H_2 area. Luxol fast blue with cresylviolet. ×89. B: H_1 area. H. & E. ×86.

FIG. 20. Histochemistry of zinc of Ammon's horn. A: Guinea pig. ×11.0. B: Magnified area indicated by arrow in A. ×25.0. C: Cat. ×25.0. D: Magnified area in C. Crosses indicate the nuclei of nerve cells. ×890. (A–D, Timm's method.) For abbreviations, see Fig. 10.

FIG. 21. SMON. Case 4 in Table 1. Superficial layer of the tongue. H. & E. ×83. For abbreviations, see Fig. 10.

FIG. 22. Green tongue of a SMON patient indicated by arrows.

cells and their dendrites but not present within their cytoplasms and dendrites (Fig. 20D).

In this regard, it may be assumed that the severe deterioration of Ammon's horn in the present example can be associated with a greater accumulation of Qf and a different amount of zinc in the same regions, although a certain discrepancy existed between the two. If it is true that diabetes of aloxantine type occasionally seen in human SMON and in experimental animals induced by Qf medication (8,9) could be ascribed to an inactivation of insulin derived by a chelation of Qf to zinc of insulin, a possibility may exist that zinc of Ammon's horn could be chelated with Qf. Actually, the 5-min autoradiogram disclosed a greater accumulation of the labeled Qf in the pancreas (Fig. 9C). In this regard, it also is emphasized that the highest concentration of zinc, the significance of which is as yet unknown, is in the choroid of the eye in a wide range of animal species (12), and, thus, it seems that this corresponds well with the highest radioactivity in the choroid (Fig. 6A–C).

Twenty-minute autoradiograms in monkeys disclosed also a higher radioactivity of the striatum, globus pallidus, and substantia nigra compatible with the activity of Ammon's horn (Fig. 7D and E). Actually, a slight-to-moderate astrocytosis with well-preserved nerve cells was frequently found in both globus pallidus and substantia nigra in humans. In this regard, it is important that the greenish pigments appearing in the urine, feces, and tongue of SMON patients comprised the iron (III) chelate of Qf, which was absorbed from the gastrointestinal tract. Thus, it may be assumed that a higher radioactivity of these nuclei can be closely associated with a higher content of iron III in these extrapyramidal motor nuclei.

However, the following questions still remain open: Why are the nerve cells of these nuclei highly resistent? Why is the Ammon's horn of SMON patients only exceptionally involved?

Green Tongue

Greenish fur occurred preferentially in the dorsocaudal portion of the tongue of SMON patients (Fig. 22), whereas it comprised histopathologically the conspicuous hyperkeratosis of superficial epithelial layers accompanied by thick coating masses (Fig. 21). Both the 5 and 20-min autoradiograms in monkeys after intravenous injection of ^{131}I-Qf disclosed precisely a greater radioactivity particularly in the circumscribed area of the dorsocaudal portion of the monkey's tongue (Fig. 9A and B). It, therefore, can be emphasized that this selective topography of high radioactivity in monkeys' tongues corresponds well with the preferential occurrence of greenish fur in the same lingual region of SMON patients (Fig. 22).

DIFFERENTIAL DIAGNOSIS, ETIOLOGY, AND PATHOGENESIS IN SMON AND SMON-LIKE DISORDERS

Certain neurotoxic and/or neurotropic agents, such as alkylmercury or alkylphosphate compounds, percamin S (local anesthetic of quinoline derivative), isoniazid, ethambutol (D-2,2′-(ethylenediimino)-di-l-butanol), chloramphenicol, etc., are compatible with Qf derivatives, since all of them could cause distribution patterns of foci similar to those of SMON. As far as the author's experiences are concerned, three agents—percamin S (16), ethambutol (5,18), and chloramphenicol (6)—are particularly noticeable. The differential diagnosis of these from SMON, however, is noteworthy because of the clearcut identification of different etiological agents in each.

Although an excess and maltreatment of Qf in quantity, time, and space comprises the most important etiological role for the SMON onset, the pathogenesis of SMON has not yet been clarified. In this regard, the following disorders, which also can cause SMON-like lesions, are worthwhile referring to. They are (a) simulating pellagra neuroradiculomyeloencephalopathy in a schizophrenic patient treated with phenothiazine derivatives for a long period of time, suggesting a pathogenesis attributable to a deficiency of pyridoxine (20,21), (b) subacute combined degeneration of the spinal cord related to pernicious anemia, considered to be deficiency disease dealing with vitamin B_{12} (20,21), (c) systemic lupus erythematous combined with myeloradiculoneuropathy presumably of collagen disease or autoimmune abnormality (20,21), and (d) different types of hepatocerebral disease, such as Wilson pseudosclerosis, Inose type and pseudoulegyric type, occasionally combined with myeloradiculoneuropathy in which certain metabolic errors, such as copper, aminoacids, and/or carbohydrate, are responsible for the occurrence of these foci (10). There, however, is no doubt that these SMON-like disorders can be precisely differentiated from SMON by considering their different clinicobiochemical and neuropathological peculiarities. It, however, is not to be overlooked that a comparative study of these with SMON can contribute a great deal to an understanding of the pathogenesis of SMON.

ACCELERATING AND/OR MODIFYING FACTORS IN THE SMON ONSET

A great majority of scientists who strongly support the Qf theory for SMON onset consider simultaneously the possibility that there may be a combination of other factors aside from Qf, and the following factors could be speculated on: (a) since a great majority of SMON patients were suffering from various preceding abdominal illnesses and often disclosed preceding surgical operations to abdominal viscera (Table 1), a malabsorption of Qf from impaired gastrointestinal tracts could cause an elevated blood concentration of Qf; (b) when the detoxicating functions of liver have been impaired due to preceding hepatic failures and/or there has existed mechanically retarded enterohepatic circulation, Qf of nonconjugated form could be elevated in the blood; (c) since preceding renal failures were found in a majority of SMON patients, an excreting process of Qf from the kidney could be retarded; and (d) a possibility exists that preceding neuropathical impairments due to isoniazid or other agents predisposed to or amplified the SMON onset. For example, a 37-year-old male suffered from pulmonary tuberculosis for 10 years and was treated with various chemotherapies including isoniazid; neurological impairments, such as paresthesia of feet and impaired gait, occurred prior to the medication of Qf. Two months after the medication of Qf for 53 days, he experienced the typical SMON syndrome and, postmortem, the typical neuropathology of SMON was identified (19); it, however, is true that the general pathology of SMON could not answer precisely for an interaction of these factors.

Considering the results of whole body autoradiographic findings mentioned above, two possibilities from the side of the nervous system could seriously be considered, i.e., easy migration of Qf into the nervous system and retarded excretion of Qf from the nervous system. In this regard, the accessory features of neuropathology of SMON, such as presenile or senile pathological changes and advanced aging processes of the nervous system, may have a certain significance in an understanding of these possibilities from the side of the host nervous system (15,17). The details of this view, however, still remain open.

CONCLUSION

From biochemical studies, the chelation of Qf to iron III now has been established, whereas the whole body autoradiographic findings could support this data indirectly. In addition, a possibility that Qf could comprise a chelating agent to zinc is suggested from the autoradiograms in certain mammalians. In this regard, whether Qf can be chelated to cobalt or not is not known, because the neuropathology of SMON closely resembles that of subacute combined degeneration of the spinal cord dealing with vitamin B_{12} deficiency.

Since a few clinical cases of SMON have been reported sporadically in other countries of the world, SMON is not restricted to one ethnic group. Two questions, whether the Japanese possess a genetic predisposition to Qf or whether a maltreatment of Qf in quantity, time, and space in the Japanese is most responsible for the SMON onset, can arise. Prior to answering to these questions, it, however, is emphasized that a comprehensive worldwide clinicoepidemiological survey of SMON is necessary.

ACKNOWLEDGMENTS

The author gratefully acknowledges the generous cooperation of the following doctors: T. Mochizuki, Department of Pathology, Toranomon Hospital, Tokyo; S. Yoshiue, Ohme City Hospital, Ohme; H. Abe, Department of Pathology, Kohnodai National Hospital, Chiba; I. Sobue, Department of Medicine, Nagoya University Medical School, Nagoya; Y. Toyokura, Department of Neurology, Institute of Brain Research, Tokyo University Medical School, Tokyo; N. Otsuka, Department of Anatomy, Okayama University Medical School, Okayama.

REFERENCES

1. Igata, A., Hasegawa, S., and Tsuji, Y. (1970): On the green pigment found in SMON patients. Two cases excreting greenish urine. *Jpn. Med. J.* 2427:25-28.

2. Imanari, T., and Tamura, Z. (1970): Detection of chinoform from green fur of the tongue of SMON patients. *Igaku no Ayumi,* 75:547-548.

3. Kaeser, H. E., and Scollo-Lavizzari, G. (1970): Akute zerebrale Störungen nach hohen Dosen eines Oxychinolinderivates. *Dtch. Med. Wochenschr.,* 95:394-397.

4. Kono, R. (1971): Subacute myelo-optico-neuropathy, a new neurological disease prevailing in Japan. *Jpn. Med. Sci. Biol.,* 24:195-216.

5. Kuribayashi, N., Utsumi, K., Oda, M., and Shiraki, H. (1972): Ueber die toxische Wirkung von antituberkulöse-Medikamenten, besonders Ethambutol und INH, auf das Nerven system: Ein Autopsie-Bericht. *Acta Pathol. Jpn.,* 22:383-390.

6. Kuroda, Sh., Tateishi, J., and Yokoyama, Sh. (1974): A case of cerebellar degeneration accompanying neuronal complication of chloramphenicol. *Clin. Neurol. (Tokyo),* 14:315-321.

7. Matsuyama, H., Ogawa, Y., Nakamura, S., and Hata, J. (1969): Pathology of paralytic illness following abdominal symptoms (Subacute myelo-optico-neuropathy, Toyokura). *Saishin Igaku,* 24:2469-2478.

8. Miyoshi, K., Ohno, F., Ohto, Y., Kawai, H., Harada, H., Tada, Y., Nakano, M., Sumitomo, T., and Kosaka, K. (1972): Diabetes mellitus or hyperglycemia observed in cases with SMON. *Shikoku Acta Medicina,* 27:164-166.

9. Miyoshi, K. (1973): Mechanism of the nervous and other tissues with quinoform. *Results of SMON Research Commission,* pp. 162-167.

10. Oda, M., and Shiraki, H. (1971): Ueber die Strangdegeneration des Rückenmarks bei hepatozerebralen Erkrankungen. *Tokyo Tanabe Quarterly,* 12:85-100.

11. Ogawa, K., Tsutsumi, K., and Motoi, Sh. (1971): The autopsy cases of SMON in Okayama area. *Reports of SMON Research Commission,* 4:18-48.

12. Prasad, A. S. (1966): *Zinc Metabolism,* p. 40. Charles C Thomas, Springfield, Ill.

13. Shigematsu, I. (1971): Review of the results of epidemiology session. *Reports of SMON Research Commission,* 12:1-2.

14. Shigematsu, T., Yanagawa, Y., Takeuchi, K., and Ishikawa, S. (1973): Actual status of SMON patients in whole territory of Japan. *Results of SMON Research Commission,* pp. 3-18.

15. Shiraki, H., and Oda, M. (1969): Neuropathology of subacute myelo-optico-neuropathy, "SMON." *Saishin Igaku,* 24:2479-2509.

16. Shiraki, H., and Fujisawa, K. (1970): Neuropathology of sensory impairments with special reference to complication after lumbar anesthesia, "SMON" and axonal dystrophy of Goll's nucleus. *Gendai Iryo,* 2:49-63.

17. Shiraki, H. (1971): Neuropathology of subacute myelo-optico-neuropathy, "SMON." *Jpn. J. Med. Sci. Biol.,* 24:217-243.

18. Shiraki, H. (1973): Neuropathology of subacute myelo-optico-neuropathy, "SMON." With special reference to etiology, particularly maladministration of chinoform, pathogenesis, modifying or

accelerating factors for disease onset and clinico-pathological relationship. *Neurol. India,* Proceeding, Supplement III:395–419.

19. Shiraki, H. (1973): Neuropathy due to intoxication with antituberculous drugs from neuropathological viewpoint. *Adv. Neurol. Sci.,* 17: 120–125.

20. Shiraki, H. (1975): An autopsy case of "SMON" complicated with the alterations of Ammon's horn. With special reference to the autoradiograms using labeled quinoform compounds. *Results of SMON Research Commission,* pp. 291–309.

21. Shiraki, H. (1975): The neuropathology of subacute myelo-optico-neuropathy, "SMON," in humans with special reference to the quinoform

intoxication. *Jpn. J. Med. Sci. Biol.,* Supplement, 28:101–164.

22. Takasu, T., Igata, A., and Toyokura, Y. (1970): On the green tongue observed in SMON patients. *Igaku no Ayumi,* 72:539–540.

23. Tateishi, J., Kuroda, Sh., Saito, A., and Otsuki, S. (1972): Experimental myelo-optic neuropathy induced by clioquinol. *Acta Neuropathol. (Berl.),* 24:304–320.

24. Tateishi, J., Kuroda, Sh., and Ikeda, H. (1975): Further study on the neurotoxicity of clioquinol in beagle dogs. *Psychiatr. Neurol. Jpn.,* 77:378–382.

25. Yoshioka, M., and Tamura, Z. (1970): On the nature of the green pigment found in SMON patients. *Igaku no Ayumi,* 74:320–322.

Neurotoxicology, edited by L. Roizin, H. Shiraki, and N. Grčević. Raven Press, New York © 1977.

Experimental Subacute Myeloopticoneuropathy

*J. Tateishi, **S. Kuroda, **H. Ikeda, and **S. Otsuki

*Department of Neuropathology, Neurological Institute, Kyushu University Medical School, 812 Fukuoka, Japan; and **Department of Neuropsychiatry, Okayama University Medical School, 700 Okayama, Japan

The long-term administration of iodochlorhyroxyquinoline (clioquinol, Entero-Vioform®) is suspected as the cause of subacute myeloopticoneuropathy (SMON) in Japan. It has been fairly well demonstrated by epidemiological studies that human SMON is an outcome of chronic intoxication of clioquinol administered to patients with digestive disorders in this country (11).

Neurotoxicity of clioquinol was not known in laboratory animals, except an occasional death from epileptic convulsions in dogs and cats that were given this drug for abdominal or skin distresses (2,6,10). We reported for the first time that oral administration of clioquinol for a long period to mongrel dogs, beagle dogs, cats, and a Japanese monkey resulted in the occurrence of a myeloopticoneuropathy in these animals (16,17). The neurological symptoms seen in these animals were well in accord with those observed in SMON patients both clinically and pathologically.

However, as the result of animal experiments made at Ciba-Geigy A.G., Switzerland, Hess et al. (3) reported that no neurological abnormalities were elicited with clioquinol.

There is also a minority opinion supporting the viral theory as the etiology of SMON (7,8). For these reasons, we repeated animal experiments on several occasions at the request of the Japanese SMON Research Commission. Results of these animal experiments and allied problems are summarized here.

CLIOQUINOL ADMINISTRATION

Long-term oral administration of clioquinol to laboratory animals reproduced the SMON syndrome with a high incidence. The number of animals that received clioquinol, the daily dose required to cause neurological symptoms, and the results of pathological examinations are summarized in Table 1.

TABLE 1. *Clioquinol administration*

Animals	No. animals	Daily dose (mg/kg)	Lesions (no. animals)	
			Spinal cord	Optic tract
Beagle dogs	17	250–400	15	14
Mongrel dogs	21	60–144	15	11
Cats	27	90–250	22(5)[a]	9
Japanese monkey	1	324	1	0

[a] Mild change.

Eight beagle dogs, four mongrel dogs, five cats, and a Japanese monkey used as controls did not show any neurological symptoms. Experiments on beagle dogs were done twice, once in 1972 and once in 1974, and the same results were obtained.

Five mongrel dogs died from acute poisoning with epileptic convulsions or general weakness. Many cats died from acute or subacute poisoning with symptoms such as loss of appetite, vomiting, diarrhea or constipation, and general weakness, suggesting low tolerance for this drug.

Fifteen beagle dogs, 13 mongrel dogs, and six cats manifested neurological signs clinically that began with side-swaying of the hips and ataxic gait followed by muscle weakness in the hindlegs. The longer the period of administration, the more severe the symptoms became. Forelegs that had remained healthy for a long period, however, developed slight weakness later. Visual acuity was also impaired in long-surviving animals.

The daily doses required to cause neurological symptoms differed much among laboratory animals. The daily dose given to our beagle dogs was three to four times larger than that given to mongrel dogs, which ranged from 60 to 144 mg/kg. The latter dose was also one and a half to seven times larger than the average dose of clioquinol (20 to 40 mg/kg) administered to many patients with SMON in Japan. These facts suggest differences in strains as well as species of animals for the neurotoxicity of clioquinol. Quantitative blood analysis by Tamura et al. (15) disclosed that the onset of neurological symptoms was more dependent on the concentration of unconjugated clioquinol, a neurotoxic form, in the blood than on the daily or total dosage. They showed that maximum levels (3.3 to 9.7 μg/ml) of unconjugated clioquinol in the blood of adult mongrel dogs that received 200 mg/kg of the drug reached a range similar (2.7 to 5.8 μg/ml) to that of men who were administered 7.4 to 9.3

mg/kg. To elevate the blood level of unconjugated clioquinol, the daily-dose-increasing method that we employed in early experiments had a great advantage. The fixed-dose method, however, also caused the same SMON syndrome in beagle dogs.

PATHOLOGICAL FINDINGS OF ANIMALS CHRONICALLY INTOXICATED

In the spinal cord, degenerative changes were most advanced in the posterior fasciculus, especially in Goll's tract in the upper cervical cord (Fig. 1), and were less severe in the corticospinal tract of the lumbar cord (Fig. 2). These changes were of a distally dominant nature, diffuse, continuous, and symmetrical, damaging axons first, then myelin sheaths. Axonal changes varied from swelling, vacuolization, and fragmentation to total disappearance. Degeneration and complete loss of myelin sheaths accompanied by neutral fat droplets occurred later. Plump and often binucleated astrocytes were seen, although proliferation of glial fibers was not marked. The severity of the degeneration depended on the duration of clinical symptoms.

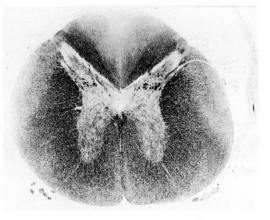

FIG. 1. Degeneration of nerve fibers mainly in Goll's tract and partly in Burdach's tract of the upper cervical cord of a beagle dog. Luxol fast blue stain. ×11.

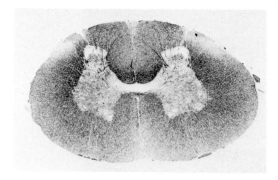

FIG. 2. Pallor of myelin sheaths in the corticospinal tract of the lumbar cord of a mongrel dog. Luxol fast blue stain. ×11.

Burdach's tract in the upper cervical cord and the proximal portion of Goll's tract at the lumbar level showed similar but milder changes later. Neither inflammatory nor vascular lesions were found among these areas.

The same advanced changes as in Goll's tract in the cervical cord occurred bilaterally in the optic tracts of long-surviving dogs and cats (Fig. 3). Similar but milder changes were seen in the chiasm and optic nerves.

The nature and distribution of these changes were specific, simulating system degeneration, composing a definite patho-logical entity, and corresponding well with those of SMON in humans (12,13).

Histological changes seen in other nervous regions, such as peripheral nerves, autonomic nerves, spinal root ganglion, ganglion cell layer of the retina, spinal roots, anterior spinal horn, brainstem, and some gray matter in the cerebrum, were occasional, mild, and nonpathognomonic.

The pathology of visceral organs in our animals was nonspecific, but intestinal abnormalities, such as invagination, volvulus, and megacolon, were noteworthy concerning the untoward abdominal effects of this substance, which follow.

ABDOMINAL SYMPTOMS

After administration of clioquinol, many SMON patients suffered from abdominal symptoms, such as abdominal pain, diarrhea and/or constipation, and vomiting, simulating ileus (14). To disclose the cause of this distress we made physiological experiments using eight mongrel dogs (4). It

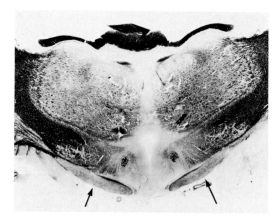

FIG. 3. Degeneration in the optic tracts (*arrow*) of a beagle dog. Luxol fast blue stain. ×3.

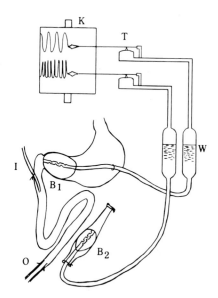

FIG. 4. *In vivo* experiment in mongrel dogs. B₁ and B₂, rubber balloon; I, small tube to pour clioquinol suspension; O, output tube; W, water manometer, K, kymograph, T, tambour.

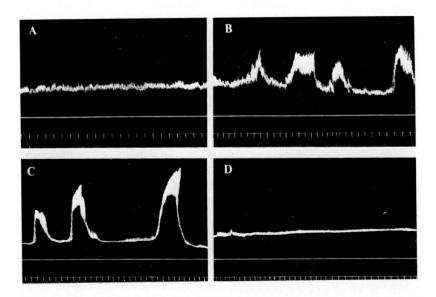

FIG. 5. *In vivo* effect of clioquinol on the intestinal movement. **A.** Before clioquinol pouring, normal peristalsis are seen. **B:** 30 min after clioquinol administration, strong constrictions occur. **C:** 60 min after cutting all splanchnic nerves, constrictions can still occur. **D:** 20 min after cut of the vagal nerve trunks, constrictions cease.

was then observed that abnormal, periodic constriction occurred in the small intestine 30 to 90 min after intraduodenal instillation of clioquinol (Fig. 4). This constriction did not disappear even when all the splanchnic nerves were severed but disappeared only when the vagal nerve trunks were cut bilaterally in the cervical region or when the animals were decerebrated in the mesencephalon (Fig. 5). Therefore, the effect of clioquinol on the intestinal tract appeared to be associated with excitation of the parasympathetic center in the diencephalon.

ORGAN DISTRIBUTION AND METABOLISM OF CLIOQUINOL

In order to know the organ distribution and metabolism of clioquinol, ^{14}C- or ^{131}I-clioquinol was administered to beagle dogs, mongrel dogs, cats, rats, and mice. Quantitative analysis of this experiment was reported by M. Ogata et al. (9). Their results were as follows: (a) Radioactivity in the whole body or blood of mice reached a steady state after 4 to 5 days of oral administration, and its level was about twice as high as that of 1 day's administration. (b) Radioactivity in the bile was about 30 to 500 times as high as that in the blood, suggesting a possible presence of "liver-intestine circulation" of this drug. (c) Among visceral organs, high uptake of clioquinol was found in the kidney, liver, pancreas, small intestine, fat tissue, lung, and spleen. Fat tissue and spleen were considered to be the main tissues where clioquinol accumulated for a long time. (d) A higher uptake in the sciatic nerve, dorsal root ganglion, hypophysis, and retina than in other nervous tissues was recognized. Half-time in the sciatic nerve was relatively longer than in the central nervous system. (e) Radioactivity in the central nervous system and dorsal root ganglion of dogs and cats was higher than in rats and mice. This result might correspond with the fact that clioquinol intoxication was more easily induced in larger animals than in smaller animals.

Autoradiographic studies in the nervous

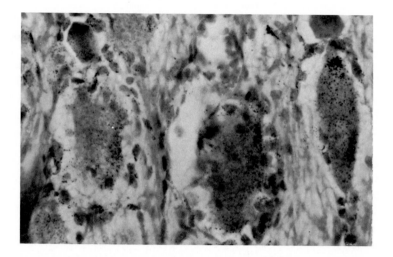

FIG. 6. Radioactive grains in ganglion cells and capsular cells in the cervical spinal root ganglion of a dog sacrificed 1½ hr after intraperitoneal injection of ^{131}I-clioquinol. ×400.

system of these animals showed marked blacking in the peripheral nerves, spinal root ganglia, spinal nerve rootlets, and retina. Blacking in the sciatic nerve was diffuse and equal in its distal and proximal portions (18).

By microautoradiography, radioactive grains were detected in the following nervous systems: nerve cells of the spinal root ganglia, spinal gray matter and nuclei in the brainstem; peripheral nerves; capsular cells of the spinal root ganglia; glial cells in the spinal cord, brainstem, and periventricular region of the cerebrum (Fig. 6 and 7). These results showed that clioquinol easily entered into the nervous tissue.

DISCUSSION

T. Yonezawa (22) observed the direct toxicity of clioquinol on the cultured

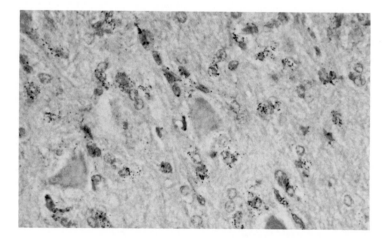

FIG. 7. Distribution of the grains in glial cells in the medullary olive in a dog sacrificed 1½ hr after intraperitoneal injection of ^{131}I-clioquinol. ×400.

nervous tissue *in vitro*. According to him, axonal mitochondria were affected directly with a high clioquinol concentration of not less than 6 ppm, a lower concentration of 0.6 to 1 ppm caused Schwann cells and myelin sheaths to degenerate slowly, and an intermediate concentration gave rise to both of the aforementioned phenomena. It was disclosed by N. Yamanaka et al. (21) that unconjugated clioquinol exerted an un-coupling action on the oxidative phos-phorylation by mitochondria *in vitro*.

As mentioned above, our repeated ani-mal experiments reproduced the SMON syndrome clinically as well as patho-logically. Similar experimental results have been obtained by many researchers in Japan (1,5,19,20).

In the summer of 1975, a Ciba-Geigy witness, testifying in the Japanese civil court dealing with the affair, admitted that pathological changes occurred in the nervous system of beagle dogs given clio-quinol with ascending dosing procedures. According to the witness, the optic tracts degenerated in nine beagle dogs (two showed doubtful change) and the spinal cord in six dogs (one was questionable) out of 26 treated dogs. The pathological changes were said to belong to an "acute dystrophic type," but their histological findings (diffuse and symmetrical changes of axons and myelin sheaths accompanied by slight increases in number of glial cells in the tracts and loss of ganglion cells as well as proliferation of glial cells in the retina) correspond well with those of our animals of shorter survival. Reproduci-bility in animals of SMON induced by clioquinol supports that this drug is re-sponsible for SMON in Japan.

SUMMARY

Long-term oral administration of clio-quinol on laboratory animals reproduced the SMON syndrome with a high incidence. The clinical signs began with side-swaying

of the hips and ataxic gait followed by muscle weakness in the hindlegs. Visual acuity was also impaired in long-surviving animals. The most marked pathological change was distal dominant degeneration in the posterior fasciculus of the spinal cord, the optic tracts, and less severely in the corticospinal tract. The clinicopatho-logical syndrome of these animals cor-responds well with that of SMON in humans. Abdominal symptoms often seen in SMON patients were also reproduced in our dogs. Distribution and metabolism of radioactive clioquinol and direct neuro-toxicity of clioquinol were discussed.

ACKNOWLEDGMENTS

Physiological studies were performed with Dr. T. Neya, and autoradiographic studies were done with the aid of Drs. M. Ogata and S. Watanabe.

ADDENDUM

Since this paper was prepared, Heywood et al. have reported the oral toxicity of clioquinol in beagle dogs (2a). Animals re-ceiving 250 and 400 mg/kg body weight per day showed disturbance in gait as well as pathological change in the posterior col-umns of the spinal cord.

REFERENCES

1. Egashira, Y. (1973): SMON. *Med. Sci.*, 1:57–63.
2. Hangartner, P. (1965): Troubles nerveux ob-servés chez le chien après absorption d'Entéro-Vioforme Ciba. *Schweiz. Arch. Tierheilkd.*, 107: 43–47.
2a. Heywood, R., Chesterman, H., and Worden, A. N. (1976): The oral toxicity of clioquinol (5-chloro-7-iodo-8-hydroxyquinoline) in beagle dogs. *Toxicology*, 6:41–46.
3. Hess, R., Keberle, H., Koella, W., Schmid, K., and Gelzer, J. (1972): Clioquinol: Absence of neurotoxicity in laboratory animals. *Lancet*, 2:424–425.
4. Ikeda, H., Neya, T., and Tateishi, J. (1975): Effects of clioquinol on the gastrointestinal peri-stalses. *Jpn. Med. J.*, 2681:26–30.

5. Kanemitsu, S., and Kasai, M. (1971): Influence of emulsifying agents mixed with clioquinol on the onset of SMON. *Igakuno Ayumi,* 79:365–367.
6. Müller, L. F. (1967): Die Mexaformvergiftung des Hundes. *Kleintierpraxis,* 12:51–52.
7. Nakamura, Y., and Inoue, Y. K. (1972): Pathogenicity of virus associated with subacute myelo-optico-neuropathy. *Lancet,* 1:223–226.
8. Nishimura, C. (1973): Cultivation of a virus associated with S.M.O.N. in chorioallantoic membranes of embryonated hen's eggs. *Lancet,* 2: 1032–1033.
9. Ogata, M., Watanabe, S., Tateishi, J., Kuroda, S., Kira, S., Hasegawa, T., and Otsuki, S. (1974): Organ distribution and metabolism of radioactive iodochlorohydroxyquinolin (clioquinol, chinoform) in animals. *Folia Psychiatr. Neurol. Jpn.,* 28:243–257.
10. Schantz, B., and Wikström, B. (1965): Suspected poisoning with oxyquinoline preparation in dogs. *Svenska Vet. T.,* 17:106–107.
11. Shigematsu, I. (1975): SMON and clioquinol. *JJPH,* 22:656–666.
12. Shiraki, H., and Oda, M. (1969): Neuropathology of subacute myelo-optico-neuropathy, "SMON." *Saishinigaku,* 24:2479–2509.
13. Shiraki, H. (1971): Neuropathology of subacute myelo-optico-neuropathy, "SMON." *Jpn. J. Med. Sci. Biol.,* 24:217–243.
14. Sobue, I., and Ando, K. (1972): Abdominal symptoms in SMON: Analysis of correlations of clioquinol medication to the onset of the neurological symptoms. *Igakuno Ayumi,* 82:354.
15. Tamura, Z., Samejima, K., Imanari, T., Ching, K., Hayakawa, K., Egashira, Y., and Kodama, H. (1974): Blood level of clioquinol and its metabolites in animals presenting SMON-like neurologic symptoms. In: *Achievements in Fiscal 1973 by the Japanese Ministry of Health and Welfare,* SMON Research Commission.
16. Tateishi, J., Kuroda, S., Saito, A., and Otsuki, S. (1971): Myelo-optic neuropathy induced by clioquinol in animals. *Lancet,* 2:1263–1264.
17. Tateishi, J., Kuroda, S., Saito, A., and Otsuki, S. (1972): Experimental myelo-optic neuropathy induced by clioquinol. *Acta Neuropathol. (Berl.),* 24:304–320.
18. Tateishi, J., Kuroda, S., Watanabe, S., Otsuki, S., and Ogata, M. (1972): Autoradiographic distribution of ^{131}I-clioquinol in canine and feline. *Folia Psychiatr. Neurol. Jpn.,* 26:159–164.
19. Tawara, J., Ichikawa, H., Sakamoto, S., and Miyoshi, A. (1972): Experimental study of SMON in dogs. *Jpn. J. Bacteriol.,* 27:527.
20. Tsubaki, A. (1973): Aetiological and clinical study on subacute myelo-optico-neuropathy (SMON). *J. Jpn. Soc. Intern. Med.,* 63:1–17.
21. Yamanaka, N., Imanari, T., Tamura, Z., and Yagi, K. (1973): Uncoupling of oxidative phosphorylation of rat liver mitochondria by chinoform. *J. Biochem.,* 73:993–998.
22. Yonezawa, T. (1973): Toxic change in nervous tissue induced by clioquinol. In: *Achievements in Fiscal 1972 by the Japanese Ministry of Health and Welfare,* SMON Research Commission.

Neurotoxicology, edited by L. Roizin, H. Shiraki,
and N. Grčević. Raven Press, New York © 1977.

Neuropathology of the Subacute Myeloopticoneuropathy (Clioquinol Intoxication) in Humans and Experimental Animals

F. Ikuta, T. Atsumi, T. Makifuchi, T. Sato, and T. Tsubaki

*Departments of Neuropathology and Neurology, Brain Research Institute, Niigata University,
Niigata City, Japan 951*

Since 1955 when the existence of a neurological disease of unknown etiology first became clear, the number of cases has increased in Japan causing more attention. In 1970 approximately 10,000 patients were publicly found. Many of these patients showed clinically subacute optic neuropathies and the motor and sensory as well as abdominal disorders. One of us (TT) (6) called this disease subacute myeloopticoneuropathy (SMON) in 1964. Since then, clinically and pathologically, we have seen extensive studies of SMON, mostly performed by the members of the SMON Research Committee (Chairman, R. Kono) of the Japanese Ministry of Health and Welfare.

SMON IN HUMANS

The following neuropathology of SMON in humans is based on our own 10 autopsy cases (Table 1) and on cases from autopsy specimens collected from all over Japan. All of them were pathologically as well as clinically diagnosed as SMON.

Like Fig. 1A, the optic nerves and tracts of most of the cases showed symmetrical degeneration, with neutral fat droplets of both the myelin and axon. By careful examination it was indicated that this degeneration was more severe in the optic

nerve and tract distal from the retina. For example, Fig. 1C is an axonal preparation of the optic nerve close to the retina, and we can still see several intact axons in it. On the other hand, Fig. 1D shows the optic tract close to the lateral geniculate body. Here the axon is almost totally destroyed. Along with this severe destruction, the neuron in the lateral geniculate body was also affected, showing definite transneuronal degeneration or loss.

When we studied the retina of such cases, the outer nuclear layer and inner nuclear layer were unchanged, whereas the ganglion cells disappeared in various degrees (Fig. 1B).

In the spinal cord, degeneration was recognized in the posterior column, dominantly in the fasciculus gracilis (Fig. 1E). This degeneration was found to be more restricted toward the upper level of the fasciculus. Corresponding to this degeneration, neuronal loss was detected in the nucleus gracilis of the medulla oblongata, which we assumed to be transneuronal degeneration. Although degeneration was seen also in the posterior nerve roots, the posterior root ganglia showed mild but definite neuronal loss with an increased number of satellite cells (Fig. 1F).

Aside from the above-noticed sym-

TABLE 1. *Human SMON autopsy cases: Brain Research Institute, Niigata University (1966–1973)*

Case no.	Name	Age, sex	Neurologic symptoms for	Clin. dx.	Duration of clioquinol and total doses	Visceral organs	Optic nerve and tracts degeneration	Spinal cord degeneration		Peripheral motor and sensory nerve degen.
								Posterior column	Lateral pyramidal tract	
1	H. Y.	71 F	4 yr	SMON	4 yr ?	Atherosclerotic heart disease Pancreas atrophy	+++	+++	+++	+
2	K. M.	67 F	2 yr 10 mo	SMON	2 yr 10 mo 1,269 g	Appendectomy	+++	+++	+++	+
3	K. K.	53 F	2 yr	SMON	? ?	Uterus cancer	++	+++	++	+
4	T. K.	42 F	11 mo	SMON?	? ?	Lung tuberculosis	++	+++	++	+
5	M. K.	68 F	2 yr 11 mo	SMON	7+α days (13 + αg)	Pancreas necrosis	+	+++	+++	+
6	M. O.	69 F	6 mo	SMON	1 mo 42 g	Necrotizing angitis in muscle	++	++	+	+
7	T. O.	62 M	1 yr 11 mo	SMON	5 mo 145 g	Lung tuberculosis amyloid angiopathy	+	++	++	+
8	M. F.	58 F	1.5 mo	Rectum cancer and paraplegia	6 mo	Postope. rectum cancer	–	++	++	+
9	T. S.	66 M	?	Stomach cancer	2 mo 72 g	Postope. stomach cancer	–	+++	+	+
10	T. K.	52 M	2 mo	SMON	2 mo 79 g	Postope. stomach cancer	–	++	+	+

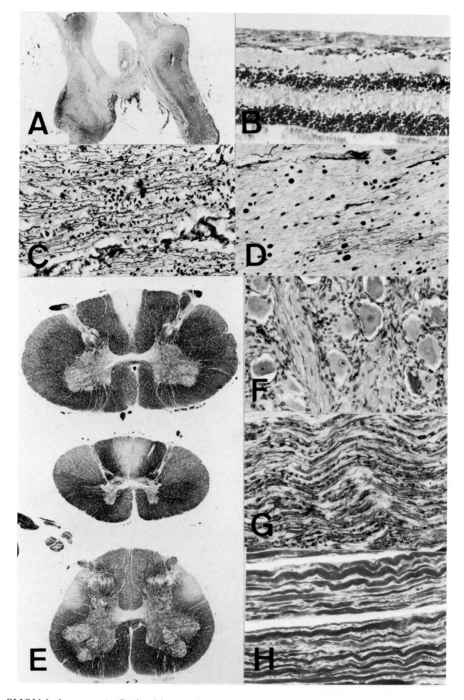

FIG. 1. SMON in humans. **A:** Optic chiasma showing complete demyelination and atrophy in a severe case. Klüver-Barrera-LFB stain. ×4. **B:** Retina showing disappearance of ganglion cells, but intact outer and inner nuclear layers. H. & E. stain. ×130. **C:** Relatively preserved axons of the optic nerve near the retina. Bodian's axonal method. ×130. **D:** Totally destroyed axons of the optic tract near the lateral geniculate body. The same case as **C.** Bodian's axonal method. ×130. **E:** Cervical, thoracic, and lumbar segments of the spinal cord showing symmetrical degeneration of the ascending and descending tracts. Klüver-Barrera-LFB stain. ×4.7. **F:** Spinal root ganglia showing mild but definite degeneration. H. & E. stain. ×150. **G:** Peripheral nerve in the gastrocnemius. PTAH stain. ×130. **H:** Gastrocnemius showing neurogenic muscular atrophy. PTAH stain. ×120.

metrical ascending tract degeneration, the corticospinal tracts also demonstrated symmetrical degeneration. The degeneration became more distinct toward the lower segments (Fig. 1E).

In the anterior horn cells, a suspicious pathological change was detectable, although this was not a constant finding. The peripheral nerves always showed definite degeneration (Fig. 1G) extending over the anterior nerve roots and accompanied by neurogenic type muscular atrophy (Fig. 1H).

It was practically impossible to point out a definite pathological alteration in the levels above the medulla oblongata of the corticospinal tracts and Betz cells.

Among these pathological alterations, the degenerations in the posterior column, in the corticospinal tracts of the spinal cord, and in the peripheral nerves were recognized in all cases, but there were cases where changes in the optic pathway were not definite.

These findings reminded us of the subacute combined degeneration. However, the vitamin B_{12} level in the blood was normal, the degeneration in the cases of SMON remained restricted to certain long tracts, and the margin was not irregular.

Then, we considered that these cases might represent intoxication due to isonicotinic acid hydrazide (INAH), antituberculosis, for some similarity can be seen in a well-documented case of INAH intoxication (M. Tanaka, *personal communication*). The cases with the INAH intoxication also show somewhat systemic degeneration of the ascending and descending tracts of the spinal cord and of the optic pathway. However, none of these SMON patients had a record of INAH intake.

Among the extensive and numerous investigations of the etiology of SMON, performed mainly from the points of view of an infectious, metabolic, or toxic disorder, Toyokura, Igata, and their group (1) particularly emphasized that tongues of SMON patients were green colored, as were their feces and urine. Then Tamura and his group (9) pointed out that the agent causing the green color was a chelate compound of a ferric ion bound to clioquinol (Fig. 2). One of us (TT) maintained that this clioquinol was a primary causative agent of the SMON (7).

This drug had been widely used, particularly in Japan, as an oral antiseptic, not only for intestinal amebiasis but also for any kind of diarrhea.

SMON IN EXPERIMENTAL ANIMALS

Thus, to see how clioquinol affects, several experiments have already been done on different kinds of experimental animals, which has led to the success in experimentally producing SMON (2,4,5).

As reported previously (8), we also performed chronic oral administration of clioquinol on four mongrel dogs and 10 beagle dogs (Table 2).

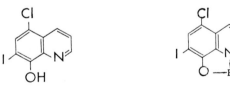

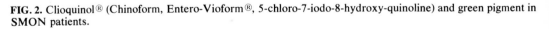

FIG. 2. Clioquinol® (Chinoform, Entero-Vioform®, 5-chloro-7-iodo-8-hydroxy-quinoline) and green pigment in SMON patients.

TABLE 2. Experimental Clioquinol Intoxication in Dog

Dog number	kg	Total dose before onset / Total dose (g/kg) / Days before Onset (12 '72 2 3 4 5 6 7 8 9 10 11)	Total experiment period (onset to autopsy) days	Histological severity
Mongrel 1	13.0		63(34) killed	6
2	10.5		68(2) dead	4
3	6.5		121(70) dead	9
4	8.0		144(113) killed	10
Beagle 1	8.7		145(30) killed	3
2	7.8		145(30) killed	3
3	9.2		183(68) killed	4
4	7.0		184(69) dead	4
5	7.5		40(0) dead	0-1
6	9.5		347(232) killed	8
7	10.0		183(134) dead	8
8	9.6		347(300) killed	10
9	9.4		145(50) killed	5
10	8.8		41(0) dead	0-1
12	7.0	Control	347 killed	0

Two other beagle dogs were used as controls, that is, Nos. 11 and 12. No. 11 has shown no suffering to the present, and No. 12 has experienced no pathological changes.

A total dose of from 2.1 to 11.9 g/kg was given to the mongrel dogs, and a total of from 7.2 to 34 g/kg was given to the beagle dogs until the onset of clinical symptoms. One hundred and sixty milligrams per kg daily was required to produce symptoms in the mongrel dogs, whereas as much as 280 to 500 mg/kg daily was needed for the beagles. This experiment continued for 347 days.

Among the 14 experimental dogs, No. 5 and No. 10, which both died within a short period, did not have any definite alteration. All of the remaining 12 dogs showed pathological changes of various degrees. These were divided into 10 grades as shown on Table 2. The changes always appeared symmetrically.

Relative to the optic pathway, distinct loss of ganglion cells in the retina was found (Fig. 3A), as was the case in human patients. An electron microscopic study showed that an alteration of the Müller cells was rather more obvious than the neuronal degeneration (8).

A change in the optic nerve and tracts was found in all 12 dogs. This change (Fig. 3B) became more severe and extensive, approaching the lateral geniculate

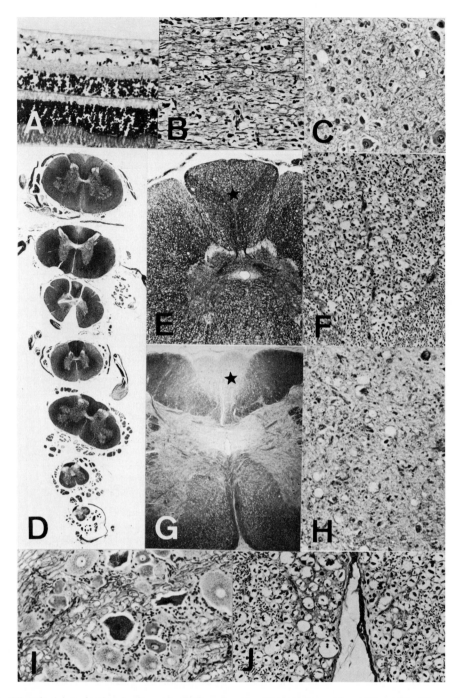

FIG. 3. Clioquinol intoxication in dogs. A: Retina showing disappearance of ganglion cells. Mongrel No. 1. Klüver-Barrera-LFB stain. ×120. B: Optic tract showing axonal degeneration. Beagle No. 8. Bodian's axonal method. ×120. C: Lateral geniculate body showing transneuronal degeneration. Mongrel No. 4. Bodian's axonal method. ×120. D: Spinal cord. Cervical to sacral segments showing obvious degeneration of the fasciculus gracilis and suspicious alteration in the descending tracts. Mongrel No. 3. Klüver-Barrera-LFB stain. ×2.8. E: Thoracic segment showing degeneration of the fasciculus gracilis (*star*). Mongrel No. 1. Klüver-Barrera-LFB stain. ×12. F: Fasciculus gracilis (*starred area* in E) showing marked axonal degeneration. Bodian's axonal method. ×120. G: Lower medulla oblongata showing marked degeneration of the nucleus gracilis (*star*). Mongrel No. 4. Klüver-Barrera-LFB stain. ×12. H: Marked transneuronal degeneration of the nucleus gracilis (*starred area* in G). Klüver-Barrera-LFB stain. ×120. I: Cervical spinal root ganglia showing mild degeneration. Mongrel No. 1. Klüver-Barrera-LFB stain. ×120. J: Descending tracts of the thoracic segment showing axonal degeneration. Beagle No. 8. Bodian's axonal method. ×120.

body, and there in the lateral geniculate body strong neuronal degeneration was recognized (Fig. 3C). The change in the axon seemed stronger than that in myelin.

Figure 3E is a thoracic segment of the No. 1 mongrel dog that didn't have very strong degeneration. However, definite myelin destruction was seen in a triangle in the posterior column, especially in the fasciculus gracilis. This change became more distinct toward the upper segments. Fig. 3G is an example of the level of the pyramidal decussation, showing the complete loss of myelin in the nucleus gracilis. In the nucleus gracilis, as seen in Fig. 3H, neurons disappeared almost completely.

Like the human cases, in the canine posterior ganglia both neuronal loss and an increase of satellite cells were detected (Fig. 3I). When the iron staining was applied here, an iron-positive substance was visible in the satellite cells and in a smaller quantity in the nuclei of neurons. This finding was also confirmed by the use of a wave-dispersive-type X-ray microanalyzer.

According to an autoradiographic study (3), a large amount of clioquinol was demonstrated in the posterior root ganglia, besides the peripheral nerve and retina.

Fig. 3J is a corticospinal tract of a cervical segment. Along with the ascending tract degeneration, the pyramidal tract of the spinal cord also revealed alteration. As well as in human cases, in all of these experimental animals the motor and sensory peripheral nerves showed stronger and more severe changes in the distal parts.

Neurogenic muscular atrophy was also definite.

In addition, a suspicious change was recognized in sympathetic ganglia such as the solar ganglion.

DISCUSSION

It seemed reasonable to conclude that SMON appearing in human cases was

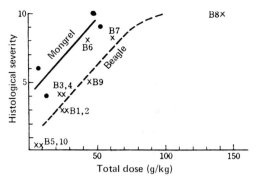

FIG. 4. Correlation between the dose of clioquinol and degree of histological severity.

identical with the clioquinol intoxication produced in experimental dogs.

Figure 4 demonstrates the dose and histological severity correlation that was noticed in these experimental animals. As seen here, mongrel dogs show considerably higher susceptibility.

Also, we saw that the severity linearly correlated with the length of the survival period (Fig. 5). B9 and B6 had been given the same doses during the same period; however, B6 was kept alive 200 days after the discontinuation of the dosage and then autopsied. Similar correlation of B1, 2 to B3, 4 also can be seen.

This evidence implies that histological

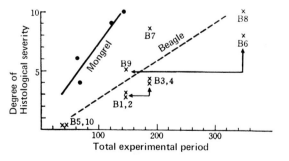

FIG. 5. Correlation of total experimental period to histological severity. B9 and B6 had been given the same doses during the same period, however, B6 was kept alive 200 days after the discontinuation of the dosage. Note similar correlation of B1, 2 to B3, 4.

changes progress in spite of the cessation of the drug.

SUMMARY AND CONCLUSION

1. Neuropathological findings of SMON in humans were identical to those of clioquinol intoxication produced in experimental dogs.

2. In addition to previous neuropathological reports on SMON (clioquinol intoxication), degeneration of the ganglion cells of the retina and marked degeneration, probably transneuronal, of the nucleus gracilis were noticed.

3. The seemingly complicated neuropathological finding obtained about SMON may be explained as a quite simple systemic degeneration. The perikaryon of either upper or lower motor neurons failed to show any obvious changes that would correspond to degeneration in corticospinal tracts and peripheral motor nerves. But with respect to the change in the optic pathway, the posterior column and peripheral sensory nerve could be explained by postulating that the ganglion cells of the retina and the neuron of the posterior ganglia undergo systemic degeneration.

REFERENCES

1. Igata, A., Takasu, T., and Toyokura, Y. (1970): Green substance in the feces and urine of SMON patients. *Igaku no Ayumi (Tokyo)* (Japanese edition), 72:539–540.
2. Jones, E. L., Searle, C. E., and Smith, W. T. (1973): Peripheral neuropathy in ageing rats fed clioquinol and a maize diet. *Acta Neuropathol. (Berl.)*, 24:256–262.
3. Takasu, T., Toyokura, Y., and Matsuoka, O. (1972): Toxicity of quinoform (5-chloro-7-iodo-8-hydroxy-quinoline) for the nervous system. I. Interstinal absorption, whole body retention and distribution of ^{131}I-quinoform in mice. *Clin. Neurol. (Tokyo)* (Japanese edition), 12:131–142.
4. Tateishi, J., Kuroda, S., Saito, A., and Otsuki, S. (1971): Myelo-optic neuropathy induced by clioquinol in animals. *Lancet*, 2:1263–1264.
5. Tateishi, J., Kuroda, S., Saito, A., and Otsuki, S. (1972): Strain-differences in dogs for neurotoxicity of clioquinol. *Lancet*, 1:1289–1290.
6. Tsubaki, T., Toyokura, Y., and Tsukagoshi, H. (1964): Subacute myelo-optico-neuropathy following abdominal symptoms: A clinical and pathological study. *J. Jpn. Soc. Intern. Med.* (Japanese edition), 53:779–784.
7. Tsubaki, T., Honma, Y., and Hoshi, M. (1971): Neurological syndrome associated with clioquinol. *Lancet*, 1:696–697.
8. Tsubaki, T. (1974): Aetiological and clinical study on subacute myelo-optico-neuropathy (SMON). *J. Jpn. Soc. Intern. Med.* (Japanese edition), 63:1–17.
9. Yoshioka, M., and Tamura, Z. (1970): Nature of green pigment in SMON patients. *Igaku no Ayumi (Tokyo)* (Japanese edition), 74:320–322.

Neurotoxicology, edited by L. Roizin, H. Shiraki, and N. Grčević. Raven Press, New York © 1977.

Neurotoxic Effects of Chinoform Studied on Nervous Tissue Maintained *In Vitro*

Takeshi Yonezawa, Takahiko Saida, Akira Nakano, and Michinori Hasegawa

Department of Pathology, Kyoto Prefectural University of Medicine, Kyoto, Japan

Subacute myeloopticoneuropathy, which is known as SMON by abbreviation, prevailed in Japan from 1960 until 1970. The main pathological alterations of this disorder were degeneration of the optic nerve, ascending degeneration of posterior column, descending degeneration of pyramidal tract of the spinal cord, and peripheral neuropathy involving both sensory and motor systems (1,4,5–7,9,11,12). Through nationwide studies made by a special research group, chinoform was found to be the causative agent for this disease. Interruption of the medication caused a dramatic decrease in outbreaks of the disorder. Our present study has been directed toward a better understanding of the neurotoxic effects of this agent using nervous tissue maintained *in vitro*.

METHODS AND MATERIAL

Dorsal root ganglia obtained from fetal rats and mice 16 to 17 days *in utero* were explanted onto collagen-coated coverslips and maintained with Maximow's double coverslip assembly (14). After myelin sheaths were fully developed, around 20 days *in vitro,* cultures were exposed to feeding media in which chinoform was diluted in concentrations of 1 to 10 μg/ml. Alterations produced in cultures were studied with light (LM) and electron microscope (EM). When needed, cultures were stained with the Bodian technique for axis cylinders, Sudan black for myelin sheaths, and Thionin ® stain for Nissl bodies.

In addition to dorsal root ganglia, cultures of sympathetic ganglia (8) and of neuromuscular junction (15) were also applied with chinoform and studied with the same techniques.

RESULTS

Since morphological changes in cultures depend on the amount of chinoform applied, results were classified into three groups — acute, subacute, and chronic.

Acute Intoxication

With a concentration of 10 μg/ml of chinoform the initial changes in the cultures were observed 3 to 4 days after the exposure and were characterized by vacuolar degeneration of axis cylinders. The alterations first appeared in the axons of nonmyelinated segment (Fig. 1) and also in axons near the node of Ranvier. Nonmyelinated nerve fibers from sympathetic ganglion seemed to be most vulnerable. Within the following few days these alterations spread into all the axons, which became

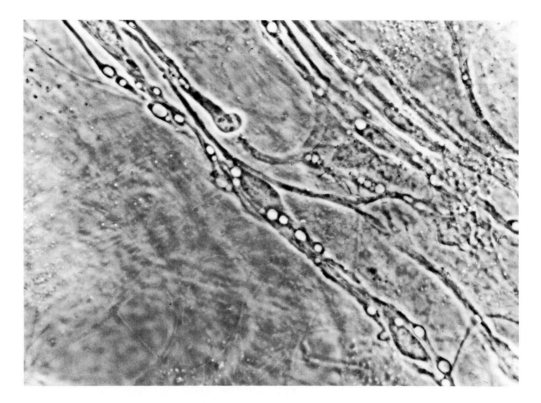

FIG. 1. Vacuolar degeneration of nonmyelinated nerve fibers 3 days after the exposure to 10 μg/ml of chinoform (living, phase contrast). Vacuolations are present inside of axons. Schwannian nucleus in the center seems unchanged.

foamy and vacuolar (Fig. 2). Myelin sheaths began to break within a few days. The changes were most often observed at the node of Ranvier and gradually advanced to the internodal region. Occasionally, continuity of the sheaths was interrupted by enlarged axonal vacuoles even in the internodal region. These alterations of myelin sheaths seemed to be secondary, being caused mechanically by the swollen axonal vacuoles.

After the axonal changes became manifest, roughly 7 to 9 days after the exposure, neuron somas began to show granular cytoplasm (Fig. 3). The granulations gradually increased in number and size. Finally these were transformed into cytoplasmic vacuolations, and the entire perikaryal cytoplasm was occupied by these vacuoles. Nuclei are slightly shrunken and deeply stained with ordinary histological staining (Fig. 4).

EM studies found that vacuolations of axis cylinders were produced by mitochondrial swelling. With enlargement of mitochondria, destruction and disappearance of cristae and inner membrane took place. In addition, the swelling further developed the disintegration of outer membrane. These changes appeared 3 to 4 days after the exposure to chinoform. Thus, axis cylinders became filled with vacuoles originating from mitochondria (Fig. 5). Neurotubules seemed less vulnerable and remained unchanged. Regarding the degeneration of neuron somas, mitochondrial swelling also seemed to be the initial change. The same alterations were found in the perikaryal mitochondria. Finally, neuron somas developed a honeycomb appearance

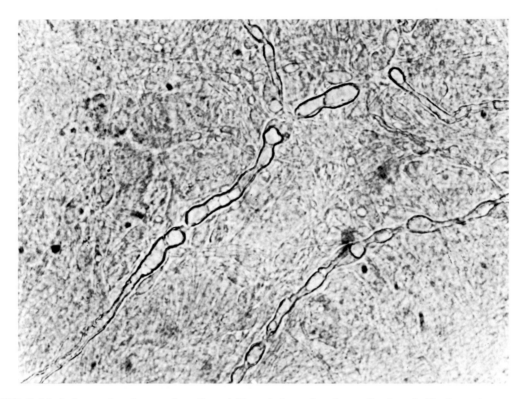

FIG. 2. Marked vacuolar change of myelinated fibers 6 days after the application of chinoform. Axons are swollen because of vacuolar and foamy changes. Occasional interruption of myelin sheaths is seen. These myelin alterations seem to be produced secondarily to swollen axons.

of the cytoplasm (Fig. 6). As shown in the illustration, satellite cells are much less sensitive to chinoform.

Subacute Intoxication

With a concentration of 5 μg/ml of chinoform, the initial changes appeared a little later than those seen in the previous group. Namely, the appearance of the earliest alteration in axons required 10 days of exposure. The mode of action, however, seemed to be identical to that described above. Axis cylinders of nonmyelinated segments and those in the vicinity of Ranvier's node were the first sites of vacuolar change. Axoplasm underneath Schwannian nucleus was found less vulnerable (Fig. 7). Within a few days these alterations were found to extend to all axons. Nerve cells also developed similar degeneration. However, in this group, different stages of alteration were seen at the same time. In other words, some of the neuron somas developed slight mitochondrial changes, whereas other cells showed honeycomb structure and intermediate forms of degeneration. Satellite cells did not show severe damage, even in the cells associated with severely damaged neurons. Myelin sheaths were disintegrated only after axons were destroyed by swollen vacuoles.

EM studies on the alterations in this group also confirmed that the granulations and vacuolations were caused by mitochondrial involvement in the same way as described in the previous group. Especially in this group, however, it was often observed that the distal portions of axis

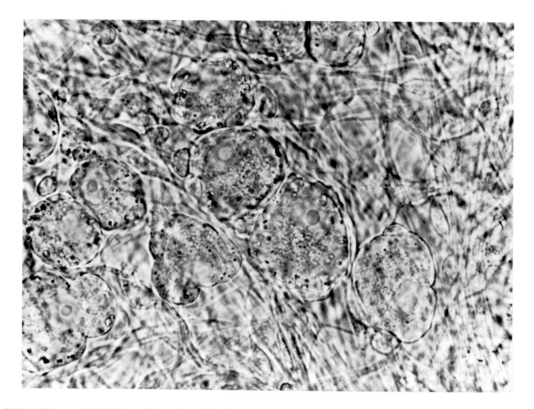

FIG. 3. Nerve cells in the ganglion culture showing granular appearance of cytoplasm 7 days after the application in amount of 10 μg/ml of chinoform.

cylinders were readily damaged compared to the proximal segments of the same nerve fibers. And the alterations advanced centropetally suggesting a dying-back type of neuropathy.

Chronic Intoxication

With a concentration of 1 μg/ml, initial changes appeared more than 20 days after the application. The alteration was mainly seen in myelinated fibers. Neuron somas, even with 1 month of exposure to chinoform, were unchanged. Myelinated fibers exhibited slowly progressing segmental degeneration of the sheaths. In the beginning of the change, the nodal gap of myelin sheaths was elongated due to the retraction of the sheaths. Splitting of myelin sheaths from exolemma and of lamellar structures gradually took place. In this group, however, mitochondrial damage was not seen. Myelin sheaths disappeared roughly 1 month after the first myelin retraction, and axons also gradually disintegrated.

Sympathetic Chain and Neuromuscular Junction Cultures

Cultures of sympathetic chain exposed to chinoform in amounts of 5 to 10 μg/ml also developed vacuolar degeneration of axis cylinders, which was identical to that found in cultures of dorsal root ganglia. The alteration in sympathetic nerve cells was vacuolation of perikaryal cytoplasm. This vacuolar degeneration in axons and perikarya was found to be produced by swelling and ballooning of mitochondria.

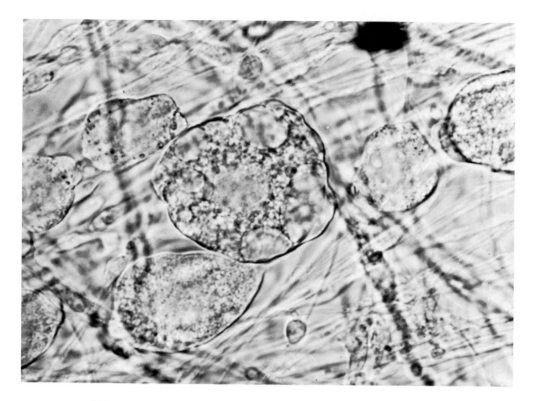

FIG. 4. Honeycomb structure of nerve cells 14 days after the application.

Cultures of neuromuscular preparation, which were developed in the co-culture of spinal cord and limb muscle, exhibited a slightly different type of vulnerability. With 5 to 10 μg/ml of chinoform, proximal segments of motor axons developed vacuolar changes as seen in other systems, whereas distal portions remained unchanged suggesting the lesser vulnerability of mitochondria in the distal motor axons.

COMMENT

Summarizing the results, the effects of chinoform on the *in vitro* nervous tissue can be classified as direct and indirect. The direct effects are characterized by vacuolar degeneration of axis cylinders and neuron somas. The mode of action seemed to be mitochondrial damage, represented by destruction of cristae and inner membrane and by ballooning of mitochondria. This change first appeared in the axons of non-myelinated nerve fibers and at the node of Ranvier. It was observed only when the cultures were treated with more than 3 μg/ml of chinoform, and it was interpreted as a direct effect. The detailed mechanism of mitochondrial alteration is uncertain. However, chinoform has a chelating action and is ready to produce chylate metal compound. Among the SMON patients, green tongue is a very common clinical sign. This discoloration was found to result from the chelating action of chinoform, producing iron chylate compound (3). This chelation seems to be a main cause of mitochondrial alteration. Chinoform also shows a similar chelating action with other metals such as zinc in the islet cells of the pancreas. However, a more detailed mechanism of this action with the

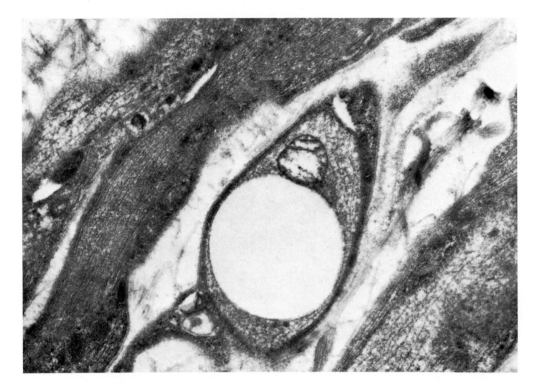

FIG. 5. Swelling and ballooning of mitochondria in the axis cylinders.

iron in the mitochondrial enzyme has not been settled. Especially Yamanaka et al. (13) emphasized the significance of the metal that was liberated by uncoupling from the chylate compound.

In this neurointoxication it is interesting to find that peripheral segments of nerve fibers were affected first, then the alteration advanced centropetally. This type of degeneration was most evident when the cultures were treated with a relatively lower doses of chinoform. The centropetal involvement of axonal mitochondria explains well the dying-back nature of chinoform neuropathy. However, this tendency could not be found in motor fibers, where mitochondria in the terminal region were exempt from degenerative changes.

Morphological similarities regarding mitochondrial involvement have been reported by Spencer et al. (10) in thallium neuropathy. Our unpublished data on thallium neuropathy also showed mitochondrial change especially in peripheral segments of sensory nerve fibers. In this respect, thallium neuropathy seems to be very much like chinoform neuropathy. However, chinoform neuropathy has never developed initial involvement in neuron somas, whereas this earlier perikaryal change can be seen in thallium intoxication when a larger dose is applied.

Regarding the indirect effect of chinoform, pathological changes in cultured nervous tissue were characterized by segmental degeneration of myelin sheaths and slowly degenerating processes of axis cylinders. This type of alteration took place only with lower doses, such as 1 μg/ml or less, and after long exposure to chinoform. No mitochondrial involvement was seen in this case. These changes seemed to be nonspecific, since similar changes could be produced by other causes such as vitamin

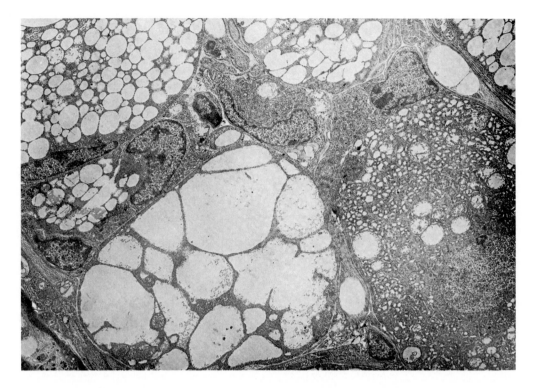

FIG. 6. Degeneration of nerve cells. Some of them simply show mitochondrial swelling, and others exhibit marked vacuolar degeneration. Intermediate stages of alteration are seen.

B_1 deficiency (14). It is probable that alterations of this type were produced by chronic metabolic disturbance of nerve cells and associated cells. Processes of action in this case, however, have not been well established.

Comparative analysis of alterations in the different nervous systems provides new information regarding the difference of vulnerability. The somatosensory system represented by cultures of dorsal root ganglia exhibited a dying-back type of neuropathy involving mainly mitochondria. Cultures of sympathetic ganglia also showed similar alterations. Since the majority of nerve fiber in this system is nonmyelinated, alterations may develop in the early stages after exposure. On the contrary, in neuromuscular cultures, mitochondria close to the axon terminal showed lower sensitivity to chinoform. In cord-ganglion-muscle culture, proximal segments of motor fibers may develop similar mitochondrial change to that of the sensory system. However, terminal axons of the same fibers remained unchanged. Presynaptic mitochondria in neuromuscular junctions were found to tolerate even high doses of chinoform. In this sense, dying-back neuropathy does not seem applicable in the motor system. The alterations described above are well correlated with clinical symptoms. The serum level of chinoform in the acute phase of SMON patients was found to be roughly 10 μg/ml, which corresponds to the amount used for the acute development of mitochondrial damage in our experimental system. Furthermore, initial clinical symptoms such as intestinal discomfort may be caused by early changes in the sympathetic nerves. Additional medication may develop further clinical manifestations involving the long

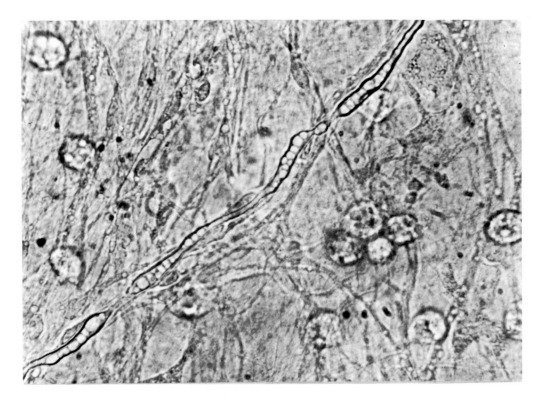

FIG. 7. Vacuolar degeneration of axis cylinders treated with 5 μg/ml of chinoform. Axons close to the Ranvier's node are much more severely altered.

tract of spinal cord and peripheral and optic nerves.

SUMMARY

Neurotoxic effects of chinoform have been studied on the cultures of dorsal root ganglia, sympathetic ganglia, and neuromuscular preparation. Morphological alterations were classified into direct and indirect effects. The former changes were characterized by mitochondrial degeneration. The latter were represented by nonspecific alterations, such as retraction of myelin sheaths from Ranvier's node and splitting of myelin lamellae.

The mitochondrial involvement was initiated by swelling, vacuolation, loss of mitochondrial cristae, and destruction of inner mitochondrial membrane. These changes first appeared in the nonmyelinated axons and in those at the node of Ranvier. With centropetal development of this degeneration, neuron somas were also involved as represented by mitochondrial swelling and vacuolation.

REFERENCES

1. van Balen, A. T. M. (1971): Toxic damage to the optic nerve caused by iodochlorhydroxyquinoline (Enterovioform). *Ophthalmologica,* 163:8.
2. Billson, F. H., Reich, J., and Hopkins, I. J. (1972): Visual failure in a patient with ulcerative colitis treated by clioquinol. *Lancet,* 1:1015–1016.
3. Igata, A., Hasebe, K., and Tsuji, T. (1971): Green substance in SMON – relation to quinoform. *Medicina (B. Aires),* 8:10.
4. Matsuyama, H., Ogawa, Y., Nakamura, S., and Hata, J. (1969): Pathology of SMON. *Recent Med.,* 24:2469–2478.
5. Onishi, A. (1972): Pathological studies on the peripheral nerves from subacute myelo-opticoneuropathy and quinoform intoxicated rabbits. (I). *Adv. Nerve Res.,* 16:914.
6. Onishi, A. (1972): Pathological studies on the

peripheral nerves from subacute myelo-optico-neuropathy and quinoform intoxicated rabbits. (II). *Adv. Nerve Res.,* 16:1095.

7. Roesch, E., Roesch, A., and Hoffter, D. (1965): Polyneuropathie durch 5-nitro-8-hydroxychinolin in Tierexperimenten. *Arch. Toxikol. (Berl.),* 20:313–322.

8. Sano, Y., Odake, G., and Yonezawa, T. (1967): Fluorescence microscopic observations of catecholamines in cultures of the sympathetic chains. *Z. Zellfors.,* 80:345–352.

9. Shiraki, H., and Oda, M. (1969): Neuropathology of SMON. *Recent Med.,* 24:2479–2509.

10. Spencer, P. C., Peterson, E. R., Madrid, A. R., and Raine, C. S. (1973): Effects of thallium salts on neuronal mitochondria in organotypic cord-ganglion-muscle combination culture. *J. Cell Biol.,* 58:79–95.

11. Tateishi, J., Kuroda, S., Saito, A., and Otsuki, S. (1972): Neurotoxicity of clioquinol in laboratory animals. *Lancet,* 2:1095.

12. Tateishi, J., Kuroda, S., Saito, A., and Otsuki, S. (1973): Experimental myelo-optic neuropathy induced by clioquinol. *Acta Neuropathol. (Berl.),* 24:304–320.

13. Yamanaka, N., Imanari, T., Tamura, S., and Yagi, K. (1973): Uncoupling of oxidative phosphorylation of rat liver mitochondria by chinoform. *J. Biochem. (Tokyo),* 73:993–998.

14. Yonezawa, T., and Iwanami, H. (1966): An experimental study of thiamine deficiency in nervous tissue, using tissue culture technics. *J. Neuropathol. Exp. Neurol.,* 25:362–372.

15. Yonezawa, T., Norman, R., Iwanami, H., and Nakatani, Y. (1971): Studies on the neuromuscular junction *in vitro. Adv. Nerve Res.,* 15:689.

Neurotoxicology, edited by L. Roizin, H. Shiraki, and N. Grčević. Raven Press, New York © 1977.

Neuronal Storage Dystrophy in Chronic Chloroquine Intoxication

Georg W. Klinghardt

Max-Planck-Institute for Brain Research, Department of Neuropathology, Frankfurt/Main, Federal Republic of Germany

Chloroquine (Resochin®) was first synthesized by Andersag et al. (5) in 1939 and is structurally related to quinacrine (Atebrin®), pamaquine (Plasmochin®), and Plasmocid®. From 1947 and for more than one decade the drug remained the most customary of the group of halogenated aminoquinoline antimalarials. When chloroquine-resistant malaria appeared, the main medical indications had already changed since the drug had been proved an anti-inflammatory substance. Chloroquine is very effective in chronic rheumatoid arthritis, in several other rheumatic diseases, and in some further groups of disease largely unrelated to malaria, such as photoallergic reactions in porphyria cutanea tarda, rosacea, and lichen ruber planus.

The therapeutic effect of chloroquine in rheumatic diseases requires high doses for several months or years. This chronic treatment led to the first observations of side effects in man, particularly in the nervous and muscular systems. All these complications of therapy are avoidable if the physician is careful. These undesirable side effects were, however, the starting point of very informative experimental model diseases (13,20,21). Some have proved closely related to natural storage diseases in man and in animals, affecting predominantly the nervous system and

mostly reducible to various inborn lysosomal enzyme defects.

These experimental model diseases and the corresponding clinical side effects may be predominantly the result of biochemical principles that are essentials of the therapeutic effects of chloroquine. This permits well-established interpretations of type and systemic selectivity of nerve cell changes occurring in chronic experimental chloroquine intoxication.

Of the intermediary mechanisms that are the basis of the pharmacodynamics of chloroquine, some may be of rather negligible and some of particular significance in the etiology and distribution of these toxic model effects. Chloroquine forms molecular complexes with DNA and inhibits DNA-dependent nucleic acid polymerase reactions *in vivo* (10). The intercalating binding of the drug to plasmodial DNA inhibits DNA synthesis in malaria schizonts, more so since chloroquine concentration in parasitized erythrocytes is much higher than in blood plasma (27). There is a reversible binding of the drug to hemoglobin (30) as is the case with some other pigments. The unlimited accumulation of chloroquine in the muscular system (15) may be the result of a reversible binding to myoglobin, as proved for quinacrine (21). Myoglobin contents and protein metabolism of type I fibers are the highest of all muscle fiber types (8) and are obviously essential conditions for the predominant affect of tonic muscle fibers (35) and red muscles (21) in chloroquine myopathy. Reversible binding of the drug to melanin is essential for changes in skin and mucous membrane pigmentation seen in man. This is the cause of drug storage in pigmented ocular tissues, especially in the chorioid of pigmented animals (6) and in man (24).

Some different pharmacodynamic aspects of chloroquine are of particular importance for an etiological explanation of the experimental neuronal storage dystrophy. The substance is one of the best investigated in the group of lysosomotropic chemotherapeutic agents (11). These drugs are accumulated selectively in lysosomes, and their pharmacological, therapeutic, toxic, and pathogenetic effects largely depend on this property. Accumulation of chloroquine in the lysosome-like autophagic vesicle and impairment of the digestive capacity of this parasite organelle were early suggested to be one of the decisive factors of the antimalarial effect of chloroquine (2,3, 28,39). The antiinflammatory effect in rheumatic diseases is also attributed to drug accumulation in lysosomes and to the dose-dependent membrane-stabilizing effect especially proved in lysosomes in many pharmacological experiments (2,4, 40). Isopycnic fractionation studies in fibroblast cultures showed that within the cells chloroquine was concentrated in the lysosomes (41). Autoradiographic studies indicated incorporation of tritium-labeled chloroquine into lysosomal residual bodies (32). Biochemical investigations in tissue cultures showed reduction of different lysosomal enzyme functions by the drug. Chloroquine is a very effective inhibitor of cathepsin B_1, a lysosomal enzyme (41). Mucopolysaccharide degradation (25) and proteolytic degradation of low-density lipoprotein (14), which also occur within

lysosomes, were prevented by exposure of the cells to the drug. These findings correspond to the variety of electron microscopical types of residual bodies (19) that substantiate the toxic neuronal storage dystrophy.

Chloroquine belongs to a group of modern chemotherapeutic agents possessing an amphophilic character (26) due to a water-repelling group in the molecule represented by aromatic rings and to a water-attracting group represented by a side chain containing a nitrogen atom protonized at physiological pH. Pharmacokinetic investigations point to various phospholipids as preferred binding sites of these drugs (33,34). This probably means a changing of the substrate character of these substances for lysosomal enzymes of regular phospholipid degradation (26). Many of these drugs are capable of inducing phospholipidosis. Chloroquine, however, is obviously the most lysosomotropic and the most effective in impairing lysosomal digestion and in producing storage of residual bodies of a different type. The quinoline derivative clioquinol contains no side chain and is not amphophilic.

Intensity and progression of experimental neuronal changes due to chloroquine depend on duration and dosage, the latter exceeding by far the therapeutic range. The pronounced lesion of ganglion cells may be due to the fact that such metabolic disturbance is rather damaging to a cell population that cannot be renewed by cell division.

The type of the experimental nerve cell affect was most distinctly realized in sensory posterior root ganglion cells. Expanded perikarya (cell bodies) and axon balloonings in ganglia and posterior roots as well as in subsequent segments of the spinal cord were caused by amassments of membranous cytoplasmic bodies (MCB). In rats and pigs these were mostly arranged in concentric layers; in rabbits, however,

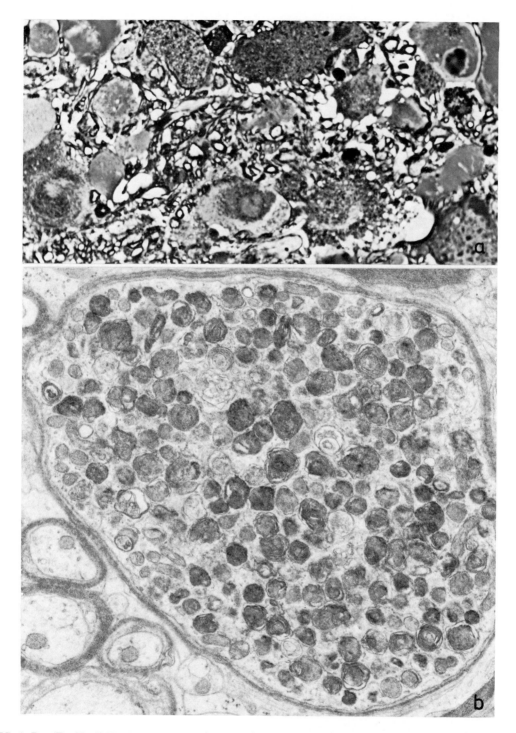

FIG. 1. Rat (Ex.-Nr.6252), 275 days of chloroquine (2.0 g/kg food). Nucleus gracilis. Glutaraldehyde fixation (perfusion), Epon. **a:** Many terminal axon balloonings mostly containing granular material equally distributed or arranged in a center and halos of different density. Myelin sheaths poor and disrupted or not distinguishable. *p*-phenylenediamine staining. Phase contrast. ×700. **b:** Granular storage material in a terminal ballooning consists of membranous cytoplasmic bodies (MCBs) of the concentric type in rather irregular membrane arrangement and in free or membrane-bound floccular material, several mitochondria, and tubular profiles. Staining according to Reynolds. ×20,000.

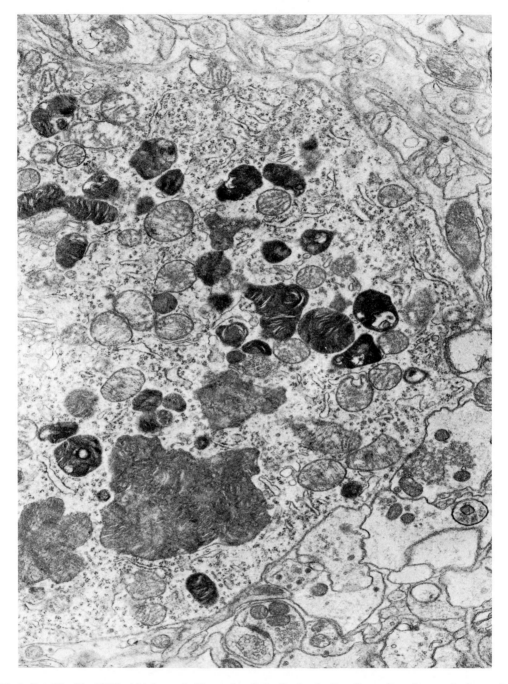

FIG. 2. Rat (Ex.-Nr. 5991), 154 days of chloroquine (2.0 g/kg food). Ganglion cell perikaryon in the nucleus gracilis containing several MCBs of different shape and size. Lamellar arrangement mostly similar to the pattern of "zebra bodies" in contrast to the concentric type in the neighboring terminal axon balloonings. Glutaraldehyde fixation, Epon. Contrast staining according to Reynolds. ×17,500.

they were arranged similarly to the pattern in zebra bodies. Another local accentuation of the nerve cell process was established in the axon terminals. There were many more axon balloonings than appropriate for age within the nucleus gracilis, and they were of enormous expansions. Characteristic balloonings also contained amassments of light microscopical granules often arranged in a "spiked ball" figure or showing a center and some halos of different granular density. In rats the granules in this location consisted of membranes arranged in rather irregular concentric layers or in dense fine granular or floccular material likewise surrounded by unit membranes (Fig. 1). The perikarya of the adjacent ganglion cells contained in contrast, if at all, only few MCB arranged in the manner of "zebra bodies" (Fig. 2).

Peripheral terminal axon manifestations of the storage dystrophy of sensory posterior root ganglion cells were evident in muscle spindles. In rats considerable dark blue granular balloonings were demonstrated by Baker's acid hematein test but only in sensory endings. The enlargement of the annulospiral terminations showed a beaded pattern also seen in Bodian's silver impregnations. Similar changes were established in amaurotic idiocy in man (23). The storage material in the experimental annulospiral balloonings consisted of abundant membranous and several rather floccular cytoplasmic bodies among mitochondria and different types of cell organelles (Fig. 3). Axon balloonings in the optic fascicle, lateral geniculate body, and anterior colliculus of rats proved the neuronal nature of the storage dystrophy of the inner ganglion cell layer in chloroquine retinopathy.

Similar to findings in amaurotic idiocy (9,22), there were also axon balloonings in peripheral motor nerve fiber endings. Preterminal axon enlargements in rats consisted of accumulations of rather irregularly arranged MCBs of the concentric type. This type of storage body was rarely seen within the axon terminals themselves. Instead, there were amassments of interconnecting tubular profiles among or in place of the synaptic vesicles as described in infantile neuroaxonal dystrophy (16,17). In this context it should be mentioned that chloroquine decreases the firing index at the endplate and eventually blocks neuromuscular transmission in nerve–muscle preparations of the frog and cat at tissue concentrations reached by therapeutic doses (7,38).

The storage regions in perikarya of posterior root nerve cells were characterized histochemically by abundant phospholipids (acid hematein test) and by a PAS-positive but water-soluble fraction (cryostat technique) of the storage material. The latter two properties are also observed in gangliosides (see Addendum).

The main purpose of this chapter is to analyze the type of ganglion cell lesion produced by the experimental intoxication. The morphological changes largely resemble the process first defined by Schaffer (32) and by Spielmeyer (36). In rats and rabbits this was by far most pronounced in posterior root and trigeminal ganglion cells. In pigs however, these changes were also very spectacular in the central nervous system. The blood-brain barrier for chloroquine is most probably less effective in this species than in rats and rabbits.

In the following, some pecularities in the distribution of lesions disclosed in the central nervous system in miniature pigs, type Göttingen, are outlined. These pigs are crossbreeds between the Vietnamese and the Minnesota miniature pig.

In contrast to the pattern of lesions in comparable natural storage diseases in man (12), considerable storage dystrophy was seen in many regions of the allocortex but none in the isocortex. There were clear differences among different fields and cell groups especially in Ammon's horn. No

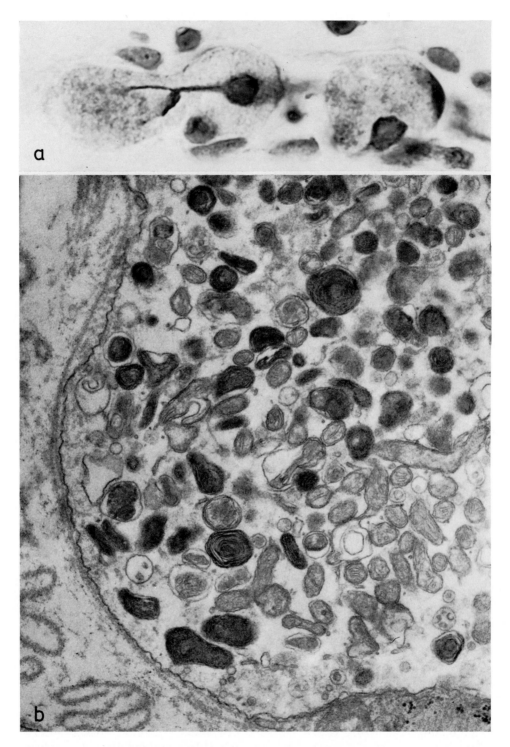

FIG. 3. a: Rat (Ex.-Nr. 5488), 159 days chloroquine (2.0 g/kg food). Beaded axon ballooning of the annulospiral ending. Granular contents of the axon enlargements (courtesy of J. Schliep from his M.D. thesis). M. lumbricalis, Bodain impregnation. ×17,500. **b:** Rat (Ex.-Nr. 5655), 136 days of chloroquine (2.0 g/kg food). Cross section of a ballooned primary sensory axon ending in a muscle spindle (m. lumbricalis). The axon contains, in the main, several MCBs of the concentric type, floccular material, small mitochondria, and vesicles of different size. Glutaraldehyde fixation (perfusion), Epon. Contrast staining according to Reynolds. ×33,000.

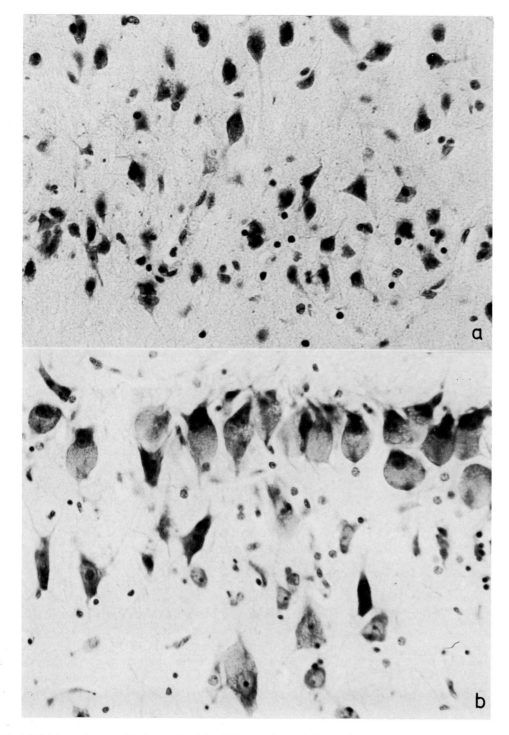

FIG. 4. Miniature pig, type Göttingen (Ex.-Nr. 6369), 142 days of chloroquine (2.0 g/kg food). Isocortex (**a**) and allocortex (**b**) on opposite sides of the fissura rhinalis. The isocortical side (**a**) exhibits no storage dystrophy in all laminae (here lamina 2 and 3); several ganglion cells are rather shrunken (formol immersion fixation). In the less differentiated allocortex (**b**) strong storage dystrophy of ganglion cells especially in the upper lamina pyramidalis is evident. Kresylviolet staining. **a:** ×450. **b:** × 400.

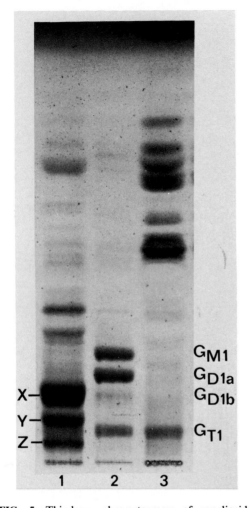

FIG. 5. Thin-layer chromatograms of ganglioside fractions from posterior root ganglia of miniature pigs, type Göttingen. Preparation of the ganglioside fractions as described by Hoffmann and Schneck (18). No. 1 shows posterior root ganglia material from chloroquine-intoxicated animal. No. 2 shows a ganglioside mixture from bovine brain containing G_{M1}, G_{D1a}, G_{D1b}, and G_{T1} (Koch-Light Laboratories). No. 3 shows posterior root ganglia material from a control pig. Adsorbent: silica gel G-60 plates from Merck. Solvent system: chloroform/methanol/2.5 N ammonia solution 60/40/9 (v/v). The lipid spots (X, Y, and Z) were visualized by anisaldehyde/sulfuric acid/acetic acid spray.

however, all perikarya were considerably ballooned. Field h3 contained only a few ganglion cells affected to a moderate degree. Fields h2 and h1 were conspicuous by storage dystrophy of many ganglion cells in the stratum oriens exclusively. The subicular cortex contained many dystrophic nerve cells, whereas in the presubicular cortex all ganglion cell perikarya were strongly ballooned due to the storage process. This degree of storage dystrophy, including several degenerated ganglion cells and satellite cells containing storage material, was seen in the entire allocortical band in all sections in frontal plains showing the fissura rhinalis. The isocortical band on the opposite side of the fissura exhibited no neuronal storage dystrophy (Fig. 4). Another striking finding was the considerable neuronal storage dystrophy in the induseum griseum and of a few cells in the fifth layer of the adjacent posterior granular cortex of the gyrus cinguli. The latter may indicate the mesocortical nature of this zone.

In the diencephalon, neuronal storage dystrophy was most pronounced in the nuclei paraventriculares and supraoptici and in the corpus mamillare. In the medulla oblongata, neighboring nuclei were affected in very different degrees. Neuronal storage dystrophy was very spectacular in several sensory nuclei, such as the nucleus vestibularis lateralis (Deiters). A moderate degree was seen in the nucleus originis nervi hypoglossi, and no storage dystrophy was established in the nucleus dorsalis nervi vagi, in the nucleus nervi abducens, and in several other motor nuclei. These histopathological differences certainly reflect premorbid metabolic differences of these ganglion cell nuclei.

Neuronal storage dystrophy in chronic chloroquine intoxication is up to now the most informative model of the type of nerve cell lesion noted in amaurotic idiocy and in various other natural storage diseases due to inborn lysosomal enzyme defects. In

storage dystrophy was seen in cells of the fascia dentata. In Rose's field h5 (29), which is known to contain different cell types, only a few ganglion cells exhibited distinct storage dystrophy. In field h4, general, the neuronal systems most severely affected in experimental intoxication may have the highest number of lysosomes and the highest lysosomal metabolism under normal conditions. Moreover the model disease offers possibilities about where different modern chemotherapeutics, related to chloroquine and of amphophilic character, may attack the central nervous system.

ADDENDUM

B. Pallmann and K. Sandhoff (Max-Planck Institute for Psychiatry, Department of Neurochemistry, Munich) were kind enough to investigate biochemically posterior root ganglia material of our miniature pigs, type Göttingen. A fivefold increase in the total amount of gangliosides without any change in other lipids was established in experimental animals. Thin-layer analysis of the ganglioside fraction (Fig. 5) revealed an increase in the amount of three lipids up to now not exactly identified. They are orcin positive and behave like gangliosides in various solvent systems. Densitometric analysis of sulfuric acid-charred thin-layer plates (18,31) showed a more than 25-fold increase of substance X. Substances Y and Z could not be quantified and are probably minor components of normal tissue.

REFERENCES

1. Abraham, R., Hendy, R., and Grasso, S. (1968): Formation of myeloid bodies after chloroquine administration. *Exp. Mol. Pathol.,* 9:212–229.
2. Aikawa, M., and Beaudoin, R. L. (1969): Effects of chloroquine on the morphology of erythrocytic stages of plasmodium gallinaceum. *Am. J. Trop. Med. Hyg.,* 18:166–168.
3. Aikawa, M. (1972): High resolution autoradiography of malaria parasites treated with ³H-chloroquine. *Am. J. Pathol.,* 67:277–284.
4. Allison, A. C., and Young, M. R. (1964): Uptake of dyes and drugs by living cells in culture. *Life Sci.,* 3:1407–1414.
5. Andersag, H., Breitner, S., and Jung, H. (1939): Verfahren zur Darstellung von in 4-Stellung basisch substituierte Aminogruppen enthaltenden Chinolinverbindungen. *Ger. Pat.,* 683–692.
6. Bernstein, H., Zvaifler, N., Rubin, M., and Mansour, A. M. (1963): The ocular deposition of chloroquine. *Invest. Ophthalmol.,* 2:384–392.
7. Chinyanga, H. M., Vartanian, G. A., Okai, E. A., and Greenberger, D. V. (1972): Chloroquine-induced depression of neuromuscular transmission. *Eur. J. Pharmacol.,* 18:256–260.
8. Citoler, P., Beniter, L., and Maurer, W. (1967): Autoradiographische Untersuchung der Protein-Synthese in roten und weissen Muskelfasern. *Exp. Cell Res.,* 45:195–205.
9. Clement, R., Gruner, J., Rameix, P., and Bretagne, J. (1953): Idiotie amaurotique de Tay-Sachs. *Presse Med.,* 61:253–255.
10. Cohen, S. N., and Yielding, K. L. (1965): Inhibition of DNA and RNA polymerase reactions by chloroquine. *Proc. Natl. Acad. Sci. USA,* 54:521–527.
11. De Duve, C., De Barsy, T., Poole, B., Trouet, A., Tulkens, P., and Van Hoof, F. (1974): Lysosomotropic agents. *Biochem. Pharmacol.,* 23:2495–2530.
12. Escolá, J. (1961): Über die Prozessausbreitung der amaurotischen Idiotie im Zentralnervensystem in verschiedenen Lebensaltern und Besonderheiten der Spätform gegenüber der Pigmentatrophie. *Arch. Psychiatr. Z. Ges. Neurol.,* 202:95–112.
13. Gleiser, C. A., Bay, W. W., Dukes, T. W., Brown, R. S., Read, W. K., and Pierce, K. R. (1968): Study on chloroquine toxicity and a drug-induced cerebrospinal lipodystrophy in swine. *Am. J. Pathol.,* 53:27–45.
14. Goldstein, J. L., Brunschede, G. Y., and Brown, M. S. (1975): Inhibition of proteolytic degradation of low density lipoprotein in human fibroblasts by chloroquine, concanavalin A, and triton WR 1339. *J. Biol. Chem.,* 250:7854–7862.
15. Grundmann, M., Mikulikova, I., and Vrublovski, P. (1972): Tissue distribution of chloroquine in rats in the course of long-term application. *Arch. Int. Pharmacodyn.,* 197:45–52.
16. Hedley-Whyte, E. T., Gilles, F. H., and Uzman, B. G. (1968): Infantile neuroaxonal dystrophy: A disease characterized by altered terminal axons and synaptic endings. *Neurology (Minneap.),* 18:891–906.
17. Herman, M. M., Huttenlocher, P. R., and Bensch, K. G. (1969): Electron microscopic observations in infantile neuroaxonal dystrophy. *Arch. Neurol.,* 20:19–34.
18. Hoffmann, L. M., and Schneck, L. (1975): Methodology: Sphingolipid analysis. In: *The Gangliosidoses,* edited by B. W. Volk and L. Schneck, pp. 223–232. Plenum Press, New York.
19. Klinghardt, G. W. (1974): Experimentelle Schädigung von Nervensystem und Muskulatur durch Chlorochin: Modelle verschiedenartiger Speicherdystrophien. *Acta Neuropathol. (Berl.),* 28:117–141.
20. Klinghardt, G. W. (1975): Chloroquine intoxication: A model of storage dystrophy. *Proc. 7th Int.*

Congr. Neuropathol., pp. 221–224. Excerpta Medica, Amsterdam.

21. Klinghardt, G. W., and Thomas, E. (1970): Experimental myoneuropathy by certain drugs of 8-amino quinoline type. In: *Proc. 6th Int. Congr. Neuropathol.,* Paris, pp. 1076–1077.

22. Krücke, W. (1959): Histologie der Polyneuritis und Polyneuropathie. *Dtsch. Z. Nervenheilk.,* 180:1–39.

23. Krücke, W., and Önol, B. (1968): Zur Histopathologie der peripheren Neurone bei amaurotischer Idiotie. *Zbl. Ges. Neurol. Psychiatr.,* 191: 133.

24. Lawwill, T., Appleton, B., and Altstatt, L. (1968): Chloroquine accumulation in human eyes. *Am. J. Ophthalmol.,* 65:530–532.

25. Lie, S. O., and Schofield, B. (1973): Inactivation of lysosomal function in normal cultured human fibroblasts by chloroquine. *Biochem. Pharmacol.,* 22:3109–3114.

26. Lüllmann, H., Lüllmann-Rauch, R., and Wassermann, O. (1973): Arzneimittel-induzierte Phospholipidspeicherkrankheit. *Dtsch. Med. Wochenschr.,* 98:1616–1625.

27. Macomber, P. B., Sprinz, H., and Tousimis, A. J. (1967): Morphological effects of chloroquine on plasmodium berghei in mice. *Nature,* 214:937–939.

28. Macomber, P. B., O'Brien, R. L., and Hahn, F. E. (1966): Chloroquine: physiological basis of drug resistance in plasmodium berghei. *Science,* 152: 1374–1375.

29. Rose, M. (1927): Der Allocortex bei Tier und Mensch. *J. Psychol. Neurol.,* 34:1–112.

30. Rubin, M., Zvaifler, N., Bernstein, H., and Mansour, A. (1965): Chloroquine toxicity. *Proc. 2nd Int. Pharmacol. Mtg., Prague 1963,* Vol. 4, pp. 467–486. Oxford University Press, Oxford.

31. Sandhoff, K., Harzer, K., and Jatzkewitz, H. (1968): Densitometrische Mikrobestimmung von Gangliosiden aus dem Gesamtlipidextrakt nach Dünnschichtchromatographie. *Hoppe Seylers Z. Physiol. Chem.,* 349:283–287.

32. Schaffer, K. (1905): cited by Spielmeyer, W. (1929). Unpublished.

33. Seiler, K. U., and Wassermann, O. (1975): Drug-induced phospholipidosis. *Naunyn Schmiedebergs Arch. Pharmacol.,* 288:261–268.

34. Seydel, J. K., and Wassermann, O. (1973): NMR-studies on the molecular basis of drug-induced phospholipidosis. *Naunyn Schmiedebergs Arch. Pharmacol.,* 279:207–210.

35. Smith, B., and O'Grady, G. (1966): Experimental chloroquine myopathy. *Neurol. Neurosurg. Psychiatr.,* 29:255–258.

36. Spielmeyer, W. (1929): Vom Wesen des anatomischen Prozesses bei der familiären amaurotischen Idiotie. *J. Psychol. Neurol.,* 38:120–133.

37. Tischner, K., and Fischer, H. A. (1975): Uptake of tritium labelled chloroquine into organized cultures of rat spinal ganglia. *Acta Neuropathol. (Berl.),* 32:353–357.

38. Vartanian, G. A., and Chinyanga, H. M. (1972): The mechanism of acute neuromuscular weakness induced by chloroquine. *Can. J. Physiol. Pharmacol.,* 50:1099–1103.

39. Warhurst, D. C., and Hockley, D. J. (1967): Mode of action of chloroquine on plasmodium berghei and P. cynomolgi. *Nature,* 214:935–936.

40. Weissmann, G. (1964): Labilization and stabilization of lysosomes. *Fed. Proc.,* 23:1038–1044.

41. Wibo, M., and Poole, B. (1974): Protein degradation in cultured cells. II. The uptake of chloroquine by rat fibroblasts and the inhibition of cellular protein degradation and cathepsin B_1. *J. Cell Biol.,* 63:430–440.

Neurotoxicology, edited by L. Roizin, H. Shiraki, and N. Grčević. Raven Press, New York © 1977.

Hexachlorophene Neurotoxicity

H. C. Powell and *P. W. Lampert

*Pathology Laboratories (Neuropathology) of the Massachusetts General Hospital, and the Department of Pathology, Harvard Medical School, Boston, Massachusetts 02115; and the *Department of Pathology, University of California, San Diego, La Jolla, California 92093*

Since it first became commercially available in 1945, hexachlorophene (HCP) has been one of the most widely used germicidal agents. Although found in products ranging from antiperspirants and toothpastes to furnace-filters, its most common use in the home and in hospitals is as a 3% emulsion (pHisoHex®, Winthrop), available since 1949 (19).

Chemical Properties and Development of HCP

HCP is a bisphenol [2,2′methylenebis (3,4,6-trichlorophenol)] (Fig. 1). It is a colorless, odorless, crystalline, nonvolatile compound that in insoluble in water, glycerine, or mineral oil but very soluble in ethyl alcohol and acetone. It emerged after a long search for a chemical agent to replace phenol, the first surgical disinfectant. In 1906 Bechhold and Ehrlich (5) found that a more effective antibacterial compound could be prepared by chemically linking two phenol molecules. When chlorine atoms were added to the phenol moieties, their germicidal properties were especially improved. In 1927 a group of industrial chemists in Germany studied this range of compounds in order to find an antimildew preparation. Their search led to the first patenting of a bisphenol in 1929. Two years later Dunning et al. (13) observed that growth of *Staphylococcus aureus* could be inhibited by thiobisphenols. HCP, which was first synthetized in 1939 (19), has the advantage of being easy to prepare commercially. Since it is insoluble in water, an emulsified form (pHisoHex®) was developed for topical use.

Correlation of Chemical Properties with Biologic Activity

The principal reasons that HCP is so effective against bacteria are its (a) lipid solubility, (b) chelative properties, and (c) interaction of hydroxyl and halogen groups with enzymes and structural proteins.

Lipid Solubility

Since the bisphenols are very lipid soluble, they are easily adsorbed by cell walls containing a high proportion of lipid. This property is closely related to its antibacterial effect (3). Once in the cell membrane, HCP interferes with structural and enzymic proteins causing a permeability change that

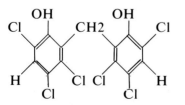

FIG. 1. Hexachlorophene 2,2′ methylene-bis (3,4,6-trichlorophenol).

allows essential cellular constituents to leak through the cell membrane, leading to cytolysis. The observations are pertinent to HCP neurotoxicity since the myelin sheath consists of a multilamellar, spirally arranged, membranous structure that is rich in lipid and protein.

Chelative Properties

Metal chelation appears to be a key antimicrobial property (1), and by chelating with copper and other metals HCP can inactivate metal-containing enzymes such as the cytochromes. Furthermore, metals liberated from protein molecules can have a toxic effect independent of the drug (22).

Interaction of Hydroxyl and Halogen Groups with Enzymes and Structural Proteins

The chlorinated bisphenols exert their effect on protein in two ways: first, they combine with thiol groups (-SH), and, second, the halogens combine with amino groups (-NH$_2$) forming chloramines. As well as denaturing structural protein, HCP can interfere with respiration by interaction with enzymes. Micromolar doses *in vitro* have been shown to uncouple oxidative phosphorylation (8). In summary, HCP acts by adsorption to the cell surface, alteration of membrane permeability, leakage of cell contents, and progressive loss of function leading eventually to death of the cells.

Absorption Metabolism and Excretion of HCP

Absorption Studies

Absorption studies with radioactive ^{14}C-labeled HCP on the skin of depilated rats showed that when HCP is applied to the body surface it is retained by the skin (41).

Once appropriate chemical techniques were developed (7) it became apparent that repeated use of HCP on the skin can lead to significant quantities in the blood stream (11,16). Blood levels of HCP recorded in infants after repeated bathing approach mean blood levels that are sufficient to produce neuropathologic changes in rats (11). Furthermore, blood levels reported in two premature infants (26,30) are equivalent to levels in rats at which spongiform changes of the myelin consistently developed.

Metabolism and Excretion

Following oral administration to rats and mice (25), HCP is incompletely absorbed and metabolized to a marked degree. The highest tissue concentrations at 24 hr are in the liver and the blood, respectively. In these animals, HCP is conjugated to glucuronide (35) and excreted in feces. In the rabbit, one-third of a given dose is excreted in the urine (46).

HCP TOXICITY: EXPERIMENTAL STUDIES

Animal Intoxication by HCP

Current interest in HCP neurotoxicity started in 1970 when scientists at the Food and Drug Administration noted that HCP was being used as a fungicide on fruit and other foods and began a series of oral subacute toxicity studies using adult rats (24). These animals were fed 25 mg/kg daily of HCP in their diet. After 2 weeks the rats showed weakness in the hindquarters progressing to paralysis in 3 to 5 weeks (24). The mean blood level in HCP-intoxicated rats on this regimen was 1.21 mg/ml (10). Microscopic examination of the central nervous system (CNS) revealed spongiform degeneration of the white matter. In an attempt to simulate clinical use of HCP in infants, newborn rhesus monkeys were washed each day with 3% HCP for 5 min and were then rinsed and dried (30). The mean blood level of HCP was 1.5 mg/ml at the end of the first week. Microscopic sections from the brains showed spongiform degeneration in the white matter of treated animals but not in controls.

Autopsy Findings

There was generalized reduction in muscle mass, fatty liver was sometimes observed, and cerebral swelling was always present. There was no staining of CNS parenchyma by Trypan blue dye injected premortem, showing that the blood-brain barrier is not affected by HCP. On sectioning the brains the corpus callosum in affected animals appeared larger than in controls, the ventricles were reduced in size, and optic tracts appeared flattened and swollen. Chemical assay showed that the HCP-intoxicated brains had significantly increased water content (27). Light micro-

scopic examination showed severe spongiform alteration of the white matter (Fig. 2). Frozen sections also showed severe spongiform alteration of the white matter indicating that the vacuolar changes of white matter are not an artifact of formalin-fixed autopsy tissue. In sections from araldite-embedded tissue that were stained with paraphenylene diamine, the myelinated axons were separated by clear spaces that occurred within myelin lamellae. In the control animals, however, the white matter contained closely packed myelinated axons (27).

Electron Microscopy

Electron microscopic examination confirmed the presence of wide intralamellar spaces within myelin sheaths (Fig. 3). These spaces developed after splits in the minor dense lines of compact sheaths. Oligodendrocytes appeared normal. Some astrocytes showed cytoplasmic swelling without increase in their mitochondrial

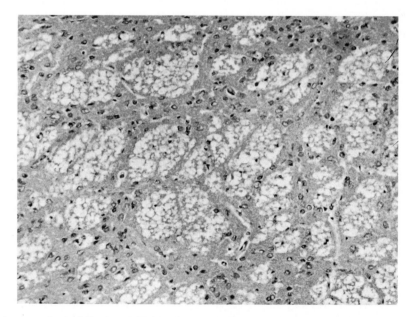

FIG. 2. Adult mouse brain following HCP intoxication. Striking status spongiosus is apparent in white matter tracts in the corpus striatum whereas the adjacent gray matter is uninvolved. Klüver-Barrera stain. ×250.

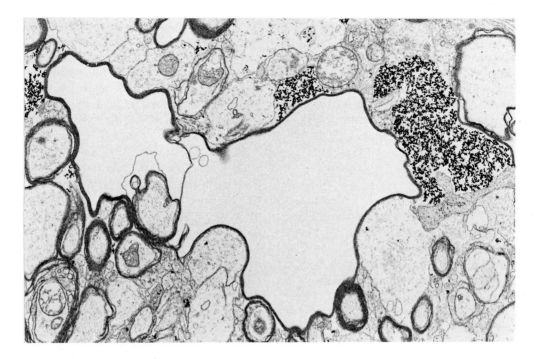

FIG. 3. HCP-intoxicated adult mouse brain 6 hr after intracerebral injection of thorium dioxide suspension (Thorotrast®). Note wide intralamellar spaces in the myelin sheath. The thorium dioxide suspension has accumulated in the extracellular spaces but does not penetrate the myelin sheath. ×75,000.

population. Mitochondrial morphology appeared generally unchanged, although focal swelling of the mitochondria was observed in some axons. Endothelial cells revealed normal tight junctions. In some animals with HCP neurotoxicity the electron-dense tracer thorium oxide suspension (Thorotrast®) was injected intracerebrally 6 hr prior to sacrifice (38). In these animals electron microscopy showed the tracer distributed within the extracellular space (Fig. 3), which was enlarged in severely affected animals. The tracer was frequently seen in heavy concentrations adjacent to the affected myelin lamellae (Fig. 3). The fact that the tracer did not penetrate the myelin sheath, even when marked intramyelinic splitting was evident, suggests that the myelin sheaths remain intact, allowing only edema fluid to pass through the myelin lamellae. One would expect this to occur in a dis-order where active energy-bound ion and water transport were inhibited and a change in membrane permeability occurred. A possible mechanism for part of this is inhibition of membrane-bound adenosine triphosphatase (ATPase) (2). Jellinger and Seitelberger (23) note that inhibition of this membrane-bound enzyme system has been observed in a variety of experimental forms of cerebral edema where there is no permeability change in the blood-brain barrier, save in advanced stages. HCP is known to uncouple oxidative phosphorylation (8), which may be important since the ion-transport membrane-bound ATPase system is especially active in the brain (6) and is particularly increased during neonatal maturation (40). However, this type of ion-transport defect may not be sufficient to account for the massive intramyelinic edema much of which may be due to a direct effect of HCP on structural proteins in the myelin sheath. Such an alteration has been suggested in reports describing red cell membrane injury by HCP (33). Miller and Buhler (33) stated that hemolysis caused by HCP was due to direct alteration in permeability of the erythrocyte membrane, that this was a dose-dependent injury, and that the rate of hemolysis and K^+ efflux was much greater than would be expected from a selective inhibition of ion-transport enzymes.

Peripheral nerves

Identical changes take place in peripheral myelin (38,43) (Fig. 4). HCP produced segmental demyelination in peripheral nerve and abnormalities at the node of Ranvier (43). Electrophysiologic studies showed reduced motor conduction velocities in the sciatic nerves (12).

Biochemic Observations in HCP Neurotoxicity

Three chemical abnormalities have been described in the CNS in HCP intoxication: (a) increased water content (9,27), (b) diminution of the chloroform-methanol-insoluble fraction, and (c) appearance of material that floats on a 0.32-M sucrose gradient (9). Diminution of chloroform-methanol-insoluble material in the brains of rats fed HCP represents a loss of approximately 10% of brain dry weight, and when HCP was removed from the diet some resynthesis of lost material occurred. The floating fraction identified on 0.32-M sucrose is similar to a fraction described in triethyltin (TET) intoxication. TET produces identical spongiform changes in the white matter of experimental animals. This fraction contained myelin lipids and proteins. No abnormalities were found during whole brain lipid analysis (9,27). The mye-

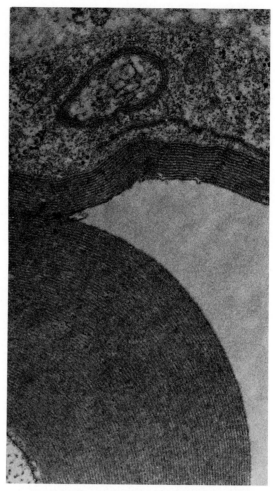

FIG. 4. Electron micrograph of sciatic nerve of HCP-intoxicated adult rat. Splitting of the myelin sheath has occurred, giving rise to a wide intralamellar space. ×180,000.

lin yield from HCP-treated rat nerve was reduced by 39% (36). HCP caused inhibition of whole nerve and myelin protein and lipid synthesis at concentrations as low as 0.5 mg/ml. Radioisotope studies using $(^{35}S)O_4$ showed normal entry of sulfate into nervous tissue but diminished formation of 3′-phosphoadenosine-5′ phosphosulfate—an important intermediary in myelin synthesis (36). When *Xenopus* tadpoles were exposed to radioactive ^{14}C-labeled HCP, the myelin fraction was subsequently found to have double the specific activity of HCP compared to the other fractions (45).

Bithionol and HCP

Bithionol, a germicide of low toxicity (15), is closely related to HCP and is also highly effective against gram-positive cocci such as *Staphylococcus aureus*. Both agents are chlorinated bisphenols, highly lipid-soluble, and are powerful chelators. When adult mice were fed similar quantities of either HCP or bithionol, the HCP-fed animals all developed spongiform myelinopathy whereas the bithionol-treated animals showed no histologic changes in the CNS. Bithionol is not presently used in commercial soaps because of its photosensitivity. Any topical use of this compound would require preparations incorporating photoprotective agents (37).

HUMAN TOXICITY OF HCP

Oral Administration

Reports of four cases of accidental ingestion were presented by Wear et al. in 1962 (44). The patients complained of anorexia, nausea, vomiting, abdominal cramps, and diarrhea, but no neurologic symptoms were described. The author suggested that 2 to

10 g of HCP would be fatal to humans. Lustig (31) described a 6-year-old mentally retarded child who drank 4 to 5 oz of 3% HCP and, despite prompt gastric lavage, became comatose at 15 min and died 9 hr later. Other fatal cases have been described recently (21,32). HCP has been given orally to Chinese patients with clonorchiasis sinensis, and neurologic side effects have been reported following 20 mg/kg daily for 5 to 6 days (29).

Topical Application

The first report of CNS involvement linked to topical toxicity involved a newborn infant that had 3% HCP applied to its skin without being washed off (20). The child later developed twitching of the arms, legs, and face that progressed to convulsions. After several days it recovered. Seizures occurred in a number of patients hospitalized for burns when HCP was applied to their skin (28). Significant amounts of HCP were present in the blood stream of six of these patients (28).

HCP Myelinopathy in Premature Infants

Spongiform changes localized to myelinated tracts (Fig. 5) were reported in seven low-birth-weight infants who had each re-

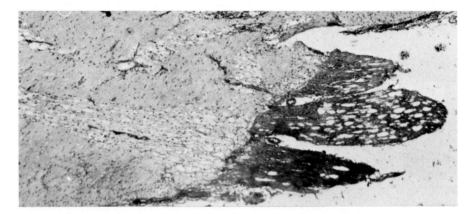

FIG. 5. Section from the brainstem of an affected infant showing pontine tegmentum and the root of the trigeminal nerve. Note status spongiosus in both the white matter and the nerve. Klüver-Barrera stain. ×60.

ceived more than three exposures to HCP (39). The disturbance was not associated with neuronal or glial changes. Electron microscopic examination confirmed the presence of wide separation of myelin lamellae. The lesions are identical to those described in experimental HCP myelinopathy, but they are less extensive because only a few myelinated tracts are present in these low-birth-weight premature infants. In this study by Powell et al. in 1973 (39) and in the more extensive series reported by Shuman et al. in 1974 (42), more mature infants with multiple exposures did not show spongiform myelinopathy. The following factors were thought to contribute to the development of spongiform myelinopathy.

1. Prematurity (gestional ages in affected infants ranged from 26 to 32 weeks)
2. Low birth weight (none of the infants with status spongiosus weighed more than 1,400 g at birth)
3. Number of exposures to HCP. Six of the seven affected infants had nine or more exposures and one infant had only four exposures (39)
4. Dermal rashes, abrasions, or wounds

Acidosis occurred during the illness of the seven reported cases. Many of the infants had hyperbilirubinemia, suggesting hepatic inability to produce adequate amounts of glucuronide. In addition, premature infants are known to have increased skin permeability (34), a factor that is pertinent to the use of topically applied agents. It should be emphasized that in none of the infants studied (39) could the cause of death be ascribed to HCP neurotoxicity. Six out of seven infants with spongiform myelinopathy had massive subependymal cerebral hemorrhage of the kind commonly seen in low-birth-weight premature infants. The remaining infant death was attributed to nonneurologic causes.

Can HCP Be Safely Used?

HCP is of particular value in the neonatal ward where epidemic *Staphylococcal* infection can cause many deaths. In recent years governmental action has restricted the use of HCP. In the United States 3% HCP can only be obtained on prescription (14), and in Britain more stringent restrictions have been applied (4). It is recommended that HCP not be used on low-birth-weight infants (34,42). Three percent HCP should never be applied to burned skin. If HCP is used during wound irrigation, it is recommended that very dilute solutions be used. The risk of introducing HCP into the blood stream during venipuncture can be minimized by prior swabbing with alcohol. Since January, 1973 the following regimen has been followed without untoward effect in the infant nursery at University Hospital of San Diego (17).

1. On admission to the nursery infants are washed in the manner described by Gluck and Wood (18).
2. On the second day the umbilical region only is washed.
3. One day later the infant receives a total body wash in 3% HCP. *Staphylococcal* colonization has been reduced to insignificant proportions when this procedure is applied (17).

ACKNOWLEDGMENT

This study was supported (in part) by USPHS training grant No. 5T1 05393 (Dr. Powell) from the National Institute of Neurological and Communicative Disorders and Stroke.

REFERENCES

1. Adams, J. B. (1958): The mode of action of chlorinated bis-phenols antibacterials. Part I. Metal chelates of hexachlorophene and thiobisdichlorophenol. *J. Pharm. Pharmacol.*, 10: 507–515.

2. Aldridge, W., and Stoner, H. (1963): Oxidative phosphorylation in liver mitochondria from cold acclimated rats. *Biochim. Biophys. Acta*, 78:736–739.

3. Allewala, N., and Riegelman, S. (1954): Phenol coefficients and the Ferguson principle. *J. Am. Pharm. Assoc.*, (Sci. Ed.) 43:93.

4. Announcement (1973): *Lancet*, 1:788.

5. Bechhold, H., and Ehrlich, P. (1906): Beziehung zwischen chemischer Konstitution und Disinfektionswirkung. *Z. Physiol. Chem.*, 47:173–199.

6. Bonting, S. L. (1964): Na-K activated ATPase and active cation transport. In: *Water and Electrolyte Metabolism*, edited by J. DeGraeff, and B. Leijnse, pp. 35–68. Elsevier, Amsterdam.

7. Browning, R., Grego, J., and Warrington, H. (1968): Gas chromatographic determination of hexachlorophene in blood and urine. *J. Pharm. Sci.*, 57:2165.

8. Cammer, W., and Moore, C. L. (1972): The effect of hexachlorophene on the respiration of brain and liver. *Biochem. Biophys. Res. Commun.*, 46:1887–1894.

9. Cammer, W., Rose, A. L., and Norton, W. T. (1975): Biochemical and pathological studies of myelin in hexachlorophene intoxication. *Brain Res.*, 98:547–549.

10. Curley, A., and Hawk, R. E. (1971): Paper. *Presented at the 161st Mtg. Am. Chem. Soc., Div. Pesticide Chemistry, Los Angeles, Calif.*

11. Curley, A., Hawk, R. E., Kimbrough, R. D., Nathenson, G., and Finberg, L. (1971): Dermal absorption of hexachlorophene in infants. *Lancet*, 2:296–297.

12. deJesus, P., and Pleasure, D. (1973): Hexachlorophene neuropathy. *Arch. Neurol.*, 29:180–182.

13. Dunning, F., Dunning, B., and Drake, W. E. (1931): Preparation and bacteriologic study of some organic sulfides. *J. Am. Chem. Soc.*, 53:3466–3469.

14. Food and Drug Administration (1972): Hexachlorophene. *FDA Consumer*, No. 9, 6:24–27.

15. Gleason, M., Gosselin, R., Hodge, H., and Smith, R. P. (1969): *Clinical Toxicology of Commercial Products*, 3rd ed. Williams & Wilkins, Baltimore.

16. Gluck, L. (1973): A perspective on hexachlorophene. *Pediatrics*, 51:400–406.

17. Gluck, L. (1976): Hexachlorophene use in the infant nursery. *(In press.)*

18. Gluck, L., and Wood, H. F. (1961): Effect of an antiseptic skin-care regimen in reducing staphylococcal colonization in newborn infants. *N. Engl. J. Med.*, 265:1177–1181.

19. Gump, W. S., and Walter, G. R. (1968): The bisphenols. In: *Disinfection, Sterilization and Preservation*, edited by C. A. Lawrence and S. S. Block, pp. 257–275. Lea & Febiger, Philadelphia.

20. Harter, W. B. (1959): Hexachlorophene poisoning. *Kaiser F. Med. Bull.*, 7:228.

21. Henry, L. D., and diMaio, V. J. (1974): A fatal case of hexachlorophene poisoning. *Milit. Med.*, 139:41–42.

22. Hugo, W. B. (1967): The mode of action of antibacterial agents. *J. Appl. Bacteriol.*, 30:17–50.

23. Jellinger, K., and Seitelberger, F. (1970): Spongy degeneration of the central nervous system. *Curr. Top. Pathol.*, 53:90–160.

24. Kimbrough, R. D., and Gaines, T. B. (1971): Hexachlorophene effects on the rat brain. *Arch. Environ. Health*, 23:114–118.

25. Kok, K. (1961): Enige onderzoekingen over de lotgevallen van hexachloropeen in het organisne. Communication, *Tweede Federatiere Vergadering van Med. Biol. Verenig., Leiden, March 27, 28.*

26. Kopelman, A. E. (1973): Cutaneous absorption of hexachlorophene in low-birth-weight infants. *J. Pediatr.*, 82:972–975.

27. Lampert, P., O'Brien, J., and Garrett, R. (1973): Hexachlorophene encephalopathy. *Acta Neuropathol. (Berl.)*, 23:326–333.

28. Larson, D. L. (1968): Studies show hexachlorophene causes burn syndrome. *Hospitals*, 42:63–64.

29. Liu, J. (1963): Hexachlorophene in the treatment of Clonorchiasis sinensis. *Chin. Med. J.*, 82:702–711.

30. Lockhart, J. (1972): How toxic is hexachlorophene? *Pediatrics*, 50:229–235.

31. Lustig, R. (1963): A fatal case of hexachlorophene (pHisoHex) poisoning. *Med. J. Aust.*, 50:737.

32. Martinez, A. J., Boehm, R., and Hadfield, M. G. (1974): Acute hexachlorophene encephalopathy: Clinico-neuropathologic correlation. *Acta Neuropathol. (Berl.)*, 28:93–103.

33. Miller, T. L., and Buhler, D. R. (1974): Effect of hexachlorophene on monovalent cation transport in human erythrocytes, a mechanism for hexachlorophene induced hemolysis. *Biochim. Biophys. Acta*, 86–96.

34. Nachman, R. L., and Esterly, N. B. (1971): Increased skin permeability in preterm infants. *J. Pediatr.*, 79:628–632.

35. Pittman, K. A. (1972): *Reports Submitted to Sterling-Winthrop Research Institute, March.*

36. Pleasure, D., Towfighi, J., Silverberg, D., and Parris, J. (1974): The pathogenesis of hexachlorophene neurotoxicity: In vivo and in vitro studies. *Neurology (Minneap.)*, 24:1068–1075.

37. Powell, H., and Lampert, P. (1973): Bithionol, a possible substitute for hexachlorophene. *Pediatrics*, 52:859–861.

38. Powell, H. C., and Lampert, P. W. (1975): Effects of hexachlorophene on the central and peripheral nervous systems. In: *Proc. VIIth Int. Cong. Neuropathol.*, Budapest, 1974. Excerpta Medica, Amsterdam.

39. Powell, H., Swarner, O., Gluck, L., and Lampert, P. (1973): Hexachlorophene myelinopathy in premature infants. *J. Pediatr.*, 82:976–981.

40. Samson, F., and Quinn, D. (1967): $Na^+ - K^+$ activated ATPase in rat brain development. *J. Neurochem.*, 14:421–427.

41. Shemano, I., and Nickerson, M. (1954): Cutaneous accumulation and retention of hexachlorophene-C^{14}. *Fed. Proc.*, 13:404.

42. Shuman, R., Leech, P., and Alvord, E. (1974): Neurotoxicity of hexachlorophene in the human. 1. Clinicopathologic study of 248 children. *Pediatrics,* 54:689–695.
43. Towfighi, J., Gonatas, N. K., and McCree, L. (1974): Hexachlorophene-induced changes in central and peripheral myelinated axons of developing and adult rats. *Lab. Invest.,* 31:712–721.
44. Wear, J. B., Shanahan, R., and Ratlif, R. (1962): Toxicity of ingested hexachlorophene. *J. Am. Med. Assoc.,* 181:587.
45. Webster, H. deF., Ulsamer, A. G., and O'Connell, M. F. (1974): Hexachlorophene induced myelin lesions in the developing nervous system of Xenopus tadpoles: Morphological and biochemical observations. *J. Neuropathol. Exp. Neurol.,* 33:144–163.
46. Wit, J., and Genderen, H. (1962): Some aspects of the fate of hexachlorophene in rabbits, rats and dairy cattle. *Acta Physiol. Pharmacol. Neerl.,* 11:123–132.

Neurotoxicology, edited by L. Roizin, H. Shiraki, and N. Grčević. Raven Press, New York © 1977.

Neurotoxicity of Actinomycin D and Related Inhibitors of RNA Synthesis: The Role of Nuclear Heterochromatinization

Harold Koenig, Rajinder Nayyar, *Panna Sanghavi, *Chung Y. Lu, and *Charles Hughes

Neurology Service, Veterans Administration Lakeside Hospital; and Department of Neurology, Northwestern University Medical School, Chicago, Illinois 60611

Mature neurons and glia feature an active turnover of RNA and protein (15,18) that is of basic importance for the biosynthetic renewal of numerous protein species necessary for normal neural structure and function. It would be expected, therefore, that any substantial interference with RNA synthesis in the nervous system would have profound neurological consequences. We have had a long-standing interest in the neurobiological effects of agents that inhibit RNA synthesis. Early studies in this laboratory explored the metabolic, neurophysiological, and neuropathological effects of certain fluorinated pyrimidines (16,17,19,20) and 6-azapyrimidines (19,20, 23,38). These pyrimidine analogs, when administered intrathecally in small doses to cats, produce striking derangements in central nervous system function. The neurotoxicity of these analogs rests on the capacity of neural cells to convert them into unnatural pyrimidine nucleotides and to block normal RNA synthesis or to elaborate analog-substituted RNAs (19,38).

We subsequently investigated the neurobiological effects of actinomycin D (AMD) and a number of related antibiotics that directly block RNA transcription without affecting pyrimidine metabolism (20–22, 24,27,28). These agents, when administered intrathecally to circumvent the blood-brain barrier, cause interesting neurophysiological disturbances and cytoplasmic lesions similar to those produced by the fluoropyrimidines. An asymptomatic "incubation" period characteristically precedes the development of these disturbances. AMD and antibiotics with similar metabolic effects, e.g., chromomycin A_3, olivomycin, and mithramycin, characteristically produce a condensation of nuclear chromatin as well as nucleolar changes early in the latent period. In correlative biochemical and morphological studies we found that the condensation of diffuse chromatin in neuronal and glial nuclei of AMD-treated tissue develops concomitantly with inhibition of RNA synthesis. Since RNA transcription occurs in diffuse chromatin, but not in dense chromatin (4,25), we reasoned that an AMD-induced heterochromatinization, i.e., conversion of diffuse chromatin to dense chromatin, might play a significant role in the repression of RNA synthesis. Our experiments support this inference.

BIOCHEMICAL AND METABOLIC OBSERVATIONS ON AMD

RNA Synthesis

[³H]AMD, injected intrathecally in cat (Figs. 1 and 2) or intracerebrally in rat

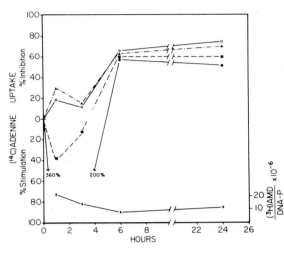

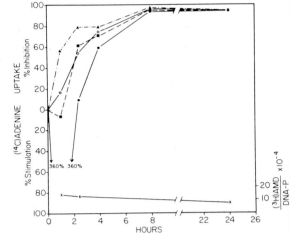

FIG. 1. Effect of [³H]AMD (5 µg) on [¹⁴C]adenine uptake into RNA in subcellular fractions of cat spinal cord as a function of time. At various times after injection of [³H]AMD into the lumbar subarachnoid space, [¹⁴C]adenine was injected via the same route, and the caudal half of the spinal cord was removed under anesthesia. The tissue was homogenized in 0.25 M sucrose and fractionated by differential centrifugation. The acid- and lipid-soluble fractions and RNA were extracted from an aliquot of the homogenate, all fractions were radioassayed for [¹⁴C] and [³H], and RNA and DNA measured by UV spectrophotometry. [¹⁴C]Adenine uptake into RNA was expressed as the relative specific (radio)activity (SA) (equals SA of RNA/SA of acid-soluble fraction) and is here given as % inhibition (or stimulation). The amount of [³H]AMD firmly bound to DNA was computed from the tritium radioactivity of the acid- and lipid-insoluble alkaline hydrolysate of purified nuclear pellets and the known SA of the [³H]AMD. ■——■, Total RNA; ▲—·—▲, nuclear RNA; ○——○, cytoplasmic RNA; ●——●, soluble RNA; X——X, [³H]AMD binding to DNA.

FIG. 2. Effect of [³H]AMD (1 mg) on [¹⁴C]adenine uptake into RNA in subcellular fractions of cat spinal cord as a function of time. Procedures were described in legend to Fig. 1. ■——■, Total RNA; ▲—·—▲, nuclear RNA; ○——○, cytoplasmic RNA; ●——●; soluble RNA; X——X, [³H]AMD binding to DNA.

(Fig. 3) and cat (Fig. 4), inhibits RNA synthesis in spinal cord and brain respectively, as measured by [¹⁴C]adenine or [¹⁴C]uridine uptake. Inhibition proceeded in two stages: (a) an initial rapid inhibition, evident at 30 to 60 min, and (b) a slow inhibition of similar magnitude extending over 6 to 7 hr. [¹⁴C]Adenine incorporation into nuclear and cytoplasmic particulate RNA was inhibited from the beginning, but labeling of the soluble RNA was initially stimulated and later inhibited. In cat cerebrum [¹⁴C]uridine uptake into RNA

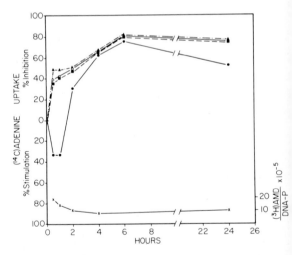

FIG. 3. Effect of [³H]AMD (10 µg) on [¹⁴C]adenine uptake into RNA in subcellular fractions of rat brain as a function of time. At various time intervals after injection of 5 µg of [³H]AMD into each cerebral hemisphere, [¹⁴C]adenine was injected via the same route 30 to 50 min before killing. Further processing was as described in the legend for Fig. 1. ■——■, Total RNA; ▲—·—▲, nuclear RNA; ○——○, cytoplasmic RNA; ●——●, soluble RNA; X——X, [³H]AMD binding to DNA.

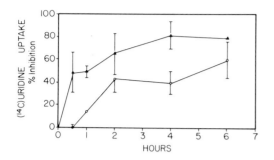

FIG. 4. Effect of [³H]AMD (120 μg) on [¹⁴C]uridine uptake into total RNA of cortex and subcortex of cat cerebrum as a function of time. At various times after injection of 20 μg of [³H]AMD into three separate sites in each cerebral hemisphere, [¹⁴C]uridine was injected into the same sites 15 min before sacrifice. White and gray matter were dissected and processed separately as described in the legend for Fig. 1. O———O, Cortex; ▲———▲, white matter.

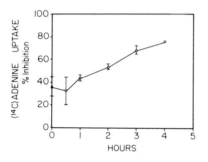

FIG. 5. Effect of varying the time of prior incubation with [³H]AMD on *in vitro* [¹⁴C]adenine uptake into total RNA of rat brain. Rat brain slices were incubated without and with [³H]AMD (5 μg, 2 μCi) for various time intervals in a physiological salt medium in a shaking incubator at 37°C under air. [¹⁴C]Adenine (5 μCi) was added to the reaction mixture 20 min before the reaction was stopped with cold trichloroacetic acid.

(Fig. 4) decreased more rapidly in subcortical white matter than in the overlying cortex. A time-dependent inhibition of RNA synthesis was also observed upon incubating rat brain slices *in vitro* in the presence of [³H]AMD (Fig. 5).

Binding of [³H]AMD

The bulk of [³H]AMD (75 to 80% of the total in rat brain, Table 1) was asso-

ciated with particulates in the various subcellular fractions in the form of acid- or lipid solvent-labile complexes. The residual [³H]AMD was recovered in an acidified alkaline hydrolysate together with RNA. This radioactivity was largely confined to the purified nuclear pellet and probably represents [³H]AMD bound firmly to DNA or to nuclear chromatin (see below). This inference was corroborated by isolating the [³H]AMD–DNA complex from rat brain by zonal centrifugation in a CsCl gradient (3). These procedures gave identical values for the molar ratio of [³H]AMD bound per mole of DNA–P.

The stoichiometry of the [³H]–DNA complex varied with the dose, ranging from 8 to 1,400 μmole of [³H]AMD per mole of DNA–P in cat spinal cord (Figs. 1 and 2), and 80 to 187 μmole of [³H]AMD per mole of DNA–P in rat brain (Fig. 3). In cat cerebrum, gray matter contained 26 to 50 μmole, and white matter 11 to 40 μmole of AMD per mole of DNA–P. It is significant that high molar ratios were present at the earliest intervals tested. *In vitro* studies with purified brain nuclei further indicate that firm binding of AMD to DNA occurs immediately upon addition of the drug.

Autoradiographs of paraffin sections of cat spinal cord made 1 to 8 days after injection of [³H]AMD revealed radioactivity, mainly nuclear in location, in glia, neurons, and other neural cells. In some neurons radioactivity also occurred in the cytoplasm. Neuronal nuclei generally exhibited much more radioactive grains than glial nuclei. Since the nuclear chromatin of neurons is largely in the diffuse or dispersed form and that of glia is largely in a dense form (see below), this suggests that AMD binds more avidly to diffuse chromatin than to dense chromatin *in vivo*. The acid- and lipid solvent-labile [³H]AMD present mostly in the cytoplasmic particulates was evidently extracted during the histological processing.

TABLE 1. *Solubility and distribution of [³H]AMD in subcellular fractions of rat brain*

| | Percent of total [³H]AMD | | | | | | | |
| | Homogenate | | Nuclear | | Cytoplasmic | | Soluble | |
Solubility	1 hr	6 hr	1 hr	6 hr	1 hr	6 hr	1 hr	6 hr
Trichloracetic acid-soluble	15.9	10.1	3.8	3.3	5.6	2.8	6.5	4.0
Lipid-soluble	64.1	64.9	35.6	36.4	22.9	16.8	5.6	11.7
Alkali-soluble	20.0	25.0	18.9	23.8	1.0	1.0	0.1	0.2
Total	100.0	100.0	58.3	63.5	29.5	20.6	12.2	15.9

[³H]AMD (10 μg, 5 μCi, 0.02 ml) was injected intracerebrally 1 and 6 hr before sacrifice. The homogenate was fractionated, the resulting fractions were extracted serially with acid and lipid solvents, and the pooled extracts were counted for tritium.

NUCLEAR CHANGES PRODUCED BY AMD

The ultrastructural and cytochemical changes are largely restricted to the nuclei of neurons and glia during the first 24 hr after AMD injection. Glia and small neurons are generally more rapidly affected than large neurons.

Light Microscopy

The distribution of DNA as seen in Feulgen preparations is congruent with that of nuclear histone, demonstrated by the fast green stain, and with that of chromatin visualized in electron micrographs. Motoneuronal nuclei of control spinal cord contain mostly sparse, fine chromatin granules embedded in a faintly colored nucleoplasm (Fig. 6G). Small spinal neurons possess abundant coarse chromatin particles, whereas medium-sized neurons exhibit an intermediate chromatin pattern. The chromatin of glial cells occurs as discrete coarse masses and as diffusely stained nucleoplasm. In AMD-treated tissues (1 mg) a coarsening of chromatin granules becomes evident in large neurons within 1 to 2 hr, and in glia in less than 30 min. The diffuse nucleoplasmic staining for DNA that represents euchromatin diminishes rapidly and disappears. By 16 to 24

hr all the chromatin of motoneurons is compacted into one or several masses that stain intensely for DNA and histone (Fig. 6H and I). Small neurons and glia exhibit comparable changes within 1 to 2 hr. Nucleoli change more slowly; they are moderately smaller and less basophilic at 4 to 8 hr, and severely shrunken and feebly basophilic by 16 to 24 hr. Two kinds of abnormal nuclear inclusions, often intimately associated, are seen in 1-μm sections of araldite-embedded tissues: (a) dense chromatin clumps that are osmiophilic and intensely basophilic; and (b) spheroidal masses, corresponding to the granular aggregates in electron micrographs, that are osmiophilic and moderately basophilic (Fig. 6J and K). The latter structures may contain lipoproteins, since they stain with Sudan black, as well as with basic and acidic dyes. Moreover, their osmiophilia is reduced by prior delipidation or bromination. These nuclear lesions develop more slowly after a small (5 μg) dose of AMD. Identical changes occur in neural nuclei of AMD-treated rat and cat cerebrum that also were closely correlated with the degree of inhibition of RNA synthesis.

Electron Microscopy

In spinal cord of control cats the large motoneurons of cat spinal cord contain

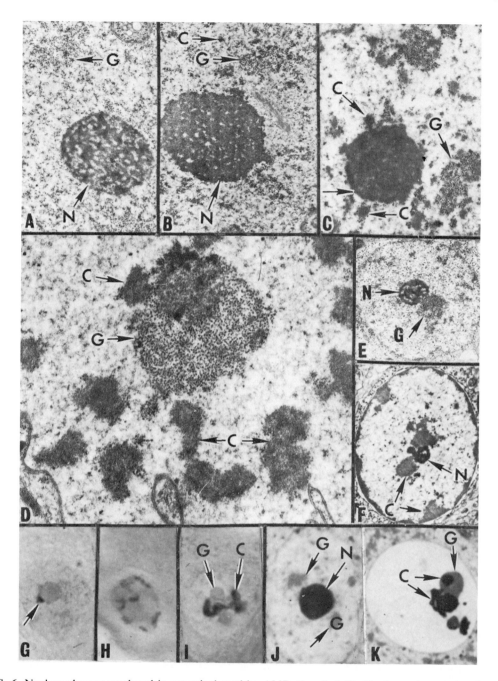

FIG. 6. Nuclear changes produced in cat spinal cord by AMD (1 mg). **A–D:** Electron micrographs of moto-neurons. **A:** Control. ×8,200. **B:** 30 Min. ×3,200. **C:** 4 Hr. ×8,200. **D:** 4 Hr. ×24,000. **E** and **F:** Electron micro-graphs of glia. ×4,500. **E:** Control. **F:** 30 Min. **G–K:** Light micrographs of motoneurons. **G–I:** Feulgen stain for DNA. ×1,280. **G:** Control showing heterochromatic Barr body (*arrow*). **H:** 8 Hr. **I:** 24 Hr. **J** and **K:** 1 μM Araldite sections stained with toluidine blue. ×2,000. **J:** Control. **K:** 24 Hr. C, chromatin; G, granular aggregates; N, nucleolus.

mostly sparse small clumps of dense chro-matin (Fig. 6A), whereas small neurons contain numerous coarse chromatin masses, and medium-sized neurons are intermediate in this respect. The nucleoplasm contains abundant osmiophilic granules from 30 to 250 Å in diameter, both scattered and in cloud-like aggregates up to 2 μm. Nucleoli reveal a granular zone with numerous 150 Å particles, a fibrous nucleolonema, and amorphous areas. Glial nuclei contain numerous coarse chromatin masses, nu-cleoli, and osmiophilic granules (Fig. 6E).

After treatment with AMD (1 mg) ultra-structural changes appear in many neuronal nuclei after 30 min, and reach major pro-portions by 8 hr (Fig. 6B–D). Small clumps of dense chromatin appear multicentrically throughout the nucleoplasm. These chro-matin clumps progressively enlarge by coalescence to form coarse, elongated, or rounded masses resembling chromosomes of mitotic cells. The granular material accumulates in large compact aggregates, and the component granules increase to 300 Å in diameter, possibly by fusion (Fig. 6D). The intervening nucleoplasm be-comes rarefied. Advanced nuclear changes appear in glia by 30 to 60 min (Fig. 6F), in small neurons by 1 to 2 hr, and in large motoneurons by 4 to 8 hr after 1 mg of AMD (Fig. 6C and D). Nucleoli of neurons and glia exhibit a loss of 150 Å granules, fragmentation and collapse of the nu-cleolonema, and segregation of these com-ponents (Fig. 6B and C). Chromatin con-denses about the nucleolus, often forming a perinucleolar envelope. After a small dose (5 μg) of AMD, moderate nuclear changes are discernible in large neurons at 1 to 3 hr, and advanced changes by 24 to 40 hr. Identical nuclear lesions occur in neurons and glia of rat and cat cerebrum, appearing as early as 10 min after the intra-cerebral injection of AMD. The early and progressive character of the AMD-in-duced condensation of chromatin is particu-larly well shown in preparations that are

selectively stained for DNA (Fig. 7A and B).

COMMENTS ON THE MODE OF ACTION OF AMD

AMD presumably acts by binding to the DNA template (7). The interaction be-tween AMD and DNA in solution has been the subject of a number of detailed studies (6,7). In the model proposed by Hamilton et al. (9) for the structure of AMD–DNA complexes, the bulky AMD molecules are hydrogen-bonded to the out-side of the DNA helix in its minor groove and according to Reich (30) interfere with the action of RNA polymerase by sterically hindering the polymerization process. Müller and Crothers (26) have recently presented evidence for another model in which the AMD chromophore is inter-calated between the base pairs in the DNA complex and the cyclic peptide rings in-teract with the DNA backbone chain, chiefly through hydrogen bonds. Dingman and Sporn (3) concluded from a study of the intracellular distribution of AMD in rat liver that DNA is the major binding site for AMD *in vivo*.

Our investigations have elicited several significant features with regard to the neurobiological activity of AMD that shed light on the mechanism of action of this agent. The first feature is that the kinetics of the AMD-induced repression of RNA transcription differ sharply from the ki-netics of AMD binding. When administered locally, [^{3}H]AMD rapidly penetrates into neural tissue, apparently through an active transport mechanism (P. Sanghavi and H. Koenig, *unpublished observations*), and a portion, approximately 20 to 25% of the total, is promptly bound in an acid- and lipid solvent-stable linkage to nuclear DNA or chromatin. However, inhibition of RNA synthesis, as measured by [^{14}C]adenine or [^{3}H]uridine uptake into nuclear RNA, is established more slowly *in vivo* and *in*

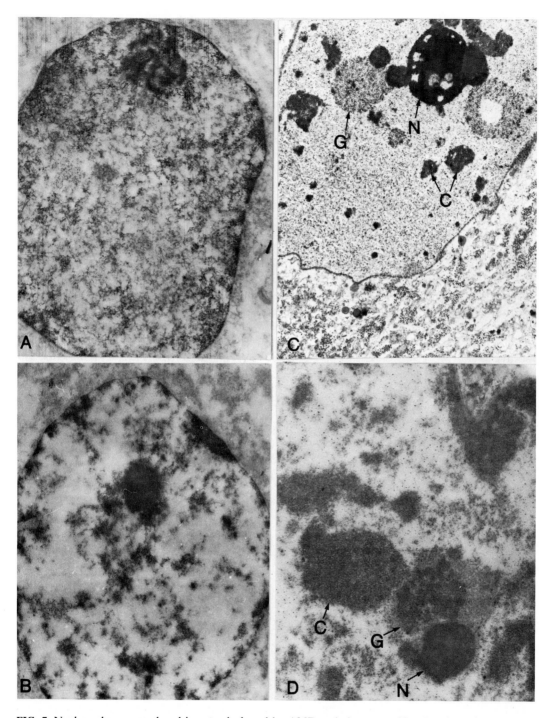

FIG. 7. Nuclear changes produced in cat spinal cord by AMD and chromopeptides. **A** and **B**: Electron cytochemical stain for DNA. Ultrathin sections were incubated with RNase and stained briefly with uranyl acetate. **A**: Control. **B**: AMD, 1 mg, 30 Min. ×15,000. **C**: Chromomycin A_3, 1 mg, 4 Hr. ×2,500. **D**: Mithramycin, 1 mg, 4 Hr. ×20,500. C, chromatin; G, granular aggregates; N, nucleolus.

vitro. This inhibition seems to occur in two stages: an initial rapid inhibition, evident at 30 to 60 min *in vivo* and 20 min *in vitro* (the earliest time intervals studied), and a slow inhibition of approximately equal magnitude, which extends over the subsequent 6 to 7 hr. Peak binding of AMD to nuclear DNA or chromatin is attained early in the period of rapid inhibition. A similar two stage increase in the inhibitory action of AMD is discernible in other biological systems, e.g., fibroblasts (see Fig. 3 in ref. 31) and developing retina (see Fig. 4A in ref. 14), but its occurrence seems to have gone unnoticed. The slow inhibition of RNA synthesis is difficult to reconcile with the steric hindrance theory (30), for according to this theory the inhibition of RNA synthesis should attain a maximum value coincident with the formation of the AMD–DNA complex. It may be concluded, therefore, that the slow inhibition, which accounts for about 50% of the total inhibition produced by AMD at 6 to 8 hr, is caused by a time-dependent process that presumably in initiated by the formation of the AMD–DNA or AMD–chromatin complex. Although this same process may also be implicated in the rapid inhibition, the available data are insufficient to exclude the possibility that steric hindrance may play a role in the latter.

A second feature is the remarkable effectiveness of AMD in repressing RNA synthesis at a low saturation level of DNA after a sufficient time interval. Thus, as little as 10^{-5} mole of AMD bound per mole of DNA–P (Fig. 1) inhibited RNA synthesis in cat spinal cord by 70% after 6 hr. Dingman and Sporn (3) found that 6.4×10^{-5} mole of AMD bound per mole of DNA–P inhibited RNA synthesis in rat liver by 88%. These *in vivo* findings are not readily explained by the steric hindrance theory, as DNA templates on the order of 10^4 to 10^5 nucleotide units in length should still be available between deoxyguanine sites occupied by AMD for the transcription process. This line of reasoning assumes

that AMD binds more or less uniformly to the DNA in the active and the inactive chromatin. It is interesting to note that the RNA polymerase reaction *in vitro* seems to be substantially less sensitive to AMD than is RNA synthesis in intact cells *in vivo*. Only about a 50% inhibition of RNA synthesis is obtained *in vitro* with a purified DNA as a primer at a concentration of 10^{-3} mole of AMD per mole of DNA–P (26,30). The differential susceptibility of gray matter and white matter to AMD is noteworthy. Although it binds less AMD, subcortical white matter of cat cerebrum exhibited an earlier and more severe inhibition of RNA synthesis than the cortex, which suggests that glia are more sensitive to the inhibitory effects of AMD than neurons. Appel (1) made similar observations in rat cerebrum, but did not measure AMD binding.

The basis for the enhanced labeling of soluble RNA by [^{14}C]adenine, which occurs soon after AMD administration, is obscure. This labeling could be partly due to terminal labeling of the cytidine-cytidine-adenine sequence, rather than to incorporation into the interior of the soluble RNA molecule. However, a similar, although less marked, increase in the incorporation of [^{3}H]uridine into soluble RNA has been observed in the AMD-treated cat spinal cord and rat brain (31a).

Our correlative studies have shown that AMD produces characteristic changes in the nuclear morphology of neural cells, namely: (a) the formation of clumps of dense chromatin through compaction of diffuse chromatin; (b) an agglomeration and enlargement of nucleoplasmic granules; (c) a rarefaction of intervening nucleoplasm; and (d) nucleolar changes leading to atrophy and loss of RNA-containing components. These changes become evident by 10 to 30 min and advance concomitantly with the slow inhibition of RNA synthesis. Although the nucleolar changes produced by AMD have attracted most of the attention of previous workers, morphological changes in nuclear chromatin after AMD treatment have been noted in certain instances, namely, in HeLa cells (8), dipteran salivary gland (33), frog embryonal cells (12), lampbrush chromosomes of amphibian oocytes (10), rat exocrine pancreas (13), rat salivary gland (11), baboon kidney cells (32), and neurons of mouse facial nucleus (35–37). These changes have been variously attributed to an apparent increase in DNA (8,32), inhibition of RNA synthesis (10), and an effect of binding of AMD to DNA (12,33). However, these alterations in nuclear chromatin have not been hitherto correlated with the metabolic effects of AMD, nor have they been invoked as a basis for the mechanism of action of AMD.

The nuclear lesions in nervous tissue are well developed prior to the abolition of RNA synthesis, at a time when the nuclear RNA content is reduced only 5 to 10%, and nuclear DNA and protein concentrations are essentially unchanged. Thus, the early nuclear alterations probably are attributable to a rearrangement of nuclear components induced directly by the binding of AMD, and not to a change in chemical composition of the nucleus. It seems likely that the interaction of AMD with the histone proteins of the nucleus makes a significant contribution to the biological action of AMD. Recent observations suggest that AMD may bind firmly to nuclear histones, rather than to DNA, when administered *in vivo* into the nervous system (C. Y. Lu and H. Koenig, *unpublished findings*).

We propose that AMD, upon binding to nuclear DNA or histones or both in the diffuse (eu)chromatin and the nucleolus, cross-links the extended nucleohistone microfibrils, thereby converting the euchromatin and nucleolar chromatin into a contracted, impervious mass of dense (hetero)chromatin that is incapable of functioning as a template for RNA transcription. AMD can cross-link DNA molecules through hydrophobic bonds between the cyclic peptide side chains (2). In contrast to the binding of AMD, which is essentially instantaneous, the cross-linking of euchromatin microfibrils *in situ* is envisaged as a time-dependent process whose velocity would vary inversely with the mean distance between the extended microfibrils. Thus, in glia and small neurons the euchromatin is contained within a small nuclear volume and would be more readily cross-linked by AMD. The euchromatin of motoneurons would be more resistant to cross-linkage because it is dispersed in a larger nuclear volume. This would account for the greater sensitivity of the glia and small neurons to AMD. Likewise the restriction of the genome for ribosomal RNA to the small compact nucleolus would facilitate its cross-linkage by AMD, thus accounting for the great sensitivity of ribosomal RNA synthesis to AMD (29).

CHROMOPEPTIDES, ANTHRACYCLINES, AND BASIC DYES

The chromopeptide antibiotics chromomycin A_3, mithramycin, and olivomycin have close structural relationships and inhibit RNA synthesis, presumably by forming a complex with DNA (5,7). The anthracycline antibiotics nogalomycin, daunomycin, and cinerubin also are structurally related and block RNA synthesis apparently by interacting with DNA (7). The basic dyes acriflavin and ethidium bromide and 4-nitroquinolin-N-oxide are likewise inhibitors of RNA synthesis and form complexes with DNA (34). These agents vary markedly in their neurotoxicity when injected into the lumbar theca of cat. The chromopeptides are the most effective inhibitors of RNA synthesis in feline spinal cord. Chromomycin A_3 is nearly as active as AMD on a weight basis, but mithramycin and olivomycin are less potent. The chromopeptides, in a 1-mg dose, produce clumping of nuclear chromatin, aggregation of nucleoplasmic granules, and nucleolar changes within 1 hr. These changes pro-

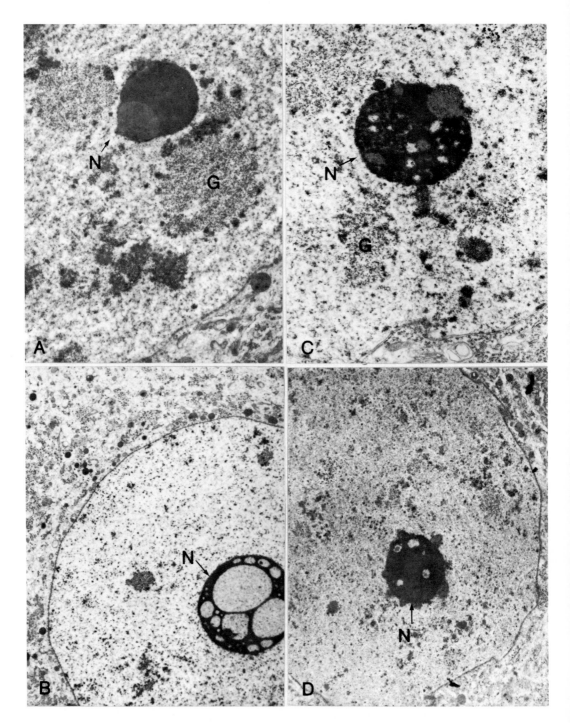

FIG. 8. Nuclear changes produced in cat spinal cord by chromopeptides and anthracyclines. **A:** Olivomycin, 1 mg, 24 hr. ×8,250. **B:** Cinerubin, 5 mg, 24 hr. × 3,750. **C:** Nogalomycin, 5 mg. 4 hr. × 11,900. **D:** Daunomycin, 5 mg, 24 hr. ×6,000. C, chromatin; G, granular aggregates; N, nucleolus.

gress with time and culminate in a severe, coarse heterochromatinization by 4 to 24 hr (Figs. 7C and D and 8A). The anthracyclines and basic dyes are less potent inhibitors of RNA synthesis in neural tissue, and in small doses may in fact stimulate RNA synthesis, and they produce less severe nuclear lesions. These agents, in a 5-mg dose, produce a finer pattern of nuclear heterochromatinization (Fig. 8B–D). Nucleolar changes range from a complete loss of the granular component with shrinkage, collapse of the nucleolonema, and sequestration of components, to nucleolar swelling and vacuolation. Glia are generally affected more rapidly and severely than neurons. The cytoplasmic morphology, including polysomal structure, is usually well preserved for 12 to 24 hr, although a mild swelling of mitochondria is occasionally seen.

These various inhibitors of RNA synthesis have been extensively used as cytological probes to correlate biochemical and ultrastructural studies of the nucleolus. Consequently, the nucleolar lesions produced by these agents have been well characterized (34). However, the interphase nucleus of eucaryotic cells appears to be somewhat more chaotic than the highly organized nucleolus, and the characteristic alterations in nuclear structure produced by these agents have been less widely recognized. Simard et al. (34) have emphasized the clumping and margination of chromatin in cells treated with these inhibitors and speculate that these changes may be related to binding to DNA. Whether or not these agents actually bind to DNA *in vivo* is difficult to ascertain, and the possibility exists that they may also bind to acidic nuclear proteins and histones. In any event, these inhibitors do bring about a heterochromatinization of the nucleus, presumably by interacting with the nuclear chromatin or some component thereof. Although we have not studied the effects of these agents on RNA synthesis in neural tissue systematically, there seems to be a general correlation between the extent of inhibition of RNA synthesis and the severity of the nuclear heterochromatinization produced by the various inhibitors. Evidently these agents, upon interacting with nuclear chromatin or a chromatin-associated component, bring about a heterochromatinization of the nucleus in much the same manner as AMD. It seems reasonable to suppose therefore that the inhibitory effect of these agents on RNA transcription may also be secondary to the structural changes that they produce in the dispersed, metabolically active chromatin.

ACKNOWLEDGMENT

This work has been supported by National Institutes Health Grants NS 06838 and NS 01456.

REFERENCES

1. Appel, S. H. (1967): Turnover of brain messenger RNA. *Nature,* 213:1253–1254.
2. Crothers, D. M., Sabol, S. L., Ratner, D. I., and Müller, W. (1968): Studies concerning the behavior of actinomycin in solution. *Biochemistry,* 7:1817–1823.
3. Dingman, C. W., and Sporn, M. B. (1965): Actinomycin D and hydrocortisone: Intracellular finding in rat liver. *Science,* 149:1251–1254.
4. Frenster, J. H. (1974): Ultrastructure and function of heterochromatin and euchromatin. In: *The Cell Nucleus,* Vol. 1, edited by H. Busch, pp. 565–581. Academic Press, New York.
5. Gause, G. F. (1975): Olivomycin, chromomycin and methramycin. In: *Antibiotics,* Vol. 3, edited by J. W. Corcoran and F. E. Hahn, pp. 197–202. Springer-Verlag, New York.
6. Gellert, M., Smith, C. E., Neville, D., and Felsenfeld, G. (1965): Actinomycin binding to DNA: Mechanism and specificity. *J. Mol. Biol.,* 11:445–457.
7. Goldberg, I. H. (1965): Mode of action of antibiotics. II. Drugs affecting nucleic acid and protein synthesis. *Am. J. Med.,* 39:722–752.
8. Goldstein, M. N., Slotnick, I. J., and Journey, L. J. (1960): *In vitro* studies with Hela cell lines sensitive and resistant to actinomycin D. *NY Acad. Sci.,* 89:474–483.
9. Hamilton, L. D., Fuller, W., and Reich, E. (1963): X-ray diffraction and molecular model building studies of the interaction of actinomycin with nucleic acids. *Nature,* 198:538–540.
10. Izawa, M., Allfrey, V. G., and Mirsky, A. E.

(1963): The relationship between RNA synthesis and loop structure in lampbrush chromosomes. *Proc. Natl. Acad. Sci. USA,* 49:544–551.

11. Jhee, H. T., Han, S. S., and Avery, J. K. (1965): A study of salivary glands of rats injected with actinomycin D. *Am. J. Anat.,* 116:631–652.

12. Jones, K. W., and Elsdale, T. R. (1964): The effects of actinomycin D on the ultrastructure of the nucleus of the amphibian embryonic cell. *J. Cell Biol.,* 21:245–252.

13. Jézéquel, A.-M., and Bernhard, W. (1964): Modifications, ultrastructurales du pancréas exocrine de rat sous l'effet de l'actinomycine D. *J. Microscopie,* 3:279–296.

14. Kirk, D. L. (1965): The role of RNA synthesis in the production of glutamine synthetase by developing chick neural retina. *Proc. Natl. Acad. Sci. USA,* 54:1345–1353.

15. Koenig, H. (1958): An autoradiographic study of nucleic acid and protein turnover in the mammalian neuraxis. *J. Biophys. Biochem. Cytol.,* 4:785–792.

16. Koenig, H. (1958): Production of injury to feline nervous system with nucleic acid antimetabolite. *Science,* 127:1238–1239.

17. Koenig, H. (1960): Experimental myelopathy produced with a pyrimidine analogue. *Arch. Neurol. (Chic.),* 2:463–475.

18. Koenig, H. (1964): RNA metabolism in the nervous system. In: *Morphological and Biochemical Correlates of Neural Activity,* edited by M. M. Cohen and R. S. Snider, chapter 3, pp. 39–56. Harper (Hoeber), New York.

19. Koenig, H. (1967): Neurobiological action of some pyrimidine analogs. In: *International Review of Neurobiology,* Vol. 10, edited by C. C. Pfeiffer and J. R. Smythies, pp. 199–230. Academic Press, New York.

20. Koenig, H. (1969): Neurobiological effects of agents which alter nucleic acid metabolism. In: *Motor Neuron Diseases: Research on Amyotrophic Lateral Sclerosis and Related Disorders,* edited by F. H. Norris, Jr. and L. T. Kurland, chapter 34, pp. 347–368. Grune & Stratton, New York and London.

21. Koenig, H., and Jacobson, S. (1966): Nuclear changes induced in neurons by actinomycin D. *J. Cell Biol.,* 31:61A.

22. Koenig, H., Lu, C. Y., and Jacobson, S. (1967): Effect of actinomycin D (AMD) and related antibiotics on biosynthetic activities and chromatin morphology in cat spinal cord. *Fed. Proc.,* 26: 291.

23. Koenig, H., Young, I. J., Wells, W., and Gaines, D. (1961): Physiologic and metabolic studies of azauridine encephalopathy. *Trans. Am. Neurol. Assoc.,* 86:219–221.

24. Koenig, H., Lu, C. Y., Jacobson, S., Sanghavi, P., and Nayyar, R. (1970): Effects of actinomycin D on RNA transcription, protein synthesis and nuclear structure. In: *Protein Metabolism of the Nervous System,* edited by A. Lajtha, chapter 24, pp. 491–515. Plenum Press, New York.

25. Littau, V. C., Allfrey, V. G., Frenster, J. H., and Mirsky, A. E. (1964): Active and inactive regions of nuclear chromatin as revealed by electron microscopy autoradiography. *Proc. Natl. Acad. Sci. USA,* 52:93–100.

26. Müller, W., and Crothers, D. M. (1968): Studies of the binding of actinomycin and related compounds to DNA. *J. Mol. Biol.,* 35:251–290.

27. Nayyar, R. P., and Koenig, H. (1971): Nuclear changes produced by agents which inhibit RNA synthesis. A light and electronmicroscopic study of neurons and glia in cat spinal cord. *Anat. Rec.,* 169:382.

28. Nayyar, R. P., and Koenig, H. (1971): Nuclear changes produced in neurons and glia by chromomycin, mithramycin and olivomycin. A light and electronmicroscopic study of cat spinal cord. *11th Annu. Mtg. Am. Soc. Cell Biol. (Abstr.),* p. 206.

29. Perry, R. P. (1963): Selective effects of actinomycin D on the intracellular distribution of RNA synthesis in tissue culture cells. *Exp. Cell Res.,* 29:400–406.

30. Reich, E. (1964): Actinomycin: Correlation of structure and function of its complexes with purines and DNA. *Science,* 143:684–689.

31. Reich, E., Franklin, R. M., Shatkin, A. J., and Tatum, E. L. (1962): Action of actinomycin D on animal cells and viruses. *Proc. Natl. Acad. Sci. USA,* 48:1238–1245.

31a. Sanghavi, P., and Koenig, H. (*In preparation*).

32. Schoefl, G. I. (1964): The effect of actinomycin D on the fine structure of the nucleolus. *J. Ultrastruct. Res.,* 10:224–243.

33. Stevens, B. J. (1964): The effect of actinomycin D on nucleolar and nuclear fine structure in the salivary gland cell of chironomus thummi. *J. Ultrastruct. Res.,* 11:329–353.

34. Simard, R., Langelier, Y., Mandeville, R., Maestracci, N., and Royal, A. (1974): Inhibitors as tools in elucidating the structure and function of the nucleus. In: *The Cell Nucleus,* Vol. 1, edited by H. Busch, pp. 447–487. Academic Press, New York.

35. Torvik, A., and Heding, A. (1967): Histological studies on the effect of antinomycin D on retrograde nerve cell reaction in the facial nucleus of mice. *Acta Neuropathol. (Berl.),* 9:146–157.

36. Torvik, A., and Heding, A. (1969): Effect of actinomycin D on retrograde nerve cell reaction. Further observations. *Acta Neuropathol. (Berl.),* 14:62–71.

37. Torvik, A., and Skjorten, F. (1974): The effect of actinomycin D upon normal neurons and retrograde nerve cell reaction. *J. Neurocytol.,* 3:87–97.

38. Wells, W., Gaines, D., and Koenig, H. (1963): Studies of pyrimidine metabolism in the central nervous system. I. Metabolic effects and metabolism of 6-azauridine. *J. Neurochem.,* 10:709–723.

Neurotoxicology, edited by L. Roizin, H. Shiraki, and N. Grčević. Raven Press, New York © 1977.

Examination of the Developing Nervous System of *Xenopus* Tadpoles with Differential Interference Microscopy: A New Assay Procedure for Neurotoxicologists

Henry deF. Webster, Takeshi Tabira, and *Paul J. Reier

*Laboratory of Neuropathology and Neuroanatomical Sciences, National Institute of Neurological and Communicative Disorders and Stroke, Bethesda, Maryland 20014; and the *Department of Anatomy, University of Maryland School of Medicine, Baltimore, Maryland 21205*

Although an extensive literature on neurotoxicology exists, the effects of most agents on cellular and subcellular components of the nervous system still are not well understood. In most current morphological studies, both light and electron microscopy are used to identify cellular lesions. When mammalian experimental animals are employed, it is a major undertaking to process, section, and study the large number of tissue blocks necessary to minimize sampling problems and preparative artifacts. Also, the distribution and evolution of lesions produced *in vivo* may depend partially on blood-brain and blood-nerve "barriers" to the agent being investigated.

Many difficulties associated with *in vivo* studies can be avoided by studying neurotoxic effects in an accessible part of the central nervous system (CNS), such as the rabbit retina (2), or in nervous tissue maintained *in vitro* (2,5,11,13). Chapters in this volume and elsewhere (11,13) illustrate how successfully these techniques have been exploited.

Recently, we have used a differential interference (Nomarski) microscope to examine the developing nervous system of *Xenopus* tadpoles *in vivo* (3,20,21) and in whole mount preparations (19,22). Here, we present observations on the lesions produced by hexachlorophene (HCP) and briefly discuss data obtained by others using mammalian experimental animals (4,6–9,17,18, and see H. C. Powell and P. W. Lampert, Chapter 40, *this volume*) and tissue cultures (13). Also, we suggest that our assay procedure deserves further trial in neurotoxicology.

MATERIALS AND METHODS

The procedures used in this study have been described (3,14,19–23). Briefly, *Xenopus* tadpoles were obtained from the Amphibian Facility (University of Michigan, Ann Arbor, Michigan) and were anesthetized with tricaine methanesulfonate at stages 53 to 55 of development (12). For observation of nerve and muscle fibers *in vivo*, each tadpole was placed on its side in a microscopic chamber. The tail was covered with immersion oil, and areas of interest were studied and photographed with a Zeiss differential interference (Nomarski) microscope equipped with a 40X long-working distance oil-immersion objective (3). To prepare whole mounts of nervous tissue, tadpoles were fixed first by intracardiac perfusion with a phosphate-buffered 2% aldehyde solution; after overnight immersion in the same solution, blocks of tissue containing regions of interest were removed and glycerinated. Then cranial nerves, ganglia, and spinal cord segments were isolated by gentle dissection and were mounted whole in glycerol on a slide with the coverslip sealed by nail polish (19,22). The whole mount preparations were studied and photographed with a Zeiss differential interference microscope (1). To study the tadpole nervous system with the electron microscope, blocks of aldehyde-fixed tissue were either glycerinated for freeze fracturing (14) or were postfixed, embedded, and sectioned according to conventional techniques (23). To study the distribution and severity of HCP lesions, tadpoles were immersed in growing solution containing 0.2 µg of HCP/ml and sacrificed after 3 and 7 days. To investigate the reversibility of lesions produced by 7 days of HCP exposure, the remaining tadpoles were transferred to control medium and sacrificed after 7 and 14 days of recovery.

RESULTS

In Vivo Observations: Peripheral Nerve and Muscle Fibers

When observed with differential interference contrast illumination, myelinated fibers in the central tail fin were easily traced from the lateral muscle mass ventrally and distally to their growing tips (3,20). Single myelinated axons suitable for serial observations were found in thinner portions of the tail (Fig. 1a). Schwann cell nuclei were usually located midway between nodes of Ranvier, which were 75 to 200 µm apart. The axons were 2 to 4 µm in diameter and were surrounded by myelin sheaths that had few irregulari-

ties. Schmidt-Lantermann clefts were not identified in these small developing fibers although there were occasional focal discontinuities in the birefringence of some sheaths.

In tail fins of tadpoles immersed in HCP (0.2 µg/ml) for 1 day, myelin internodes contained focal collections of vacuoles located within the myelin sheath (Fig. 1b). Similar lesions were present after 3 days (Fig. 1c), and a few of the vacuoles were quite large. In tadpoles studied after 5, 6, or 7 days of immersion in HCP, the same type of alteration was found in a small proportion of myelin internodes. Only a few of these were reexamined after 1 to 3 days of additional immersion; their lesions were either unchanged or larger (23).

Muscle fibers of *Xenopus* tadpoles can also be observed *in vivo* (21) using differential interference contrast illumination (Fig. 1d). Relatively few muscle fibers of HCP-intoxicated tadpoles were surveyed. Their sarcomeres, mitochondria, and end-plate regions appeared normal.

Whole Mounts: Optic Nerves, Spinal Cord, Trigeminal Nerve, and Ganglion

In whole mount preparations of optic nerves from control tadpoles, myelinated fibers measuring 2 to 5 µm in diameter could be traced for long distances (Fig. 2a). The myelin sheaths were generally smooth in contour, but occasionally there were groups of small ovoids (19). In optic nerves of tadpoles immersed in HCP for 3 (Fig. 2b) and 7 days, most myelin sheaths were vacuolated and split. Slight recovery was apparent in some nerves 3 days after the tadpoles were transferred to control medium. After 7 days of recovery, fewer myelin sheaths were vacuolated, and most lesions were smaller. Most myelinated fibers in nerves from tadpoles that had recovered for 14 days appeared normal (Fig. 2c). Reactive changes were slight; only a few lipid-

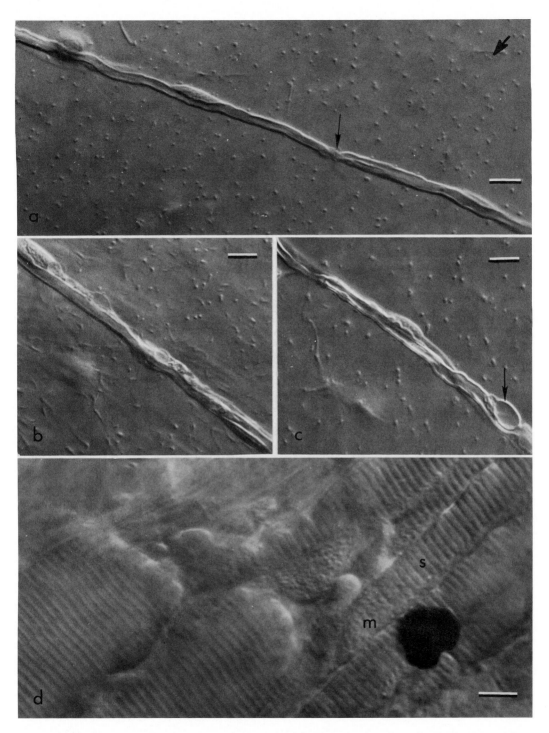

FIG. 1. Myelinated peripheral nerve (**a–c**) and muscle (**d**) fibers observed *in vivo* with differential interference contrast illumination. In a control tadpole tail fin (**a**) there are two normal myelin segments and a node of Ranvier (*arrow*). After 1 day in HCP, 0.2 μg/ml, a few myelin internodes like the one shown in (**b**) contain small vacuoles and a few ovoids. A much larger vacuole (*arrow*) is located in a myelin sheath exposed to HCP for 3 days (**c**). In control muscle fibers examined *in vivo* (**d**), the sarcomeres (s) and mitochondria (m) are well shown and appear normal. Upper right arrow in (**a**) shows direction of shear. Scale bars, 10 μm.

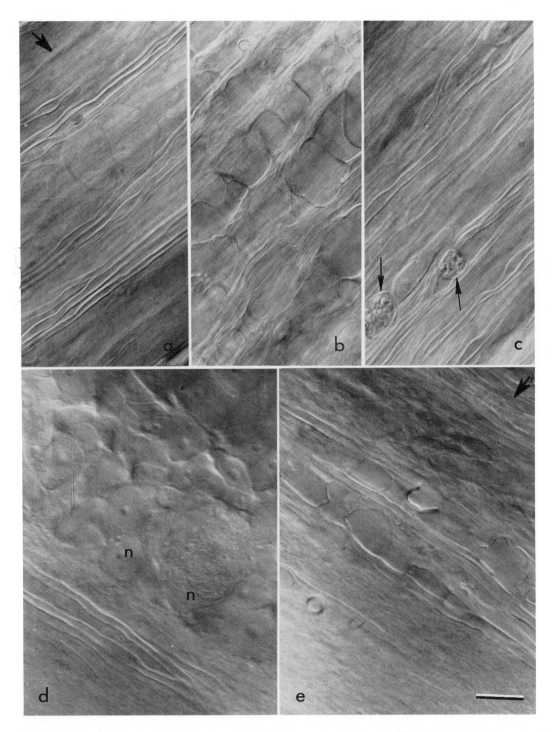

FIG. 2. Right optic nerve **(a–c)** and spinal cord **(d, e)** whole mounts viewed with differential interference contrast illumination. In an optic nerve from a control tadpole **(a)**, there are glial nuclei between normal myelin sheaths that appear as if they were longitudinally sectioned. After 3 days of HCP 0.2 μg/ml, myelin sheaths are severely vacuolated **(b)**. After 7 days of exposure to HCP and 14 days of recovery in control medium **(c)**, the appearance of most myelin sheaths is normal. Very few areas contain lipid-filled macrophages (*arrows*). In the spinal cord from a control tadpole **(d)**, neurons (n) and myelin sheaths appear normal. After 7 days of HCP **(e)**, vacuolation of myelin is less severe than in the optic nerves. Arrows in **(a)** and **(e)** show direction of shear. Scale bar, 10 μm.

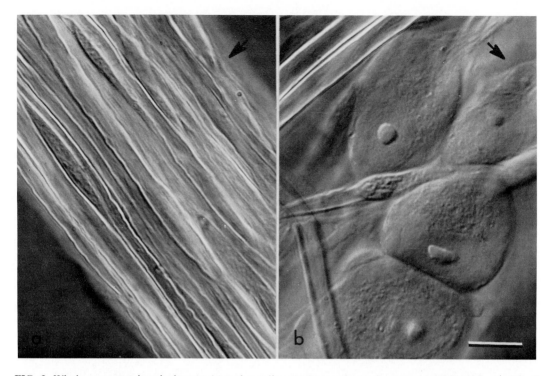

FIG. 3. Whole mounts, trigeminal nerve (**a**) and ganglion (**b**) from tadpoles immersed in HCP, 0.2 μg/ml for 7 days. The myelin sheaths illustrated in (**a**) and (**b**) are smooth in contour; no vacuoles or other alterations are present. There are no abnormalities apparent in the neurons shown in (**b**). Arrows show the direction of shear. Scale bar, 10 μm.

filled macrophages were found. Thus, under the conditions of these tests, HCP produced little demyelination even though vacuolation of myelin was severe. The rapid recovery we observed was associated with removal of vacuolar fluid and the reestablishment of the compact structure of existing sheaths. Since demyelination did not occur, remyelination was not observed.

Myelinated fibers, neurons, and glia were well visualized in whole mounts of spinal cords from control tadpoles (Fig. 2d). When the myelin lesions in a tadpole's spinal cord and optic nerves were compared, those in the spinal cord were smaller and less numerous after 3 and 7 days (Fig. 2e) of HCP exposure. After only 7 days of recovery in control medium, almost all spinal cord myelinated fibers appeared normal. As noted above, optic nerves of these tadpoles still contained many lesions.

Peripheral myelinated fibers in the trigeminal nerve and ganglion were larger, and in whole mount preparations it was easy to identify Schwann cell nuclei, nodes of Ranvier, and Schmidt-Lantermann clefts. During HCP exposure, no lesions were observed in these myelinated fibers or in the trigeminal ganglion neurons (Fig. 3a and b).

Electron Microscopic Observations

In electron micrographs of thin sections, the HCP-induced vacuoles are found within myelin sheaths (Fig. 4a), and the splitting of myelin lamellae occurs at the less dense, intraperiod lines (6–8,13,14,17,18,23). Bleb-like collections of membranous profiles were present at the margins of some vacuoles. Very few lesions were found in axons or glial cells. Recently, Reier et al.

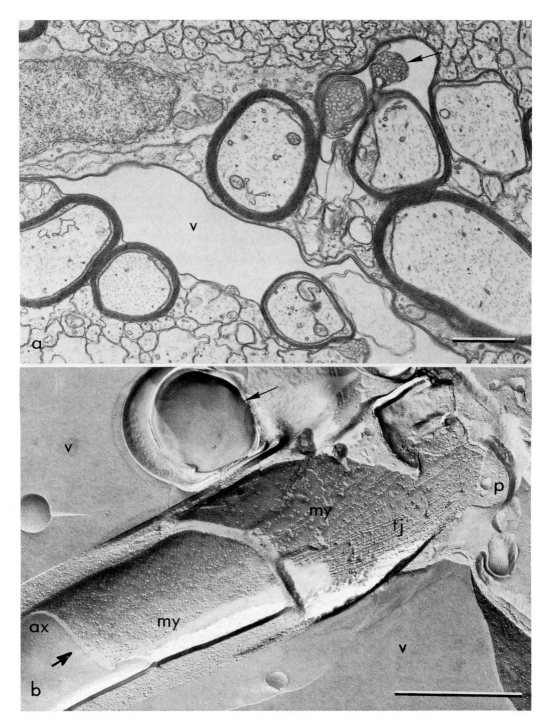

FIG. 4. Electron micrographs of transversely sectioned optic nerve (**a**) and a freeze fracture replica of an optic nerve (**b**) from tadpoles immersed for 6 to 7 days in HCP, 0.2 μg/ml. In (**a**), several myelin lamellae surround a large vacuole (v). Above, a smaller vacuole contains a membrane-bound bleb (*arrow*). In (**b**) an axon (ax), myelin lamellae (my), and a vacuole (v) are fractured longitudinally. A bleb (*arrow*) protrudes into the vacuole. Below and to the right, there are rows of particles that form tight junctions (tj) between the outer myelin layer and the olidodendrocyte's tongue process (p). Scale bars, 1 μm.

(14) studied the distribution of intramembranous particles in replicas of freeze-fractured optic nerves from HCP-intoxicated tadpoles. In Fig. 4b there is a myelin lesion similar to that illustrated in Fig. 4a. Surfaces of large vacuoles arising from layers of compact myelin were indented by blebs similar to those noted above. Also linear arrays of particles corresponding to tight junctions between outer tongue processes of oligodendrocytes and the outermost layer of myelin spirals were similar to those observed in control preparations.

DISCUSSION

The results presented here and in other studies (3,14,15,19–23) demonstrate several advantages of the developing tadpole nervous system for investigating cellular effects of neurotoxic substances. Compared to other experimental animals or cultures of nervous tissue, tadpoles are less expensive and easier to maintain in the laboratory. When immersed in dilute solutions of substances like HCP, absorption is prompt and the concentration in the nervous system rises rapidly (23). Test solutions can also be injected easily near structures of interest like the optic nerve (19,22). Rapid diffusion is observed and lack of "barriers" allows even macromolecules to enter the parenchyma of the nervous system within a few hours (15).

The tadpole nervous system is especially well suited for morphological studies that attempt to define the distribution and time course of cellular alterations. With differential interference contrast illumination, muscle and peripheral nerve fibers have been observed *in vivo* and selected regions were studied at intervals to define a sequence of changes occurring during development (3) or HCP intoxication (23). To characterize HCP lesions elsewhere in the nervous system, we prepared whole mounts of spinal cord, cranial nerves, and ganglia and sectioned them optically with differential interference contrast illumination (19). Using this procedure, many regions containing undehydrated myelinated fibers, neurons, and glia were studied with substantially less effort than is required to prepare and survey areas of comparable size in stained microscopic slides. A final advantage of *Xenopus* tadpoles for morphological studies was the relative ease of achieving good cellular preservation by perfusion fixation. Since the distribution of vascular clearing can be observed directly, success is apparent immediately. Many blocks from large numbers of animals did not have to be processed in order to find areas in freeze fracture replicas or thin sections that were suitable for electron microscopic study.

Although brains of tadpoles are small, they can be removed and studied biochemically. After tadpoles were immersed in 0.1 or 0.2 μg of HCP/ml, the whole body and brain content of HCP rose rapidly. Also, when subcellular fractions of brain were prepared and studied, HCP was found in all fractions, and its concentration (per mg of protein) was highest in myelin (23).

The toxicity of HCP and its use as an antibacterial agent are described in Chapter 40 and have been reviewed recently (7). The mechanism of the HCP effect on myelin and other membranes has also been extensively investigated (7,13). Our results and other biochemical evidence (4,8,9,13) suggest that HCP affects myelin directly, perhaps by altering components responsible for the apposition of the less dense intraperiod lines. Although the gap between these lines is continuous with extracellular space and swells when exposed to hypotonic solutions (16), tracers such as horseradish peroxidase (14,17) and microperoxidase (17) do not penetrate vacuoles produced by HCP. Zonulae occludentes between myelin layers probably form the barrier to tracer entry and in freeze fracture preparations appear to be unaffected by HCP (14). These junctional complexes (10) may also play a role in limiting the size of vacuoles, preventing demyelination, and reestablishing the apposition of myelin's intraperiod lines during recovery.

In conclusion, we suggest that the developing nervous system of *Xenopus* tadpoles is a relatively simple *in vivo* model that deserves further trial in neurotoxicology, particularly by investigators interested in using our whole mount technique (19) to study the distribution and time course of cellular lesions.

ACKNOWLEDGMENT

The authors wish to thank Maureen O'Connell and Kathyrn Winchell for their excellent technical assistance.

REFERENCES

1. Allen, R. D., David, G. B., and Nomarski, G. (1969): The Zeiss-Nomarski differential interference equipment for transmitted-light microscopy. *Z. Wiss. Mikr.*, 69:193–221.
2. Ames, A., III., and Pollen, D. A. (1969): Neurotransmission in central nervous tissue: A study of isolated rabbit retina. *J. Neurophysiol.*, 32:424–442.
3. Billings-Gagliardi, S., Webster, H. deF., and O'Connell, M. F. (1974): In vivo and electron microscopic observations on Schwann cells in developing tadpole nerve fibers. *Am. J. Anat.*, 141:375–391.
4. Cammer, W., Rose, A. L., and Norton, W. T. (1975): Biochemical and pathological studies of myelin in hexachlorophene intoxication. *Brain Res.*, 98:547–559.
5. Crain, S. M. (1975): Physiology of CNS tissues in culture. In: *Metabolic Compartmentation and Neurotransmission*, edited by S. Berl, D. D. Clarke, and D. Schneider, pp. 273–303. Plenum, New York.
6. Kimbrough, R. D., and Gaines, T. B. (1971): The effect of hexachlorophene on the rat brain: Study of high doses by light and electron microscopy. *Arch. Environ. Health*, 23:114–118.
7. Kimbrough, R. D. (1976): Hexachlorophene: Toxicity and use as an antibacterial agent. In: *Essays in Toxicology*, Vol. 7, edited by W. J. Hayes, Jr., pp. 99–120. Academic Press, New York.
8. Lampert, P., O'Brien, J., and Garrett, R. (1973): Hexachlorophene encephalopathy. *Acta Neuropathol. (Berl.)*, 23:326–333.
9. Matthieu, J.-M., Zimmerman, A. W., Webster, H. deF., Ulsamer, A. G., Brady, R. O., and Quarles, R. H. (1974): Hexachlorophene intoxication: Characterization of myelin and myelin related fractions in the rat during early postnatal development. *Exp. Neurol.*, 45:558–575.
10. Mugnaini, E., and Schnapp, B. (1974): Possible role of zonula occludens of the myelin sheath in demyelinating conditions. *Nature*, 251:725–727.
11. Murray, M. R. (1965): Nervous tissues *in vitro*. In: *Cells and Tissues in Culture*, edited by E. N. Willmer, pp. 373–455. Academic Press, London.
12. Nieuwkoop, P. S., and Faber, J. T. (1967): *Normal Table of Xenopus Laevis (Daudin). A Systematical and Chronological Survey of the Development from the Fertilized Egg till the End of Metamorphosis.* North-Holland Publ., Amsterdam.
13. Pleasure, D., Towfighi, J., Silberberg, D., and Parris, J. (1974): The pathogenesis of hexachlorophene neuropathy: In vivo and in vitro studies. *Neurology (Minneap.)*, 24:1068–1075.
14. Reier, P. J., Tabira, T., and Webster, H. deF. (1977): A freeze-fracture and tracer analysis of hexachlorophene-induced myelin lesions in *Xenopus* tadpole optic nerves. *J. Neurol. Sci.* (In press.)
15. Reier, P. J., Tabira, T., and Webster, H. deF. (1976): The penetration of fluorescein-conjugated and electron-dense tracer proteins into *Xenopus* tadpole optic nerves following perineural injection. *Brain Res.*, 102:229–244.
16. Robertson, J. D. (1958): Structural alterations in nerve fibers produced by hypotonic and hypertonic solutions. *J. Biophysic. Biochem. Cytol.*, 4:349–364.
17. Towfighi, J., and Gonatas, N. K. (1977): The distribution of micro and horseradish peroxidase in the sciatic nerves of developing normal and hexachlorophene (HCP) intoxicated rats. *J. Neurocytol.* (In press.)
18. Towfighi, J., Gonatas, N. K., and McCree, L. (1974): Hexachlorophene-induced changes in central and peripheral myelinated axons of developing and adult rats. *Lab. Invest.*, 31:712–721.
19. Tabira, T., Webster, H. deF., and Wray, S. H. (1976): In vivo test for myelinotoxicity of cerebrospinal fluid. *Brain Res.* (In press.)
20. Webster, H. deF., and Billings, S. M. (1972): Myelinated nerve fibers in *Xenopus* tadpoles: *In vivo* observations and fine structure. *J. Neuropathol. Exp. Neurol.*, 31:102–112.
21. Webster, H. deF., Billings, S. M., and Guth, L. (1973): Muscle fibers and their innervation in *Xenopus* tadpoles: Fine structure, histochemistry and *in vivo* observations. In: *Basic Research in Myology*, Part 1, edited by B. K. Kakulas, pp. 19–25. Excerpta Medica, Amsterdam.
22. Webster, H. deF., Reier, P. J., Kies, M. K., and O'Connell, M. F. (1974): A simple method for quantitative morphological studies of CNS demyelination: Whole mounts of tadpole optic nerves examined by differential-interference microscopy. *Brain Res.*, 79:132–138.

23. Webster, H. deF., Ulsamer, A. G., and O'Connell, M. F. (1974): Hexachlorophene induced myelin lesions in the developing nervous system of *Xenopus* tadpoles: Morphological and biochemical observations. *J. Neuropathol. Exp. Neurol.*, 33:144–163.

Neurotoxicology, edited by L. Roizin, H. Shiraki, and N. Grčević. Raven Press, New York © 1977.

Fine Structure of Sciatic Nerves in Nitrofurantoin Neuropathy Induced in Rats

Albert J. Behar, Nelly Livni, and Dov Soffer

Department of Pathology, The Hebrew University—Hadassah Medical School, Jerusalem, Israel

Nitrofurantoin (NF), an effective antiseptic widely used in the treatment of urinary tract infections, has for some time now been known to be potentially neurotoxic and to cause peripheral neuropathy in patients, with both reversible and irreversible symptoms (1,2,4,5,8–10,12–15). Previously we have described the electrophysiological and light microscopy changes in NF polyneuropathy experimentally induced in rats (1).

In the present chapter we have attempted to elucidate the ultrastructural alterations occurring in sciatic nerves of rats, in an acute experiment in which animals were given NF during a short-term period. To the best of our knowledge no electron microscopy study of NF neuropathy has yet been reported.

MATERIALS AND METHODS

Adult albino rats (body weight 300 g) were used, three in the experimental group and three in the control one. Each of the experimental animals was given a single daily p.o. dose of 100 mg/kg 1-(5-nitrofurfurilideneamino) hydantoin (Urantoin®, Rafa Pharmaceutical Co., Jerusalem) for a period of 8 days. With this dose, mean plasma NF levels estimated by the phenyhydrazone method of Buzard et al. (3), 2 hr after administration of the drug, were 15 mg/ml as found in our previous experiments (1). These levels were four times

higher than the highest ones measured in patients with renal insufficiency 2 hr after they were given an oral dose of 100 mg NF (5).

On the day following withdrawal of the drug the animals were put into light anesthesia by subcutaneous injection of sodium pentothal, the sciatic nerves were exposed by incision through the muscles, and a segment just above the popliteal fossa was excised. Small samples of each nerve were fixed for electron microscopy in 3% glutaraldehyde with 0.1 M phosphate buffer at pH 7.3 for 3 hr, then postfixed in 2% osmium tetroxide for 2 hr at 4°C and embedded in Epon 812 by standard methods. Thick sections (1 μm) stained with toluidine blue were examined under the light microscope. Thin sections stained with uranyl acetate and lead citrate were examined with a Phillips 300 electron microscope.

RESULTS

No animal died during NF treatment, but all three showed definite sluggishness of movement. None lost weight.

Light Microscopy

Epon-embedded sections (1 μm thick) of the nerves of the NF-treated animals showed segmental loss of myelin sheath as well as undulation and irregular thickenings

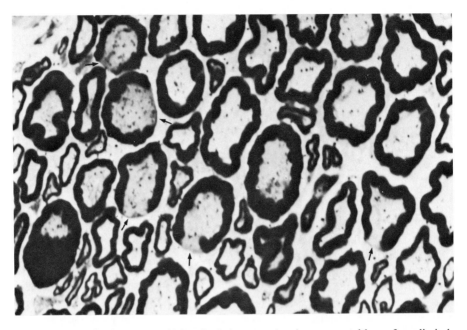

FIG. 1. Epon-embedded section (1 μm thick) of sciatic nerve showing segmental loss of myelin in large fibers alone. Toluidine blue. ×800.

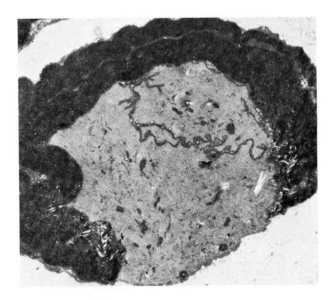

FIG. 2. Cross section of a nerve fiber. Segmental breakdown of the myelin sheath with denudation of axon and proliferation of membranes into the axoplasm. ×11,200.

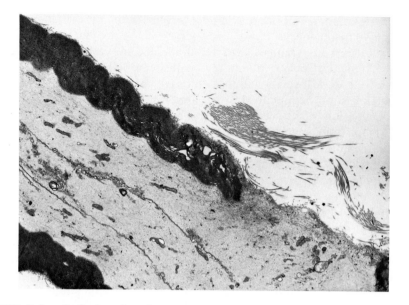

FIG. 3. Longitudinal section of a nerve fiber with same changes as in Fig. 2. ×9,000.

of the sheath, protruding into the axoplasm (Fig. 1). Only the largest fibers were affected by loss of myelin, and comprised roughly 10% of all large fibers. Careful study showed no demyelination of medium and small nerve fibers. No inflammatory cellular exudate was present.

Electronmicroscopy

Nerves of the treated rats showed many granule-studded mast cells as well as free mast cell granules in the interstitial tissues, but, again, no inflammatory cells. Endothelial cells of the vessels as well as

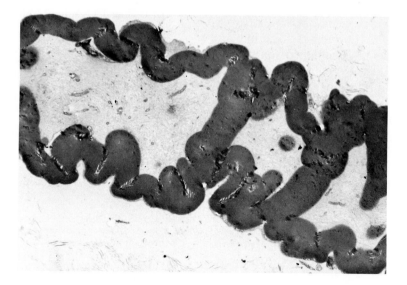

FIG. 4. Myelin masses protruding into axoplasm and forming "bridges" across the nerve fiber. ×7,800.

Schwann cells revealed no noticeable alterations. Nonmyelinated nerve fibers appeared normal. Marked changes were observed in myelinated fibers of large calibers. These consisted of segmental loss of the entire thickness of the myelin sheath resulting in denudation of the axoplasm (Figs. 2 and 3). In other segments distortion, separation, rupture, and homogenization of myelin lamellae were evident. Large masses of homogenized myelin sheath material often protruded into the axoplasm, occasionally forming "bridges" across the axis cylinder (Fig. 4) or replacing it completely. In demyelinated fibers there was a marked proliferation of membranes of linear, twisted, or annular configuration. They appeared to arise from disrupted innermost myelin lamellae.

Samples of control nerves showed no alteration under the light and electron microscopes.

DISCUSSION

Histopathological findings in peripheral nerves of human cases of NF neuropathy have included demyelination, Wallerian degeneration, and swelling of the axis cylinders (4,6,9,12,14). In a previous work dealing with experimental NF polyneuropathy in rats we described sausage-like and bulbous segmental swelling of axis cylinders as revealed by light microscopy of paraffin sections stained with the Bielschowsky method, but we then were unable to demonstrate convincing demyelination, using the Weil–Weigert method for paraffin sections, and the Marchi method for frozen sections (1).

The present study provides definite evidence of pathological alterations affecting both myelin sheaths and axoplasm of peripheral nerves in NF neuropathy. It also corroborates our previous electrophysiological studies in rat NF polyneuropathy.

Proliferation of cell membranes as observed in the present study in the axoplasm of affected nerve fibers has been described in the cerebellum of rats given long-term dosage of diphenylhydantoin (11). This abnormality is intriguing since both diphenylhydantoin and NF are hydantoin compounds. Evidence of peripheral nerve damage may appear in patients treated with diphenylhydantoin, but no direct causal relationship has been found between an abnormal folate metabolism and neuropathy (7). It has been suggested that vitamin C deficiency may be the causative agent of both the neuropathy and the abnormal folate metabolism following administration of a hydantoin compound such as NF. However, recent studies have failed to show evidence of vitamin C deficiency in patients before, during, or after treatment with NF (5). The pathogenetic mechanism of NF neuropathy appears to be unknown for the present.

REFERENCES

1. Behar, A. J., Rachmilewitz, E., and Rachamimoff, R. (1965): Experimental nitrofurantoin polyneuropathy in rats. Early histological and electrophysiological alterations in peripheral nerves. *Arch. Neurol.,* 13:160–163.
2. Briand, P., and Tygstrup, I. (1959): Polyneuropathy after therapy with nitrofurantoin (Furadantin). *Ugeskr. Laeger,* 121:664–666.
3. Buzard, L. A., Brabic, D. M., and Paul, F. M. (1956): Colorimetric determination of nitrofurazone, nitrofurantoin and furazolidone in plasma. *Antibiot. Chemother.,* 6:702–704.
4. Ellis, F. G. (1962): Acute polyneuritis after nitrofurantoin therapy. *Lancet,* 2:1136–1138.
5. Felts, J. H., Hayes, D. M., Gergen, J. A., and Toole, J. F. (1971): Neural hematologic and bacteriologic effects of nitrofurantoin in renal insufficiency. *Am. J. Med.,* 51:331–339.
6. Herndon, R. F., and Fox, G. E. (1966): Polyneuropathy due to nitrofurantoin. *Ill. Med. J.,* 129:164–166.
7. Horwitz, S. J., Klipstein, F. A., and Lovelace, R. E. (1968): Relation of abnormal folate metabolism to neuropathy developing during anticonvulsant drug therapy. *Lancet,* 1:563–564.
8. Loughridge, L. W. (1962): Peripheral neuropathy due to nitrofurantoin. *Lancet,* 2:1133–1135.
9. Morris, J. S. (1966): Nitrofurantoin and peripheral

neuropathy with megaloblastic anaemia. *J. Neurol. Neurosurg. Psychiatry,* 29:224–228.

10. Rubenstein, C. J. (1964): Peripheral polyneuropathy caused by nitrofurantoin. *JAMA,* 187:647–649.

11. Snider, R. S., and del Cerro, M. (1972): Diphenythidantoin: Proliferating membranes in cerebellum resulting from intoxication. In: *Antiepileptic Drugs,* edited by D. M. Woodbury, J. K. Penry, and R. P. Schmidt, pp. 237–245. Raven Press, New York.

12. Suchenwirth, R., and Dahl, P. (1968): Nitro-furantoin-polyneuritis. *Fortschr. Neurol. Psychiatr.,* 36:100–115.

13. Toole, J. F., and Parrish, M. L. (1973): Nitrofurantoin polyneuropathy. *Neurology (Minneap.),* 23:554–559.

14. Uesu, C. T. (1962): Peripheral neuropathy due to nitrofurantoin: Case report and review of literature. *Ohio State Med. J.,* 58:53–56.

15. Vogelsang, H., and Danke, F. (1971): Nitrofurantoin polyneuropathy. *Dtsch. Med. Wochenschr.,* 96:72–74.

Neurotoxicology, edited by L. Roizin, H. Shiraki, and N. Grčević. Raven Press, New York © 1977.

Degeneration of Choroid Plexus Epithelium Induced by Some Tertiary Amines

Seymour Levine

Pathology Department, New York Medical College Center for Chronic Disease, Bird S. Coler Hospital, Roosevelt Island, New York 10044

In 1968 Benitz and Kramer (1) reported a hydropic vacuolization of choroid plexus epithelium after ingestion of piperamide maleate [4'-(4-(3-dimethylaminopropyl)-1-piperazinyl) acetanilide dimaleate] in the diet. Piperamide was one of several substituted piperazines synthesized by Tomcufcik et al. (9) and found to have chemotherapeutic activity against *Trypanosoma cruzi*. Tomcufcik found that the substituted piperazine part of the molecule, but not the acetanilide, was essential for antitrypanosomal activity. Piperazine is a saturated six-member ring structure, with nitrogens instead of carbons at the 1 and 4 positions. In unsubstituted piperazine, both nitrogens are secondary amines (two bonds to carbons and one bond to hydrogen). However, both nitrogens in the piperazine of piperamide are completely substituted; inasmuch as all three bonds from the nitrogens are attached to carbons, they are classified as tertiary amines. Furthermore, the aliphatic side chain of piperamide contains still another tertiary amine. In view of these chemical considerations, we studied a series of compounds with one, two, or three tertiary amines. All of them contained a cyclic structure, either saturated (piperazine, piperidine, cyclohexane) or unsaturated (naphthyridine, pyridine, benzene, etc.). We found that a remarkable number of tertiary amines of diverse structure were capable of reproducing the piperamide lesion in choroid plexus.

METHODS

The chemical compounds were dissolved in saline or occasionally in peanut oil, or suspended in 0.5% aqueous carboxymethylcellulose. A single dose of drug was given to Lewis male or female rats by subcutaneous injection or by gavage. The rats were killed 1 day later by exsanguination from the neck vessels while under ether anesthesia. Brains and other organs were fixed in Bouin's fluid. Frontal section at the level of the median eminence contained the first three choroid plexuses, and a section from the caudal half of the cerebellum included the fourth plexus. The slices were embedded in paraffin, sectioned, and stained with hematoxylin–eosin. Vacuolation was scored on a scale of 1 to 4, graded from barely detectable at 100 times magnification to maximum effect, easily visible at 40 times.

RESULTS

Correlations with Chemical Structure

Four piperazine derivatives caused choroid plexus vacuolation, in addition to piperamide (Table 1 and Fig. 1). Com-

TABLE 1. *Hydropic degeneration of choroid plexus of rats caused by tertiary amines*

| | Degree of hydropic degeneration[a] | | | | | | | |
| | Subcutaneous dose (mg/kg body weight) | | | | Oral dose (mg/kg body weight) | | | |
Compound[b]	200	400	800	1,200	200	400	800	1,200
1. Piperamide		1	4			0	2	3
2. S37875-4		0	2	3		0	1	1
3. S36081-3		3	D	D		3	D	D
4. N,N'DMP	0	0	4	D		0	2	4
5. S35524-0		1	1	0		0	0	D
6. CL65703	0	3				0	2	
7. S34598-9		3	4	4		4	4	D
8. S34177-0		0	3	4		1	2	D
9. S43259-8	1	2	2		1	2	3	
10. 15005-3	0	2	4		0	0	D	
11. S38793-2	1	2	3		1	3	D	
12. S35496-1		2	4	D		1	D	D
13. S36462-2	0	3	4		0	4	D	
14. WR4206AD	0	D	D				3	
15. Chloroquine	0	D	D		0	0	0	1
16. BL20803	0	0	0			0	0	2
17. S55872-9		2	3	4		2	3	4
18. S34583-0	2	4	4	4	2	D	D	D
19. S41028-4	0	1	2		0	0	1	
20. S34223-8	1	D	D		0	1	D	
21. RC12	0	0	1		0	0	1	

[a] Scores from 1 to 4 based on histologic evaluation of all four choroid plexuses in one or more rats killed 1 day later. A score of 1 indicates vacuolation was barely detectable at ×100 magnification, and 4 indicates it was easily visible at ×40. D, died and therefore not studied histologically.

[b] Identified by name, code, or catalog number. Chemical formulas in Fig. 1, except see ref. 8 for compounds 15 and 21, and ref. 7 for compound 16. Sources: compounds 1 and 6, Lederle Laboratories; Compound 4, Jefferson Chemical Co.; Compounds 14 and 21, Walter Reed Army Institute of Research; Compound 15, Sterling Winthrop Research Institute; Compound 16, Bristol Laboratories; all others, Aldrich Chemical Co.

pounds 2 and 3, like piperamide, contained three tertiary amine groups (two piperazine nitrogens and the side chain nitrogen). Compound 4, the smallest and simplest active molecule, was merely a piperazine both of whose nitrogens were tertiary amines by virtue of methyl substituents on each. Compound 5 was weakly active perhaps because it had only one tertiary amine (one of the two piperazine nitrogens and the side chain nitrogen were not completely substituted). Piperazine, the parent compound, had no tertiary amine due to absence of substitutions, and it was inactive.

Piperidine is a saturated six-member ring that includes only one nitrogen. The active compounds 6 through 9 contained two tertiary amines in the form of two substituted piperidine rings or one substituted piperidine plus a side chain tertiary amine. Compounds 10 through 13 were equally active despite possession of only a single tertiary amine, either in the piperidine or in the side chain.

Compounds 14, 15, and 16 differed from the foregoing by the aromatic (unsaturated) rings instead of piperazine or piperidine. Each had a tertiary amine group in the side chain. Although their activity was weak, it added to the evidence that one tertiary amine was sufficient to affect the plexus.

Compounds 17 through 21 also had unsaturation in or adjacent to the rings. Unlike any of the foregoing, each had two or three identical tertiary amine side chains

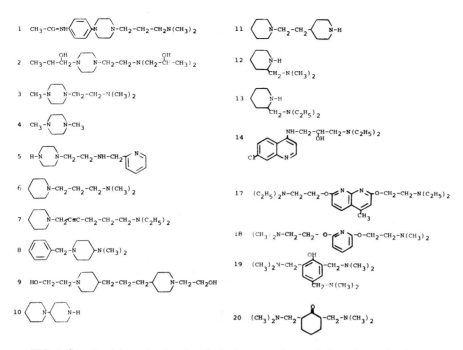

FIG. 1. Structural formulas for chemicals that caused vacuolation of choroid plexus.

symmetrically disposed about the rings. The pyridine and naphthyridine derivatives (compounds 18 and 17) had relatively good activity.

Morphology

Benitz and Kramer (1) observed slight vacuolation after 2 days of feeding piperamide in the diet, moderate changes after 4 days, and marked lesions after 8 or more days. We observed the same changes, even the most extreme vacuolation, as early as 1 day after oral or subcutaneous administration of a single large dose of drug (Figs. 2 and 3). Hydropic degeneration affected all of the choroid plexuses, but there was a tendency to milder involvement of the third ventricular plexus. In moderate or severe lesions, every choroidal epithelial cell was involved, albeit to differing degrees. One or several severely vacuolated cells were often seen adjoining one or several mildly affected cells, with an abrupt transition. The vacuoles varied from the size of the nucleus down to the limit of visual resolution. The vacuoles did not stain with periodic acid-Schiff in paraffin sections after formalin or alcohol fixation or with Sudan black in whole mounts fixed with formalin. In very severe cases, every choroidal cell was greatly swollen and the nuclei were displaced basally. The increased mass of choroidal villi often obliterated the ventricular lumen. Choroidal stroma, vessels, ependyma, and brain parenchyma had no abnormalities.

Electron microscopic study by Wenk revealed that the vacuoles were optically empty except for membranous fragments.

Similar changes were seen with all the active chemicals listed in Table 1, and after oral or subcutaneous administration. Compounds 1 and 6 were tested by intraperitoneal route and both were effective, but the intravenous route for compound 1 was lethal.

Benitz and Kramer observed evidence of recovery 16 days after the termination of

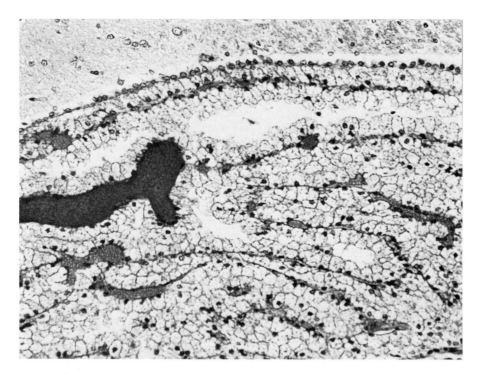

FIG. 2. Severe vacuolation. Swelling of choroidal epithelial cells has obliterated most of the lateral ventricular lumen. The dark structures are veins and capillaries filled with erythrocytes. H. & E. ×205.

a 2- or a 50-week course of dietary treatment (1). We also found that the lesion was reversible. A single dose of 500 mg/kg i.p. or 750 mg/kg s.c. of piperamide gave peak vacuolation of choroid plexus after 1 day, slight regression after 2 days, and complete recovery after 7 days.

Cyclophosphamide produces in rats a choroid plexus lesion characterized by a fibrin rich edema of the stroma (3). It was of interest to produce both lesions simultaneously. Rats were given 750 mg/kg piperamide preceded by 250 mg/kg cyclophosphamide 2 days earlier or accompanied by 125 mg/kg, at separate subcutaneous sites (the 250 mg/kg dose was lethal if given at the same time as piperamide). The distinctive vacuolation of the epithelium due to piperamide was observed in rats killed 1 or 2 days later, but the stroma, instead of being inconspicuous, was markedly edematous and contained large amounts of fibrin, as in the cyclophosphamide plexitis.

It was remarkable that the epithelial and stromal lesions could be produced separately or simultaneously at will.

Pathogenesis

It occurred to me that the unique affinity of piperamide for the choroid plexus might depend in some manner on the specialized secretory function of the plexus or on some peculiarity of its blood supply. Therefore, fourth ventricular plexuses of six Lewis rats were implanted beneath the left renal capsule of six other (histocompatible) Lewis rats as described elsewhere (see ref. 4). Three weeks later, the recipients were treated with piperamide intraperitoneally and sacrificed 2 days after treatment. The grafts appeared viable and had the typical hydropic vacuolation, equal, in fact, to the vacuolation in the recipients' own choroid plexuses. Inasmuch as plexus grafts are not likely to function normally

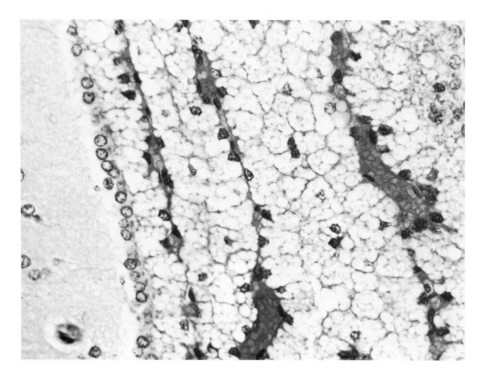

FIG. 3. Higher magnification of Fig. 2. The vacuoles have displaced the nuclei basally. The ependyma and adjacent brain parenchyma (*left*) are normal; the slight separation between them is an artifact. H. & E. ×450.

and have acquired a completely new blood supply, the piperamide lesion is more likely based on chemical affinity for some constituent of the plexus rather than on its function or blood supply. It is of interest that renal tubules in immediate juxtaposition to the plexus grafts had no trace of vacuolation.

None of the foregoing experiments gave any indication whether biotransformation was required before the tertiary amines acquired the ability to cause vacuolation. In order to elucidate this problem, one of the active compounds (compound 17) was implanted directly into the right lateral ventricle of eight rats, thereby achieving direct contact with the choroid plexus. The chemical was mixed with an equal weight of graphite which facilitated formation of a pellet and its expulsion from a Pitkin spinal puncture needle, as described elsewhere (see ref. 6), and which also served as a marker for the implant site in histologic sections. The rats were killed 1 day after implantation, and the brains were fixed and sectioned horizontally. Microscopic examination revealed slight to moderate vacuolation in the choroid plexus on the side of the implant, and no vacuolation on the opposite side. Surprisingly, three of the rats also had slight vacuolation in the fourth ventricular plexus. Five rats implanted only with pure graphite had no vacuolation in any of the plexuses, therefore the changes cannot be ascribed to trauma alone. The results favor the concept that tertiary amines cause hydropic degeneration by direct chemical interaction with choroid plexus. However, it is not yet proven that vacuolation after intraventricular implantation is of identical ultrastructural character or of identical chemical specificity as that which follows systemic administration.

DISCUSSION

Many compounds did not cause hydropic degeneration even though they contained piperazine or piperidine rings and one, two, or even three tertiary amine groups (negative compounds listed in ref. 5). These negative results are of limited significance because the range of doses may not have been sufficiently broad to detect weak activity. In addition, some features of these molecules may have prevented absorption or caused rapid metabolism or excretion, thereby preventing effective contact with the choroid plexus. Despite these caveats, it is of interest that the activity of compound 18 was not shared by a related compound, S34663–2, in which only one of the two tertiary amine side chains is present (5). This comparison adds to the evidence in Table 1 that a second tertiary amine group, although not essential, may increase the tendency of a compound to cause plexus degeneration.

All of the results presented here are based on examinations 1 day after a single dose of drug. This could be another cause of false negative results if certain compounds require repeated doses and a more protracted schedule before there is sufficient absorption or biotransformation to cause vacuolation of the plexuses. We have studied one drug in which the dose schedule was critical. This agent is tilorone [2,7-bis-(diethylaminoethoxy)fluoren 9-one hydrochloride]. One dose of this drug caused important histologic changes in lymphoid tissue in 1 day (2), but it had no effect on the choroid plexus (5). It should be noted that tilorone has a complex unsaturated ring system (fluorene) to which are attached two identical tertiary amine side chains. Compound 17 has the same two side chains, but it differs from tilorone by possessing the unsaturated naphthyridine ring system which is heterocylic and smaller than fluorene. In view of its close resemblance to compound 17 and in view

of the diversity of tertiary amines that are capable of damaging the choroid plexus, it would not be surprising if tilorone had similar activity. The interesting feature was the necessity for repeated doses of tilorone over a period of several days in order to elicit this activity (5). One can speculate that a longer exposure was needed for the relatively large tilorone molecule to penetrate the plexus, to interact with a hypothetical receptor, or to undergo biotransformation into a smaller molecule with heightened penetrability or affinity.

There is another intriguing relationship between tilorone and the compounds described herein. Tilorone and its analogs have a unique ability to deplete lymphocytes of the thymus-derived category from spleen, lymph nodes, and Peyer's patches in 1 day after a single dose (2). Most of the tertiary amines in Table 1 have exactly the same ability, albeit to a lesser degree (5). It is difficult to explain the coincidence of drug effects on two cell types of such disparate structure, function, and embryogenesis as lymphocytes and choroidal epithelium. However, brain and lymphoid tissue do share a common tissue antigen called "theta," so there is a precedent for these unusual observations.

SUMMARY

Vacuolar degeneration of choroid plexus epithelium of the rat was produced in 1 day by a single oral or parenteral dose of certain tertiary amines. Active compounds contained one, two, or three tertiary amine groups as parts of the saturated piperazine or piperidine rings or as side chains attached to these rings or to naphthyridine, pyridine, or other aromatic rings. Vacuolization affected all cells of all plexuses, even after transplantation to an ectopic site. The lesion was reversible. A similar lesion was produced locally by direct implantation of an active chemical into the ventricle. It is probable that the lesion results from chemical affinity between the tertiary amines and some component of the choroid plexus epithelium.

ACKNOWLEDGMENTS

I am indebted to R. Sowinski for assistance with the experiments, to the Kroc Foundation for grant support, and to Lederle Laboratories, Jefferson Chemical Co., Walter Reed Army Institute of Research, Sterling Winthrop Research Institute, and Bristol Laboratories for materials specified in Table 1, and to M. Moritz for the photomicrographs.

REFERENCES

1. Benitz, K.-F., and Kramer, A. W. (1968): Piperamide-induced morphological changes in the choroid plexus. *Fd. Cosmet. Toxicol.*, 6:125–133.
2. Levine, S., Gibson, J. P., and Megel, H. (1974): Selective depletion of thymus dependent areas in lymphoid tissue by tilorone. *Proc. Soc. Exp. Biol. Med.*, 146:245–248.
3. Levine, S., and Sowinski, R. (1973): Choroid plexitis produced in rats by cyclophosphamide. *J. Neuropathol. Exp. Neurol.*, 32:365–370.
4. Levine, S., and Sowinski, R. (1975): Choroid plexus isografts in rats. *J. Neuropathol. Exp. Neurol.*, 34:335–339.
5. Levine, S., and Sowinski, R. (1977): T-lymphocyte depletion and lesions of choroid plexus and kidney induced by tertiary amines. Toxicol. Appl. Pharmacol., 40:147–159.
6. Levine, S., Zimmerman, H. M., Wenk, E. J., and Gonatas, N. K. (1963): Experimental leukoencephalopathies due to implantation of foreign substances. *Am. J. Pathol.*, 42:97–117.
7. Siminoff, P., Bernard, A. M., Hursky, V. S., and Price, K. E. (1973): BL-20803, a new, low-molecular-weight interferon inducer. *Antimicrob. Agents Chemother.*, 3:742–743.
8. Thompson, P. E., and Werbel, L. M. (1972): *Antimalarial Agents. Chemistry and Pharmacology.* Academic Press, New York.
9. Tomcufcik, A. S., Hewitt, R. I., Fabio, P. F., Hoffman, A. M., and Enwistle, J. (1965): N^4-substituted N'-(3-dimethylaminopropyl)-piperazines: A new series of compounds active against *Trypanosoma cruzi* infections in mice. *Nature*, 205:605–606.

Neurotoxicology, edited by L. Roizin, H. Shiraki, and N. Grčević. Raven Press, New York © 1977.

Industrial Neuropathies

Peter S. Spencer and Herbert H. Schaumburg

Departments of Pathology and Neuroscience, Saul R. Korey Department of Neurology, and the Rose F. Kennedy Center for Research in Mental Retardation and Human Development, Albert Einstein College of Medicine, Bronx, New York 10461

Among the agents responsible for recent outbreaks of nervous system disease in industry are the vinyl monomer acrylamide and the hexacarbon solvents *n*-hexane and methyl *n*-butyl ketone (1,5–8). Individuals exposed for prolonged periods of time to relatively low levels of these compounds develop a largely reversible sensory-motor polyneuropathy — sensory symptoms being prominent with acrylamide and motor signs dominating the clinical picture with the hexacarbons. Sensory abnormalities characteristically commence in a stocking-and-glove distribution with weakness, which is always more pronounced in the lower extremities beginning distally and affecting more proximal muscles with time. Commonly, the neuropathy worsens for a short time after the individual's departure from the toxic environment but eventually remits, and recovery is usually complete.

EXPERIMENTAL STUDIES

The present study has used acrylamide (10 mg/kg daily) and four chemically and biologically related straight chain hexacarbons, *n*-hexane (500 ppm), methyl *n*-butyl ketone (300 mg/kg daily, s.c.), 2,5-hexanedione, and 2,5-hexanediol (as 0.5% drinking solutions), to study in approximately 100 cats and rats the pattern and spatial–temporal distribution of nervous system degeneration. These studies have demonstrated that all six compounds produce a typical peripheral neuropathy characterized clinically by slowly developing hindlimb weakness. Unlike the clinical expression of the disease, pathological changes are not confined to the peripheral nervous system, but occur concurrently in both the central and peripheral nervous system as axonal degeneration of the dying-back type.

It has been suggested that in the dying-back process, there is a malfunction of vulnerable central and peripheral neuronal perikarya that results in a gradual decrease in the production of materials required for the maintenance of axonal integrity. On the basis of this theory, extremities of the axon would suffer first from a reduction of

TABLE 1. *Causative agents of some industrial neuropathies (1–3) and related hexacarbons (4,5)*

1. Acrylamide	$CH_2CHCONH_2$
2. *n*-Hexane[a]	$CH_3CH_2CH_2CH_2CH_2CH_3$
3. Methyl *n*-butyl ketone[a]	$CH_3COCH_2CH_2CH_2CH_3$
4. 2,5-Hexanedione[a]	$CH_3COCH_2CH_2COCH_3$
5. 2,5-Hexanediol[a]	$CH_3CHOHCH_2CH_2CHOHCH_3$

[a] Hexacarbon compounds

essential materials exported from neuronal perikarya, since proximal regions would be adequately nourished. Axonal degeneration would commence at the terminals of the longest axons and show a temporal, seriate progression of change proximally along the axon *pari passu* with increasing perikaryal impairment. Cavanagh and his colleagues (2–4) clearly established that certain toxic chemicals could be utilized to produce animal models of dying-back disease. The hexacarbon compounds offer important advantages for the further study of experimental dying-back disease since an initial pathological event consists of giant axonal swelling with secondary changes in the myelin sheath. These studies have led to a reappraisal of the dying-back concept and the pathologic mechanisms that might underly this type of nervous system disease.

The distribution of giant axonal swellings in the central nervous system of rats with hexacarbon neuropathy was characteristic of a dying-back disease. Early in the neuropathy, when slight hindlimb weakness was noted, giant axonal swellings were found symmetrically in the distal regions of long ascending and descending tracts located in the spinal cord, medulla oblongata, and cerebellum. As the neuropathy became more pronounced, axonal swellings were found in more proximal regions of affected nerve tracts, whereas the distal regions had undergone complete fiber breakdown with concomitant loss of myelin. Within the dorsal columns of the medulla oblongata, axons located in the long gracile tracts seemed to be more vulnerable than adjacent axons in the shorter cuneate tracts. Thus, when the neuropathy was severe and hindlimb paralysis was present, axons within the cuneate tract were undergoing giant axonal swelling in the medulla, whereas the wave of swelling in the gracile tracts had moved caudally to involve thoracic and lumbar regions.

The distribution of peripheral nerve fiber change was studied principally within the sciatic/tibial/plantar nerve complex and associated muscles of the rat. By sampling proximal and distal branches of these nerves, it was possible to examine the role of axon length and diameter in determining the differential vulnerability of nerve fibers in these toxic neuropathies. These findings were correlated with studies in the cat where sensory and motor nerve terminals in the hindfeet were sampled repetitively throughout the development of neuropathy. These studies revealed differences between the distribution of axonal degeneration produced by the hexacarbons compared with that produced by acrylamide (10). The plantar sensory nerves were much more vulnerable to acrylamide than to the hexacarbons. Pacinian corpuscles and muscle spindle primary afferents within the hindfeet of cats intoxicated with acrylamide commenced axonal degeneration before adjacent motor nerve terminals supplying extrafusal muscle fibers. By contrast, pacinian corpuscles in the hindfeet of cats intoxicated with the hexacarbon methyl *n*-butyl ketone showed a remarkable resistance to damage and degenerated long after hindlimb weakness was profound. Perhaps the most surprising finding in both acrylamide- and hexacarbon-treated animals was the special vulnerability of the very large diameter fibers that exit from the tibial nerves in branches to the calf muscles. Giant axonal degeneration commenced later within the smaller diameter fibers supplying the plantar nerves in the hindfeet of rats. This resulted in two, independent ascending waves of giant axonal degeneration—the initial wave commencing in the tibial branches to the calf muscles and ascending the sciatic nerve and a later wave commencing in the plantar nerves and ascending the posterior tibial nerve. With time, giant axonal degeneration was found in lumbosacral dorsal and ventral roots, but corresponding sensory and motor neurons were largely unaffected morphologically by the degenerative process.

The pattern and evolution of nerve fiber degeneration was studied by sampling vulnerable calf muscle branches at various stages in the development of the neuropathy (9). One of the earliest features of the disease process was the production of multifocal, giant axonal swellings in distal but nonterminal regions of such large myelinated fibers. Axonal swellings first appeared on the proximal sides of multiple paranodes and subsequently at facing paranodes and internodal loci. Proximal paranodal swelling occurred concomitantly with shrinkage and corrugation of the adjacent distal internodes. Enlarged nodal and paranodal axons seemed to displace the paranodal myelin sheath producing naked, giant axonal swellings within the vicinity of nodes of Ranvier. Ultrastructural examination of swollen axons showed that they were composed principally of accumulated 10-nm neurofilaments. Proximal paranodal giant axonal swellings were associated with distal accumulations of axonal mitochondria and complex profiles believed to represent a process of selective adaxonal Schwann cell sequestration and phagocytosis of axonal organelles (11).

Examination of long lengths of single nerve fibers removed from animals with hexacarbon neuropathy emphasized the multifocal distal degenerative process. Denuded axons became associated with numerous Schwann cells and presumably underwent local shrinkage before remyelination commenced. It was also apparent in nerve fibers supplying the calf muscles that proximal portions could be more severely affected than distal regions of the same fiber. When neuropathy was advanced, nerve fiber breakdown and ovoid formation was observed to commence distal to an especially prominent giant axonal swelling. There was no suggestion of a centripetal spread of degeneration in individual fibers, and, indeed, proximal regions frequently displayed ovoid formation before more distal regions of the same fiber. It was likely, therefore, that once a swollen interface had been established, the entire distal portion of the axon underwent a simultaneous degeneration analagous to Wallerian degeneration. It also seemed probable that such swollen interfaces later attenuated to form the positions from which axonal regeneration was observed, a phenomenon that occurred during the maintenance of intoxication.

CONCLUSION

This interpretation of the evolution of nerve fiber degeneration in these toxic neuropathies differs radically from previous concepts of the sequence of pathological events in analagous, toxic dying-back diseases. One implication of the term 'dying-back' was that degeneration commenced in the nerve terminal and, with time, proceeded *seriatim* up the nerve fiber toward the neuron cell body. The present study challenges these opinions since it demonstrates that within the affected distal lengths of single fibers there is: (a) a simultaneous, multifocal, apparently random occurrence of giant axonal swelling; (b) commonly, a greater degree of damage proximal to the nerve terminal than at the position of the nerve terminal; and (c) an approximately simultaneous formation of ovoids distal to a swollen interface during the later phases of degeneration. Taken in concert, these observations force a revision of the classic concept of the evolution of dying-back diseases: although it seems clear that the term 'dying-back' remains a useful description of the overall centripetal, temporal spread of damage within nerve trunks, it does not reflect accurately the evolution of change within individual nerve fibers. Furthermore, it is unresolved whether there is any net retrograde spread of damage along individual fibers or whether different fibers within the affected nerve trunk commence degeneration at different times and at progressively increasingly proximal levels as the neuropathy evolves. It is clear, however, that the diameter of the axon is equally as important as the length of the axon in determining the vulnerability of a nerve fiber.

These observations seem to indicate that the favored hypothesis to account for the dying-back process—progressive impairment of neuron perikaryal metabolism—is unlikely to be entirely responsible for distal axonal degeneration. The presence of a distal distribution of multifocal axonal change is equally compatible with a theory of local axonal action of these toxic substances. The initial change of giant axonal swellings on the proximal sides of nodes of Ranvier suggests that the node may be especially vulnerable to the action of these neurotoxic compounds. It is conceivable that this results in partial blockade of anterograde axonal transport at nodal regions that restricts the volume of material passing along the fiber. This would account for the swellings on proximal sides of nodes of Ranvier and the axonal attenuation and myelin corrugation of adjacent, distal internodes. The simultaneous formation of ovoids distal to an axonal swelling might then result from a complete blockade of anterograde transport at that site.

ACKNOWLEDGMENTS

This work was supported by research grants OH–00535, NS–08952, and NS–03356 from the National Institutes of Health; and by grants from the Alfred P. Sloan Foundation, Tennessee Eastman Co., American Cyanamid Co., Dow Chemical Co., Vistron Co., Nalco Chemical Co., and Exxon Corporation.

Dr. Spencer is the recipient of a Joseph P. Kennedy, Jr. Fellowship in the Neurosciences.

REFERENCES

1. Allen, N., Mendell, J. R., Billmaier, D. J., Fontaine, R. E., and O'Neill, J. (1975): Toxic polyneuropathy produced by the industrial solvent methyl n-butyl ketone. *Arch. Neurol.*, 32:209.
2. Cavanagh, J. B. (1963): Organophosphorus neurotoxicity: A model "dying-back" process comparable to certain human neurological disorders. *Guys Hosp. Rep.* 112:303.
3. Cavanagh, J. B. (1964): The significance of the "dying-back" process in experimental and human neurological disease. *Int. Rev. Exp. Pathol.*, 3:219.
4. Cavanagh, J. B. (1973): Peripheral neuropathy caused by chemical agents. *CRC Crit. Rev. Toxicol.*, 2:365.
5. Garland, T. O., and Patterson, M. W. H. (1967): Six cases of acrylamide poisoning. *Br. Med. J.*, 4:134.
6. Graveleau, J., Loirat, P., and Nusinovici, V. (1970): Polynévrite par l'acrylamide *Rev. Neurol.* (Paris), 123:62.
7. Herskowitz, A., Ishii, N., and Schaumburg, H. (1971): n-Hexane neuropathy: A syndrome occurring as a result of industrial exposure. *N. Engl. J. Med.*, 285:82.
8. Inoue, T., Takeuchi, Y., Takeuchi, S., Yamada, S., Suzuki, H., Matsushita, T., Miyagaki, H., Maeda, K., and Matsumoto, T. (1970): A health survey on vinyl sandal manufacturers with high incidence of n-hexane intoxication. *Jpn. J. Ind. Health*, 12:73.
9. Spencer, P. S. and Schaumburg, H. H. (1977): Ultrastructural studies of the dying-back process. III. The evolution of experimental peripheral giant axonal disease. *J. Neuropathol. Exp. Neurol.*, 36:276.
10. Spencer, P. S. and Schaumburg, H. H. (1977): Ultrastructural studies of the dying-back process. IV. Differential vulnerability of selected PNS and CNS fibers in experimental central distal axonopathies. *J. Neuropath. Exp. Neurol.*, 36:300.
11. Spencer, P. S. and Thomas, P. K. (1974): Ultrastructural studies of the dying-back process. II. The sequestration and removal by Schwann cells and oligodendrocytes of organelles from normal and diseased axons. *J. Neurocytol.*, 3:763.

Neurotoxicology, edited by L. Roizin, H. Shiraki, and N. Grčević. Raven Press, New York © 1977.

Tri-Ortho-Cresyl Phosphate Neurotoxicity

A. Bischoff

Neurology Department, University of Berne, Medical School, Inselspital, 3010 Berne, Switzerland

The neurotoxicity of tri-ortho-cresyl phosphate (TOCP) was already recognized at the beginning of the century because of peripheral neuropathies accompanying the treatment of pulmonary tuberculosis by phosphocreosote. In the 1920s the epidemic occurrence of ginger paralysis in the southern states of the United States pointed out this potential hazard dramatically (16,30). Owing to this experience and another major outbreak of a similar neurological disorder in Morocco in 1959 caused by TOCP that led to the paralysis of some 10,000 persons, the characteristic clinical picture of TOCP neurotoxicity became obvious (31,32). The intake of an individually variable amount of the toxic oily substance (about 1 g) was followed, approximately 12 hr later, by a prodromal gastrointestinal disturbance. Then, after an interval of 8 to 14 days, a flaccid paresis developed distally in the legs accompanied by aches and tingling paresthesias. Depending on the dose a predominant motor paresis spread to the intrinsic muscles of the hands and the thighs and to the muscles of the pelvic girdle. As a rule, it stopped short of com-

plete quadriplegia, and cranial nerves remained intact. Sensory loss was scanty. However, at the same time, signs of spinal cord damage such as spasticity and ataxia became apparent when remission of the neuropathy progressed (10).

The intoxication has been extensively studied in experimental animals for biochemistry and histology, particularly in chicken (5,9,14), cats (10,27), and baboons (17).

BIOCHEMISTRY AND METABOLISM

TOCP is an aryl phosphate that is derived from the phosphorylation of phenols. It is a small molecule with a molecular weight of 368 which is soluble in lipds and lipid solvents.

Today, it is mainly used as a plasticizer and high temperature lubricant. It has the same chemical base as organophosphorus compounds employed as insecticides.

As the latter are potent inhibitors of esterases and particularly of cholinesterase and in part have a delayed neurotoxic effect in hens similar to that produced by TOCP,

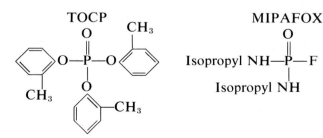

suggestions on the neurotoxicity of TOCP were focused mainly on its binding reaction with esterase enzymes (1,2,17,19,21). Other studies concentrated on phosphorus metabolism of the nervous tissue, originally basing their work on the erroneous premise that the structural damage caused by TOCP was primarily demyelination of the nerve fiber (3,24,26,33).

It is thought that TOCP is converted by the liver. This has been suggested by Aldridge (1), Casida et al. (7), and Eto et al. (13) in rats and chickens. Aldridge (1) showed that only after passing through a conversion stage does TOCP become a potent cholinesterase inhibitor, whereas a highly purified specimen of TOCP turned out to be inactive against serum cholinesterase *in vivo* unless previously incubated with liver tissue. Casida et al. (8) and Eto et al. (13) were able to isolate a metabolite synthesized from liver microsomes of TOCP-intoxicated rats that was a very powerful cholinesterase inhibitor and more effective in inducing paralysis in chickens than was the parent compound. The finding was confirmed by Morazain and Rosenberg (24) who found that liver minces from chicken and rats were very active in converting 5 μmoles of TOCP to a potent cholinesterase inhibitor, whereas spinal cord and sciatic nerve were inactive in converting the TOCP to the anticholinesterase metabolites that could not be detected in the nervous tissue.

As to the inhibitory action of the TOCP molecule, it was thought to have occurred because of phosphorylation of the active esteratic site of the enzyme, i.e., it depends on the presence of the phosphoric acid ester.

However, in the serum of TOCP-poisoned animals only a temporary inhibition of pseudocholinesterase not of true cholinesterase was found (12,28). In a recent study, however, Hern (17) found a marked depression of true cholinesterase activity also in addition to an almost complete inhibition of pseudocholinesterase activity in baboons intoxicated by TOCP. The action of the organophosphorus compound was potentiated by the polysorbate 80 "Tween 80" (17). In that experimental animal the grade of true cholinesterase inactivation corresponded reasonably to the severity of acute cholinergic effects evidenced by diarrhea, vomiting, and muscle fasciculations. The diarrhea persisted for 2 to 3 days, but only after a delay of 8 to 14 days did a progressive neurologic damage similar to human disease become apparent. Although this event seems very suggestive regarding the mechanism of action of the initial and early signs of TOCP intoxication, it is unlikely that the cholinesterase inhibition shares any relationship with the delayed neurotoxic effect (2,19).

In previous studies the possibility of structural abnormalities of the nervous tissue due to TOCP intoxication has been discussed. Most of this work concentrated on phospholipid metabolism. Webster (33) showed that despite TOCP poisoning the incorporation of the radioactive precursors containing ^{32}P into the phospholipids was normal. In addition, no major changes could be observed in the distribution of the lipids of the nervous tissue (29) or in the proportions of the various fatty acids (18).

On the other hand, some biophysical changes seem to occur in the major structural phospholipids of peripheral nervous tissue in TOCP-intoxicated chickens (24). There is a two- to threefold increase in hydrolysis of phospholipids from TOCP-poisoned chicken sciatic nerves exposed to phospholipidases in 1 mg/ml venom for 30 min. The increase is already evident on day 8 after administration of TOCP and is not present in chicken brain.

PATHOLOGY

Histological studies on patients intoxicated by TOCP did not clarify the nature of the neurotoxic damage. More information was gained from investigations into experimental animals. As to the site of the toxic lesion, they revealed that not only do the long tracts of the spinal cord and certain cerebellar systems show obvious degenerative lesions but also the peripheral nerve fibers do as well (3,4,9,14,15,22). Hern (17), carrying out extensive experimental studies in intoxicated baboons and squirrel monkeys, definitively demonstrated that the primary histological lesion was axonal degeneration initially present only in the distal ends of the longest motor nerve fibers. No segmental demyelination was visible. Morphological features consistent with Wallerian degeneration occurred only in progressed stages of clinical disorder. Thick myelinated nerve fibers were not more affected than thin myelinated ones. Similar alterations had been seen also in the long tracts of the spinal cord in birds (11) as well as in squirrel monkeys (17).

Electron microscopic observations have been reported first by Bischoff (5). In chickens of mixed breed weighing between 1.5 and 3.5 kg to which 1 ml/kg body weight of pure TOCP was administered by stomach tube, a single fiber degeneration became visible as soon as 1 day after the appearance of clinical signs. The myelin sheath being intact, an accumulation of vesicles and tubular profiles was apparent in the axon giving some suggestion of a hypertrophic reaction form of the endoplasmic reticulum. It coincided with an aggregation and disintegration of neurofilaments (Fig. 1). Myelinated nerve fibers were predominantly affected, but unmyelinated nerve fibers obviously were also abnormal. In the progressed stages, the axoplasmic organelles became replaced by irregular patterns of granular material or they were dissolved.

Similar changes could be observed in the long tracts of the spinal cord (6). In about 10% of the nerve fibers a swelling and proliferation of the vesicular elements of the agranular endoplasmic reticulum could be observed (Fig. 2) together with a disintegration and disappearance of the neurofilamentous organelles which were subsequently replaced by granular masses. The mitochondria remained structurally intact. At the 16th day some axons appeared devoid of normal organelles. In the gray matter the majority of the diseased presynaptic terminals appeared distinctively distended and densely packed with clusters of small vesicles or multimembraneous complexes, or both (Figs. 3 and 4). In some cases the terminals were filled with tangles of filaments or a granular web of more amorphous material (Fig. 5).

The most striking initial pathological feature however could be observed in the axon endings. In approximately 10 to 20% of the axosomatic synaptic knobs a marked swelling and deterioration of synaptic vesicles was visible (Fig. 6). The alteration had to be ascribed to the synaptic complex with spherical vesicles and an asymmetric synaptic cleft, which according to Bodian corresponds to excitatory synapses, whereas the synapses with flattened vesicles, the F type, representing inhibitory activity, did not show this alteration. Functionally this finding was interpreted as a primary defect of excitatory influences and otherwise exaggerated inhibitory influences by partial deafferentation of motor cells which themselves showed only minor pathological changes.

In a further experiment TOCP intoxication was applied to immature animals. The study aimed to clarify whether the axonal degeneration might represent a primary defect of the neuron, although axon flow measurements had not revealed any change in the rate of axoplasmic transport of protein in the ventral and dorsal roots of cats intoxicated by TOCP (25). Furthermore, it had been suggested by various authors that there exists an insusceptibility of immature animals to organophosphorus neurotoxic effects in correlation with a relative resistance to anoxic damage (10,24), an

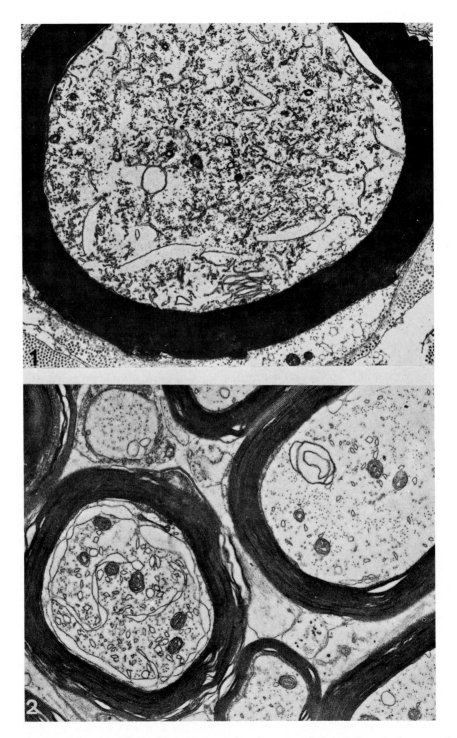

FIG. 1. Transverse section through a peripheral nerve, 1 day after onset of clinical signs. An increase of vesicular and tubular elements of the endoplasmic reticulum is apparent in the axoplasm.×12,200.

FIG. 2. Transverse section through the ventromedial tract in chicken spinal cord. Single fiber degeneration (*left*) with dilatation of axoplasmic vesicular organelles is shown. ×18,300.

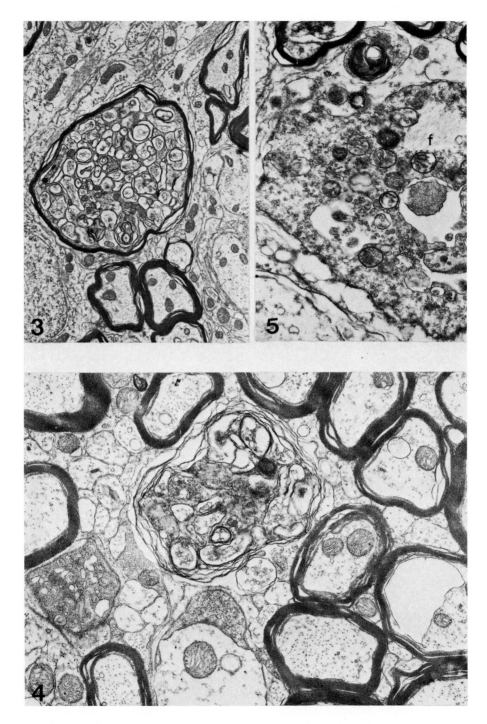

FIG. 3. Transverse section through the dorsal column of chicken spinal cord. An axonal ending shows extention and accumulation of membraneous structures. ×8,000.

FIG. 4. Transverse section showing single fiber degeneration with disappearance of normal axoplasmic organelles. ×18,300.

FIG. 5. Presynaptic nerve ending showing an increased granularity as well as fibrillar (f) material. ×16,700.

assumption refuted by results in a toxicity test using the chick embryo technique in which it had been shown that hatched chicks developed paralysis 2 to 6 weeks after hatching (23).

The study was carried out according to the techniques described by McLaughlin et al. (23). One hundredth of a milliliter of undiluted TOCP was injected into the yolk sac of fertile eggs prior to incubation. The dose provided that about 30% of the chick embryos hatched, whereas 70% decayed during embryonic development. The living chick embryos were sacrified at the 14th, 16th, 18th, and 20th day of incubation, and the sciatic nerve was prepared for electron microscopy. A reliable number of control eggs were treated in the same way. Electron microscopic examination revealed no evidence of a damage or loss of ganglion cells in the spinal cord. Nor was a clear-cut depletion of axons seen as might be expected in the case of a primary cellular lesion (Table 1). However, as early as 16 days after the onset of incubation some axonal degeneration comparable to the findings in adult hens was apparent (Fig. 7). However, the diseased nerve fibers were not as numerous as in adult intoxicated chickens nor was the degree of disintegration as severe.

ISOTOPE STUDIES

There exist some reports on investigations into the phosphorus metabolism of TOCP-poisoned animals that were substantiated by studies of the incorporation of radioactive tracers, particularly of ^{32}P (22,26,33). They concentrated on the problem of whether TOCP causes abnormalities of the biosynthesis rates of labeled precursors into the phospholipid compound of the nervous tissue. As mentioned above, they failed to bring any evidence of inhibition of the uptake of ^{32}P in the intoxicated animals in either spinal cord or nerves (22,26, 33). With regard to *in vivo* phosphorus incorporation into normal chicken phospholipid the results suggested that this is slow since the relative specific activities of ^{32}P did not reach a maximum at 72 hr. The rate of the incorporation of the isotope into chicken sciatic nerve was faster than that into cord.

In order to study the fate of TOCP in experimental animals we investigated the *in vivo* incorporation of TOC-^{32}P. Oral administration of tri-[ortho-cresyl-T(G)] phosphate (0.5 mC; for every 2 ml/kg body weight) was carried out on adult chickens. The animals were sacrified at 2,6, and 10 days. Samples of spinal cord, sciatic nerve, and other tissues such as liver and spleen were prepared by dissolution in chloroform–methanol and by freezing and homogenizing. The concentration of ^{32}P was determined by liquid scintillation counting. The accumulation rate of ^{32}P in the lipid fraction of the examined spinal cord and sciatic nerve shows a gradual rise in concentration during the first 10 days (Table 2). The increase in radioactivity is greater in the sample of chicken sciatic nerve than in spinal cord. The rates of uptake of ^{32}P expressed as relative specific activities are in remarkable agreement with those for the incorporation of nontoxic ^{32}P as reported by Webster (33).

In a second experiment we investigated the incorporation of TOCP with ^{32}P by *autoradiography*. Ten days after intoxication sections of the lumbar spinal cord and sciatic nerve were prepared for autoradiography. Reduced grains of emulsion can be recognized over intraspinal nerve fibers (Fig. 8) and the peripheral nerve and also over the motoneuron to a lesser degree. Their site of deposition corresponds to the membraneous structures and the myelin sheath in particular.

CONCLUSIONS

There is wide agreement today that TOCP intoxication in experimental ani-

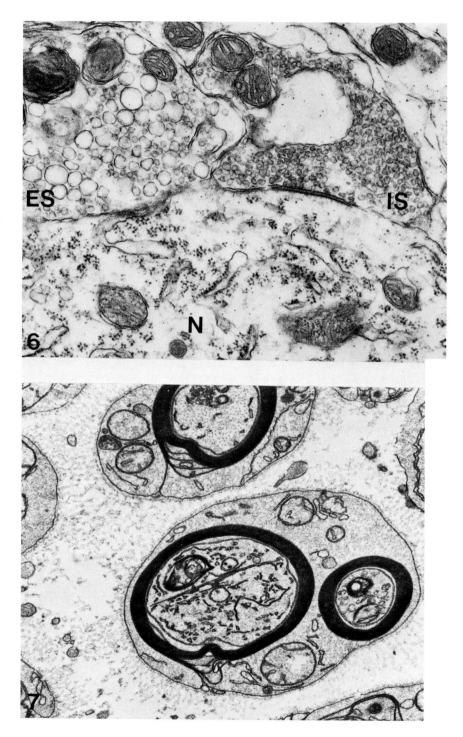

FIG. 6. Axosomatic synaptic knobs of the S type (spherical vesicles) (ES) and of the F type (flattened vesicles) (IS). The S-type synapse shows markedly inflated vesicles. N, neuron. ×20,000.
FIG. 7. Chick embryo sciatic nerve with sparse single fiber degeneration. ×20,000.

TABLE 1. *Diameter histogram of myelinated and unmyelinated nerve fibers/mm² of fascicular area of sciatic nerve of TOCP-poisoned chick embryos and age-matched controls*

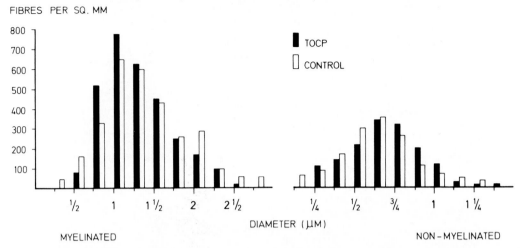

mals produces a primary axonal degeneration. Disintegration of the myelin sheath definitively must be understood to be of secondary nature in the sense of Wallerian degeneration. The pathological changes in the peripheral nerve apparently become visible around the eighth day after intoxication, and their appearance correlates well with the onset of clinical signs of paresis. At the same time with the pathological alterations in the peripheral nerve, definite lesions can also be observed in the spinal cord. Here they are confined to the longest tracts and initially affect the nerve endings in the same way as in the peripheral nerve.

Qualitatively, at the ultrastructural level,

TABLE 2. *Radioactivity in spinal cord and sciatic nerve following administration of TOC-³²P in adult chicken.*

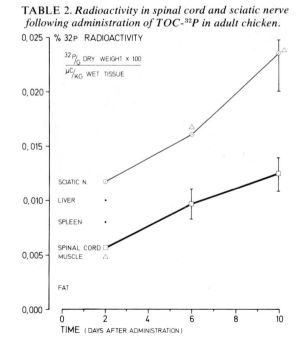

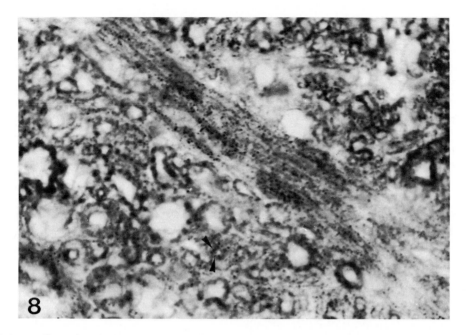

FIG. 8. Autoradiography of spinal cord of chicken intoxicated with TOC-^{32}P at the 10th day after administration of the toxic radioactive tracer. ×400.

the structural changes are characterized by a marked proliferation and distention of vesicular elements of the endoplasmic reticulum (ER) and a coinciding disintegration of the filamentous and tubular organelles. The presynaptic nerve terminals and boutons terminaux seem to be particularly affected in TOCP intoxication. As a most striking feature, an inflation of the synaptic vesicles which is confined to the spherical vesicles becomes apparent. The spherical vesicles of the axosomatic synapses being the site of excitatory transmitter effect, the suggestion of exaggerated inhibitory influences on the motoneurons could explain the early flaccid paresis by neuronal deafferentiation.

As to the neurotoxicity of TOCP, it is evident from a review of the literature that most of the authors believe an essential early step in the neurotoxic effect might be an inhibition of a particular esterase due to phosphorylation by the TOCP molecule. The concept is based on some hard facts that TOCP, like other organophosphorus compounds, likely is passing into a conversion system in the liver and that its metabolites exert an active inhibition of pseudocholinesterase and cholinesterase as well, producing a cholinergic crisis in humans and susceptible animals like chicken and cats. As a temporary inhibition of the suggested esterase by carbamates provides some protection against the neurotoxic effect of organophosphorus compounds (19,20), a pathogenetic significance of the so-called neurotoxic esterase seemed obvious not only for the cholinergic action but also for the delayed neurotoxicity. However, the anticholinesterase activity of TOCP which shows its maximum in the first 48 hr after the uptake of the compound hardly explains the delayed neurotoxicity.

A hypothesis proposed to account for the delayed neurotoxic effect suggests a biochemical lesion in certain neuronal perikarya (19), an assumption that actually is not supported by morphological and axon-flow studies (6,25).

The newest findings presented and interpreted above would favor a concept that TOCP exerts a direct effect on the axon by altering some structural components, particularly of the axon and synaptic vesicle membrane. Some ultrastructural findings such as the vesicular proliferation would indicate a breakdown of the permeability barrier. Hypothetically, normal structural phosphates might be replaced by the TOCP molecule with the consequence of a steric reorientation of phospholipids in the membranes. The results of the autoradiographic and recent metabolic studies are in reasonable agreement with a hypothesis that states that the rather inert molecule in part is not converted in the liver but rather is incorporated into some structural lipid elements of the nervous system. This assumption again considers the fact and fits in with the statement of Morazain and Rosenberg (24) that they could not detect the anticholinesterase metabolites in the spinal cord or sciatic nerve of TOCP-poisoned chickens.

ACKNOWLEDGMENTS

I wish to thank Dr. H. Roesler, head of the Department of Nuclear Medicine of the University of Berne, Medical School, who carried out the isotope measurements.

The investigations were supported by the Swiss National Fund (grants No. 3503, 4527, and 3.302.–0.74).

REFERENCES

1. Aldridge, W. N. (1954): Tricresyl phosphates and cholinesterase. *Biochem. J.,* 56:185–189.
2. Aldridge, W. N., and Barnes, J. M. (1961): Neurotoxic and biochemical properties of some triaryl phosphates. *Biochem. Pharmacol.,* 6:177–188.
3. Barnes, J. M., and Denz, F. A. (1953): Experimental demyelination with organophosphorus compounds. *J. Pathol. Bacteriol.,* 65:597–605.
4. Beresford, W. A., and Glees, P. (1963): Degeneration in the long tracts of the cords of the chicken and cat after tri-ortho-cresyl phosphate poisoning. *Acta Neuropathol. (Berl.),* 3:108–118.
5. Bischoff, A. (1967): The ultrastructure of tri-

6. Bischoff, A. (1970): The ultrastructure of tri-ortho-cresyl phosphate poisoning in the chicken. II. *Acta Neuropathol. (Berl.),* 15:142–155.
7. Casida, J. E., Eto, M., and Baron, R. L. (1961): Biological activity of a tri-ortho-cresyl phosphate metabolite. *Nature,* 191:1396–1397.
8. Casida, J. E., Baron, R. L., Eto, M., and Engel, J. L. (1963): Potentiation and neurotoxicity induced by certain organophosphates. *Biochem. Pharmacol.,* 12:73–83.
9. Cavanagh, J. B. (1954): The toxic effects of tri-ortho-cresyl phosphate on the nervous system. An experimental study in hens. *J. Neurol. Neurosurg. Psychiatry,* 17:163–172.
10. Cavanagh, J. B. (1963): Organo-phosphorus neurotoxicity: A model "dying back" process comparable to certain human neurological disorders. *Guys Hosp. Rep.,* 112:303–319.
11. Cavanagh, J. B., and Patangia, G. N. (1965): Changes in the central nervous system in the cat as a result of tri-ortho-cresyl phosphate poisoning. *Brain,* 7:165–180.
12. Earl, C. J., and Thompson, R. H. S. (1952): The inhibiting action of tri-ortho-cresyl phosphate on cholinesterases. *Br. J. Pharmacol. Chemother.,* 7:261–269.
13. Eto, M., Casida, J. E., and Eto, T. (1962): Hydroxylation and cyclization reactions involved in the metabolism of tri-ortho-cresyl phosphate. *Biochem. Pharmacol.,* 11:337–352.
14. Glees, P. (1961): Experimentelle Markscheidendegeneration durch Tri-ortho-kresyl Phosphat und ihre Verhütung durch Cortisonazetat. *Dtsch. Med. Wochenschr.,* 86:1175–1178.
15. Glees, P., and Janzik, H. (1965): Chemically (TCP) induced fibre degeneration in the central nervous system, with reference to clinical and neuropharmacological aspects. *Prog. Brain Res.,* 14:97–121.
16. Harris, S., Jr. (1930): Jamaica ginger paralysis (peripheral polyneuritis) *South. Med. J.,* 23:375–380.
17. Hern, J. E. C. (1967): Inhibition of true cholinesterase in TOCP poisoning with potentiation by "Tween 80." *Nature,* 215:963.
18. Joel, C. D., Moser, H. W., Majno, G., and Karnovsky, M. L. (1967): Effects of bis-(mono-isopropylamino)-fluorophosphine oxide (mipafox) and of starvation on the lipids in the nervous system of the hen. *J. Neurochem.,* 14:479–488.
19. Johnson, M. K. (1969): Delayed neurotoxic action of some organophosphorus compounds. *Br. Med. Bull.,* 25:231–235.
20. Johnson, M. K. (1970): Organophosphorus and other inhibitors of brain "neurotoxic esterase" and the development of delayed neurotoxicity in hens. *Biochem. J.,* 120:523–531.
21. Johnson, M. K. (1972): An approach to the study of the mechanism of organophosphorus delayed neurotoxicity. *Proc. R. Soc. Med.,* 65:195–196.
22. Majno, G., and Karnovsky, M. (1961): A biochemical and morphological study of myelination

and demyelination. III. Effect of an organo-phosphorus compound (mipafox) on the biosynthesis of lipid by nervous tissue of rats and hens. *J. Neurochem.*, 8:1–16.

23. McLaughlin, J., Marliac, J.-P., Verret, M. J., Mutchler, M. K., and Fitzhuh, O. G. (1963): The injection of chemicals into the yolk sac of fertile eggs prior to incubation as a toxicity test. *Toxicol. Appl. Pharmacol.*, 5:760–771.

24. Morazain, R., and Rosenberg, P. (1970): Lipid changes in tri-ortho-cresyl phosphate induced neuropathy. *Toxicol. Appl. Pharmacol.*, 16:461–474.

25. Pleasure, D. E., Mischler, K. C., and Engel, W. K. (1969): Axonal transport of proteins in experimental neuropathies. *Science*, 166:524–525.

26. Porcellati, G., and Mastrantonio, M. A. (1964): Phospholipid metabolism of peripheral nerves during demyelination by organo-phosphorus compounds. *Ital. J. Biochem.*, 13:332–352.

27. Prineas, J. (1969): The pathogenesis of dying back polyneuropathies. Part 1. An ultrastructural study of experimental tri-ortho-cresyl phosphate intoxication in the cat. *J. Neuropathol. Exp. Neurol.*, 28:571–597.

28. Roger, J.-C., Chambers, H., and Casida, J. E. (1964): Nicotinic acid analogs: Effect on response of chick embryos and hens to organophosphate toxicants. *Science*, 144:539–540.

29. Sheltawy, A., and Dawson, R. M. C. (1969): The metabolism of phosphoinositides in hen brain and sciatic nerve. *Biochem. J.*, 111:12–18.

30. Smith, M. I., and Lillie, R. D. (1931): The histopathology of tri-ortho-cresyl phosphate poisoning. *Arch. Neurol. Psychiatry*, 26:976–992.

31. Smith, H. V., and Spalding, J. M. K. (1959): Outbreak of paralysis in Morocco due to ortho-cresyl phosphate poisoning. *Lancet*, 2:1019–1021.

32. Svennilson, E. (1960): Studies of tri-ortho-cresyl phosphate neuropathy. Morocco 1960. *Acta Psychiatr. Scand. (Suppl.)*, 150:334–340.

33. Webster, G. R. (1954): The distribution and metabolism of phosphorus compounds in normal and demyelinating nervous tissue of the chicken. *Biochem. J.*, 57:153–158.

Neurotoxicology, edited by L. Roizin, H. Shiraki, and N. Grčević. Raven Press, New York © 1977.

Kepone Poisoning: Cliniconeuropathological Study

*A. Julio Martinez, **John R. Taylor, **Sidney A. Houff, and **Edward R. Isaacs

*Departments of Pathology (Neuropathology) and **Neurology, Medical College of Virginia, Virginia Commonwealth University, Richmond, Virginia 23298

Since the occurrence of "Minamata disease" in Japan reported in 1962 caused by methyl mercury poisoning (24), there has been increased interest in diseases produced by exposure to organic chemicals, which parallel the development of industrialization and pollution of our environment. Recent striking examples in humans are the discovery that a polyneuropathy is caused by acrylamide (6), that n-hexane, used as a cement solvent, is neurotoxic to peripheral nerves (8,12,15), that ortho-cresyl phosphate was implicated in the production of a polyneuropathy in workers exposed to glue used in the shoe industry (29), and that methyl-n-butyl Ketone used in plastic-coated and color-printed fabrics provoked a distal polyneuropathy (1). Iatrogenically induced neuropathy is exemplified by the use of isoniazid in the treatment of pulmonary tuberculosis (20, 23). In addition experimental production of peripheral neuropathies or degenerative changes in CNS structures in animals has been reported by using the same chemicals or drugs (10,13,17,22,27).

Our chapter concerns a previously unknown neurological disorder that appeared during the summer of 1975 in workers of a chemical plant in Hopewell, Virginia. Epidemiological and clinical studies indicated that chlordecone (Kepone®) was the responsible agent (Fig. 1). Chlordecone is a chlorinated, organic insecticide used in the control of leaf-eating insects, ants, and larvi of flies. The widespread used of the chemical has caused some concern regarding reproduction in mice (7,14) and quail (4,16). Patients with prolonged occupational exposure to the chemical developed tremors, chest pains, weight loss, arthralgia, skin rash, mental changes, opsoclonus, muscle weakness, gait ataxia, incoordination, and slurred speech (Table 1). In addition, semen analysis in four of these patients revealed severe impairment of spermatogenesis (Table 2). The presence of chlordecone in several body fluids and tissues (Table 3) was established by the method of Griffith and Blanke (9). Electromyograms and nerve conduction velocities revealed nonspecific changes (Table 4). The severity of the neurological symptoms appears to be directly proportional to the dose and duration of exposure. Although the biochemical basis for this syndrome is obscure (2,5,11), and neither the site of toxic action nor the precise mechanism of nervous system damage is known, its toxicity may be related to the ability of chlordecone to bond to lipids. The pathological changes in peripheral nerves and skeletal muscles are essentially nonspecific (Table 5).

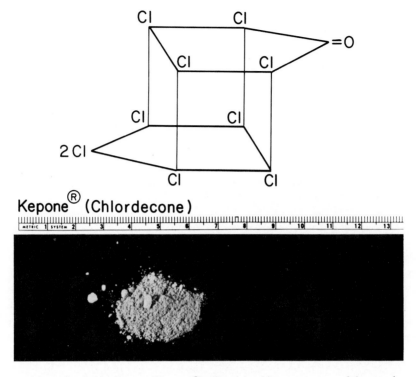

FIG. 1. Structural formula of chlordecone (Kepone®). Grayish-white appearance of the powder can be seen at bottom.

The purpose of this chapter is to elucidate the peripheral nerve and skeletal muscle involvement in six patients with prolonged occupational exposure to chlordecone and to describe the clinical features of the intoxication.

MATERIAL AND METHODS

Five sural nerve and six gastrocnemius muscles from six patients poisoned with chlordecone were studied by routine light microscopy (LM), enzyme histochemistry (EZ), and electron microscopy (EM). Biopsy specimens of sural nerve, approximately 1 cm in length, were obtained from the postmaleolar or midcalf areas. Muscle biopsies were taken from gastrocnemius or deltoid muscles.

Specimens from nerves and skeletal muscles for routine LM were fixed in 10% formalin and embedded in paraffin. Transverse and longitudinal sections were cut and stained by hematoxylin and eosin, myelin stain, Bodian and Masson trichrome techniques.

Two specimens for teasing of fibers (cases 1 and 4) were fixed for 15 min in 4% glutaraldehyde in cacodylate buffer (pH 7.4) and stained with 1% osmium tetroxide for 4 hr, then placed in the buffer for 3 hr, washed four times in the buffer, and placed in a mixture of glycerine and buffer (2:1, v/v). The individual nerve fibers were mounted in glycerin, and the edges of the coverslip were sealed with nail polish and studied by LM (3).

Fragments for EM were fixed by immersion in cold (4°C) 4% glutaraldehyde in cacodylate buffer (pH 7.4) for 4 hr followed by "postfixation" in 1% osmium tetroxide. The samples were dehydrated in graded

TABLE 1. *Clinical data in six patients*

Case number Patient's initials Age/race/sex	1 NS 24wm	2 DG 34wm	3 EM 37wm	4 KR 37wm	5 DW 30wm	6 MR 24wm
Duration of exposure to chlordecone (months)	4	6	4	8	8	6
Tremors	+++	+++	++	++	+++	+
Opsoclonus	+++	++	+	0	+++	+
Mood changes	+++	++	++	+	++	+
Hallucinations	++	0	0	+	0	0
Incoordination	++	+	+	0	+	0
Gait ataxia	+	0	+	0	++	0
Slurred speech	+	+	+	0	0	0
Weight loss (lbs)	10	40 plus	25	0	40	0
Chest pain	++	++	++	0	++	+
Arthralgia	++	+	+	0	+	+
Skin rash	++	++	++	0	+	+
Decreased libido	+	+	+	+	+	0
Abdominal pain	++	+	+	0	+	0
Conjunctivitis	+	0	+	0	+	0
Stretch reflexes	+	+	+	+	+	+
Babinski	0	0	0	0	0	0
Sensory loss	0	0	0	0	0	0

(Leftmost row label for the signs rows: Clinical signs and symptoms)

+, Mild; ++, moderate; +++, marked; 0, absent.

alcohol series, cleared in propylene oxide, and embedded in Epon 812. Cross sections of some fascicles were cut with glass knives at approximately 1 μm thick, stained with 1% toluidine blue, and examined by conventional LM. The semithin sections were photographed on a Zeiss ultraphot photomicroscope II. The chosen areas were then cut with a diamond knife in a Sorval Porter Blum MT2 ultramicrotome. Ultrathin sections of gray interference color were mounted in 240-hole uncoated copper grids, double stained with uranyl acetate and lead citrate, and then examined in an Hitachi H-S8-F2 electron microscope.

Muscle biopsies were obtained shortly after admission. Portions of the biopsy material were immediately frozen in isopentane that had been cooled in liquid nitrogen. Cryostat sections were made at 8 to 10 μm thick. The enzymes investigated were NAD-H tetrazolium reductase and myofibrillar ATPase after preincubation at pH 4.6 and 9.4. In addition, Sudan black, oil red 0, and the modified Gomori trichrome method were also used.

TABLE 2. *Semen analysis*

Case number Patient's initials	1 NS	2 DG	3 EM	4 KR	5 DW	6 MR
Volume/ml	4.6	2.7		6.1		1
Count/cc	2,150,000	Only 2 dead spermatozoa seen		12,000,000		129,000,000
Motility	None	None	Vasectomy	90% actively motile At 12 hr: 65% motile At 24 hr: Stationary motile	Vasectomy	25% motile At 6 hr: 20–25% motile
Morphology Normal Dark head Double head Double tail Micro head Large head	4% 80% 2% 7% 4%	No spermatozoa seen		44% 49% 1% 1% 4%		65% 34% 1%

MORPHOLOGICAL FINDINGS

LM

On LM examination of the five sural nerves it was found that all the specimens contained increases in endoneurial and perineurial connective tissues. A relative decrease in the number of small myelinated and unmyelinated axons was noted when compared with controls. The myelin sheaths showed no significant abnormalities. Occasionally segmental fusiform swelling of axons cylinders was encountered. There was no evidence of myelin breakdown or of myelin phagocytosis. In 1 μm-thick sections of sural nerves there was hypertrophy of Schwann cell cytoplasm in some fibers associated with an accumulation of elongated metachromatic

TABLE 3. *Toxicological data*

Case number Patient's initials	1 NS	2 DG	3 EM	4 KR	5 DW	6 MR
Blood	++++	+++	+++	++	+++	+++
CSF	+	+	+	*	*	*
Skeletal muscle	+++	*	*	*	*	*
Subcutaneous fat	*	*	*	++	*	*
Sural nerve	*	*	*	*	*	*

Gas chromatographic method using electron capture detector of Griffith and Blanke (9). Chlordecone in ppb or ng/ml or ng/g is indicated as follows: +, less than 100; ++, 100–1,000; +++, 1,000–10,000; ++++, more than 10,000. *, examination not performed.

TABLE 4. *Electrodiagnostic data*

Case number Patient's initials	1 NS	2 DG	3 EM	4 KR	5 DW	6 MR
Nerve conduction time	Normal	Normal	Normal	Normal	Normal	Normal
Electromyogram	Slightly increased number of polyphasic potentials	Increased number of polyphasic potentials	Normal	Normal	Normal	Slightly increased number of polyphasic potentials

cytoplasmic inclusions (Fig. 2A and B). The skeletal muscle had slightly increased in lipochrome pigment.

EM (Table 5)

The lesions consisted of:

1. Redundant Schwann cell cytoplasmic folds, often interdigitated in a complex manner and enveloping bundles of collagen fibrils to form "collagen pockets" (Fig. 3);

2. increases in interstitial collagen and occasional axonal degeneration (Fig. 4);

3. accumulation of elongated crystalloid rods and short, laminated, and comma-shaped membranous bodies within Schwann cell cytoplasm with a definite periodicity (the dark lines measure 30 nm on the average, whereas the light bands measure 15 nm) (Fig. 8A–D);

TABLE 5. *Ultrastructural pathology in sural nerves*

Case number Patient's initials	1 NS	2 DG	3 EM	4 KR	5 DW	6 MR
Endoneurial collagen	++	+	+++	++	++	
Schwann cells Reich bodies (π granules) Elzholz bodies (μ granules of Reich)	+++	+	++	++	+	
Axons (Clusters of dense bodies, membranous structures, vacuoles in axoplasm, condensed tubules, & filaments)	++	+	++	+	+	*
Myelin sheaths (Focal demyelination, myelin bodies, interlamellar splitting)	++	+	++	+	+	

+, Minimal number; ++, moderate number; +++, numerous; *, biopsy not performed.

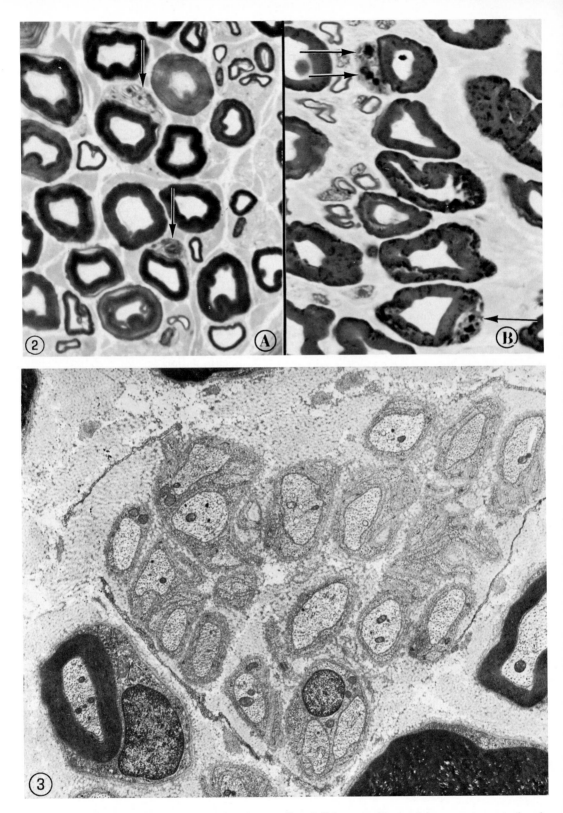

FIG. 2. A: One-micrometer cross section of sural nerve. Case 1. Schwann cells containing numerous cytoplasmic inclusions (*arrows*). Toluidine blue. ×1,500. **B:** Schwann cells are hypertrophic with cytoplasmic inclusions (*arrows*). Case 4. ×1,500.
FIG. 3. Schwann cell cytoplasmic processes, which became hypertrophied, showing an increased tendency to encircle connective tissue forming collagen pockets. Case 2. ×9,000.

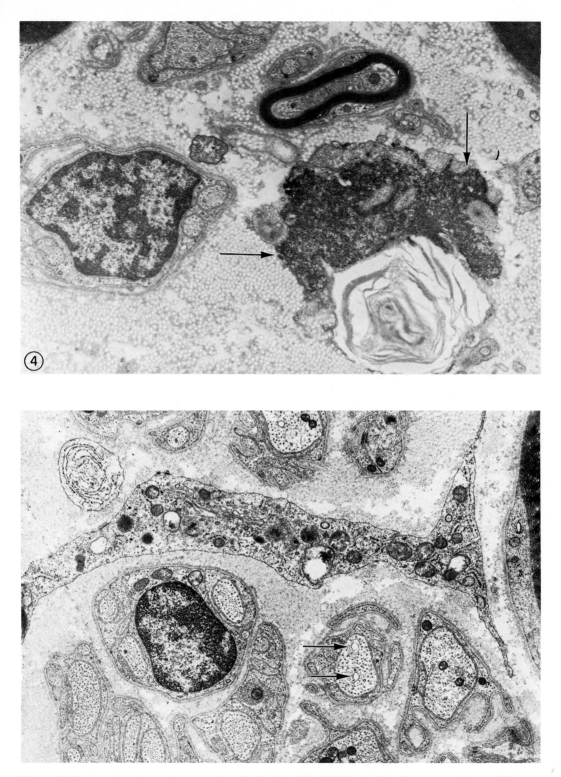

FIG. 4. Sural nerve showing an increase of endoneurial collagen, degeneration of an axon with no evidence of myelin, and the presence of a large amount of dense granular material probably within a degenerated Schwann cell (*arrows*). The concentric membranous structures are compatible with a disintegrating myelin sheath. Case 3. ×13,950.

FIG. 5. Prominent fibroblastic cytoplasm within endoneurial collagen. Note the large numbers of dense bodies. There are clusters of unmyelinated fibers with prominent stacks of Schwann cell cytoplasmic processes. Note empty vesicles within axoplasm of unmyelinated fibers (*arrows*). Case 2. ×14,000.

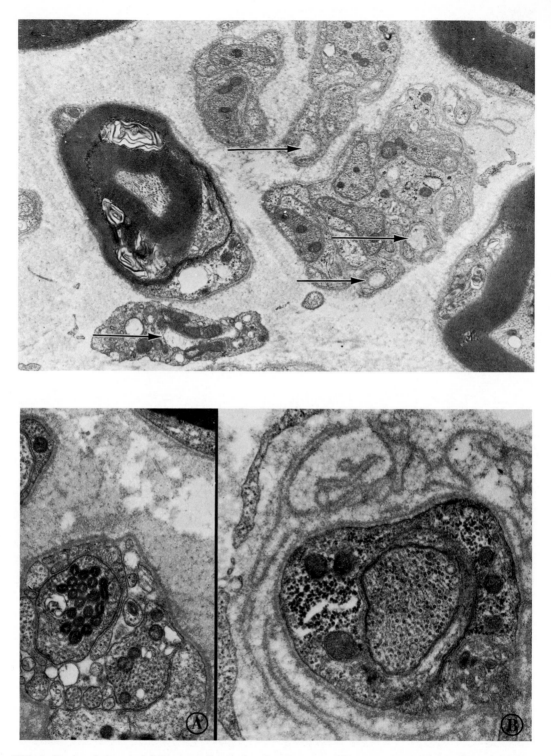

FIG. 6. Stacks of elongated Schwann cell cytoplasmic processes with empty spaces, compatible with former sites of axons (*arrows*). The large myelinated fibers disclose splitting of myelin sheath. Case 1. ×14,000.

FIG. 7. A: Transverse section from sural nerve. There are a group of excessively small axon cylinders and an aggregate of dense bodies within unmyelinated axoplasm. Case 1. ×24,750. B: Schwann cell encompassing a demyelinated axon. The basement membrane is redundant and shows numerous, collapsed infolding. Case 3. ×38,250.

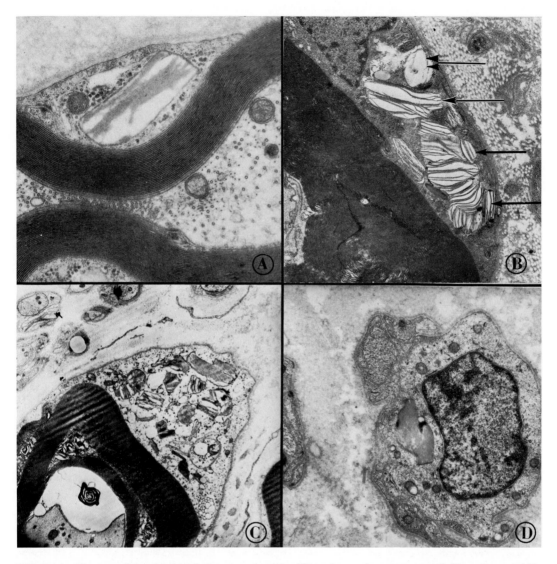

FIG. 8. A: Electron photomicrograph from sural nerve. There is an elongated crystalloid structure within Schwann cell cytoplasm. The myelin sheath is intact except for some blurring artifacts. There are sparse neurofilaments, some dense bodies, and swelling mitochondria. Case 3. ×38,350. **B:** Schwann cell inclusion compatible with π granules of Reich (*single-head arrows*) and μ granule of Reich or Elzholz body (*double-head arrows*). Case 3. ×10,200. **C:** Hypertrophic Schwann cell containing numerous electron dense inclusions. Case 2. ×10,200. **D:** Unmyelinated fibers showing an irregular electron dense crystalloid structure within Schwann cell cytoplasm. Case 3. ×14,400.

4. focal degeneration of axons containing condensed neurofilaments, neurotubules, and clusters of dense bodies, whereas others contained evenly dispersed neurotubules and neurofilaments with occasional dense mitochondria (Fig. 9A–D);

5. adaxonal infolding of myelin sheath due to detachment from axolemma (Fig. 9A and B);

6. focal splitting of myelin lamellae at the interperiod line in small myelinated fibers with occasional formation of "myelin bodies" (Fig. 6);

7. increases of endoneurial collagen

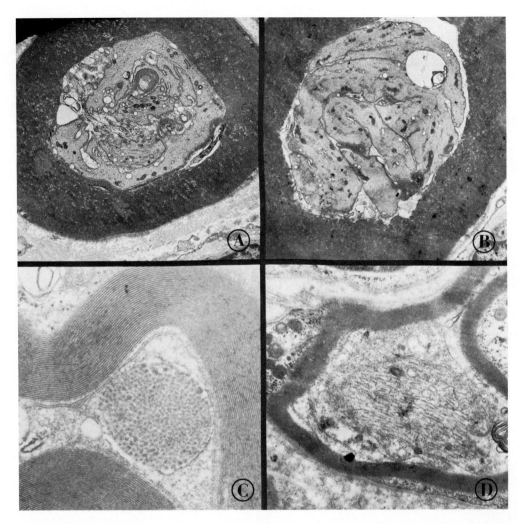

FIG. 9. A: Compact axoplasm with numerous irregular membranous structures, arising from the inner mesaxon. Case 1. ×5,300. **B:** Large myelinated fiber with abnormal densely packed neurotubules and neurofilaments. Irregular membranes, vacuoles, and dense bodies are prominent. Case 3. ×5,400. **C:** Collection of electron dense, spherical particles membrane bound, within axoplasm of large myelinated fiber. Case 2. ×41,000. **D:** Prominent collection of neurotubules within an apparently abnormal axoplasm of a partially collapsed myelinated fiber. Case 3. ×20,400.

with occasional mast cells and fibroblasts;

8. vacuolization of axons of unmyelinated and small myelinated fibers, associated with redundant interdigitation of Schwann cells, forming stacks of cytoplasmic processes (Fig. 5);

9. Schwann cell cytoplasmic vacuoles, dense bodies, π bodies of Reich, and Elzholz bodies; and

10. occasional small unmyelinated axons with conspicuous dense bodies and re-

dundant basement membranes (Fig. 7A and B). The skeletal muscle revealed increases in lipofuscin pigment and lipid-like droplets in subsarcolemmal areas and intermyofibrillar spaces (Figs. 10 and 11).

Teased Fiber Studies

In the sural nerve of two patients (cases 1 and 5), no demyelinated fibers were seen in multiple strands of the nerve tissue ex-

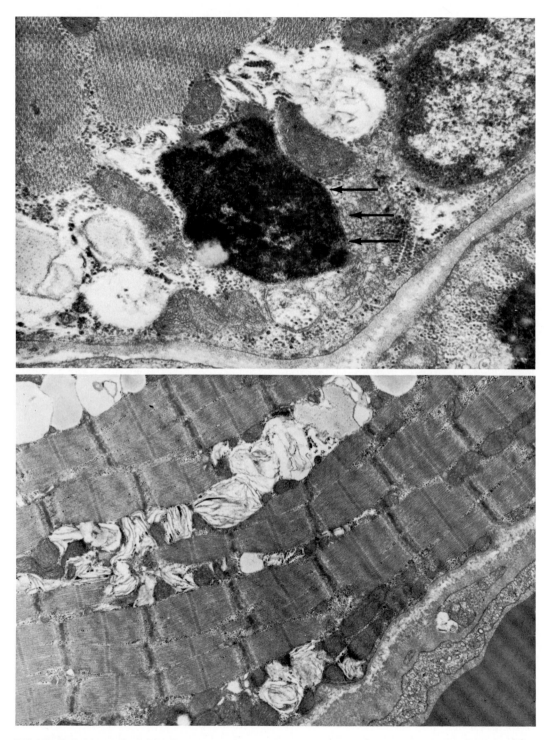

FIG. 10. Skeletal muscle, left gastrocnemius. Showing irregular mitochondria, abundant subsarcolemmal glycogen, and large clump of dense lipofuscin-like material (*arrows*). There are also collections of less dense lipid-like material. Case 3. ×45,000.

FIG. 11. Skeletal muscle, left gastrocnemius, showing collections of electron-dense, laminated structures within myofilament bundles. Case 1. ×13,950.

amined, but occasional myelin ovoids of various sizes were noted. The qualitative evaluation of internode length and its variability in teased fibers fell within the range of normal values.

DISCUSSION

The sural nerve is predominantly a sensory nerve with some autonomic functions (19). Unmyelinated and small caliber axons subserve pain modalities (21). Some of the unmyelinated fibers are components of the peripheral autonomic nervous system (19).

In chlordecone neuropathy there is predominance of involvement of unmyelinated and smaller myelinated fibers, therefore explaining in part the clinical symptomatology and the electrophysiological and electromyographic features. A distinctive finding under LM and EM is the presence of an excessive number of dense rods, crystalloid structures, and lipid-like droplets in aggregate or diffusely distributed within Schwann cell cytoplasm (Figs. 3A, B and 9A–C).

The moderately increased amount of interstitial collagen, redundant folds of Schwann cell cytoplasm, and presence of occasional crystalloid inclusions and lipid-like deposits suggest that the changes in nerves may be due to factors disturbing or altering the metabolism of Schwann cells, or both, (23,26,30) and that the toxicity is perhaps due to a metabolite, rather than to a direct action on the nerve fibers or to cellular elements of nerves. The degenerative changes are essentially, however, nonspecific and similar to those described after other toxic polyneuropathies (6,8,12, 13,24,25,27–29).

The mode of action of these various agents is not clear, but some may effect the adhesive properties of the myelin lamella at the intraperiod line (27); others, the membranes between the terminal myelin loops and the axolemma in the paranodal region (20); and yet others may have a direct toxic effect on the Schwann cell (17,23,26).

The presence of dense granules of Reich has been reported in isoniazid neuropathy (20,23). It has been suggested that they originated from lysosomes of Schwann cell, but their true significance is obscure. The presence of an excessive number of Reich bodies and Elzholz bodies in our cases is considered abnormal. These inclusions are very similar to the protagon (π) granules of Reich and μ granules of Reich or Elzholz bodies. They measure between 1 and 2 μm in length. They are metachromatic granules when stained with toluidine blue, thionin, and methylene blue. Their true significance is obscure, but they appear in larger number in these cases than expected in a normal nerve. In any case they may indicate a response of the Schwann cell to injury by a toxic substance or its metabolite. These inclusions either may suggest a reparative process in which the Schwann cell is trying to get rid of an abnormal, useless, or harmful substance or may indicate perhaps a nonspecific cell reaction and a sign of "focal degradation." In addition, "lysosomal-like" structures have been reported in hepatocytes of experimental animals intoxicated with chlordecone (2).

These granules contain lipids (phospholipid or cerebrosides), phosphatide, or sulphatide and are associated with acid phosphatase, therefore they can be classified as lysosomes (18). They have been observed accumulating with increasing age. They are analogous to lipofuscin granules, and they are not degradation products of myelin (26); however, Thomas and Slatford (25) considered them involved in myelin metabolism.

SUMMARY

In 1975, several workers at a chemical plant in Virginia developed an insidious neurological disorder characterized by tremors, chest pain, weight loss, mental changes, arthralgia, skin rash, opsoclonus, muscle weakness, gait ataxia, and incoordination. Chlordecone (Kepone®), an insecticide, was identified as the cause. A total of 62 verified cases was detected on screening 148 employees — 22 patients had disabling neurological symptoms, 7 had mild clinical symptoms, and 33 had no objective neurological findings. Skeletal muscle and sural nerve biopsies were done in six patients.

The significant findings in peripheral nerves consisted of: (a) accumulation of elongated, crystalloid and electron-dense rods and short, laminated and parallel membranous inclusions within Schwann cell cytoplasm (π and μ granules of Reich and Elzholz bodies); (b) redundant Schwann cell cytoplasmic folds; (c) prominent endoneurial collagen pockets; (d) vacuolization of unmyelinated fibers associated with interdigitation of stacks of Schwann cell cytoplasmic processes; (e) focal degeneration of axons characterized by condensation of neurofilaments, neurotubules, dense mitochondria, and clusters of dense bodies; (f) focal interlamellar splitting of myelin sheath and occasional formation of "myelin bodies"; (g) complex infolding of inner mesaxonal membranes into axoplasm; and (h) decreased number of unmyelinated fibers. The skeletal muscles disclosed an increase in lipofuscin pigment and lipid-like droplets in subsarcolemmal areas and intermyofibrillar spaces.

The results of this study suggest that chlordecone is a neurotoxic agent involving predominantly the Schwann cells of myelinated and unmyelinated fibers of peripheral nerves, associated with marked decreases in density of unmyelinated fibers and relative sparing of the larger myelinated fibers. These findings may explain the clinical symptoms and the electrophysiological and the electromyographic features and suggest the presence of a derangement of metabolism in Schwann cells.

ACKNOWLEDGMENTS

We are indebted to Dr. J. G. dos Santos, who performed the semen analysis, and Dr. Saul Kay and Dr. William Still for performing the ultrastructural studies of testis and liver biopsies reported elsewhere. Morphometric values of myelinated and unmyelinated fibers from nerves of patients 1,2,3,4, and 5 were obtained by Dr. Peter James Dyck, Neurology Department, Mayo Clinic, Rochester, Minnesota and will be the subject of a subsequent publication. Also our thanks to Francis D. Giffith, Jr., Pesticide Laboratory, Division of Consolidated Laboratories, Commonwealth of Virginia, who under the supervision of Robert V. Blanke, Ph.D. performed the toxicological studies, and to Dr. Robert S. Jackson, State of Virginia Epidemiologist, for providing the epidemiological data.

REFERENCES

1. Allen, N., Mendell, J. R., Billmaier, D. J., Fontained, R. E., and O'Neill, J. (1975): Toxic polyneuropathy due to methyl b-butyl ketone. *Arch. Neurol.*, 32:209–222.
2. Atwal, O. S. (1973): Fatty changes and hepatic cell excretion in avian liver. An electron microscopical study of Kepone toxicity. *J. Comp. Pathol.*, 83:115–124.
3. Dyck, P. J. (1975): Pathological alterations of the peripheral nervous system of man. In: *Peripheral Neuropathy*, Vol. I, edited by P. J. Dyck, P. K. Thomas, and E. H. Lambert, pp. 296–301. Saunders, Philadelphia.
4. Eroschenko, V. P., and Wilson, W. O. (1975): Cellular changes in the gonads, livers and adrenal glands of Japanese quail as affected by the insecticide Kepone. *Toxicol. Appl. Pharmacol.*, 31:491–504.
5. Gaines, T. B., and Kimbrough, R. D. (1970): Oral toxicity of Mirex® in adult and suckling rats. *Arch. Environ. Health*, 21:7–14.
6. Garland, T. O., and Patterson, M. W. H. (1967): Six cases of acrylamide poisoning. *Br. Med. J.*, 4:134–138.
7. Good, E. E., Ware, G. W., and Miller, D. F. (1965): Effects of insecticides on reproduction in the laboratory mouse: I. Kepone. *J. Econ. Entomol.*, 58:754–757.
8. Goto, T., Matsumura, M., Inoue, N., Murai, Y., Shida, K., Santa, T., and Kuroiwa, Y. (1974):

Toxic polyneuropathy due to glue sniffing. *J. Neurol. Neurosurg. Psychiatry,* 37:848–853.

9. Griffith, F. D., and Blanke, R. V. (1974): Microcoulometric determination of organochlorine pesticides in human blood. *J. Assoc. Off. Anal. Chem.,* 57:595–603.
10. Haymaker, W., Ginzler, A. M., and Ferguson, R. L. (1946): The toxic effects of prolonged ingestion of DDT* on dogs with special reference to lesions in the brain. *Am. J. Med. Sci.,* 212:423–431.
11. Hendrickson, C. M., and Bowden, J. A. (1975): The in vitro inhibition of rabbit muscle lactate dehydrogenase by Mirex and Kepone. *J. Agric. Food Chem.,* 23:407–409.
12. Herskowitz, A., Ishii, N., and Schaumburg, H. (1971): N-hexane neuropathy. A syndrome occurring as a result of industrial exposure. *N. Engl. J. Med.,* 285:82–85.
13. Herman, S. P., Klein, R., Talley, F. A., and Krigman, M. R. (1973): An ultrastructural study of methyl mercury-induced primary sensory neuropathy in the rat. *Lab. Invest.,* 28:104–118.
14. Huber, J. J. (1965): Some physiological effects of the insecticide Kepone in the laboratory mouse. *Toxicol. Appl. Pharmacol.,* 7:516–524.
15. Korobkin, R., Asbury, A. K., Sumner, A. J., and Nielsen, S. L. (1975): Glue-sniffing. *Neuropathy Arch. Neurol.,* 32:158–162.
16. McFarland, L. Z., and Lacy, P. B. (1974): Physiologic and endocrinologic effects of the insecticide Kepone in the Japanese quail. *Toxicol. Appl. Pharmacol.,* 15:441–450.
17. Miyakawa, T., Deshimaru, M., Sumiyoshi, S., Teraoka, A., Udo, N., Hattori, E., and Tatetsu, S. (1970): Experimental organic mercury poisoning—pathological changes in peripheral nerves. *Acta Neuropathol. (Berl.),* 15:45–55.
18. Noback, C. R. (1953): The protagon (π) granules of Reich. *J. Comp. Neurol.,* 99:91–99.
19. Pick, J. (1970): *The Autonomic Nervous System,* pp. 357–358. Lippincott, Philadelphia.

20. Ochoa, J. (1970): Isoniazid neuropathy in man: Quantitative electron microscopy study. *Brain,* 93:831–850.
21. Sweet, W. H. (1959): Pain. In: *Handbook of Physiology,* Vol. 1, edited by J. Field, H. W. Magoun, U. E. Hall, pp. 459–506. American Physiological Society, Washington, D.C.
22. Spencer, P. S., and Schaumburg, H. H. (1974): A review of acrylamide neurotoxicity. Part II. Experimental animal neurotoxicity and pathologic mechanisms. *Can. J. Neurol. Sci.,* 1:152–169.
23. Schroder, J. M. (1970): Zur Pathogenese der Isoniazid-Neuropathie. I. Eine feinstrukturel differenzierung gegenuber der Wallerschen Degeneration. *Acta Neuropathol. (Berl.),* 16:301–323.
24. Takeuchi, T., Morikawa, N., Matsumoto, H., and Shirishi, Y. (1962): A pathological study of Minamata disease in Japan. *Acta Neuropathol. (Berl.),* 2:40–57.
25. Thomas, P. K., and Slatford, J. (1964): Lamellar bodies in the cytoplasm of Schwann cells. *J Anat.,* 98:691.
26. Tomonaga, M., and Sluga, E. (1970): Zur Ultrastruktur der π-Granula. *Acta Neuropathol. (Berl.),* 15:56–69.
27. Towfighi, J., Gonatas, N. K., and McCree, L. (1973): Hexachlorophene neuropathy in rats. *Lab. Invest.,* 29:428–436.
28. Towfighi, J., Gonatas, N. K., Pleasure, D., Cooper, H. S., and McCree, L. (1976): Glue sniffer's neuropathy. *Neurol.,* 26:238–243.
29. Vora, D. D., Dastur, D. K., Braganca, B. M., Parihar, L. M., Iyer, C. G. S., Fondekar, R. B., and Prabhakaran, K. (1962): Toxic polyneuritis in Bombay due to ortho-cresyl-phosphate poisoning. *J. Neurol. Neurosurg. Psychiatry,* 25:234–242.
30. Weller, R. O., and Herzog, I. (1970): Schwann cell lysosomes in hypertrophic neuropathy and in normal human nerves. *Brain,* 93:347–356.

Neurotoxicology, edited by L. Roizin, H. Shiraki, and N. Grčević. Raven Press, New York © 1977.

Parathion-Induced Alterations in Acetylcholinesterase of the Rat Nervous System: A Histochemical, Biochemical, and Isozyme Study

R. H. Brownson, *H. D. McDougal, **D. B. Suter, and V. K. Vijayan

*Department of Human Anatomy, School of Medicine, University of California, Davis, California 95616; *Department of Anatomy, Eastern Virginia Medical School, Norfolk, Virginia 23507; and **Department of Biology, Eastern Mennonite College, Harrisonburg, Virginia 22801*

Parathion (E605; *O,O*-diethyl *O-p*-nitrophenyl phosphorothioate) is one of a large group of chemically active insecticides that directly or indirectly resulted from the work of Gerhard Schrader in Germany (29). These organophosphorus compounds may be identified by a common pharmacological property—the ability to interfere with the function of a group of enzymes that catalyze the hydrolysis of esters of choline, such as acetylcholine (ACh). *In vivo,* parathion is converted into its more toxic oxygen analog, paraoxon (E600; *O,O*-diethyl *O-p*-nitrophenyl phosphate), which poisons an enzyme present in the tissues of most animals (10,13). Since parathion is rapidly hydrolyzed after application and does not appear to accumulate in the earth or in human tissue, there has been widespread commercial use of it as an insecticide. Unfortunately, the properties which account for parathion's outstanding value as an insecticide also render it extremely toxic to mammals. The withdrawal of chlorinated hydrocarbons such as DDT from domestic and most agricultural use in the United States and abroad has greatly increased the use of the organophosphorus compounds, including parathion, as an alternate means for pest control (28).

A preliminary histochemical study of parathion-induced changes in mammalian brain in our laboratory disclosed marked changes in acetylcholinesterase (AChE) activity (31). These changes were characterized by a dramatic decrease in brain AChE following intraperitoneal (i.p.) administration of parathion. Furthermore, it was noted that 15-day-old animals were more sensitive than 30-day-old animals. The inhibition of AChE activity in brain tissue occurred rapidly (within minutes) after injection of parathion. It was also noted that the dosage of 2.5 mg/kg, i.p., of parathion was lethal within 15 min to all 15-day-old and most 30-day-old animals, whereas 1.25 mg/kg was not lethal to any group.

These initial observations made on the effects of parathion on the mammalian nervous system prompted further investigations including an examination of histochemical, biochemical, and isozyme reactions. The results of some of these studies are presented in this chapter.

MATERIALS AND METHODS

Experimental 15- and 30-day-old Sprague-Dawley rats of both sexes were used. Parathion (Staufer Chemical Co., 99.2% active) in carbowax (polyethylene glycol 300) was administered intraperitoneally to the experimental animals. The dosage of parathion was 2.5 or 1.25 mg/kg body weight in 1 ml of carbowax. Control animals were treated in the same manner but without parathion. The technical procedures leading to the final tissue preparation varied with the method of analysis. The following techniques were utilized.

Histochemistry

Animals 15 and 30 days of age were decapitated 15 min, 1, 4, 12, and 24 hr following administration of 2.5 or 1.25 mg/kg body weight of parathion, and the brain and diaphragm were quickly removed. Slices of fresh unfixed brain and diaphragm were quenched in isopentane, chilled in liquid nitrogen, and transferred to a cryostat for sectioning. The remaining tissue slices were fixed in formal-ammonia-sucrose for a minimum of 2 hr or overnight and then sectioned at 10 μm. Standard histochemical procedures were carried out for acid phosphatase, cytochrome oxidase, and succinic dehydrogenase and simple esterases. The El-Badawi and Schenk (11) procedure was implemented for the AChE reaction, and the usual control procedures were utilized throughout.

Electron Microscopy

Experimental animals 30 days of age were administered parathion (1.25 mg/kg), anesthetized with sodium pentobarbital, and terminated by perfusion fixation at 1, 4, 12, and 24 hr. The perfusate consisted of 1% paraformaldehyde and 2% glutaraldehyde buffered with cacodylate (pH 7.2, 0.07 M, 600 to 620 mOsm/kg). Small cubes of tissue less than 1 mm^3 were removed from caudate-putamen (NCP) and brainstem (BS), rinsed, and stored in buffer overnight at 4°C.

The tissues were incubated in a medium, after Karnovsky and Roots (19). Standard

inhibitors were used to confirm the AChE reaction and inhibit cholinesterase (ChE). Tissues were postfixed 1 hr in 1% buffered osmium. After fixation the tissues were dehydrated, embedded in Epon, and sectioned. Thick sections (1 μm) were stained with methylene blue (0.5%). Thin sections were unstained or lightly stained with uranyl acetate and examined for fine structure.

Biochemistry

Experimental animals 30 days of age received parathion, i.p. (1.25 mg/kg), and were decapitated at 15 min, 1, 2, and 4 hr; 1, 3, 7, and 14 days. The olfactory bulb (OB) and NCP were dissected bilaterally on an ice-cooled glass plate. The tissues were rinsed several times in cold saline, blotted, and the wet weights determined. Ten milliliters of phosphate buffer (pH 8.0, 0.1% Triton X-100) was added to each gram of OB tissue and 30 ml of buffer per gram of NCP tissue prior to homogenizing. The inhibitor tetraisopropylpyrophosphoramide (iso-OMPA, 8×10^{-5}M) was included in the solutions as a selective irreversible inhibitor of ChE. The tissues from each animal were separately homogenized in glass (1,200 rpm, 1 min). Homogenates from each time period and brain area were reacted with acetylthiocholine iodide (0.075 M) as substrate and dithiobisnitrobenzoic acid (DTNB, 0.01 M) as chromogen. The AChE activity of the homogenates was measured spectrophotometrically (12).

Electrophoresis

Experimental female animals 30 days of age received parathion, i.p. (1.25 mg/kg), and were decapitated at 2, 4, and 24 hr. Brain areas examined were OB, NCP, BS, and cerebellum. Brains were removed as rapidly after death as possible and rinsed in ice cold saline. Samples were weighed and homogenized in 0.1% Triton X-100 in Tris-hydrochloride buffer (pH 8.5, 0.038 M Tris) at a dilution of 1:6, w/v. Homogenates were centrifuged (40,000 g for 90 min, 4°C) and supernatants collected (34).

Electrophoresis was carried out using a vertical flat-bed polyacrylamide gel cast at pH 8.4. The separating gel consisted of 7.5% polyacrylamide containing Triton X-100 at 0.1% final concentration. The tissue supernatants were diluted 1:1 with Tris-buffered 80% sucrose, and 15 to 30 μl of this diluted material was introduced into wells cast in a 7.5% polyacrylamide layer over the separating gel. Power for the separation was provided by pulsed constant power supply, and the separation was carried out at room temperature for approximately 2 hr. Following the separation the gels were stained and quantitated for AChE activity (34).

RESULTS

Behavioral Response at 1.25 and 2.5 mg/kg

Most experimental animals injected with 2.5 mg/kg of parathion showed signs of poisoning within 5 to 9 min. These typical signs were hypersensitivity, shivering salivation, grinding of teeth, gasping movements, and hyperextension. At the lower dose many of the identical signs were observed but with much less severity. Animals receiving only carbowax demonstrated no behavioral change.

Histochemical Observations at 2.5 mg/kg

No effect of parathion poisoning could be detected in acid phosphatase or succinic dehydrogenase activity. There was a slight decrease in activity of cytochrome oxidase; however, it was too small to be significant.

The most marked change was in AChE (Fig. 1A–D) in which there was a greater reduction in young than in old and females than males. AChE reduction characterized

both cell soma and neuropil; furthermore, the light background staining normally seen in controls was absent from experimental tissue thus making neurons more visible. In the cerebellum the loss of staining was almost complete. Loss of AChE was almost complete in the cerebral cortex and hippocampus. In the BS it was noted that a small cluster of cells, often large multipolar neurons, did not completely lose the staining reaction (Fig. 2C–F).

Selective use of inhibitors demonstrated that, in addition to AChE, ChE and simple esterases were inhibited during parathion poisoning. The loss in ChE was primarily in blood vessels. Esterase reduction was generalized, both as to brain region and tissue components.

Histochemical Observations at 1.25 mg/kg

The motor end plate in diaphragmatic muscle of 30-day rats gave a heavy, well-localized AChE reaction. Fifteen minutes after parathion administration motor end plates exhibited a rapid depletion of AChE reaction product. By 1 hr there were signs of recovery of the AChE reaction, and by 4 hr the reaction in motor end plates had returned to the control level (Fig. 3).

The effects of parathion on AChE activity in the NCP and BS were principally related to the extracell compartment and large multipolar neurons. Neuroglial and endothelial cells were negative. Little reaction product was found associated specifically with the synapses in these regions. Light microscopic observations of the NCP and BS (Figs. 3 and 4A–F) showed a decrease in AChE activity by 15 min after administration of parathion. This change was principally in the neuropil, with little or no involvement of the large neurons (Figs. 3 and 4B). Within 1 hr maximum effects were noted in the neuropil and moderate changes in the large neurons (Figs. 3 and 4C). By 24 hr (Fig. 4F) the activity in

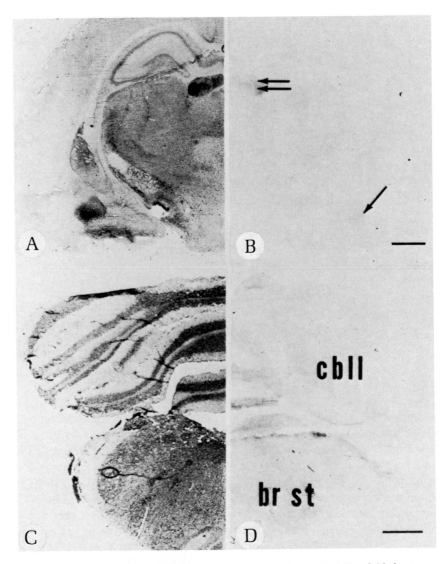

FIG. 1. Hemisections through mid-diencephalon (**A,B**) and cerebellum-BS (**C,D**) of 30-day rats, stained for AChE. **A** and **C**: normal; **B** and **D**: 15 min after 2.5 mg/kg. AChE activity is completely inhibited in **B** except for the nucleus habenularis (*double arrow*) and nucleus amygdaloideus basalis (*single arrow*); slight activity remains in BS and median ventral portion of cerebellum (CBll). Scale: 1.0 mm.

the neuropil equaled or exceeded the control.

These observations were extended by fine structure studies on NCP and BS (Fig. 5). The AChE reaction product on limiting membrane surfaces of large neurons extended into the extracellular spaces (Fig. 5A). Also the reaction product was located in the cisternae of rough endoplasmic reticulum (Fig. 5C,D). Neurotubules of some axons and dendrites were observed to be reactive. The majority of the remaining cytoplasmic organelles as well as myelin were essentially negative (Fig. 5B–D).

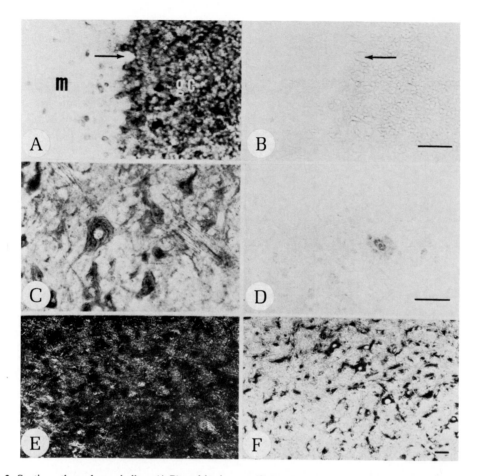

FIG. 2. Sections through cerebellum (**A,B**) and brainstem (**C–F**) of 15-day rats. **A–D** stained for AChE; **E** and **F** stained for nonspecific esterases. **A, C,** and **E**: normal; **B, D,** and **F**: 10 min after 2.5 mg/kg. Note in control **A** that the molecular layer (**M**) and Purkinje cells (*arrow*) are almost negative for AChE, while the glomeruli of granule cell layer (**GC**) show a heavy reaction; the corresponding parathion-treated section (**B**) is entirely negative. Scale: 50 μm.

Biochemistry at 1.25 mg/kg

The homogenates of OB and NCP were examined colorimetrically for AChE activity following parathion (1.25 mg/kg) during a series of recovery periods.

Not all animals exhibited signs of poisoning at the dose. However, if these signs occurred, they appeared 15 to 30 min following the injection. The signs of poisoning paralleled the fall of AChE activity as it dropped below 45% of control levels (Fig. 6). To compare the OB and NCP the data were expressed as percent of the mean activities of paired controls of each time period. Each value was plotted as the best estimate of the standard deviation of the mean $\left(Sx = \dfrac{s}{\sqrt{N}} \right)$. The fall and rise of AChE activity with time appeared to occur in four phases. In *phase I* (0 to 2 hr) the AChE activity in both OB and NCP dropped rapidly, OB to 15% of control and NCP to 30% of control (Fig. 6). *Phase II* recovery (2 to 4 hr) was represented by a rapid rise in AChE activity to 65 to 85%

PARATHION-INDUCED ALTERATIONS
IN ACETYLCHOLINESTERASE[1]

RESPONSE TIME	BRAIN STEM		MUSCLE
	CELL[2]	EXTRACELL[3]	END-PLATE[4]
	(A)	(B)	(C)
CONTROL	+++	+++	++++
5 min	+++	+++	++++
15 min	++	+±	+
1 hr	+	±	++±
4 hrs	++	+	++++
12 hrs	+++	++	++++
24 hrs	++++	+++±	++++

FIG. 3. A histochemical comparison of light microscopic changes in AChE activity of BS (medullopontine reticular formation) and motor end plates following parathion (1.25 mg/kg). BS neurons, ventromedial reticular, pontis caudalis, and gigantocellularis. (1), histochemical study; (2), neurons of the reticular formation; (3) including synapse; (4) diaphragm.

of control values. By 4 hr symptoms of poisoning had markedly diminished or were absent. *Phase III* (4 to 24 hr) was represented by a diminution in the rate of recovery of activity. *Phase IV* recovery period (1 to 14 days) displayed an overshoot of and gradual return to control levels.

Electrophoresis

In the 30-day female rat, three zones of AChE activity were apparent in all brain areas examined. Of these, isozyme zone 3 was relatively cathodal in position and constituted more than 50% of the total isozyme activity.

At 2 hr after parathion administration, the total isozyme activity was inhibited to 50% of the control levels in OB, NCP, BS, and cerebellum. There were no regional differences in the degree of this response. In all regions, moreover, a differential isozyme

inhibition could be noted, with maximum depression exhibited by the major AChE zone—zone 3. In all brain areas, the isozyme inhibition was maximum at 2 hr after the injection; considerable isozyme recovery was observed at 4 hr; and the recovery was complete at 24 hr following the administration of parathion (Fig. 7).

DISCUSSION

The rapid effects of parathion are well documented, and the signs or symptoms of poisoning occur when its metabolic by-product, paraoxon, inhibits tissue AChE activity below a critical level.

Investigators have reported on the localization of AChE activity in the nervous system of the rat (5,15,20,21,23,24). The majority of these studies dealt with the normal adult animals and were not concerned with inhibition of AChE activity by organophosphorus compounds. Initial studies of parathion at a dosage of 2.5 mg/kg were found too lethal for chronic studies. In these studies AChE activity was essentially extinguished within 5 to 10 min (Figs. 1 and 2). Consequently, additional testing established a dosage of 1.25 mg/kg as a base for the chronic studies. In this investigation all techniques demonstrated depression of AChE activity within 15 min following intraperitoneal administration of parathion.

Histochemical observations were in agreement with quantitative biochemical data within the time frames studied. The AChE reaction in the nervous system began to decrease by 15 min (Figs. 3, 4B, and 6) and reached minimal levels by 1 to 2 hr (Figs. 3, 4C, 6, and 7). Partial recovery of AChE activity occurred within 2 to 4 hr (Figs. 3, 4D, 6, and 7) and reached or exceeded the control levels by 24 hr (Figs. 3, 4F, 6, and 7).

Small neurons were essentially negative in AChE activity; however, large neurons stained very intensely (Fig. 4A). Large neurons appeared to retain the AChE re-

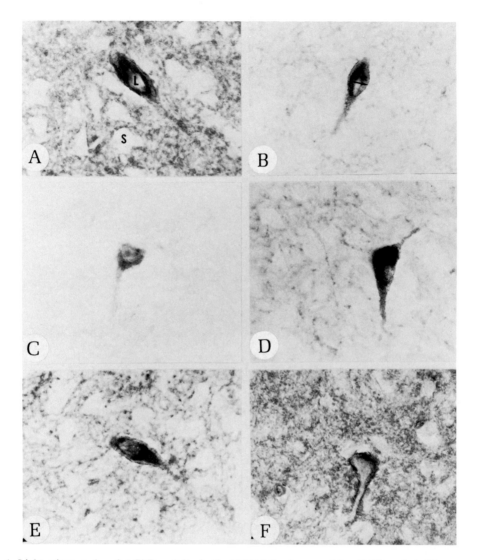

FIG. 4. Light micrographs of AChE activity in the NCP following parathion (1.25 mg/kg). The response of AChE activity was at: **A:** control; **B:** 15 min; **C:** 1 hr; **D:** 4 hr; **E:** 12 hr; and **F:** 24 hr. Note activity in the neuropil, large neuron (L), and plasma membrane (*arrow*). The small neuron (S) is essentially nonreactive. ×1,200.

action product in the cytoplasm (Fig. 4), specifically in cisternae of rough endoplasmic reticulum, Golgi, and nuclear envelope as reported by others (26,30) and demonstrated only minimal loss of this activity by the first hour (Fig. 5C,D). These findings suggest that the reaction product of the large neuron cell soma was protected from the toxic effects of a sublethal dose of parathion. However, this dose level was

sufficiently toxic to severely reduce the AChE reaction on the membranes facing the extracellular space. The sites of AChE reaction have not been clearly defined in the synaptic cleft membranes by others (5). The biochemical and histochemical data closely correspond during the 1-day recovery phase. These data indicate that there is an overshoot of AChE activity above control levels. This phenomenon was observed

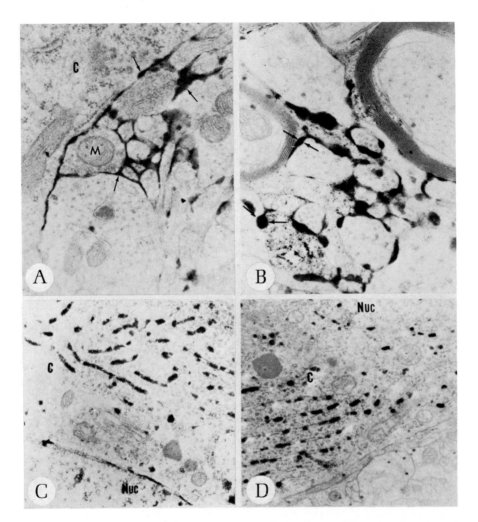

FIG. 5. **A:** Electron micrograph of AChE activity in control. Note staining in the extracellular space (*arrows*), cytoplasm of neuron (C), and mitochondrion (M). ×40,000. **B:** Electron micrograph of AChE activity in experimental (1.25 mg/kg) after 24-hr recovery. Note the regions of expanding, balloon-shaped, extracellular space (*arrows*). ×50,000. **C:** Electron micrograph of AChE activity in control. Note activity in cisternae of rough endoplasmic reticulum. Nucleus (Nuc) at bottom. ×22,000. **D:** Electron micrograph of AChE activity in experimental (1.25 mg/kg) after 24-hr recovery. Note reaction in rough endoplasmic reticulum. Nucleus (Nuc), upper right; neuropil, lower right. ×22,000.

at the fine structure level and may be described as a ballooning of the membranes of the extracellular spaces (Figs. 5B, 6, and 7). The presence of activity in the extracellular space other than the synaptic sites has been noted by other authors (4,32) and suggested to them that the ACh–AChE system is not limited solely to neural transmission functions in the central nervous system.

The AChE activity of poisoned motor end plates in diaphragmatic muscle essentially paralleled that of brain with the possible exception of an earlier depression and subsequent recovery (Fig. 3).

Decreased AChE activity leads to an accumulation of ACh through impairment of the normal deactivation mechanism and occurs in both the peripheral and central nervous systems. It has been observed that

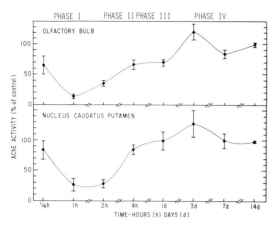

FIG. 6. Time course of AChE activity following parathion (1.25 mg/kg). The elapsed time following parathion was plotted on the abscissa and the AChE activity as a percent of the paired control means on the ordinate. The standard deviation of the mean for each experimental group was plotted. Note the rapid fall of activity within the first 2 hr (*phase I*) followed by a rapid recovery starting at the 2-hr period (*phase II*). After the 4-hr observation a slower recovery rate was observed until the 1-day observation (*phase III*). Following the 1-day observation, a gradual increase over control values occurred with eventual stabilization at control levels within 14 days (*phase IV*). The administration of parathion is represented by time zero.

taneous reactivation or dissociation may occur prior to the aging of the inhibited AChE (1,2,8,9). Whether or not the early symptomatic recovery from a moderate dose of parathion is a result of dissociation or dephosphorylation of the paraoxon–AChE complex or new synthesis of AChE to control levels is not presently known (27). One author reported that the recovery of AChE activity in adult animals proceeded slowly until the fourth day of recovery (60% of control), then proceeded at a much slower rate (8).

It has been suggested that there may be more than one AChE isozyme (4). This suggests one AChE isozyme may recover more rapidly than another. This supposition may be represented by *phases I* and *II* and a more slowly recovering AChE isozyme in *phases III* and *IV* (Fig. 6).

The early reversibility of parathion inhibition of AChE (whole brain) has been demonstrated in adult rats (10). These investigators reported that AChE levels were depressed but returned to 97% of controls within 4 hr. In the present study young

a rise in ACh resulting from parathion exposure is closely allied to central nervous system increases in cortical discharge that are evidenced as tremors and convulsions when the level of total brain ACh has risen by 60% or more over normal values (18). If exposure to parathion is not lethal, as in the present study, symptomatic recovery appears to be complete within 24 hr. Other authors have observed symptomatic recovery from a sublethal dose of parathion within 24 to 48 hr (14,27). The inhibited paraoxon–AChE complex following "aging" is believed to be irreversible, and then the return of activity must occur through the resynthesis of AChE (17). Aging is the apparent increase in the association of the AChE and paraoxon molecules forming a complex that appears to occur in a matter of hours. However, some spon-

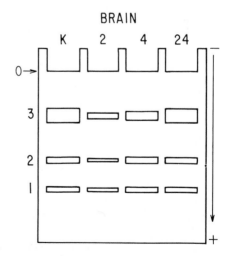

FIG. 7. Course of AChE isozyme inhibition by parathion (1.25 mg/kg) in the BS (pons) of 30-day female rats. K represents control animal; 2, 4, and 24 represent the activities of isozymes at time intervals in hours following the administration of the inhibitor. Origin is at 0; isozymes are numbered 1 to 3.

female rats received only one-fourth of the dose given in the above study, and AChE activity required 1 to 3 days to equal or exceed control levels and 7 to 14 days to stabilize. Whether the rate of reversibility of the paraoxon–AChE complex is related to the age of the animal in question is not known. It has been noted that recovery of AChE (in man) in the synapse is rapid and that symptoms of poison disappeared within 24 hr (31). It was suggested that early recovery of AChE activity is probably due to replacement by new synthesis rather than reactivation (27). The observations by others that there are symptomatic levels is consistent with the present study.

These observations may be explained in one or more ways, the first by the presence of isozymes, one of which may recover more rapidly than the others. In the present study the short, rapid recovery (*phase II*) may be explained by the dissociation of the "unaged" paraoxon–AChE complex. The slower rate of recovery (*phase III*) may be related to the location of the AChE, that is, its protection from complete inhibition by isolation within the interstices of the intracellular compartment and then the release of this reserve enzyme. *Phase IV* or the overshoot of control levels and eventual stabilization may be explained by new synthesis and is consistent with studies of turnover times of nucleic acids and proteins in the central nervous system (22).

Inhibition of multiple forms of AChE or isozymes demonstrated in this study and reported previously (35) could be attributed to the well-known anticholinesterase property of the insecticide parathion *in vivo*.

The present report is one of the few investigations of alterations in multiple forms of AChE resulting from organophosphorus poisoning. Davis and Agranoff (7) demonstrated differential recovery of retinal AChE isozyme of the rat following inhibition by di-isopropylphosphofluoridate. In the present study, the maximum inhibition was revealed by the major AChE isozyme,

a slow-moving diffuse zone close to the origin. This may be the result of a special sensitivity of isozyme 3 to the metabolite of parathion, paraoxon (E600; O, O-diethyl O-p-nitrophenyl phosphate). However, *in vitro* inhibition studies using paraoxon failed to demonstrate this property of isozyme 3 (34). In light of this finding, the alternate possibility of increased accessibility of isozyme 3 to paraoxon needs to be considered. Electron microscopic studies in NCP and BS indicate a greater inhibition of the enzyme in the neuropil than of the intracellular enzyme (6,25). When this finding is correlated with the results of the isozyme study, it is tempting to postulate that the AChE isozyme 3 may represent the enzyme present in the neuropil of the NCP and BS tegmentum and therefore may be more accessible to intravascular paraoxon than the intracellular enzyme. Location and availability of AChE isozymes within the brain of the housefly have been shown to be major factors influencing their susceptibility to organophosphates (33). The recovery of multiple forms of AChE following parathion poisoning was not examined in detail in this study. However, the sequence of reappearance of the bands 1 to 3 at 4 and 24 hr after injection suggests the possibility that the major AChE zone 3 may recover at a slower rate than the isozyme zones 1 and 2.

In recent years, differential alterations in AChE isozymes have been demonstrated in denervated skeletal muscles (16), in deafferentation of the cerebellum (3), and in cerebellar mutation (36). These observations strengthen the possibility of *in vivo* occurrence of multiple forms of AChE in the mammalian nervous system.

ACKNOWLEDGMENTS

Much of the work described herein was submitted by H. D. McDougal and V. K. Vijayan in partial fulfillment of the requirements for the degree of Doctor of Philosophy in Anatomy at the University of California, Davis. This study was supported by extramural funds from the National Institutes of Health #1 FO3 ES13065-11 and intramural funds from the University of California, Davis, #D540. D. B. Suter is a National Institutes of Health Postdoctoral Fellow under contract #1 FO3 ES13065-01.

REFERENCES

1. Aldridge, W. N. (1953): The inhibition of erythrocyte cholinesterase by tri-esters of phosphoric acid. 3. The nature of the inhibitory process. *Biochem. J.*, 54:442–448.
2. Aldridge, W. N., and Davison, A. N. (1953): Mechanism of inhibition of cholinesterase by organophosphorus compounds. *Biochem. J.*, 55:763–765.
3. Bajgar, J., and Pařizek, J. (1973): Changes of acetylcholinesterase and esterase isoenzymes in isolated cerebellar cortex of the rabbit. *Brain Res.*, 57:299–305.
4. Bernsohn, J., and Barron, K. D. (1964): Multiple molecular forms of brain hydrolases. *Int. Rev. Neurobiol.*, 7:297–344.
5. Bloom, F. E., and Barrnett, R. J. (1967): The fine structural localization of cholinesterases in nervous tissue. *Ann. NY Acad. Sci.*, 144:626–645.
6. Brownson, R. H., Suter, D. B., Vijayan, V. K., and McDougal, H. D. (1974): Parathion-induced alterations in acetylcholinesterase activity of brain—depression and recovery. *J. Neuropathol. Exp. Neurol.*, 33:177.
7. Davis, G. A., and Agranoff, B. W. (1968): Metabolic behaviour of isoenzymes of acetylcholinesterase. *Nature*, 220:277–280.
8. Davison, A. N. (1955): Return of cholinesterase activity in the rat after inhibition by organophosphorus compounds. *Biochem. J.*, 60:339–346.
9. Davison, A. N. (1953): Return of cholinesterase activity in the rat after inhibition by organophosphorus compounds. 1. Diethyl-p-nitrophenyl phosphate (E600, Paraoxon). *Biochem. J.*, 54:583–590.
10. Dubois, K. P., Doull, J., Salerno, P. R., and Coon, J. M. (1949): Studies on the toxicity and mechanism of action of p-nitrophenyl diethyl thionophosphate (parathion). *J. Pharmacol.*, 95:79–91.
11. El-Badawi, A., and Schenk, E. A. (1967): Histochemical methods for separate, consecutive and simultaneous demonstration of acetylcholinesterase and norepinephrine in cryostat sections. *J. Histochem. Cytochem.*, 15:580–588.
12. Ellman, G. L., Courtney, K. D., Valentino, A., and Featherstone, R. M. (1961): A new and rapid colorimetric determination of acetylcholinesterase activity. *Biochem. Pharmacol.*, 7:88–95.
13. Fukuto, T. R., and Metcalf, R. L. (1969): Metabolism of insecticides in plants and animals. *Ann. NY Acad. Sci.*, 160:97–111.
14. Golz, H. H., and Shaffer, C. B. (1960): *Parathion Poisoning—A Brief Review: Toxicological Information on Cyanamid Insecticides*, p. 41. American Cynamid Company, New York.
15. Hajos, F., Priymak, E., and Kerpel-Fronius, S. (1970): The electron microscopic demonstration of acetylcholinesterase activity in some cholinergic and non-cholinergic synapses of the rat brain. *Acta Histochem. (Jena)*, 35:114–122.
16. Hall, Z. W. (1973): Multiple forms of acetylcholinesterase and their distribution in endplate and non-endplate regions of rat diaphragm muscle. *J. Neurobiol.*, 4:343–361.
17. Hobbiger, F. (1963): Reactivation of phosphorylated acetylcholinesterase. In: *Handbuch der Experimentellen Pharmakologie Ergünzungswerk*, Vol. 15, edited by G. B. Koelle, pp. 921–988. Springer-Verlag, Berlin.
18. Holmstedt, B., Härkönen, M., Lundgren, G., and Sundwall, A. (1967): Relationship between acetylcholine and cholinesterase activity in the brain following an organophosphorus cholinesterase inhibitor. *Biochem. Pharmacol.*, 16:404–406.
19. Karnovsky, M. J., and Roots, L. (1964): A "direct-coloring" thiocholine method of cholinesterase. *J. Histochem. Cytochem.*, 12:219–221.
20. Kasa, P. (1968): Acetylcholinesterase transport in the central and peripheral nervous tissue: The role of tubules in the enzyme transport. *Nature*, 218:1265–1267.
21. Kasa, P., and Csillik, B. (1968): AChE synthesis in cholinergic neurons: Electron histochemistry of enzyme translocation. *Histochemie*, 12:175–183.
22. Koenig, H. (1958): An autoradiographic study of nucleic acid and protein turnover in the mammalian neuraxis. *J. Biophysic. Biochem. Cytol.*, 4:785–809.
23. Kokko, A., Mautner, H. G., and Barrnett, R. J. (1969): Fine structural localization of acetylcholinesterase using acetyl-β-methylthiocholine and acetylselenocholine as substrates. *J. Histochem. Cytochem.*, 17:625–640.
24. Lewis, P. R., and Shute, C. C. D. (1964): Demonstration of cholinesterase activity with the electron microscope. *J. Physiol.*, 175:5–7.
25. McDougal, H. (1973): Parathion Induced Alterations in Acetylcholinesterase Activity of Rat Brain: A Biochemical, Light and Electron Histochemical Study. Ph.D. Thesis, University of California, Davis.
26. Mori, S., Maeda, T., and Shimizu, N. (1964): Electronmicroscopic histochemistry of cholinesterase in the rat brain. *Histochemie*, 4:65–72.
27. Namba, T. (1971): Cholinesterase inhibition by organophosphorus compounds and its clinical effects. *Bull. WHO*, 44:289–307.
28. Ruckelshaus, W. D. (1972): Opinion and order of the administrator, Environmental Protection Agency Director, Consolidated DDT Hearing. *Fed. Reg.*, 37:13369–13376.
29. Schrader, G. (1963): Unpublished speech given to Agricultural Faculty, University of Bonn, De-

cember 2, 1959. Quoted in: *Readings in Pharma-cology,* edited by B. Holmstedt and G. Liljestrand, pp. 376–379. Macmillan, New York.

30. Shimizu, N., and Ishii, S. (1966): Electron microscopic histochemistry of acetylcholinesterase of rat brain by Karnovsky's method. *Histochemie,* 6:24–33.

31. Suter, D. B., and Brownson, R. H. (1971): Parathion-induced changes in enzyme activity in rat brain. *Anat. Rec.,* 169:440.

32. Torack, R. M., and Barrnnett, R. J. (1962): Fine structural localization of cholinesterase activity in the rat brain stem. *Exp. Neurol.,* 6:222–244.

33. Tripathy, R. K., and O'Brien, R. D. (1973): Effects of organophosphates in vivo upon acetyl-cholinesterase isoenzymes from housefly head and thorax. *Pestic. Biochem. Physiol.,* 2:418–424.

34. Vijayan, V. K., and Brownson, R. H. (1974): Polyacrylamide gel electrophoresis of rat brain acetylcholinesterase: Isoenzymes of normal rat brain. *J. Neurochem.,* 23:47–53.

35. Vijayan, V. K., and Brownson, R. H. (1975): Polyacrylamide gel electrophoresis of rat brain acetylcholinesterase: Isoenzyme changes following parathion poisoning. *J. Neurochem.,* 24:105–110.

36. Vijayan, V. K., and Wilson, D. B. (1977): Acetyl-cholinesterase activity in the cerebellum of the lurcher (Lc) mutant mouse. (*In preparation.*)

Neurotoxicology, edited by L. Roizin, H. Shiraki, and N. Grčević. Raven Press, New York © 1977.

Cerebral Changes in Paraquat Poisoning

Nenad Grčević, Dubravka Jadro-Šantel, and *Stanko Jukić

*Department of Neuropathology, University of Zagreb, Clinical Medical Center Rebro, Zagreb; and *General Hospital Vinkovci, Yugoslavia*

Paraquat (1,1'-dimethyl 4,4'-bipyridylium dichloride, Gramoxan®, Weedol®) is a potent and widely used herbicide. Since its introduction (43), it has come into use in more than 130 countries (42). Its high toxicity to man was recognized soon after its introduction (5), and numerous cases of poisoning have been reported in the literature (1–5,8,11,13–15,19,20,27–30,34, 35,37,42,44). According to Teare (42), 232 fatal cases of poisoning had been reported in the 10 years before his paper, with accidental and suicidal cases equally represented.

Pathological changes produced by paraquat and considered responsible for its high toxicity have been studied in numerous human cases (1–5,8,11,13,14,19, 20,35,37,42,44), but the most important contributions to this problem derive from animal experiments (6,7,9,10,12,16–19,21, 23–26,31–33,36,38,39–41,45). These pathological changes are dominated by severe involvement of lungs, kidneys, and liver, but changes have also been described in myocardium, testes, adrenal glands, intestines, pancreas, and stomach. Changes in the lungs are best known; they include degeneration of the alveolar cells of Type I with impairment of alveolar surfactant, edema, congestion, hyaline membranes, intraalveolar hemorrhage, atelectasis, severe changes in the interstitial vessels, and interstitial fibrosis (1,5,8–11,15,19,20,23–25,27,28,33–35,39,40,42). As far as kidneys are concerned, the main change seems to be necrosis of proximal tubules and changes in the vessels (5,8,9,15,17,35). Changes in the liver are less typical, the most frequent finding being centrilobular necrosis and congestion, with jaundice as a frequent clinical sign of poisoning (29,32, 33,37,42).

In spite of clinical signs of effects on the nervous system in many cases of poisoning, practically no information on pathological changes in the central nervous system exists in the literature, except some general observations of edema, congestion, and "nonspecific" changes (10,20,27).

We have had the opportunity to examine the brains of two patients who died of paraquat poisoning, and since they showed certain pathological changes that might indicate the direct or indirect neurotoxicity of this compound, we considered them interesting for presentation and discussion.

MATERIALS AND METHODS

Our material for study consisted of the brains of two patients who survived acute intoxication with paraquat for 9 and 11 days, respectively.

Case 1 was a 49-year-old man who swallowed, by accident, about 50 ml of paraquat solution. After initial vomiting, a severe clinical picture developed, with nausea, vomiting, abdominal pains, dizziness, and general malaise, followed on the third day by jaundice and signs of renal insufficiency. The jaundice progressed rapidly with renal failure. On the seventh day after ingestion of paraquat, tremor of the hands and psychomotor disturbances began that also deteriorated on the following day when the patient developed respiratory distress, went into stupor and coma, and died on the ninth day after intoxication.

Case 2 was a 45-year-old man who swallowed a similar amount of paraquat and developed a clinical picture similar to the patient of case 1. In addition to nausea, vomiting, and dizziness, this patient also had difficulty in swallowing due to direct necrotic effects on pharyngeal and esophageal mucosa. Jaundice, which occurred on the third day, was followed by signs of renal failure. He also

had tremor of the hands developing on the eighth day when the patient also began to show some mental disturbances. Respiratory difficulties began on the ninth day, and the whole clinical picture began to deteriorate rapidly, with coma and death on the 11th day after ingestion of paraquat.

The brains of both patients were fixed in 10% formaline. For gross examination the brains were cut in consecutive coronal sections. Light microscopic investigations were carried out on large hemispheral sections of blocks imbedded in paraffin. The sections were stained by hematoxilin-eosin (H.&E.), cresylviolet, Luxol fast

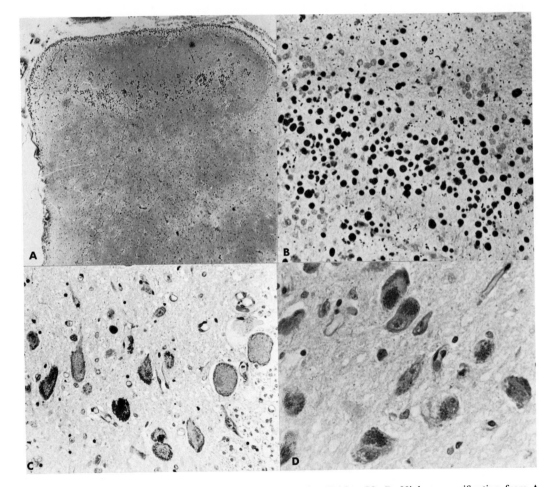

FIG. 1.A: Temporal cortex. Large amounts of amyloid bodies. PAS. ×80. B: Higher magnification from A. Amyloid bodies of various sizes in deeper layers of cortex. PAS. ×300. C: Lipofuscin and central chromatolysis in the trigeminal nucleus. PAS. ×380. D: Lipofuscin in the lateral geniculate body. PAS. ×450.

blue, Heidenhain, Mallory, Gömöri, PAS, Sudan Black B, Bodian, and Gross-Bielschowsky. Material for electron microscopic study was taken from all representative areas of the brain. After postfixation in 5% paraformaldehyde-glutardialdehyde solution and treatment in 1% osmium tetroxide, the blocks were imbedded in Epon and cut on Reichert OmU2 ultramicrotome. The sections were postcontrasted with 4% uranylacetate.

Paraffin blocks of lungs, kidneys, liver, pancreas, myocardium, and testis were also examined.

RESULTS

Light Microscopic Examination

Case 1

Gross examination of the brain, besides edema and congestion, did not show any abnormality.

Histological examination, in addition to severe edema and congestion, showed a number of quite marked morphological changes. The most striking was a very pronounced accumulation of lipofuscin-like material in the ganglion cells throughout the brain, but most marked in the pallidum, interlaminary nuclei of thalamus, corpus geniculatum laterale, substantia nigra, dentate and fastigial nuclei of the cerebellum, Purkinje cells, nuclei of the motor cranial nerves, and inferior olivary nucleus. Stained by H. & E., one portion of this material showed a brownish color like typical lipofuscin, but large amounts of it became visible only by PAS staining (Fig. 1C and D). Some of this granular material was Sudan Black positive. This PAS-positive material in the most affected cells not only occupied the perikaryon, but the same material could also be seen in the proximal parts of the cell processes. Some cells were so filled with this material that a storage-effect phenomenon appeared. Similar material was

also found in some endothelial cells, microglia, and even oligodendroglia as well as free in the perivascular spaces. In these extraneuronal locations no brownish pigmentation was present. The other, equally pronounced, phenomenon was central chromatolysis with swelling of cell bodies in the dentate nucleus, substantia nigra, locus ceruleus, oculomotor nuclei, motor trigeminal nucleus, facial and hypoglossal nuclei, and, to much lesser degree, the pallidum and lateral geniculate body (Fig. 1C). These changes appeared as an axonal reaction to some distal injury, a dying-back phenomenon. In many cells storage of lipofuscin clearly coincided with the central chromatolysis. Many ganglion cells showed swellings of proximal parts of the processes, which sometime appeared like "neuroaxonal dystrophy." Purkinje cells displayed marked changes that included torpedo-like structures (Fig. 2C and D). Another peculiar finding was an unusually large amount of amyloid bodies. They not only occupied their usual sites, but also were scattered in the gray matter, often close to the ganglion cells. They varied in size from the usual ones to the very small round granular bodies (Fig. 1A and B). This could be seen especially in the cerebellar cortex in the Purkinje layer, where large amounts of such PAS-positive round bodies and granules were found around ganglion cells and their processes, intermixed with the amyloid bodies of normal size (Fig. 2A and B). It looked as though the amyloid bodies and smaller granular bodies represented the same process in various stages of development. An increase of astroglia was found in the cerebellum, especially the Bergmann glia, but a slight increase in glial nuclei was also found in the pallidum, lateral geniculate body, and thalamus. No conspicuous change in astroglia was seen in the cortex; there was no marked activity of microglia. In the stroma of choroid plexuses of the lateral ventricles some calcium deposits were found.

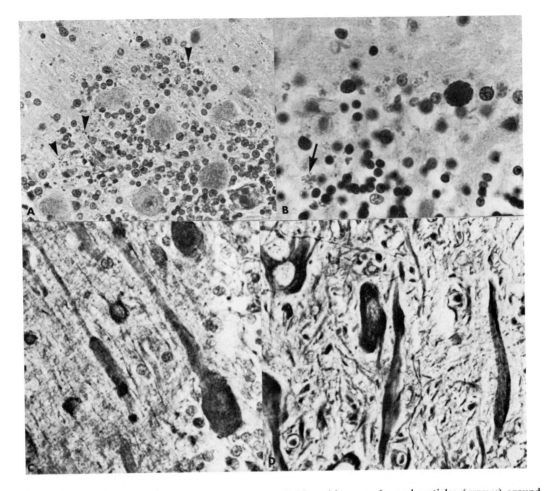

FIG. 2.A: Proliferation of Bergmann glia and numerous PAS-positive granules and particles (*arrows*) around Purkinje cells. PAS. ×450. **B:** Amyloid bodies of various sizes and small PAS-positive granules at the edge of granular layer of cerebellar cortex (*arrow*). PAS. ×540. **C:** Axonal swelling and torpedo formation in the Purkinje cells. Bielschowsky-Gross. ×680. **D:** Torpedo formations in the processes of Purkinje cells. Bodian. ×680.

Histological examination of blocks from visceral organs showed what could be considered typical pathology of paraquat poisoning, as repeatedly described in the literature. Most marked were the changes in the *lungs,* with hemorrhage, congestion, degeneration of alveolar lining, hyaline membranes, and interstitial proliferations. *Kidneys* showed typical necrotic changes in the proximal tubules, but there were also changes in the glomeruli, with shrinkage and increased cellularity. There were also calcium deposits in the interstitium. The *liver* showed the most severe changes in the bile ducts and bile capillaries, with obliteration and bile stasis. There were also some degenerative changes in the hepatic parenchyma, but this was rather difficult to interpret because of steatosis and incipient interstitial fibrosis with some lymphocyte infiltration of an obviously preexisting nature. The *pancreas* exhibited widespread foci of necrosis with saponification. In the *hypopharynx* and *esophagus* there were large areas of necrotic mucosa and sub-mucosa.

Case 2

Gross and histological examination of the brain showed a strikingly similar picture to that of case 1. Here also the most pronounced pathological change was an accumulation of PAS-positive, mostly granular, partly brownish, lipofuscin-like material in the ganglion cells, with the same pattern of predilection as in the previous case. As in case 1, this material was often found not only in the perikaryon but also in the proximal parts of the processes, and similar material could also be seen in some endothelial and glial cells, as well as free in the perivascular areas. Coinciding with this in similar or the same places, pronounced central chromatolysis of ganglion cells was found, suggesting, as in the previous case, an axonal reaction. Axonal swellings, at times not unlike neuroaxonal dystrophy, were also encountered, but strikingly similar also was the phenomenon of accumulation of small PAS-positive granules around Purkinje cells described in detail in case 1. Torpedo structures were also found. There were large amounts of amyloid bodies throughout the brain, similar to case 1.

Histological examination of the blocks from *visceral* organs revealed changes very similar to those described in case 1. It may be worth noting that here, too, glomerular changes in the kidneys were found in addition to the necrosis of the proximal tubules and that calcium deposits were seen in the interstitium of the pyramids. The findings in the liver differed from the previous case by the lack of steatocirrhosis; the main pathology was represented by changes in the bile capillaries and hepatic cells, as commonly seen in paraquat poisoning. The pancreas showed scattered slight necrosis and interstitial proliferation of fibrous tissue. Plaques of necrosis in the mucosa and submucosa of the esophagus were also found.

Electron Microscopic Examination

As mentioned before, only material from the brain was available for electron microscopic examination, which was done on a large number of blocks from all representative areas. This examination revealed that great similarity existed between the two cases, with a number of outstanding features repeating themselves in both cases and in the corresponding areas. We therefore describe the electron microscopic findings of these two cases together.

First, there were numerous morphological changes obviously due to autolysis and standard formalin fixation, factors that certainly decreased the precision of our observations and the possibility of defining all abnormal phenomena that we saw. We review here those changes that we consider most conspicuous in both cases.

In the cytoplasm of ganglion cells large amounts of osmium-dense, lipofuscin-like material were found (Figs. 3 and 4). This material showed variable concentration and distribution, affecting not only the perikarya of the cells but also cellular processes, the axons, and the dendrites (Fig. 3C). Similar material was also found in the cytoplasm of some oligodendroglial cells as well as in the endothelial and perithelial cells of the capillaries and small blood vessels (Figs. 8B and 9B). It seemed that the cells retained their integrity and shape even if they were densely packed with storage material. This material consisted of aggregates of membrane-bound, mostly granular particles of variable electron density. Some contained lamellar structures (Fig. 3C). Electron-dense lipid particles alternated with fenestrated areas and electron-lucent parts. This material appeared as lipofuscin in various stages of autophagic or heterophagic activity. Among these lipofuscin-like particles, especially in the cells with pronounced central chromatolysis, aggregates of condensed rough endoplasmatic reticulum with plump ribosomal branches were found (Fig.

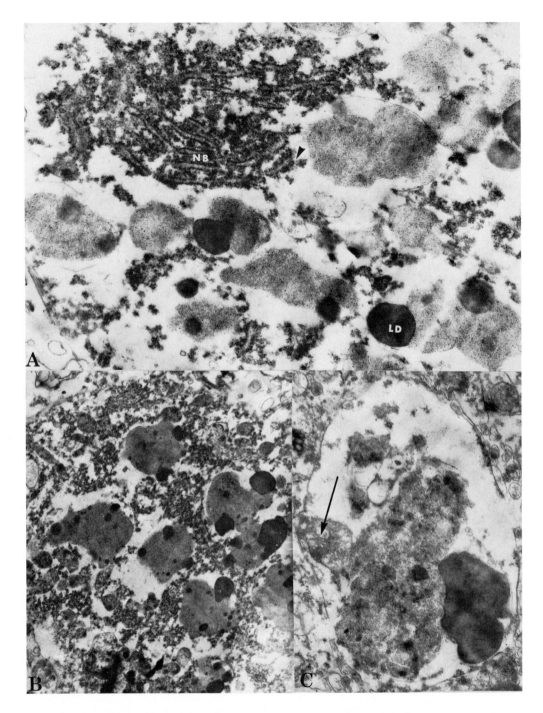

FIG. 3.A and **B:** Osmium-dense pleiomorphic membrane-bound bodies in the cytoplasm of ganglion cells. Within these lipofuscin-like elements lipid droplets (LD) were also found. Rough endoplasmatic reticulum (NB) is condensed and plump with pronounced ribosomal branches (*arrow*). **A:** ×49,400; **B:** ×26,950. **C:** A dendritic process filled with the same material, which at some places shows lamellated structure (*arrow*). The dendrite seems to be before disintegration. ×52,250.

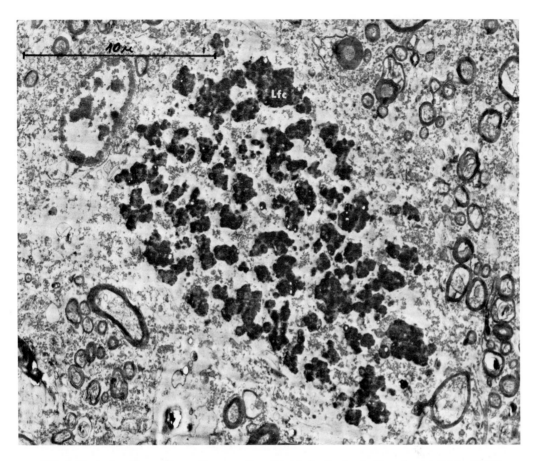

FIG. 4. Typical stuffing of the perikaryon of a cell with the lipofuscin-like material (Lfc). ×8,550.

3A). In addition, in the perikaryon and processes of many ganglion cells, agglomerations of pleiomorphic cytolysosomes were found in which electron-dense material similar to that described above was seen incorporated in the multilamellar, as well as concentric structures (Fig. 5A and B). In such places mitochondrion-like organelles with double membranes and foamy osmium-dense inclusions could also be seen (Fig. 5A). Both these organelles also showed various stages of digestion and were in some cells so abundant that the whole cytoplasm was packed with them. Osmium-dense material of the same type as described above was found in the neuropil. Aggregates of lipofuscin-like material were also detected in the perivascular spaces

(Fig. 9). Some oligodendroglial cells contained, in their cytoplasm, particles of similar appearance, and, as described later, capillary endothelium in many areas showed changes in which similar material was found.

Various specimens from both brains revealed severe changes in the myelinated axons. This was especially marked in the white matter distal from the cells. These changes were characterized by the occurrence of vacuolar and vesicular structures that appeared to lie within the sheath pushing the axon away. Some of these vesicular, membrane-bound bodies were situated clearly in the area of the inner mesaxon (Fig. 6A). In such places "compressed" axons seemed to contain increased amounts

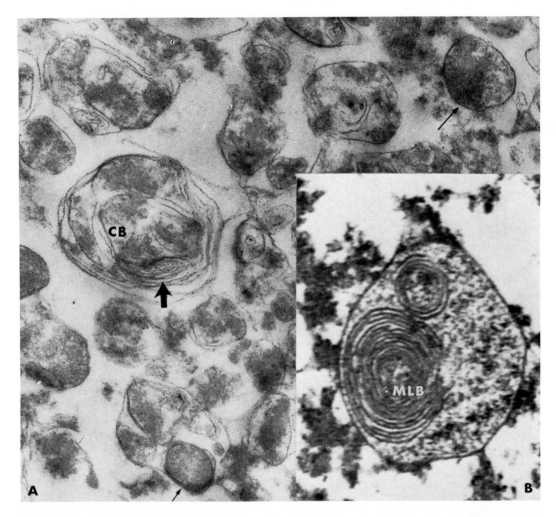

FIG. 5.A: Beside lipofuscin-like bodies in many cells and their processes, cytosomal organelles were found. They were in various stages of digestion and contained multilamellated, sometimes concentric structures (*large arrow*), as well as osmium-dense granular elements bound by double membrane (*small arrow*). ×38,000. **B:** A membrane-bound typical lysosome containing two multilamellar bodies (MLB). ×33,250.

of axoplasmic organelles (Fig. 6A and B). There were also irregular formations produced by peeling of the lamellae or splitting of the myelin structure on the outer or inner zones of the myelin sheath (Fig. 6C).

As in histological preparations, a remarkable quantity of pleiomorphic amyloid body structures were also found in the electron microscopic preparations (Fig. 7). They were found in the neuropil, sometimes attached to the myelinated or unmyelinated nerve fibers. They were also

FIG. 6.A: Accumulation of vesicular pseudocrystalline osmium-lucent material in the area of inner mesaxon. The axon is compressed to one-third of its normal thickness (*arrow*). ×52,250. **B:** Cross-section through a similar place (*long arrows*). ×57,000. **C:** Beneath another axon with similar changes there is an amyloid body (AB) containing osmium-dense material (*short arrows*). ×47,500.

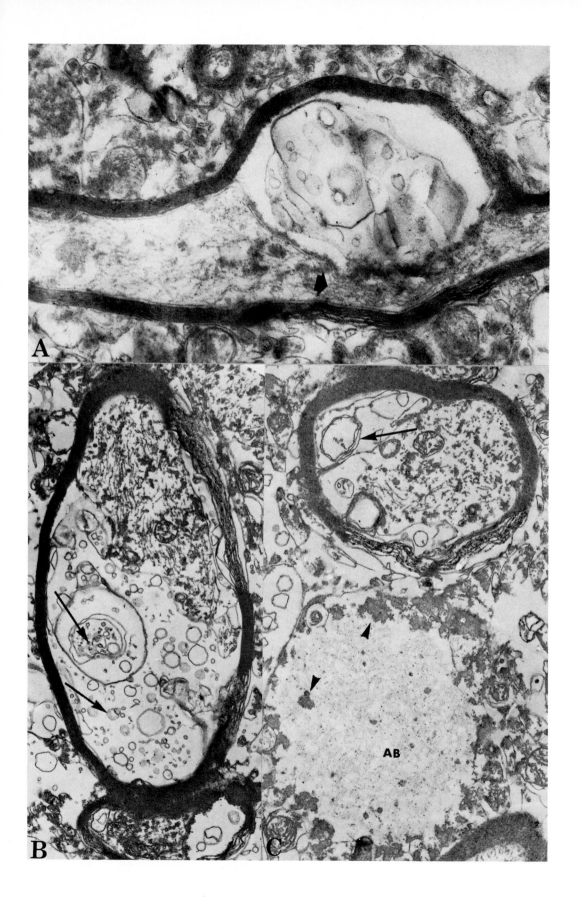

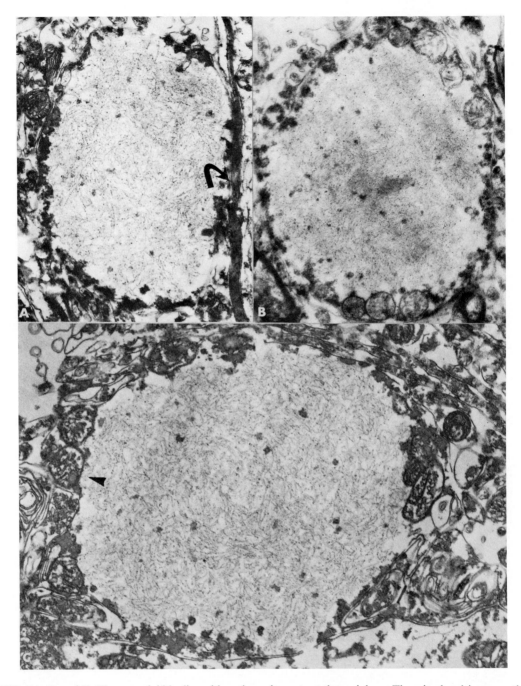

FIG. 7.A, B, and **C:** Three amyloid bodies with various elements at the periphery. The mitochondria are partly normal and partly abnormal and swollen, with longitudinal cristae and inclusions of osmium-dense material similar to that found in the ganglion cells (**C,** *arrow*). The amyloid body at **A** is intimately attached to a myelinated nerve fiber (*arrow*). **A:** ×42,750; **B:** ×71,250; **C:** ×80,750.

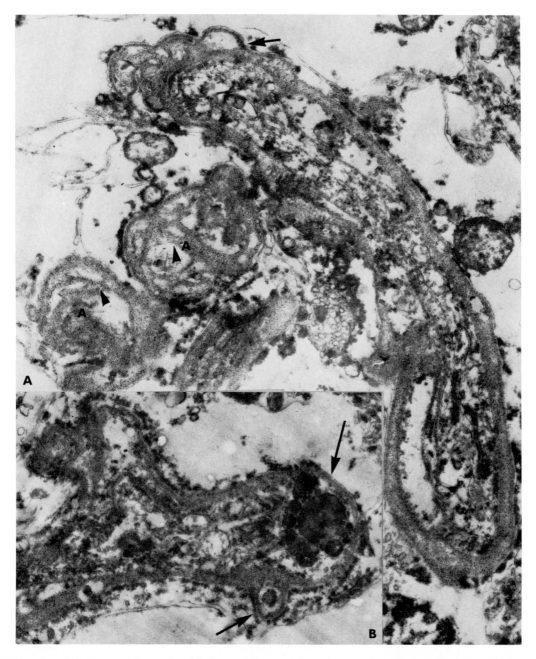

FIG. 8.A and **B:** Two small vessels with degenerative changes at the basal membrane. Markedly thickened membrane (**A**) shows splitting, resulting in fenestrations and buddings, which gives the impression of aneurysmatic protrusions. In a fenestration at **B** intramural (within the basal membrane) accumulations of osmium-dense, lipofuscin-like material were found (*arrows in* **B**). **A:** ×22,050; **B:** ×22,050.

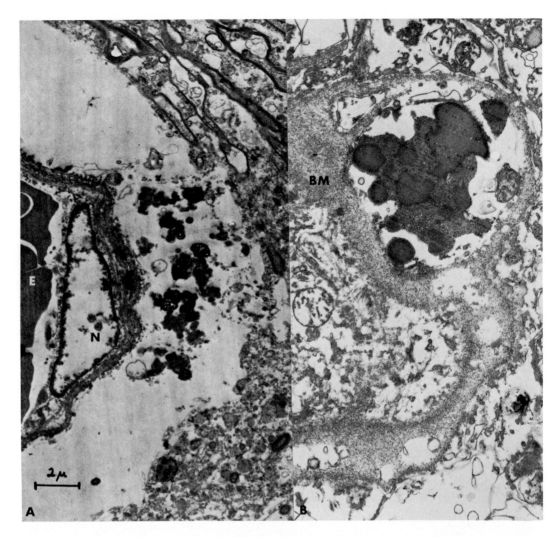

FIG. 9.A: Aggregates of lipofuscin-like material around a vein in the pons. The basal membrane at this place does not show degenerative changes as severe as those observed in smaller vessels and capillaries. **A:** ×8,550. E, erythrocyte; N, nucleus of endothelial cell. **B:** A detail from the wall of a capillary showing enormously swollen basal membrane with fenestrations one of which is filled with lipofuscin-like material. **B:** ×9,500. BM, basal membrane.

found within the dendritic processes, axons, and even in the cytoplasm of ganglion cells. They varied in size, sometimes being extremely small, whereas in other instances they were of normal size. Some contained dense osmiophylic particles, especially at the periphery (Figs. 6C and 7C). In some of them, an increased amount of mitochondria was found at the periphery (Fig. 7B and C). In some places similar material

without the formed shape of a body was found in the neuropil in aggregations without membrane.

Another interesting finding was a peculiar process in the capillaries and small vessels throughout both brains. First, many vessels showed tortuous aneurysmatic deformities of the lumen, with protrusions and evaginations (Fig. 8). The basal membrane of many capillaries was swollen and undergoing degenerative changes with splitting and fenestrations that resulted, in places, in formation of intramural cavitations. In such places deposits of osmium-dense material in droplets or in lysosome-like, membrane-bound organelles were often found (Figs. 8B and 9B). Morphological features of this material were similar to those of the lipofuscin-like material found in the ganglion cells. Due to the changes of the walls, the lumen of such vessels was often reduced or even obliterated (Fig. 8).

DISCUSSION

Our attempt to undertake neuropathological studies of the brains of these two patients who died of paraquat poisoning was justified first by the fact that practically no information existed in the literature on the condition of the CNS in such poisoning. We also believed that a relatively long survival in both cases offered a chance of finding some morphological abnormalities that require time to develop, especially since it is known that some visceral changes in paraquat poisoning develop rather late. Finally, both patients had a clinical history of quite certain neurological and mental disturbances with terminal coma, which indicated the possibility of brain involvement. We are aware that postmortem material, especially as far as electron microscopic examination is concerned, substantially decreased the accuracy and reliability of our observations due to the interference of autolytic processes. Because of this, our conclusions are made with certain reservations, and this chapter should be considered a preliminary report requiring further experimental confirmations.

As described above, the most outstanding feature in both of our cases was an unusual amount of lipofuscin-like, lipid material aggregated in the ganglion cells, their processes, but also in the capillary endothelium, some oligodendroglial and microglial cells, and even free in the neuropil.

Histologically, only part of it showed brownish pigmentation, and none of the extraneuronally located particles was pigmented. In the electron microscopic preparations this PAS-positive material displayed a wide range of variations both in osmium density and morphological structures, which included multilammelar and circular bodies, cytolysosomes, mitochondrial inclusions, and even fat-like droplets. The amount and pleiomorphism of this material, together with the fact that it occurred in an almost equal manner in the brains of two unrelated middle-aged men who were spatially separated, logically indicated the probability that paraquat intoxication played a certain role in the development of this phenomenon in our cases.

Neuronal lipofuscin is one of the most common findings in the aging brain, but can also occur in increased quantities in younger individuals due to known (vitamin E deficiency, hypoxia, retrograde degeneration, various intoxications) or unknown causes (22). Several details concerning its significance, formation, location, and subcellular variations have not yet been clarified or generally agreed upon. The fact of its constant presence in the CNS and its pathological increase under various conditions should not, however, cause it to be discarded as some nonspecific and therefore nonimportant phenomenon for various disease processes. This only means that various conditions may pathogenetically include a mechanism that triggers the process of lipofuscin formation in quantities that could be considered pathological. In this context, lipofuscin, or, rather, metabolic disturbance due to which lipofuscin-like material is being pathologically produced, may also belong to the picture of paraquat poisoning. It is of interest that similar lipid material has been described in both human and experimental paraquat poisoning in the pulmonary alveolar cells and capillary endothelium (3,4,19,24,39,40,45), as well as in the kidneys (17). This suggests a process typical for a certain toxic action, although so pronounced a predilection for the CNS in our cases may also suggest that some additional mechanisms might have aggravated the picture. One of such mechanisms may be retrograde degeneration (dying-back) due to some injury to the distal axon. As described before, in both of our cases central chromatolysis was quite conspicuous and had the same pattern of predilection. Many of the subcortical gray nuclei in which the ganglion cells showed such axonal reaction were also the sites of the most pronounced storage of the lipofuscin-like material. Our material was not suitable for further exploration of this phenomenon, but there are several reports of experimentally induced storage of lipofuscin as a result of retrograde degeneration (22). Our observations may only bring us to presume, at this moment, that the axonal reaction in our cases was due to some distal axonal injury that may have been produced by intoxication directly or through some local or general metabolic changes induced by degenerative processes in the liver, kidneys, or somewhere else in the visceral system. Hypoxia has also been indicated by some authors as a possible cause of excessive production of lipofuscin (22). Pathological changes in the lungs of our cases, as well as in many cases from the literature, seemed to have developed rather late in the course of the disease, with blockage of alveolar space being produced mostly by acute hemorrhages and hyaline membranes. Clinically, both of our patients developed breathing difficulties quite terminally. Thus, one would presume that hypoxia of respiratory origin could not have played a decisive role in influencing formation of lipofuscin-like material in our cases.

Unusually large amounts of amyloid bodies and granular bodies similar to them in the CNS of both of our cases was another feature of the histological and electron microscopical picture. Of special interest are those small amyloid body-like structures found in close relation to the ganglion cells. The abundance of such particles in the Purkinje layer was especially pronounced. The impression was gained that the small and large amyloid bodies are related to these very small particles as if an active process of their production were in course. Many of the amyloid structures, especially those that lay within the processes of the ganglion cells, contained osmium-dense material similar to that found in the lipofuscin. Formation of amyloid bodies is a nonspecific and frequent phenomenon in the CNS. However, the fact stressed above of such diverse sizes and granules suggesting a rapid formation of amyloid bodies in our cases, as well as the fact that the same finding existed in two unrelated men without any known pre-existing illness, should keep our attention until the experimental data are available.

Changes in the capillaries and small vessels observed in electron microscopic preparations in both of our cases deserve special attention. Similar changes were described in the lungs of human and experimental cases of paraquat intoxication (20,34), and vascular changes of other types have repeatedly been described in the lungs (23,24,41) and in the kidneys (17) as an integral part of the pathological process. Our findings in the cerebral vessels clearly indicate the intracerebral action of paraquat, bringing further evidence toward connecting paraquat and the above-described neuronal pathology. This can be further substantiated by peculiar intraendothelial (intramural) deposition of lipid material in pathologically altered capillaries and small vessels in the brain of our cases. Finally, the mural changes produced such alterations of vascular lumina that the impairment of microcirculation in those areas could logically be presumed. This could have contributed to the development of relative hypoxia and edema in the affected areas, which topographically corresponded also to the areas of pronounced lipofuscinosis.

Regarding the changes in the nerve fibers, which were characterized by peculiar vesicular phenomena in the myelin sheaths and some axonal changes, it is difficult to draw any definite conclusion because of severe postmortem artifacts. However, within the scope of the whole complex described above, with axonal reaction as a pronounced phenomenon, we believe that these changes, too, have to be recorded and further investigated.

In conclusion, we would like to underline certain facts pertinent to our observations and to the problem of neurotoxicity in general. At this moment, when neuropathology is entering the field of neurotoxicology on a wider front, the possibility certainly arises that some rather nonspecific changes may be overemphasized and that conclusions may be drawn too quickly about the morphological correlates of certain toxic actions. However, there is an equal danger that some morphological phenomena of great importance might be rejected as typical for a given drug or agent just because similar phenomena are encountered in other conditions. Morphological correlates of neurotoxicity will probably seldom be specific, just as correlates of infection, mechanical injury, and even oxygen deficiency are not specific in many instances, especially on the subcellular level. It is by combination of "nonspecific" changes that we shall probably be able to build and define the morphological *complexes* typical for a certain toxic agent or group of agents. These combinations are obviously very complicated, or, rather, they are correlates of quite complicated, interrelated mechanisms, some of which will be due to the toxic agent *per se*, whereas others will be due to metabolic disturbances arising in pathological changes elsewhere in the body. The present state of our knowledge on the neuropath-

ology of toxic injury requires careful recording of everything that may be observed in human cases of poisoning as well as in the animal experiments. Only collection of such data will help clarify problems by offering solutions and by opening hypotheses necessary for further studies.

REFERENCES

1. Almong, C. H., and Tal, E. (1967): Death from paraquat after subcutaneous injection. *Br. Med. J.,* 3:721.
2. Bescol-Liversac, J. (1975): Ultrastructural study of a renal biopsy in a patient poisoned by paraquat. *Eur. J. Toxicol. Environ. Hyg.,* 8:236–246.
3. Borchard, F. (1974): Ultrastrukturelle und licht mikroskopische Befunde bei drei protrahiert todlich verleufenen paraquat Vergiftungen. *Pneumonologie,* 150:185–189.
4. Borchard, F., Grabensee, B., Jax, W., and Huth, F. (1974): Morphologische Befunde bei Paraquatvergiftungen. *Klin. Wochenschr.,* 52:657–671.
5. Bullivant, C. M. (1966): Accidental poisoning by paraquat: Report of two cases in man. *Br. Med. J.,* 1272–1273.
6. Bus, J. S., Aust, S. D., and Gibson, J. E. (1974): Superoxide and singlet oxygen-catalysed lipid peroxidation as a possible mechanism for paraquat toxicity. *Biochem. Biophys. Res. Commun.,* 58:749–755.
7. Calderbank, A. (1968): The dipyridylium herbicides. *Adv. Pest. Contr. Res.,* 8:127–235.
8. Campbell, S. (1968): Death from paraquat in a child. *Lancet,* 7534:144.
9. Clark, D. G., Mc Elligott, T. F., and Hurst, E. W. (1966): The toxicity of paraquat. *Br. J. Ind. Med.,* 23:126–132.
10. Conning, D. M., Fletcher, K., and Swan, A. A. B. (1969): Paraquat and related bipyridyls. *Br. Med. Bull.,* 25:245–249.
11. Copeland, G. M., Kolin, A., and Shulman, H. (1974): Fatal pulmonary intra-alveolar fibrosis after paraquat injection. *N. Engl. J. Med.,* 291:290–292.
12. Daniel, J. W., and Gage, J. I. (1966): Absorption and excretion of diquat and paraquat in rats. *Br. J. Ind. Med.,* 23:133–136.
13. Douze, J. M. (1975): Paraquat poisoning in man. *Arch. Toxicol. (Berl.),* 34:129–136.
14. Eisenmenger, W. (1974): Clinical and pathologic-anatomical findings in paraquat poisoning. *Beitr. Gerichtl. Med.,* 32:262–266.
15. Fennelly, J. J., Gallagher, J. T., and Carroll, R. J. (1968): Paraquat poisoning in a pregnant woman. *Br. Med. J.,* 3:722–723.
16. Ferguson, M. D., Etherton, J. E., and Hayes, M. S. (1969): Mitochondrial increase after

long-term feeding of morfamquat. *Nature,* 224: 83–84.

17. Fowler, B. A., and Brooks, R. E. (1971): Effects of the herbicide paraquat on the ultrastructure of mouse kidney. *Am. J. Pathol.,* 63:505–520.

18. Gardiner, T. H. (1976): Effect of paraquat-induced lung damage on permeability of rat lungs to drugs. *Proc. Soc. Exp. Biol. Med.,* 151:288–292.

19. Gaultier, M., Bescol-Liversac, J., Frejaville, J. P., Leclerc, J. P., and Guillan, C. (1973): Anatomo-clinical and experimental study of paraquat poisoning. Ultrastructural lesions. *Sem. Hop. Paris,* 49:1972–1987.

20. Hardt, H. von der, and Cardesa, A. (1971): Die histopathologischen Fruhveranderungen nach Paraquat-Intoxikation. *Klin. Wochenschr.,* 49:544–550.

21. Harland, W. A. (1970): Paraquat poisoning. *J. Pathol.,* 100:vi.

22. Hasan, M., and Glees, P. (1972): Genesis and possible dissolution of neuronal lipofuscin. *Gerontologia,* 18:217–236.

23. Kimborough, R. D., and Gaines, T. B. (1970): Toxicity of paraquat to rats and its effects on rat lungs. *Toxicol. Appl. Pharmacol.,* 17:679–690.

24. Kimborough, R. D., and Linder, R. E. (1973): The ultrastructure of the paraquat lung lesions in the rat. *Environ. Res.,* 6:265–273.

25. Malmquist, E., Grassmann, G., Ivemark, B., and Robertson, B. (1973): Pulmonary phospholipids and surface properties of alveolar wash in experimental paraquat poisoning. *Scand. J. Respir. Dis.,* 54:206–214.

26. Manktelow, B. W. (1967): The loss of pulmonary surfactant in paraquat poisoning: A model for the study of the respiratory distress syndrome. *Br. J. Exp. Pathol.,* 48:366–369.

27. Masterson, J. G., and Roche, W. J. (1970): Fatal paraquat poisoning. *J. Irish Med. Assoc.,* 63:261–264.

28. Matthew, H., Logan, A., Woodruff, M. F. A., and Heard, B. (1968): Paraquat poisoning, lung transplantation. *Br. Med. J.,* 3:759–763.

29. McDonough, B. J., and Martin, J. (1970): Paraquat poisoning in children. *Arch. Dis. Child.,* 45:425–427.

30. McKean, W. I. (1968): Recovery from paraquat poisoning. *Br. Med. J.,* 3:292.

31. Modee, J., Ivemark, B. J., and Robertson, B.

(1972): Ultrastructure of the alveolar wall in experimental paraquat poisoning. *Acta Pathol. Microbiol. Scand.* [*A*], 80:54–60.

32. Murray, R. E., and Gibson, J. E. (1972): A comparative study of paraquat intoxication in rats, guinea pigs and monkeys. *Exp. Mol. Pathol.,* 17:317–325.

33. Murray, R. E., and Gibson, J. E. (1974): Paraquat disposition in rats, guinea pigs and monkeys. *Toxicol. Appl. Pharmacol.,* 27:283–291.

34. Nieuhans, H., and Ehrenfeld, H. (1971): Zur Pathogenese der Lungenerkrankung durch Paraquat. *Beitr. Pathol.,* 142:244–267.

35. Oreopoulos, D. G., Soyannwo, M. A. O., Sinniah, R., Fenton, S. S. A., McGeown, M. G., and Bruce, J. H. (1968): Acute renal failure in case of paraquat poisoning. *Br. Med. J.,* 1:749–750.

36. Osten, van G. K., and Gibson, J. E. (1974): Effect of paraquat on the biosynthesis of deoxyribonucleic acid, ribonucleic acid and protein in the rat. *Food Cosmet. Toxicol.,* 13:47–54.

37. Ramachandran, S., Rajapakse, C. N. A., and Perera, M. V. F. (1974): Further observations on paraquat poisoning in man. *Forensic. Sci.,* 4:257–266.

38. Robertson, B. (1971): Experimental respiratory distress induced by paraquat. *J. Pathol.,* 103:239–244.

39. Robertson, B., Grassmann, G., and Ivemark, B. (1976): The alveolar lining layer in experimental paraquat poisoning. *Acta Pathol. Microbiol. Scand.* [*A*], 84:40–46.

40. Smith, P., and Heath, D. (1974): Ultrastructure and time sequence of the early stages of paraquat lung in rats. *J. Pathol.,* 114:177–184.

41. Smith, P., and Heath, D. (1974): Paraquat lung: A reappraisal. *Thorax,* 29:643–653.

42. Teare, R. D. (1976): Poisoning by paraquat. *Med. Sci. Law,* 16:9–12.

43. Thomson, W. T. (1967): *Agricultural Chemical, Book II: Herbicides,* 1967 rev., pp. 138–140. Thomson Publ., Davis, Cal.

44. Tompsett, S. L. (1970): Paraquat poisoning. *Acta Pharmacol. Toxicol.* (*Kbh.*), 28:346–358.

45. Vijeyeratnam, G. S., and Corrin, B. (1971): Experimental paraquat poisoning: A histological and electron optical study of the changes in the lungs. *J. Pathol.,* 103:123–129.

Neurotoxicology, edited by L. Roizin, H. Shiraki, and N. Grčević. Raven Press, New York © 1977.

Ultrastructural Observations on the Cytoplasmic Inclusions of Nervous Tissues and the Peripheral Neuropathy Induced in Suckling Mice by Chlorphentermine Administration

A. P. Anzil, H. Herrlinger, and K. Blinzinger

Max-Planck Institute for Psychiatry, Munich 40, Federal Republic of Germany

Chlorphentermine hydrochloride (*p*-chloro-$\alpha\alpha$-dimethyl phenethylamine hydrochloride) is an appetite suppressant with a structural formula consisting of a chlorinated benzene ring with a side chain carrying a positively charged nitrogen ion.

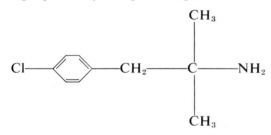

The drug belongs to a large series of chemical compounds known to induce cytoplasmic bodies of varied morphology in most, if not all, tissues of small laboratory mammals (for reviews, see references 8 and 13). Recently, one of these compounds has been shown to cause a peripheral neuropathy in young rats (16). In this chapter we review our observations on chlorphentermine-induced cytosomes in the nervous tissues of the suckling albino mouse (4) and report our findings on chlorphentermine neuropathy.

MATERIALS AND METHODS

Chlorphentermine hydrochloride (Tropon Werke, Cologne, Federal Republic of Germany) was administered subcutaneously to newborn albino mice for 13 or 14 days in a daily dose of 100 mg/kg of body weight. At the end of the second week, the animals were killed and appropriate specimens of the retinae, the brain and spinal cord, the craniospinal sensory ganglia, and the sciatic nerves were placed in 3% glutaraldehyde, postfixed in 1% osmium tetroxide, and embedded in epoxy resin. Ultrathin sections were stained with uranyl acetate and lead citrate and examined with a Zeiss EM 9A electron microscope. Semithin sections were prepared from selected blocks of tissue, stained with paraphenylenediamine and viewed with a phase microscope. One or two littermates from each group of experimental animals were left untreated, and the corresponding tissues were prepared in the same manner as indicated above and studied as controls.

RESULTS

Clinical Observations

About 10% of the animals died during the experimental period. At the end of the second week chlorphentermine-treated mice weighed less and showed less spontaneous activity than control littermates. Upon handling, they moved about slowly and only for a short run; deambulation was somewhat unsteady, particularly at the level of the hindlegs.

Phase Contrast Microscopy

Sections of the spinal cord showed isolated neurons loaded with cytoplasmic granules of varying size (Fig. 1). Preparations of craniospinal sensory ganglia revealed numerous neurons teeming with cytoplasmic granulations (Fig. 2). Sections of sciatic nerves demonstrated scattered foci of fine and coarse granularity (Fig. 3) and demyelinated nerve fibers (Fig. 4).

Electron Microscopy

A number of discrete changes were found throughout the central nervous system in addition to a plethora of cytoplasmic bodies. In the following discussion, only the cytoplasmic bodies will be dealt with in detail together with findings in the peripheral nervous system. For the sake of convenience, we will report our observations first on the cytoplasmic bodies and then on the peripheral neuropathy.

Cytoplasmic Bodies

Cytoplasmic bodies of diverse morphology were found at all levels of the central and peripheral nervous system, in all tissues making up the different anatomic structures and in all cell types entering in the composition of these tissues. Differences concerned the morphology of the cytosomes as well as the frequency with which all types of cytosomes were found in the different anatomic structures and the frequency with which a certain type of cytosome occurred either in the different cell types or in the cells of one and the same type. Regarding the morphology of the cytosomes, two major types could be observed: a membranous type and a honeycomb-like type of body. The membranous type consisted of roughly parallel membranes having a more or less straight or a concentric course. Bodies containing stacks of parallel-layered membranes were not common in the experimental material and were occasionally found in the control material. Much more frequent throughout the tissues of the experimental animals were the concentric membranous bodies (CMB) (Figs. 5–7). They appeared as unicentric or multicentric bodies of variable electron density. They measured up to 2 μm in diameter, although the diameter of the average body lay below this figure. Multicentric bodies seemed to form by fusion of unicentric bodies. They consisted of concentric layers of smooth membranes surrounded by a somewhat thicker limiting membrane. These membranes were generally loosely arranged but often showed variably extensive areas of dense packing and periodic organization. Some of the bodies contained a dense granular core and a variable proportion of granular matrix along their periphery. The second major type of cytoplasmic body showed a honeycomb-like structure resulting in a fine crystalline pattern (Fig. 8) or in a more loosely reticular organization (Fig. 9). Honeycomb-like bodies (HLB) were of medium electron density and had about the same size as CMB. They showed little tendency to fuse together, and they occurred isolatedly or in small groups. Collections of more than 10 bodies per cell were never seen. Single cytosomes showing, side by side, two types of internal organization were not uncommon (Fig. 9). Cytosomes with a transitional area of intermediate character suggesting some kind of development from one type to the other type of organization were occasionally encountered. A consistent spatial relationship to a class of cell organelles was not detected. Profiles of small dense elongated organelles (primary lysosomes ?) merging at one end with a cytosome were observed from time to time. Cytosomes indenting the contour

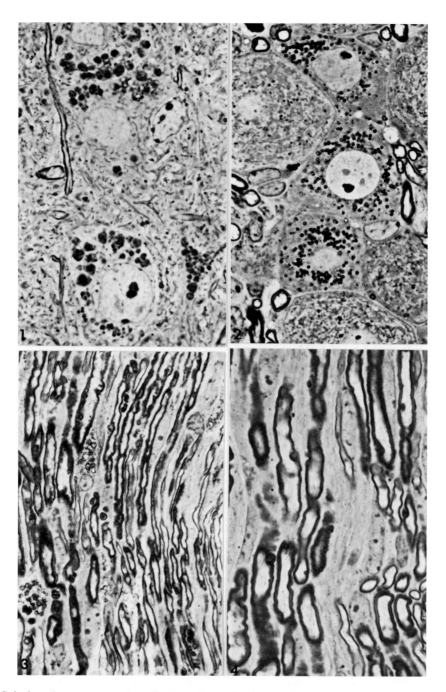

FIG. 1. Spinal cord neurons contain collections of cytoplasmic granules. Epon-embedded, 1-to-2-μm-thick section stained with paraphenylenediamine. ×1,540.

FIG. 2. Nerve cells of trigeminal ganglion crowded with cytoplasmic granules. Epon-embedded, 1-to-2-μm-thick section stained with paraphenylenediamine. ×1,200.

FIG. 3. Fine and coarse granulations in some cells and nerve fibers of sciatic nerve. Epon-embedded, 1-to-2-μm-thick section stained with paraphenylenediamine. ×770.

FIG. 4. Demyelinated nerve fibers are best seen in this section of sciatic nerve. Epon-embedded, 1-to-2-μm-thick section stained with paraphenylenediamine. ×1,200.

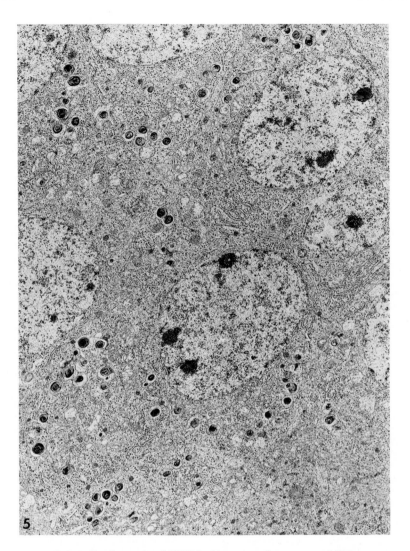

FIG. 5. Small groups of CMB in hippocampal neurons. ×4,000.

of an axon or bulging into a dilated cisterna of endoplasmic reticulum were exceptionally encountered.

Quantitative studies were not carried out with regard to the frequency of the different cytosomes in the different tissues. However, it was our impression that cytosomes of all types were more frequent in the gray, including the peripheral ganglia, than in the white matter, including the peripheral nerves. Furthermore, we felt that HLB were more prevalent in the peripheral than in the central nervous system. In fact, it seemed that HLB were the characteristic bodies of the myelin cell, the central but especially the peripheral cell; whereas, CMB were the characteristic bodies of the nerve cell, the central but apparently more so the peripheral cell. As for the astrocyte, a rare cell of this type was seen containing an isolated CMB. Numerous CMB were seen in cells in and around the vascular

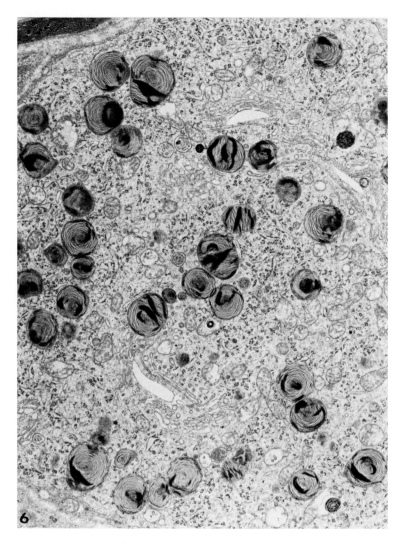

FIG. 6. Numerous CMB in a nerve cell of trigeminal ganglion. ×11,000.

walls and in so-called M cells (microglia). Great variation existed in the frequency of a given type of cytosome among cells of the same type. For instance, a large number of cerebral cortical neurons appeared to be free of CMB, at least in the plane of section; others, on the contrary, were filled to capacity with them. Control tissues contained only an occasional membranous body and then almost exclusively of the parallel-layered type. HLB were never seen in any tissues of the control mice.

Peripheral Neuropathy

Another change observed in chlorphentermine-treated mice was a rather severe form of peripheral neuropathy of the demyelinating type. The degree of involvement varied somewhat from animal to

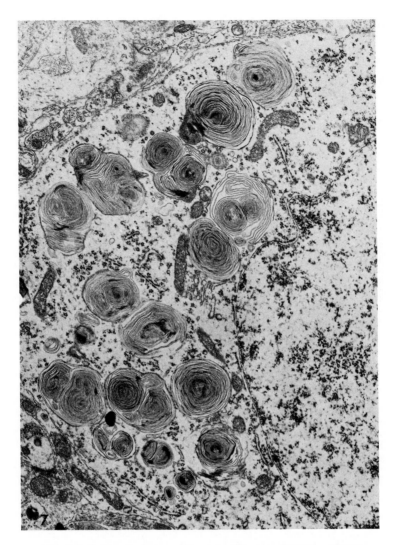

FIG. 7. Spinal cord neuron with a rich collection of CMB. ×15,000.

animal, so that the following is a description of the most prominent features found in the average sample of examined material. A few necrotic cells, possibly Schwann cells, were found in all animals. Myelin ovoids (Figs. 10–12) occurred isolatedly or in short rows in many internodes; larger collections of them were seen in about 10% of the Schwann cell population either at the perinuclear or paranodal region. Myelin spheroids had a high electron density and often showed a well-preserved periodicity. Occasionally, loose whorls of concentric myelin lamellae in various stages of degeneration occurred side by side with the more compact ovoids. Infolding of groups of myelin lamellae into the inner or outer Schwann cell cytoplasm was a common finding. Splitting of myelin lamellae at the intraperiod line was often associated with various forms of focal myelin fragmentation. Some myelin sheaths had lost their usual compactness and high electron density. Few nodes were entirely

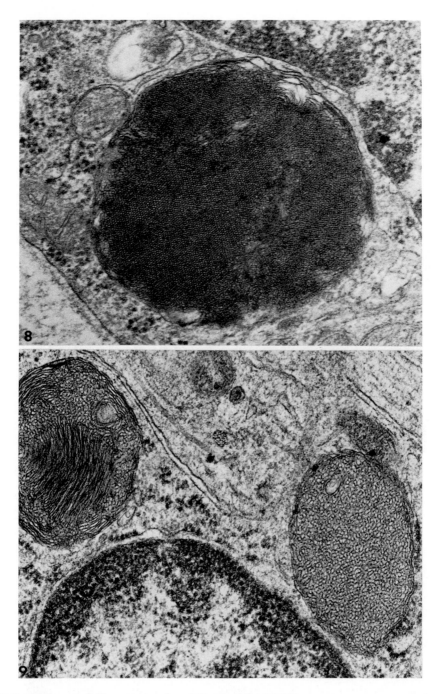

FIG. 8. HLB with fine crystalline structure in a Schwann cell. ×54,000.
FIG. 9. HLB with a reticular pattern in a Schwann cell. One of the two cytosomes shows two different patterns side by side. ×54,000.

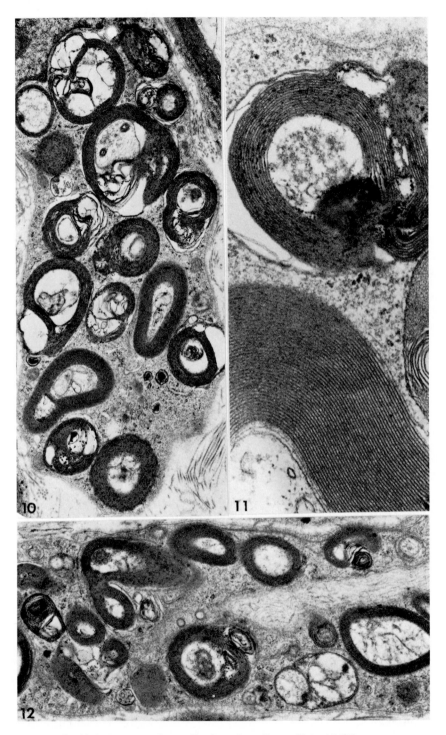

FIG. 10. Schwann cell with large paranuclear collection of myelin ovoids. ×14,500.
FIG. 11. Isolated myelin ovoid in a Schwann cell outer cytoplasm some place along the internode. ×45,000.
FIG. 12. Section of Schwann cell cytoplasm containing many well-preserved myelin spheroids and a small segment of demyelinated axon. ×18,000.

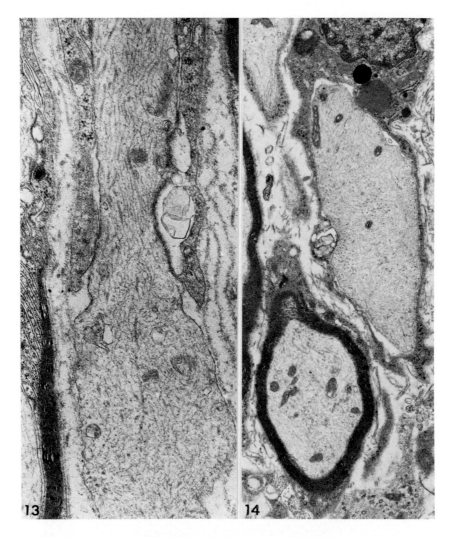

FIG. 13. Normal arrangement at one side and loss of Schwann cell cytoplasm and myelin-sheath-covering at the opposite side of a node of Ranvier along the course of this nerve fiber. Lengths of redundant basal lamina and part of a normal node are also included in this electron micrograph. ×24,000.
FIG. 14. Large demyelinated axon in a Schwann cell. ×8,500.

normal; many of them disclosed instead a number of degenerative changes affecting chiefly the paranodal myelin. Variably long stretches of axoplasm lay bare, being covered only by the axolemma and neurolemma (Fig. 13). Retraction of myelin at either one or both sides of the node resulted in lengthening of the nodal gap. Segments of demyelinated nerve fibers were not uncommon (Fig. 14). Isolated axons appeared swollen and filled up with degenerating mitochondria, membrano-vesicular bodies, and other kinds of dense circular profiles. Many Schwann cells had abundant dense cytoplasm containing dilated cisternae of endoplasmic reticulum. Lengths of loose basement membrane lay free in the extracellular space (Fig. 13) or clung to a shrivelled up outline of Schwann cell cytoplasm. Macrophages featured profiles of dense amorphous or lamellar material with electron-lucent inclusions em-

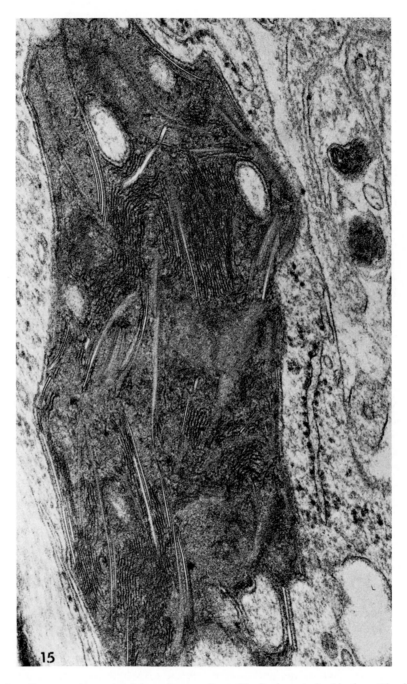

FIG. 15. Section of a macrophage containing a large variegated body characterized by long thin electron-lucent inclusions. ×54,000.

bedded in them (Fig. 15). Many endoneurial fibroblasts had giant vacuolated endoplasmic reticulum. Mononuclear cells probably of hematogenous origin but difficult to identify were seen a few times. A few plasma cells were identified in the vicinity of an endoneurial vessel. Myelination, on the whole, seemed to lag behind that seen in control material; however, no particular attention was paid to this detail of our experimental material. Control sciatic nerves were unremarkable except for the occurrence of many minor irregularities of the internodal and paranodal myelin and of a rare ovoid at the paranodal region of an occasional Schwann cell.

DISCUSSION

Chlorphentermine shares with many drugs the ability to induce the formation of cytosomes in nervous tissues as well as in other tissues of common laboratory animals. As for the biologic dignity of the cytosomes of different morphology, it would seem that HLB have the highest and the stacks of parallel-layered membranes the lowest. At the same time, one wonders whether it is correct to lump together the two main morphologic types of cytosomes and to treat them as if they both had the same composition and formal pathogenesis. However, if one overlooks this point, there is almost general agreement that drug-induced cytosomes contain a large proportion of phospholipids (6,19), and that tissues harboring these bodies have a higher than normal phospholipid content (6,14), the increment resulting apparently from a lower rate of degradation rather than a higher rate of synthesis of these molecules (7). The question then arises why phospholipids are sequestered into lysosomal structures and why the segregated phospholipids resist digestion. In answer to this, it may be recalled that *in vitro* studies have shown that chloroquine has a stabilizing effect on lysosomal membranes (18) and an inhibitory effect on certain lysosomal enzymes (5,11), whereas AY9944 has no direct effect on many lysosomal enzymes (9). Corresponding studies *in vivo* have yielded conflicting results (1,2,6, 9,10). In summary, there is no compelling evidence that the drugs of this group interfere with the formation and fusion of primary lysosomes or inhibit lysosomal

enzymes in the tissues of experimental animals. Therefore, it is tempting to speculate that these drugs, perhaps because of their amphipathic character (12), may have a higher affinity to phospholipid molecules than to other molecules. For triparanol (19) and chloroquine (17) there is evidence to suggest that both drugs are enriched in the cytosomal population. As for chlorphentermine, *in vitro* binding to phospholipids is well documented (15). If one is to accept that these compounds bind to the phospholipids of the cytocavitary system altering the physicochemical properties of this class of molecules, one must assume that the resulting complexes can be metabolized only with difficulty and can stimulate, if anything, the autophagic processes that go on normally in the cell. In conclusion, our studies on chlorphentermine and a review of the pertinent literature lead us to believe that the drug complexes the cell's phospholipids prior to their segregation in the cytosomal bodies. The chlorphentermine–phospholipid complexes in turn, being poorly amenable to normal catabolic breakdown, are enriched in a progressively increasing number of secondary lysosomes by focal cytoplasmic degradation and autophagic sequestration (8).

The problem of the peripheral neuropathy merits a separate comment. We have demonstrated that chlorphentermine, like AY9944 (16), can cause a peripheral neuropathy in young rodents. It is a demyelinating process in which the Schwann cell and its myelin sheath product are recognized as the main seat of the disorder. Although suppression of cholesterol biosynthesis has been looked on as the determining factor in AY9944 neuropathy (16), the observation of a chlorphentermine neuropathy suggests to us a more general mechanism, possibly related to the main cytologic effect shared by these compounds. If chlorphentermine on complexing the cell's phospholipids is sequestered into countless cytosomes, then it creates, on the one hand, a membrane-bound accumulation of physiologically inert phospholipids and, on the other hand, a relative depletion of the pool of freely available molecules of this kind. This intracellular shift with attending relative scarcity of critical molecules may go unnoticed in most cells; or, it may cause a reduction of cytomembranes in some cortical neurons (*personal unpublished observations*); or, it may eventually prove incompatible with the normal function and structure of other cells (3), including the peripheral myelin-forming cells, especially at a time of sustained high demand for such molecules. In conclusion, it is possible that this drug-induced form of Schwann cell disorder may be due to a relative lack of structural molecules leading eventually to myelin breakdown and to a form of demyelinating neuropathy.

REFERENCES

1. Abraham, R., and Hendy, R. (1970): Effects of chronic chloroquine treatment on lysosomes of rat liver cells. *Exp. Mol. Pathol.,* 12:148–159.
2. Abraham, R., and Hendy, R. J. (1970): Irreversible lysosomal damage induced by chloroquine in the retina of pigmented and albino rats. *Exp. Mol. Pathol.,* 12:185–200.
3. Adachi, M., Tsai, C. Y., Wellmann, K. F., and Volk, B. W. (1974): Ultrastructural alterations of liver, lungs, pancreas and CNS of mice induced by chlorphentermine. *Fed. Proc.,* 33:607.
4. Anzil, A. P., Herrlinger, H., and Blinzinger, K. (1975): Lamellar and crystalloid inclusions in central and peripheral nervous tissues of chlorphentermine-treated mice. In: *Proc. VIIth Int. Congr. Neuropathol.,* Vol. 2, edited by St. Környey, St. Tariska, and G. Gosztonyi, pp. 395–398. Excerpta Medica, Amsterdam and Akadémiai Kiadó, Budapest.
5. Cowey, F. K., and Whitehouse, M. W. (1966): Biochemical properties of antiinflammatory drugs. VII. Inhibition of proteolytic enzymes in connective tissue by chloroquine (resochin) and related antimalarial, antirheumatic drugs. *Biochem. Pharmacol.,* 15:1071–1084.
6. de la Iglesia, F. A., Feuer, G., McGuire, E. J., and Takada, A. (1975): Morphological and biochemical changes in the liver of various species in experimental phospholipidoses after diethylaminoethoxyhexestrol treatment. *Toxicol. Appl. Pharmacol.,* 34:28–44.
7. Hildebrand, J., Thys, O., and Gérin, Y. (1973): Alterations of rat liver lysosomes and smooth endoplasmic reticulum induced by the diazafluoranthen derivative AC-3579. II. Effects of the drug on phospholipid metabolism. *Lab. Invest.,* 28:83–86.
8. Hruban, Z., Slesers, A., and Hopkins, E. (1972): Drug-induced and naturally occurring myeloid bodies. *Lab. Invest.,* 27:62–70.
9. Igarashi, M., Suzuki, K., Chen, S. M., and Suzuki, K. (1975): Changes in brain hydrolytic enzyme activities in rats treated with cholesterol biosynthesis inhibitor, AY9944. *Brain Res.,* 90:97–114.
10. Kalina, M., Lopez, M. L., and Bubis, J. J. (1973): Effect of triparanol (Mer 29) on rat liver lysosomes: Cytochemical and biochemical study. *Histochemie,* 36:5–14.
11. Lie, S. O., and Schofield, B. (1973): Inactivation of lysosomal function in normal cultured human fibroblasts by chloroquine. *Biochem. Pharmacol.,* 22:3109–3114.
12. Lüllmann, H., Lüllmann-Rauch, R., and Wassermann, O. (1973): Arzneimittel-induzierte Phospholipidspeicherkrankheit. *Dtsch. Med. Wochenschr.,* 98:1616–1625.
13. Lüllmann, H., Lüllmann-Rauch, R., and Wassermann, O. (1975): Drug-induced phospholipidoses. *CRC Crit. Rev. Toxicol.,* 4:185–218.
14. Schmien, R., Seiler, K. U., and Wassermann, O. (1974): Drug-induced phospholipidosis. I. Lipid composition and chlorphentermine content of rat lung tissue and alveolar macrophages after chronic treatment. *Naunyn Schmiedebergs Arch. Pharmacol.,* 283:331–334.
15. Seydel, J. K., and Wassermann, O. (1973): NMR-studies on the molecular basis of drug induced phospholipidosis. I. Interaction between chlorphentermine and phosphatidylcholine. *Naunyn Schmiedebergs Arch. Pharmacol.,* 279:207–210.
16. Suzuki, K., and De Paul, L. (1972): Myelin degeneration in sciatic nerve of rats treated with hypocholesteremic drug AY9944. *Lab. Invest.,* 26:534–539.
17. Tischner, K., and Fischer, H. A. (1975): Uptake of tritium labelled chloroquine into organized cultures of rat spinal ganglia. An electron microscope autoradiographic study. *Acta Neuropathol. (Berl.),* 32:353–357.
18. Weissmann, G. (1964): Labilization and stabilization of lysosomes. *Fed. Proc.,* 23:1038–1044.
19. Yates, R. D., Arai, K., and Rappaport, D. A. (1967): Fine structure and chemical composition of opaque cytoplasmic bodies of triparanol treated Syrian hamsters. *Exp. Cell. Res.,* 47:459–478.

Neurotoxicology, edited by L. Roizin, H. Shiraki, and N. Grčević. Raven Press, New York © 1977.

Neurotoxic Effects of Chlorphentermine on Rats

M. Adachi, L. Schneck, and B. W. Volk

Neuroscience Center, Isaac Albert Research Institute of the Kingsbrook Jewish Medical Center, Brooklyn, New York 11203

Chlorphentermine, known as an anorexic drug, induces cytoplasmic alterations in the central nervous system of rodents (see Chapter 51 by Anzil et al., *this volume,* and refs. 2–5,7). Although the cytoplasmic inclusion bodies in this model have been considered the experimental counterpart of a lipidosis of man, our study showed that the cytoplasmic changes are due to cytotoxic effects, rather than to true experimental lipidosis.

MATERIAL AND METHODS

The experimental animals were divided into three groups. The first group consisted of 12 pregnant rats at 10 days gestation weighing 300 g, which were injected with a single daily s.c. dose of 80 mg/kg body weight, of chlorphentermine hydrochloride. Since all baby rats were stillborn and showed autolysis of the tissues, the material obtained from these animals was not studied.

In the second group, 12 pregnant rats at 10 days gestation received a single subcutaneous daily injection of 40 mg/kg body weight of the drug. In control animals, three pregnant rats received a single subcutaneous daily dose of saline solution. Since the majority of the litters of group 2 died within 2 days after delivery, six newborn rats and three control animals had to be sacrificed at 1 day after birth. Samples of the central nervous system tissue were taken from the frontal cortex and white matter, basal ganglia, the cerebellar cortex and white matter, and spinal cord.

In the third group, 30 pregnant rats were injected with a single subcutaneous daily dose of 10 mg/kg body weight, of chlorphentermine. In order to get a continuous effect on the babies, the same dose was given to the nursing mothers until 3 weeks after delivery. Thereafter, these infant rats received the same injection schedule until 12 weeks of age. In a control study for this group, five pregnant rats and 32 delivered babies received the same dose of normal saline solution. The 40 surviving experimental animals and the 32 control rats were scarificed at intervals of 1 to 12 weeks.

Electron microscopic and biochemical studies on the specimens were carried out according to previously described standard techniques (1,9).

RESULTS

The neurons in the brain and spinal cord of the 1-day-old rats in the second experimental group showed abnormal inclusion bodies in the cytoplasm which were membrane-bound and consisted of concentrical membranous structures (Fig. 1). No changes were observed in the glial cells.

In the control animals of group 2, similar alterations were not seen in the neurons or glial cells.

497

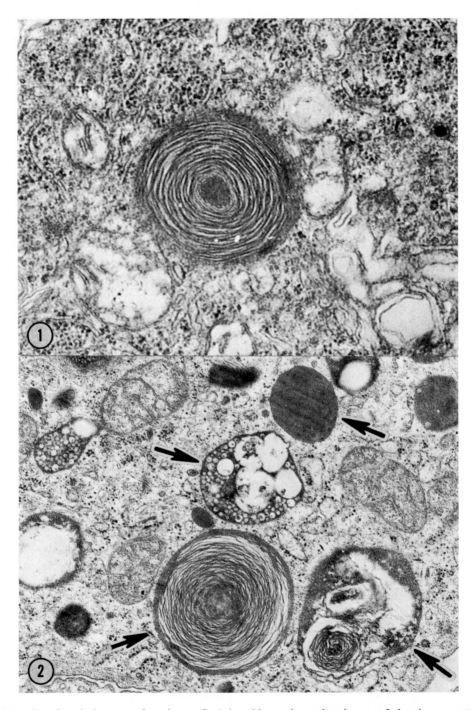

FIG. 1. Portion of cortical neuron of cerebrum of a 1-day-old experimental rat in group 2 showing concentrically arranged membranous bodies in cytoplasm. ×49,000.
FIG. 2. Portion of frontal neuron at 8 weeks in group 3 exhibiting various stages of alterations within lysosomes (*arrows*). ×30,300.

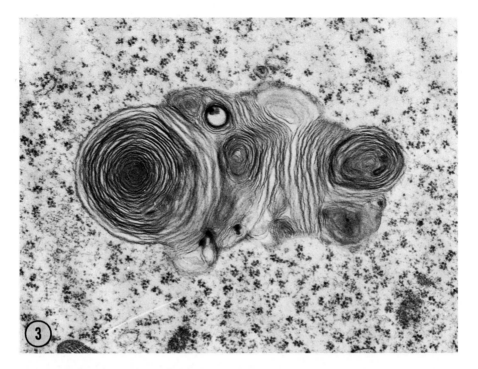

FIG. 3. At 12 weeks cerebral neuron showing pleomorphic inclusion bodies in cytoplasm which contain irregular membranous structures. ×30,300.

In the third group, the experimental rats displayed membranous structures within lysosomes in the neurons during the fourth to eighth week (Fig. 2). At 12 weeks, there was a significant increase in the number of membranous cytoplasmic bodies in the neurons, astrocytes, and oligodendroglial cells some of which were pleomorphic (Fig. 3). Despite the involvement of the oligodendroglial cells, myelination of the animals during the experimental period was histochemically and ultrastructurally normal.

None of the control rats in the third group showed similar changes.

Biochemical studies showed a slight increase of total sialic acid in the brains of the 12-week-old rats as compared with the controls (Table 1). Although thin-layer chromatograms of the brains obtained at 12 weeks exhibited normal major ganglioside fractions, analysis of the total N-acetyl neuraminic acid showed an approximately 46% increase of G_{M1}-ganglioside in the brains at 12 weeks when compared with the controls (Table 2). The total and frac-

TABLE 1. *Lipid-bound sialic acid[a]*

Experimental brain	Control brain
0.078	0.076

[a] Expressed as percent dry weight.

TABLE 2. *Cerebral ganglioside pattern[a]*

	Experimental brain	Control brain
G_{M1}	90.0	44.0
G_{D1a}	6.64	33.1
G_{D1b}	0.97	9.9
G_T	1.27	9.9
G_0	0.22	3.1

[a] Expressed as percent of total N-acetyl neuraminic acid.

tions of phospholipids in the brain of 12-week-old rats were within normal limits, except for a moderate increase of phosphatidic acid. Myelin lipids were within normal limits.

Enzyme studies showed normal β-galactosidase activities in the experimental brains.

DISCUSSION

Although myelin alterations in the peripheral nervous system in this experimental model have been reported (see Chapter 50 by Anzil et al., *this volume*), the effects of chlorphentermine on the central nervous system myelin are unknown. The present histochemical and ultrastructural studies showed normal myelination in the central nervous system during the 12 weeks of the experiments. This was substantiated by the biochemical studies. These findings seem to be of interest since the drug was administered in the pre- and postnatal periods during the time of myelination.

Since the ultrastructural features of the lamellar inclusion bodies were similar to those seen in cases of lipidoses (6,10), the mechanism and the evaluation of these changes were thought to be either inhibition of certain enzymes or formation of undigestable substances by biochemical and pharmacological interactions of the drug (?). The present study showed an increase of G_{M1}-ganglioside in the experimental animals. Enzyme studies, however, elicited normal β-galactosidase.

Therefore, the accumulation of the cytoplasmic inclusion bodies in the present study seems to be due to a metabolic disturbance of the cell membranes rather than an impairment of the degrading enzyme. These observations were in accordance with our previous studies in which active

neuronal degeneration was noted in the central nervous system when the dose of the drug administered was increased (3).

Furthermore, the cytotoxic effects of this chemical compound were noted in the Schwann cells which were accompanied by various stages of demyelination (see Chapter 50 by Anzil et al., *this volume*). These demyelinating changes in the peripheral nervous system due to cytotoxicity are supported by our additional studies on rats that received larger doses of chlorphentermine (120 to 140 mg/kg body weight) and displayed oligodendroglial inclusion bodies as well as active degeneration of myelin lamellae in the central nervous system.

REFERENCES

1. Adachi, M., Torii, J., Schneck, L., and Volk, B. W. (1971): The fine structure of fetal Tay-Sachs disease. *Arch. Pathol.*, 91:48–54.
2. Adachi, M., Tsai, C.-Y., Greenbaum, M., Mask, B., and Volk, B. W. (1976): Ultrastructure and biochemical studies of rat CNS and viscera after subcutaneous injection of chlorphentermine. In: *Current Trends in Sphingolipidoses and Allied Disorders,* edited by B. W. Volk and L. Schneck, pp. 429–451. Plenum Press, New York.
3. Adachi, M., Tsai, C.-Y., Wellmann, K. F., and Volk, B. W. (1974): Ultrastructural alterations of liver, lungs, pancreas and CNS of mice induced by chlorphentermine. *Fed. Proc.*, 33:607.
4. Anzil, A. P., Herrlinger, H., and Blinzinger, K. (1974): Lipidose des Nervensystems nach Chlorphentermin-Applikation. *Naturwissenschaften*, 61:35–36.
5. Anzil, A. P., Herrlinger, H., and Blinzinger, K. (1975): Lamellar and crystalloid inclusions in central and peripheral nervous tissue of chlorphentermine-treated mice. In: *VIIth Int. Congr. Neuropathol.*, Vol. 2, edited by St. Környey, St. Tariska, and G. Gosztony, pp. 395–398. Excerpta Medica, Amsterdam.
6. Gonatas, N., and Gonatas, J. (1965): Ultrastructural and biochemical observations on a case of systemic late infantile lipidosis and its relationship to Tay-Sachs disease and gargoylism. *J. Neuropathol. Exp. Neurol.*, 24:318–340.
7. Lüllmann-Rauch, R. (1974): Lipidosis-like alterations in spinal cord and cerebellar cortex of rats treated with chlorphentermine or with tricyclic antidepressants. *Acta Neuropathol. (Berl.)*, 29:237–249.

8. Lüllmann-Rauch, R., Reil, G. H., Rossen, E., and Seiler, K. U. (1972): The ultrastructure of rat lung changes induced by an anoretic drug (chlorphentermine). *Virchows Arch.* [*Zellpathol.*], 11:167–181.

9. Schneck, L., Adachi, M., and Volk, B. W. (1972): The fetal aspects of Tay-Sachs disease. *Pediatrics,* 49:342–351.

10. Terry, R. D., and Weiss, M. (1963): Studies on Tay-Sachs disease. II. Ultrastructure of the cerebellum. *J. Neuropathol. Exp. Neurol.,* 22: 18–55.

Neurotoxicology, edited by L. Roizin, H. Shiraki, and N. Grčević. Raven Press, New York © 1977.

Alcohol–Drug Interactions

Cedric M. Smith

Research Institute on Alcoholism, New York State Department of Mental Hygiene, and Department of Pharmacology and Therapeutics, State University of New York at Buffalo, Buffalo, New York 14203

Interest in interactions between ethanol, in the form of beverages, and other drugs altering the nervous system stems from three different areas of concern. First, the frequency and degree with which alcohol is used by members of our society means that most, if not all, other drugs are used with appreciable frequency before, after, or with alcohol; in fact, many alcoholic beverages are classed as foodstuffs rather than as drugs. This extensive combined use raises clinical and epidemiological concerns about alterations in action through changes in the intensity or nature of the effects of either the drug or the alcohol and about the frequency of occurrence of such combined actions as well as the societal import of the use of such combinations. Of course, the prime issue, among these components, is the nature and frequency of increased toxicity.

The second concern addresses the potential for increased understanding that can be derived about the nature of either the drug or the alcohol's actions from studies of the interactive effects of two or more agents.

The third concern deals with the possible influence of effects or experiences with one agent on the probability of using a second. For example, does caffeine (or amphetamine or cocaine) ingestion during the day predispose to the use of alcohol or sleeping pills in the evening? Does extensive experience with alcohol intoxication during maturation or adolescence predispose the individual to explore or adopt other means of intoxication? Reference is made to the reviews and bibliographies of Kissin (36), Polacsek et al. (49), Forney and Hughes (12), Maling (39), Forney (10), Milner (44), and Gruber (22).

With respect to the first concern, the *clinical* import of alcohol–drug interactions, there is little to add to the previous compilations other than generalizations that are relatively common knowledge among the lay as well as the professional. In general, among the various psychoactive drugs, including the so-called drugs of abuse, on acute administration all produce at least the combined effects of the two agents, both qualitative and quantitative. Thus, from a clinical point, they are all "additive," and their combination results in the combined effects of both.

Moreover, I am aware of no instances of striking antagonism—such as that seen between naloxone and morphine. Of recent interest are reports of antagonism between chlordiazepoxide and alcohol, when both are ingested in moderate doses (6–8,24,26, 35). Conversely, marked potentiation of an active drug or alcohol by a relatively inactive one is rarely observed either. Recently, there are reports of extensive animal research demonstrating exaggerated toxicity with certain combinations of amphetamine and alcohol (16,51). I can add that, in spite of reports to the contrary, Ernest Abel of our Institute has recently tested the interaction of naloxone and ethanol and could find no antagonism of ethanol by naloxone, even though the brain Ca^{++}-depleting effects of ethanol are antagonized by naloxone.

Moreover, over rather broad dose ranges, drugs that depress a given function tend to be synergic, and within narrow physiological limits, depressants may antagonize certain stimulant effects. For example, the induction of sleep by a barbiturate is delayed in an individual who has received amphetamine, and mutual antagonism between low doses of pentobarbital and caffeine has been detected (e.g., ref. 13). However, the use of these agents and combinations has failed to reveal any neural or biochemical processes not observable in the undrugged individual. To date, there are no known specific or competitive antagonists of ethanol (or of the inhalational or barbiturate anesthetics as well).

With respect to interactions with either the drug or the alcohol when either or both have been present for an appreciable time prior to the other agent, a variety of clinical concerns can be identified. These factors are so complex in their impact that an analysis of the usual clinical situation is nearly impossible; thus, practically speaking, such time-confounded interactions are not predictable! Among identifiable time-related outcomes are the following:

1. *An additive outcome* in which the effects sum qualitatively and quantitatively as usually observed with simultaneous administration.

2. *An outcome of acute acquired, functional tolerance,* which is observable with most, if not all, sedative hypnotics and ethanol. The time course for onset of acute tolerance to ethanol is 3 hr or more (i.e., within the usual acute administration situation), and its magnitude is dose-related so that up to some 2 to 4 times the previously effective dose is required to produce a given effect (see reviews in refs. 21,28,32,37,42,45). The acute toler-

ance varies in degree with the dose, the agent, the time of testing, and, very importantly, the system and function used to measure the drug effect.

3. *A postulated outcome of an "acute withdrawal syndrome"* following recovery from the acute sedative effects of a single dose of ethanol or of barbiturates during the "common" hangover period. The large physiological alterations characteristic of severe hangovers make assessment of drug effects during that period difficult, although the nervous system is obviously altered.

The postulated acute withdrawal syndrome has been suggested in some animal studies. It has not been clearly described in man except in the sustained alterations in sleep patterns observed after single doses of hypnotics or benzodiazepines (see, e.g., refs. 3 and 47) or possibly ethanol, in epileptic patients (41).

4. *Various possibilities with chronic administration for functional and dispositional tolerance, cross-tolerance, sensitization, and physical dependence* denoted by withdrawal syndromes. Included among these possibilities are alterations in ethanol metabolism, its induction, alterations in barbiturate and other drug metabolism, and complex alterations in metabolism consequent to acute or chronic liver disease. The extensive literature and the recent important findings of groups coordinated by Kalant, Israel, Khanna, and Lieber are not reviewed here (see, e.g., refs. 31 and 34). In addition, other extraneuronal interactions may be important with alcohol; for example, its oral administration alters absorption of many agents, including barbiturates and diazepam (e.g., refs. 58,59). Distribution of a second drug would also be expected to be altered if for no other reason than because of vasodilation and diuresis (see, e.g., ref. 1).

Among the sedative hypnotics and ethanol there is also marked chronic, acquired functional tolerance and cross-tolerance. On withdrawal a *withdrawal syndrome,* whose intensity depends on prior dose, frequency, and duration, occurs that may be fully reversed by administration of any of the sedative hypnotics; during withdrawal apparent sensitivity to such drugs decreases (e.g., ref. 48).

Stimulants, such as amphetamine, tend to antagonize partially the somnolence and sedation of depressants as well as to aggravate the withdrawal syndrome, although this latter effect has been little studied. Although no antagonism or synergy was found between ethanol and amphetamine by measuring lethal effects in mice (30), Rech (51) has found extensive and complex interactions between large doses of these two agents (see also ref. 16).

An area of appreciable confusion exists around the effects of sedative hypnotics on the withdrawal syndrome to opiates and *vice versa.* Although this has not been extensively studied in either man or experimental animals, some of the results obtained are relatively plausible and predictable and can be summarized by saying that the agents continue to have their characteristic effects, such that the hyperactivity and anxiety, for example, of mild withdrawal from opiates is partially alleviated by sedatives or alcohol (24). The reverse, i.e., the treatment of alcohol or barbiturate withdrawal with an opiate, has been less studied. Goldstein and Judson (20) were unable to precipitate an abstinence syndrome with naloxone in alcohol-dependent animals.

A specific combination of interest is marihuana and alcohol. The subject is complex since the acute interaction of modest doses appears to be a mixture of the two syndromes, such that there is both qualitative and quantitative combined additive effects. As a generalization, when subjects receiving both are queried regarding the experience about the effects of either agent alone, they report that it is "different, bigger, and better." Chronic

experimental studies demonstrate complex interactions in the dispositional and metabolic aspects of both the active tetrahydrocannabinols and ethanol; cross-tolerance also occurs (see refs. 4,11,27,38; also refs. 34,40, and 60). Much is made of the differences between potentiation and addition, and the distinction is important when it can be drawn from precise dose-effect determinations, such as those of Gessner and Cabana (18) or Gebhart et al. (17). However, it is important to observe precisely what the dose-effect curves with ethanol and such agents actually detect and measure. In man such dose "effect" relationships usually entail little more than assessment of the effect of two doses in which it is a complex mixture of actions on various neuronal systems. Frequently these are demonstrably different neural systems, such as those involved in sleep versus those involved in motor coordination. Thus, what is being detected with various doses is not only an increase in action on a given cell but also the appearance of actions on other cells. Thus, the terms "addition" or "synergy" or "potentiation" in most central nervous system agents is not helpful. In addition, most studies on interaction confound time course of action with intensity, and very few control for possible alterations in distribution.

What has been referred to above as "additive" might, on close examination with isobolographic techniques, exhibit more than quantitative addition—and thus be "potentiated" interactions; however, the point being made is that such potentiation is not marked in any of the combinations of drugs of concern. Such combinations may well be hazardous to life, and this fact, as well as the unpredictability of large single or combination doses, needs continuing awareness by the public.

5. *Long-term chronic toxicity of combined drug–alcohol use.* Perhaps more significant, but less well recognized, are

the interactions among drugs, alcohol, the individual, and toxic agents that take place over time spans of months and years. Certainly, senile dementia and the chronic brain syndromes commonly associated with alcohol need much further study (see ref. 50) in relation to other significant events, including drugs, trauma, and infectious disease.

From the clinical management point of view, it becomes academic to nitpick over the terminology of quantitative aspects. All of the studies stress the finding that the drugs act as combinations [as just one of many examples, the study of Morland et al. (46) on combinations of diazepam and ethanol]. Only rarely can these syndromes be described as antagonistic, such as that reported between chlordiazepoxide and alcohol with respect to behavioral endpoints and possible utility in anesthesia (e.g., refs. 6–8,19,26,29).

A variety of brief reports has appeared on interactions between ethanol and various drugs (49), but how these can be assessed is difficult to state. For example, Smith (62) reports that alcoholics are remarkably resistant to the effects of 200 to 400 μg of LSD administered orally.

Wiberg et al. (64) appropriately emphasize that the unidimensional categorization of the terms "additive" or "synergistic" does not help clarify understanding of the effects of combinations of drugs.

[Results with the subjective rating scales employed by the Lexington group raise the question of perhaps the converse of antagonism, i.e., there are overlaps between the various drugs, such as barbiturates and amphetamines in terms of feeling better or of relief from worry (See, e.g., Martin, W. R. et al. (1974): *Clin. Pharm. Ther.*, 15:623–630). Are there, perhaps, common threads of actions that are positively reinforcing, and are these what underlie certain patterns of self-administration? In addition, not only are the amphetamines and barbiturates or benzodiazepines (and probably alcohol) not direct antagonists, but also the subjective effects of the two taken simultaneously are detectably different from either

alone or even what might have been predicted (55)].

The second of the previously mentioned primary concerns is the opportunity to deduce possible sites or mechanisms of action of various agents by examining quantitative interrelationships of the effects of various concentrations of two or more agents. As part of his extensive studies on peripheral nerve and red cell permeability, Seeman (e.g., refs. 56,57) found that three different classes of blocking agents were simply additive in their actions over wide concentration ranges: the anesthetics including ethanol, the amine local anesthetics such as procaine, and tetrodotoxin. Each agent appeared to act by altering action potential generation and passive sodium permeability.

The fact that ethanol, anesthetics including barbiturates, and even hypoxia (cf. refs. 52,63) are usually approximately additive in their effects on a given isolated neural or behavioral system in many varied investigations leads to one or more of the following conclusions:

1. each agent or chemical class of an agent has a different site(s) of action — on the same or on different neurons; AND/OR
2. even if there may be common receptor sites, the concentration of receptor sites probably is far in excess of the relative concentration of the agents, such that there is no detectable competition between agents or evidence for saturation of sites; AND/OR
3. the number of receptor sites that must be occupied for the given or maximal drug action is far less than the total number available. (The maximum may well be limited by the appearance of other effects, e.g., the assessment of drug-induced depression of spinal reflexes that becomes confounded by cardiorespiratory failure.)

These possible inferences are analogous to a variety of treatments of theories of biochemical kinetics.

Note may be made that it is *not* concluded that alcohol or any of its synergists or antagonists act "nonspecifically." Alcohols and general anesthetics neither produce an identical syndrome nor act on all excitable cells with the same intensity or action. Nevertheless, there are no specific, competitive antagonists of alcohol or the sedative hypnotic agents, even of some of the barbiturates that exhibit a degree of stereospecific binding characteristics (see ref. 5).

The relevant action of alcohol, related drugs, or antagonists is the alteration in a specific synaptic system. To date none of such synaptic systems has been examined for the nature of interactions between synergists and antagonists of ethanol, with perhaps the exception of the neuromuscular junction. The specification of site and mechanism of action is clearly being established at this site (see ref. 2). The neuromuscular junction is not a particularly applicable model of central synaptic systems, but extensive studies point to methodology and approaches that may prove fruitful (14,15,33).

[With respect to mechanism of action of alcohol and anesthetics, much is made of correlations between passive distribution of agents in lipid or water phases and potency or translocation kinetics. But I would continue to emphasize that, although such factors are of critical and necessary importance, they are not sufficient to explain anesthetic, sedative, or antianxiety action any more than the demonstration of stereospecific blocking or binding constitutes isolation of the receptor.]

A variety of curious or incidental interactions among these drugs have been reported. One of the more intriguing is the reports of Ross (53) on calcium levels in cerebral tissue. Both alcohol and morphine, separately, evoke a marked decrease in brain calcium; this effect is blocked or reversed by naloxone. Further, this depletion exhibits tolerance and cross-tolerance between ethanol and morphine! Whether the calcium depletion is related to the central nervous system depression or is secondary to other phenomena remains to be determined. The absence of antagonism of acute ethanol effects by naloxone suggests that the calcium depletion is not critical for alcohol's action. Reference is made to extensive interactions between ethanol, morphine, and naloxone detailed by Ho et al. (24).

The third area of concern mentioned previously is of great importance but can be dealt with quickly because of the paucity of information. Alcoholic beverages and sedative hypnotics are used and abused by many people, they say, to produce relaxation, sleep, or relief from anxiety, worry, and insomnia. Clinically, self-treatment of manic states with alcohol may be an important factor in alcohol abuse. It is further conceivable that in some individuals such internal manic or anxiety states might indeed be induced by another drug, e.g., caffeine, cocaine, or amphetamines (51a). The seesaw of stimulant and depressant drug use is a frequently described clinical situation. However, recent studies have failed to find any increase in ethanol consumption in rats treated with caffeine (9,23). Whether or not the alternate drug use is causally or strongly related is not known and constitutes an important area for future study. The degree to which one drug may predispose to the use of another in man remains to be determined. [Relevant animal models are just beginning to be defined (see ref. 43).]

The interaction of dependence aspects of addictive drugs from different classes is just beginning to be addressed, e.g., in a recent symposium in New York (4,11,16,24,27,35,38,51). It should be noted that Roizin et al., some 7 years ago, reported (65) that heroin addicts on methadone maintenance who subsequently became dependent on ethanol had an extra-ordinarily high mortality rate.

Recently, the possibility that opiates might serve to substitute for ethanol received support from rat and mouse studies. A single injection of morphine, methadone, acetylmethadol, or levorphanol significantly suppressed volitional consumption of ethanol solutions (25,54,61). That this effect is due to narcotic agonist activity seems clear from the inactivity of dextrorphan or naloxone.

As an extension of these studies, Ho et al. (24) report that withdrawal from ethanol is significantly more severe in animals that have experienced a period of neonatal addiction to morphine or methadone.

Whether these intriguing interaction studies hold important clues to mechanisms of drug action or dependency awaits further painstaking investigation. Without doubt, they are important relative to the human risks.

REFERENCES

1. Coldwell, B. B., Wiberg, G. S., and Trenholm, H. L. (1970): Some effects of ethanol on the toxicity and distribution of barbiturates in rats. *Can. J. Physiol. Pharmacol.*, 48:254–264.
2. Colquhon, D. (1975): Mechanisms of drug action at the voluntary muscle endplate. *Annu. Rev. Pharmacol.*, 15:307–325.
3. David, J., Grewal, R. S., and Wagle, G. P. (1974): Persistent electroencephalographic changes in rhesus monkeys after single doses of pentobarbital, nitrazepam and imipramine. *Psychopharmacologia*, 35:61–75.
4. Dewey, W. L. (1976): Interactions of active constituents of marihuana with other drugs in the neuron, edited by M. Braude and E. Vesell. *Ann. N.Y. Acad. Sci.*, 281:190–197.
5. Downes, D. A., Woods, J. H., and Llewellyn, M. E. (1975): The behavioural pharmacology of addiction: Some conceptual and methodological foci. In: *Biological and Behavioural Approaches to Drug Dependence*, edited by S. L. Lambert, pp. 53–73. House of Lind, Ontario, Canada.
6. Dundee, J. W., and Isaac, M. (1970): Interaction between intravenous alcohol and some sedatives and tranquillizers. *Br. J. Pharmacol.*, 39:199–200.
7. Dundee, J. W., and Isaac, M. (1970): Interaction of alcohol with sedatives and tranquillizers (a study of blood levels at loss of consciousness fol-

lowing rapid infusion). *Med. Sci. Law*, 10:220–224.
8. Dundee, J. W., and Isaac, M. (1971): Interaction between intravenous alcohol and some sedatives and tranquillizers. *Med. Sci. Law*, 11:49–50.
9. Eriksson, K., Pekkanen, L., Forsander, O., and Ahtee, L. (1975): The effect of dietary factors on voluntary ethanol intake in the albino rat. In: *The Effects of Centrally Active Drugs on Voluntary Alcohol Consumption*, Vol. 24, edited by J. D. Sinclair, and K. Kiianmaa, pp. 15–26. Finnish Foundation for Alcohol Studies, Finland.
10. Forney, R. B. (1972): The interactions of alcohol and other drugs including psychotomimetics. *Drug Information J.*, January/June:59–63.
11. Forney, R. B. (1977): Marihuana and alcohol interactions, edited by M. Braude and E. Vesell. *Ann. N.Y. Acad. Sci.*, 281:162–170.
12. Forney, R. B., and Hughes, F. W. (1970): Interaction between alcohol and psychopharmacological drugs. In: *International Encyclopedia of Pharmacology and Therapeutics*, Vol. II, edited by J. Tremolieres. Pergamon Press, New York.
13. Forrest, W. H., Jr., Bellville, J. W., and Brown, B. W., Jr. (1972): The interaction of caffeine with pentobarbital as a nighttime hypnotic. *Anesthesiology*, 36:37–41.
14. Gage, P. W., McBurney, R. N., and Schneider, G. T. (1975): Effects of some aliphatic alcohols on the conductance change caused by a quantum of acetylcholine at the toad end-plate. *J. Physiol.* (Lond.), 244:409–429.
15. Gage, P. W., McBurney, R. N., and VanHelden, D. (1974): Endplate currents are shortened by octanol: Possible role of membrane lipid. *Life. Sci.*, 14:2277–2283.
16. Garattini, S. (1977): Interactions of various drugs with amphetamine, edited by M. Braude and E. Vesell. *Ann. N.Y. Acad. Sci.*, 281:409–425.
17. Gebhart, G. F., Plaa, G. L., and Mitchell, C. I. (1969): The effects of ethanol alone and in combination with phenobarbital, chlorpromazine, or chlordiazepoxide. *Toxicol. Appl. Pharmacol.*, 15:405–414.
18. Gessner, P. K., and Cabana, B. E. (1970): A study of the interaction of the hypnotic effects and of the toxic effects of chloral hydrate and ethanol. *J. Pharmacol. Exp. Ther.*, 174:247–259.
19. Goldberg, L. (1966): Interaction between alcohol and tranquilizing agents. In: *Proc. 4th Int. Conf. Alcohol and Traffic Safety*, edited by R. N. Harger. Indiana Univ. Press, Bloomington.
20. Goldstein, A., and Judson, B. A. (1971): Alcohol dependence and opiate dependence: Lack of relationship in mice. *Science*, 172:290–292.
21. Greizerstein, H. B., and Smith, C. M. (1973): Development and loss of tolerance to ethanol in goldfish. *J. Pharmacol. Exp. Ther.*, 187:391–399.
22. Gruber, C. M., Jr. (1955): A theoretical consideration of additive and potentiated effects between drugs with a practical example using alcohol and barbiturates. *Arch. Int. Pharmacodyn.*, 102:17–32.

23. Hederra, A., Aldunate, J., Segovia-Riguelme, N., and Mardones, J. (1975): Effect of caffeine on the voluntary alcohol intake of rats. In: *The Effects of Centrally Active Drugs on Voluntary Alcohol Consumption,* Vol. 24, edited by J. D. Sinclair and K. Kiianmaa, pp. 9–14. Finnish Foundation for Alcohol Studies, Finland.

24. Ho, A. K. S., Chen, R. C. A., and Morrison, J. M. (1976): Potential interactions between narcotics and narcotic antagonists with ethanol during acute, chronic and withdrawal states, edited by M. Braude and E. Vesell. *Ann. N. Y. Acad. Sci.* 281:297–310.

25. Ho, A. K. S., Chen, R. C. A., and Morrison, J. M. (1975): Potential interactions between narcotics and narcotic antagonists with ethanol during acute, chronic and withdrawal states. *Presented at the Fall Pharmacology Society Meeting, Davis, California, August, 1975.*

26. Hoffer, A. (1962): Lack of potentiation by chlordiazepoxide (Librium) of depression or excitation due to alcohol. *Can. Med. Assoc. J.,* 87:920–921.

27. Hollister, L. E. (1977): Interactions of Δ⁹-tetrahydrocannabinol with other drugs, edited by M. Braude and E. Vesell. *Ann. N.Y. Acad. Sci.,* 281:212–218.

28. Hug, C. C. (1972): Characteristics and theories related to acute and chronic tolerance development. In: *Chemical and Biological Aspects of Drug Dependence,* edited by S. J. Mulé and H. Brill. CRC Press, Cleveland.

29. Hughes, F. W., Forney, R. B., and Richards, A. B. (1965): Comparative effect in human subjects of chlordiazepoxide, diazepam, and placebo on mental and physical performance. *Clin. Pharmacol. Ther.,* 6:139–145.

30. Iverson, F., Coldwell, B. B., Downie, R. H., and Whitehouse, L. W. (1975): Effect of ethanol on toxicity and metabolism of amphetamine in the mouse. *Experientia,* 31:679–680.

31. Kalant, H., Khanna, J. M., Lin, G. Y., and Chung, S. (1976): Ethanol—a direct inducer of drug metabolism. *Biochem. Pharmacol.,* 25:337–342.

32. Kalant, H., LeBlanc, A. E., and Gibbins, R. J. (1971): Tolerance to, and dependence on, some non-opiate psychotropic drugs. *Pharmacol. Rev.,* 23:135–191.

33. Kennedy, R. D., and Galindo, A. (1974): Comparative site of action of various anesthetics at the mammalian myoneural junction. *Fed. Proc.,* 33:579.

34. Khanna, J. M., Kalant, H., Yuvonne, Y., Chung, S., and Siemens, A. J. (1976): Effect of chronic ethanol treatment on metabolism of drugs *in vitro* and *in vivo. Biochem. Pharmacol.,* 25:329–335.

35. Killam, K. F. (1976): Evaluation of narcotic and narcotic antagonist interactions in primates, edited by M. Braude and E. Vesell. *Ann. N.Y. Acad. Sci.* 281:331–335.

36. Kissin, B. (1974): Interactions of ethyl alcohol and other drugs. In: *The Biology of Alcoholism,* Vol. 3, edited by B. Kissin, and H. Begleiter. Plenum Press, New York.

37. LeBlanc, A. E., Kalant, H., and Gibbins, R. J. (1975): Acute tolerance to ethanol in the rat. *Psychopharmacologia,* 41:43–46.

38. Lemberger, L. (1976): Interactions of psychopharmacologic agents with marihuana, edited by M. Braude and E. Vesell. *Ann. N.Y. Acad. Sci.* 281:219–228.

39. Maling, H. M. (1970): Toxicology of single doses of ethyl alcohol. In: *International Encyclopedia of Pharmacology and Therapeutics,* Vol. II, edited by J. Tremolieres. Pergamon Press, New York.

40. Manno, J. E., Kiplinger, G. F., Scholz, N., and Forney, R. B. (1971): The influence of alcohol and marihuana on motor and mental performance. *Clin. Pharmacol. Ther.,* 12:202–211.

41. Mattson, R. H., Sturman, J. K., Gronowski, M. L., and Goieo, H. (1975): Effect of alcohol intake in non-alcoholic epileptics. *Neurology (Minneap.),* 25:361.

42. Maynert, E. W., and Klingman, G. I. (1960): Acute tolerance to intravenous anesthetics in dogs. *J. Pharmacol. Exp. Ther.,* 128:192–200.

43. Mello, N. K. (1973): A review of methods to induce alcohol addiction in animals. *Pharmacol. Biochem. Behav.,* 1:89–101.

44. Milner, G. (1970): Interaction between barbiturates, alcohol and some psychotropic drugs. *Med. J. Aust.,* 1:1204–1207.

45. Mirsky, I. A., Piker, P., Rosenbaum, M., and Lederer, H. (1941): "Adaptation" of the central nervous system to varying concentrations of alcohol in the blood. *Q. J. Stud. Alcohol,* 2:35–45.

46. Morland, J., Setekleiv, J., Haffner, J. F. W., Stromsaether, C. E., Danielson, A., and Wethe, G. H. (1974): Combined effects of diazepam and ethanol on mental and psychomotor functions. *Acta Pharmacol. Toxicol. (Kbh.),* 34:5–15.

47. Oswald, I. (1968): Drugs and sleep. *Pharmacol. Rev.,* 20:273–303.

48. Patel, G. J., and Lal, H. (1973): Reduction in brain gamma; aminobutyric acid and in barbital narcosis during ethanol withdrawal. *J. Pharmacol. Exp. Ther.,* 186:625–629.

49. Polacsek, E., Barnes, T., Turner, N., Hall, R., and Weise, C. (1972): *Interaction of Alcohol and Other Drugs: An Annotated Bibliography,* 2nd ed., revised. Addiction Research Foundation, Toronto, Ontario, Canada.

50. Rankin, J. G. (1975): *Alcohol, Drugs and Brain Damage.* Addiction Research Foundation, Toronto, Ontario, Canada.

51. Rech, R. H. (1977): Interactions between amphetamine and alcohol and their effect on rodent behavior, edited by M. Braude and E. Vesell. *Ann. N.Y. Acad. Sci.,* 281:426–440.

51a. Reich, L. H., Davies, R. K., and Himmelhoch, J. M. (1974): Excessive alcohol use in manic-depressive illness. *Am. J. Psychiatry,* 131(1):83–86.

52. Roseler, P. (1961): Observations and Investigations on the Interaction of Alcohol and Carbon monoxide. Dissertation, Faculty of Medicine of

the Free University of Berlin, West Germany.

53. Ross, D. H. (1976): Selective action of alcohol on cerebral calcium levels. *Ann. N.Y. Acad. Sci.,* 273:280–294.

54. Ross, D., Hartmann, R. J., and Geller, I. (1976): Ethanol preference in the hamster: Effects of morphine sulfate and naltrexone, a long-acting morphine antagonist. *Presented at Proc. Western Pharmacology Society Meeting, San Francisco, 1976.*

55. Rushton, R., Steinberg, H., and Tomkiewicz, M. (1973): Effects of chlordiazepoxide alone and in combination with amphetamine on animals and human behavior. In: *The Benzodiazepines,* edited by S. Garattini, E. Mussini, and L. O. Randall. Raven Press, New York.

56. Seeman, P. (1972): The membrane actions of anesthetics and tranquilizers. *Pharmacol. Rev.,* 24:583–655.

57. Seeman, P. (1975): The membrane expansion theory of anesthesia. In: *Progress in Anesthesiology,* Vol. 1, edited by B. R. Fink. Raven Press, New York.

58. Sellman, R., Kanto, J., Raijola, E., and Pekkarinen, A. (1975): Human and animal study on elimination from plasma and metabolism of diazepam after chronic alcohol intake. *Acta Pharmacol. Toxicol. (Kbh.),* 36:33–38.

59. Sellman, R., Pekkarinen, A., Kangas, L., and Raijola, E. (1975): Reduced concentrations of plasma diazepam in chronic alcoholic patients following an oral administration of diazepam. *Acta Pharmacol. Toxicol. (Kbh.),* 36:25–32.

60. Siemens, A. J., Kalant, H., and deNie, J. C. (1976): Metabolic interactions between Δ^9-tetrahydrocannabinol and other cannabinoids in rats. In: *The Pharmacology of Marihuana,* edited by M. C. Braude and S. Szara, pp. 77–92. Raven Press, New York.

61. Sinclair, J. D., Adkins, J., and Walker, S. (1973): Morphine-induced suppression of voluntary alcohol drinking in rats. *Nature,* 246:425–527.

62. Smith, C. M. (1958): A new adjunct to the treatment of alcoholism: The hallucinogenic drugs. *Q. J. Stud. Alcohol,* 19:406–417.

63. Stewart, R. D. (1975): The effects of carbon monoxide on humans. *Annu. Rev. Pharmacol.,* 15:409–423.

64. Wiberg, G. S., Coldwell, B. B., and Trenholm, H. L. (1970): Toxicity of ethanol barbiturate mixtures. *J. Pharm. Pharmacol.,* 22:465.

65. Roizin, L., Helpern, M., Baden, M., Kaufman, M., Hashimoto, S., Liu, J. C., and Eisenberg, B. (1972): Methadone fatalities in heroin addicts. *Psychiatr. Q.,* 46:393–410.

Neurotoxicology, edited by L. Roizin, H. Shiraki, and N. Grčević. Raven Press, New York © 1977.

Food and Drug Interactions

C. Jelleff Carr

Life Sciences Research Office, Federation of American Societies for Experimental Biology, Bethesda, Maryland 20014

In the United States Federal Food, Drug and Cosmetic Act (9) any food substance generally recognized as safe, or considered GRAS, is exempt from the premarketing clearance required for other food additives. As stated in the Code of Federal Regulations, GRAS means general recognition of safety by experts qualified by scientific training and experience to evaluate the safety of substances on the basis of scientific data derived from the published literature. The Code indicates that expert judgment is to be based on the evaluation of results of creditable toxicological testing or, for those substances used in foods prior to January 1, 1958, on a reasoned judgment founded in experience with common food use, and is to take into account reasonably anticipated patterns of consumption, cumulative effects in the diet, and safety factors appropriate for the utilization of animal experimental data. As a footnote, the Code recognizes further that it is impossible to provide assurance that any substance is absolutely safe for human consumption.

According to these guidelines a select committee of qualified scientists has been reviewing the several hundred substances on the GRAS list, evaluating the known information, and arriving at a conclusion on the health aspects of these substances for the past 4 years. This committee, organized by the Life Sciences Research Office of the Federation of American Societies for Ex-perimental Biology, has repeatedly encountered serious questions of food and drug interactions. Because so few guidelines have been developed on this subject and because the issue is a critical toxicological matter of international import, an outline of the facts and examples are presented.

It is noteworthy that the provisions of the Code of Federal Regulations do not stipulate concern about the metabolic fate of food additives or about the possible effects of untoward reactions in patients taking therapeutic drugs. Creditable toxicological testing and long use in foods are the two major factors considered originally in selecting those food additives to be included in the GRAS list. Based on the requirement to reassess all the GRAS compounds, the Food and Drug Administration Bureau of Foods is evaluating the health aspects of all 300 to 400 of these substances including food items such as antioxidants, gums, inorganic salts, acidulants, and preservatives. In addition, an estimated 1,200 food flavors, including many synthetic organic compounds, are being evaluated for their safe use in foods.

As a result of our work on the review of the GRAS substances for FDA, it became evident that attention needed to be directed to the issue of food and drug interactions. Physicians customarily consider the influence of food in the gastrointestinal tract on the absorption and utilization of therapeutic drugs given orally. Pharmacology texts review the issues of gut diffusion, lipid solubility, and absorption of drugs from the alimentary tract, and pharmacokinetic studies include consideration of absorption factors influencing plasma levels of drugs especially where the plasma concentration must be kept within a narrow range. The presence of food in the stomach and the small intestine prevents the inactivation of some drugs by the low gastric pH or by destruction from digestive enzymes. These are relatively elementary facts related to efficient drug therapy and wisely observed by the careful physician (10). Metabolic changes and tissue interactions at target cell sites of drug actions are more arcane and frequently not recognized, indeed, are often not known.

FACTORS INFLUENCING GASTROINTESTINAL ABSORPTION

Even though the issues are of wide clinical concern, relatively few investigators pursue studies to develop the necessary background knowledge to enhance our understanding of gastrointestinal absorption, and basic research in this field is limited. The bioavailability of various sources of dietary iron as influenced by phytates in cereal foods via the formation of insoluble iron phytates is a classic example of a well-known but little understood problem in gastrointestinal physiology and nutrition (13).

Absorption of L-DOPA is slower and peak blood levels are lower when a drug is ingested with food (4). Parkinson's disease patients receiving 3 to 8 g daily of L-DOPA administered with food had average plasma levels of approximately 1 mcg/ml with a very wide range between patients and in the same patient on different occasions. Although the relationship of L-DOPA's plasma levels to its clinical effects has not been determined, the short duration of improvement that occurs

after each dose and that disappears within 5 hr demands a better understanding of the factors influencing absorption. How foods that are administered along with L-DOPA modify this important clinical factor is unknown. The numerous serious side effects of L-DOPA therapy might be controlled if the facts that control gastrointestinal absorption were known. The example cited is but one of many psychopharmacological agents that might be utilized more efficiently in therapy if we had better knowledge of the food–drug absorption interactions.

HIGH-FIBER DIETS AND DRUG ABSORPTION

Recent enthusiasm for high-fiber diets may carry a special challenge for drug therapy. Colloidal laxatives and fiber-bulking agents might reduce the toxicity, absorption, or pharmacological effects of drugs. Essential elements and/or food additives such as the salts of magnesium, zinc, or tin are covalently bound by fiber. Indeed, it is possible to produce zinc deficiency in animals or man by feeding high soybean protein diets. Fiber can be shown to hold the inorganic ion in a clathrate matrix that prevents absorption of the metal from the gut.

EFFECT OF FOODS ON BIOCHEMICAL TRANSFORMATION OF DRUGS

Living cells have a remarkable capacity to chemically modify drug molecules. This biochemical transformation frequently achieved by the nonspecific enzymes present in the microsomes of liver cells is one of the chief oxidative pathways drug molecules undergo. These are usually hydroxylation reactions leading to detoxification of the drug. More polar metabolites are formed and hence are less capable of penetrating the lipid target cell barrier.

The result is subsequent excretion of the less toxic metabolite.

However, not all enzymic reactions of drugs in liver cells produce less toxic metabolites—some are more toxic. The insecticide parathion is changed by metabolism to the more toxic paraoxon and is an example of this kind of enhanced toxicity.

Following the prolonged administration of numerous drugs or chemicals, hepatic microsomal enzymes may be stimulated, and the process of induction takes place (5). The implications of microsomal enzyme induction are just beginning to be appreciated by clinicians. Indeed, this phenomenon explains why repeated drug dosage may lead to decreased therapeutic effectiveness. The detoxification mechanisms of the liver become more efficient in metabolizing the drug, and larger doses are required to elicit the desired pharmacologic effects. Microsomal enzymes can also be induced in such tissues as the intestine, lung, adrenals, and kidney, although less is known about these extrahepatic systems. The increased liver size, total protein content, and weight as a result of enzyme induction are the most prominent signs.

Food chemicals have been shown to induce hepatic microsomal enzymes. Butylated hydroxytoluene, 2,6-di-*tert*-butyl-*p*-cresol (BHT) and the closely related butylated hydroxyanisole (BHA), used as antioxidants in many foods, also cause an increase in liver weights in experimental animals fed these compounds and a substantial increase in drug metabolizing enzymes (6–8). Several studies suggest that the metabolism of BHT and BHA in man is similar to that in some experimental animals (2). Although very high doses of either BHT or BHA must be fed to produce a rise in liver mitochrondrial enzymes in experimental animals, the effects of prolonged, low dosage are not known for human subjects. The

consensus seems to be that the effect is reversible and likely without toxicological significance (11,12).

Some workers regard the liver hypertrophy as an adaptive mechanism (11,14); and this may be correct. The significant fact remains that if other therapeutic drugs are simultaneously administered that also are metabolized by these same hepatic microsomal enzymes, adaptation may fail. The question concerning the challenge to fully adapted livers by drugs that also raise the level of microsomal enzymes thus takes on added significance.

The example of ingestion of the food antioxidant BHT with the resulting liver hypertrophy followed by ingestion of an oral steroid contraceptive illustrates the situation described. If ingestion of BHT or similar compounds reaches a point at which adaptation fails, a new condition is created, and injury could follow. In view of the wide use of food antioxidants and steroid hormones, information should be available on the effect of challenging fully adapted livers with compounds that are themselves metabolized by microsomal hydroxylases. Fortunately, these experiments can be conducted in experimental animals that have a high predictive value for man. The studies have not been done. It would appear that further clarification of the ramifications of this type of food–drug interaction should be sought.

SPECIAL ENZYME-RELATED INTERACTIONS

The ingestion of food containing tyramine, such as cheese, and the hypertensive crisis produced in patients taking the antidepressive drug tranylcypromine is a classic example of a food–drug interaction. Tyramine-containing foods apparently stimulate the release of norepinephrine, which likely results in the sharp elevation in blood pressure. The norephinephrine release is also accelerated by the drug itself, a monoamine oxidase inhibitor. According to the *Medical Letter on Drugs and Therapeutics,* the following foods contain tyramine and may produce similar food–drug interactions: Chianti wines, beer, sherry, pickled herring, yeast extracts, chicken liver, chocolate, broad beans, sour cream, canned figs, raisins, and soy sauce (1). It would be suprising if there were not many more examples of unrecognized cases of enzymic changes produced by usual dietary items that elicit subsequent adverse drug responses. Patients receiving the monoamine oxidase inhibitors are now cautioned to avoid foods that have been recognized to contain high amounts of tyramine as a result of this well-publicized interaction. One is tempted to speculate, however, how many other instances there are that are not detected.

INTERRELATIONSHIPS OF NUTRITION AND DRUG METABOLISM

The metabolism of foreign compounds and drugs depends on the nutritional status of the organism. Basu and Dickerson (3) have reviewed the salient factors related to malnutrition, disease states that cause nutritional imbalance, and the fate of foreign compounds, drugs, food additives, pesticides, and toxic plant foodstuffs in the body. Food faddism can produce hypo- or hypervitaminosis, malnutrition, or a severely unbalanced diet as easily as disease. As a consequence, normal drug metabolizing pathways are disturbed, and detoxification mechanisms are less efficient. The result may be acute or chronic toxicity from a drug dosage that would be considered optimal in a well-nourished person.

There are many inconsistencies however. Low-protein diets although usually decreasing enzyme activity and hence making various drugs more toxic do not increase the toxicity of all drugs. Some foreign chemical compounds are less toxic to young animals fed protein-free diets for only 7 days. The exact cause of these results remains unknown but may be an adaptive enzyme response.

Mineral or vitamin deficiencies are known to change the toxicity of numerous drugs, and ascorbic acid is presumed to have a significant role in drug metabolism. Thus, these nutrition elements must be included in any consideration of food–drug interactions. By the same process therapeutic drugs influence the safety of food additives, and foods often determine the therapeutic effectiveness of drugs.

It is unfortunate that a food history is not part of the information usually obtained by physicians treating patients. If this information were elicited from the patient, in many cases a superior therapy could be provided. If nutritional biochemists, basic and clinical toxicologists, and pharmacologists representing the various fields interested in these issues were to mount the studies needed to assess the importance of food–drug interactions, a significant contribution could be made to patient care. The Organizing Committee of The First International Symposium on Neurotoxicology should collaborate with the Society of Toxicology and the American College of Clinical Toxicology to develop a plan for subsequent studies with the able workers in the field of nutrition, and symposia can explore these possibilities.

REFERENCES

1. Anonymous (1973): Adverse interactions of drugs. *Med. Lett. Drugs. Ther.,* 15:80.
2. Astill, B. D., Fassett, D. W., and Roudabuch, R. L. (1960): The metabolism of phenolic antioxidants. 2. The metabolism of butylated hydroxyanisole in the rat. *Biochem. J.,* 75:543–555.
3. Basu, T. K., and Dickerson, J. W. T. (1974): Interrelationships of nutrition and the metabolism of drugs. *Chem. Biol. Interact.,* 8:193–206.
4. Calne, D. B., and Reid, J. L. (1972): Antiparkinsonian drugs pharmacological and therapeutic aspects. *Drugs,* 4:49–72.
5. Conney, A. H. (1967): Pharmacological impli-

cations of microsomal enzyme induction. *Pharmacol. Rev.*, 19:317–366.

6. Creaven, P. J., Davies, W. H., and Williams, R. T. (1966): The effect of butylated hydroxytoluene, butylated hydroxyanisole, and octyl gallate upon liver weight and biphenyl-4-hydroxylase activity in the rat. *J. Pharm. Pharmacol.*,18:485–489.

7. Feuer, G., and Granda, F. (1970): Antagonistic effect of foreign compounds on microsomal enzymes of the liver of rats. *Toxicol. Appl. Pharmacol.*, 16:626–637.

8. Gilbert, D., and Goldberg, L. (1965): Liver weight and microsomal processing of drug metabolism enzymes in rats treated with butylated hydroxytoluene or butylated hydroxyanisole. *Biochem. J.*, 97:28P–29P.

9. Office of the Federal Register, General Services Administration. (1975): *Code of Federal Regulations,* title 21, parts 121.101, pp. 315–327. US Govt. Printing Office, Washington, D.C.

10. Prescott, L. F. (1974): Gastrointestinal absorption of drugs. *Med. Clin. North Am.,* 58:907–916.

11. Schaffner, F., and Raisfeld, I. H. (1969): Drugs and the liver: A review of metabolism and adverse reactions. *Adv. Intern. Med.,* 15:221–251.

12. Takanaka, A., Kato, R., and Omori, Y. (1969): Effect of food additives and colors on microsomal drug-metabolizing enzymes of rat liver. *Shokuhin Eiseigaku Zasshi,* 10:260–265.

13. Waddell, J. (1973): The bioavailability of iron sources and their utilization in food enrichment. Fed. Proc., 33:1779–1783.

14. Wattenberg, L. W. (1975): Effect of dietary constituents on the metabolism of chemical carcinogens. *Cancer Res.,* 35:3326–3331.

Neurotoxicology, edited by L. Roizin, H. Shiraki, and N. Grčević. Raven Press, New York © 1977.

Some Observations on the Neurological Effects of Alcohol Intoxication and Withdrawal

Maurice Victor

Department of Medicine (Neurology), Cleveland Metropolitan General Hospital, and Case-Western Reserve University, School of Medicine, Cleveland, Ohio 44109

The abuse of alcohol gives rise to a wide variety of neurological disorders. However, the mechanism by which alcohol produces its effect is quite different in each of them. One group of symptoms is due to the toxic effects of alcohol *per se;* another, to the withdrawal of the drug after a period of prolonged inebriation; and still others, to the effects of malnutrition or derangements of liver function. The failure to appreciate these fundamental distinctions among the alcoholic neurological disorders has led to a great deal of confusion and contradictory statements about them in medical writings. In particular, there has been a failure to distinguish clearly between effects of alcohol intoxication and the effects of withdrawal of alcohol following a period of chronic intoxication.

Why delirium tremens and related disorders were ever confused with the effects of alcohol intoxication is difficult to understand. A moment's reflection indicates the basic differences between these syndromes. It is obvious that the symptoms of toxicity, consisting of slurred speech, uninhibited behavior, staggering gait, stupor, and coma are in themselves distinctive and different from the symptom complex of tremor, hallucinations, fits, and delirium. The former group of symptoms is associated with an elevated blood alcohol level, whereas the latter become evident only when the blood alcohol level is reduced.

Finally, the toxic symptoms increase in severity as more alcohol is consumed (the drowsy patient becomes stuporous, for example), whereas tremor, hallucinosis, and similar symptoms are suppressed by the administration of alcohol.

The manifestations of acute alcohol intoxication are so commonplace that they hardly require elaboration. These manifestations and the mechanisms by which they are produced do not differ essentially from those of many other sedative-hypnotic drugs and anesthetic agents. For these reasons little more is said of them here, and the remainder of this discussion is concerned with the alcohol withdrawal syndrome.

GENESIS OF DELIRIUM TREMENS AND RELATED SYMPTOMS

It is now generally agreed that the one indispensable factor in the genesis of delirium tremens and related symptoms is the withdrawal of alcohol following a period of chronic intoxication (20). The precise mechanism(s) by which the withdrawal of alcohol produces symptoms is far from clear, however. It is a matter of common observation that the states of chronic intoxication and withdrawal are associated frequently with disturbances of water and electrolyte balance, glucose metabolism, blood gases, liver function, and so forth, and all of these have been incriminated at one time or another in the genesis of the withdrawal syndrome. Of these many abnormalities, two in particular — hypomagnesemia and respiratory alkalosis — have proved in our experience to be consistently associated with all but the mildest withdrawal symptoms and are probably important in their causation. Our investigations of these factors have been the subject of several articles (18, 20,25,26) to which the reader is referred for a more complete account than can be given here. The following is a brief summary of our observations.

Early in the course of our studies we be-

came aware that patients with "rum fits" were remarkably sensitive to photic stimulation. This sensitivity took the form of coarse clonic movements of the muscles of the face and neck, spreading to involve the trunk and limbs, without loss of consciousness (photomyoclonus), or a major tonic-clonic seizure with loss of consciousness (photoconvulsion). A systematic investigation of large numbers of hospitalized alcoholics disclosed that photomyoclonus or photoconvulsions, or both, could be induced in about half of the patients during the early stages (8 to 60 hr) of alcohol withdrawal, whether or not there had been spontaneous seizures. In contrast, this

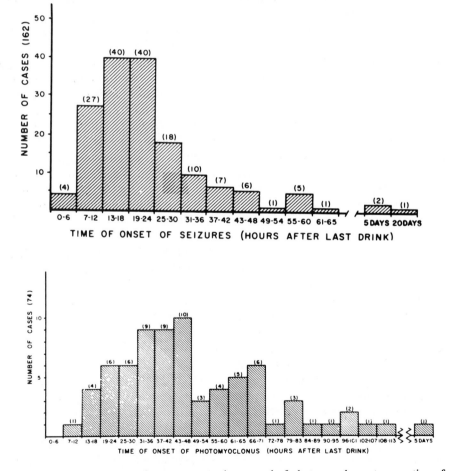

FIG. 1. Relation of the occurrence of spontaneous seizures and of photomyoclonus to cessation of drinking. (From Wolfe and Victor, ref. 25.)

type of photic response could practically never be induced in normal individuals and only rarely in nonalcoholic patients with idiopathic epilepsy (7,18,21).

Photomyoclonic responses in patients with alcohol withdrawal symptoms proved to have much the same temporal relationship to the cessation of drinking as did spontaneous seizures (Fig. 1). The characteristic myoclonic and convulsive responses could often be induced over a period of several hours or even days, and, for long stretches of time (30 to 60 min), stimulation could be repeated at intervals of 5 min without significantly altering the seizure threshold (the number of flashes per second and the duration of the stimulus required to produce myoclonus), provided the patient was allowed to rest for a few minutes between tests. Thus, for the first time, we were provided with an experimental means of assessing: (a) the patients' vulnerability to seizure activity (photic threshold) in the withdrawal period and (b) the effects of administration of a variety of agents on the seizure (photomyoclonus) threshold.

ROLE OF HYPOMAGNESEMIA

Our attention was directed initially to the possible role of magnesium in the genesis of alcohol withdrawal symptoms. We had been impressed, as had others, with the frequent occurrence of hypomagnesemia in the alcohol withdrawal states (2,4,11,13). Our preliminary observations suggested that the administration of magnesium has a salutory effect on tremulousness and vulnerability to photomyoclonus in the early phases of the withdrawal period. These observations prompted a more careful study of these relationships (25). Eighteen alcoholic patients who were free of hepatic or renal disease, diabetes mellitus, hypocalcemia, or malabsorption were subjected to stroboscopic stimulation at the time of their admission to the hospital, and at 8-hr intervals thereafter until the symptoms of

alcohol withdrawal had abated. Ten of these patients responded with photomyoclonus; five of the 10 patients who responded in this way also had spontaneous seizures, and three of them went on to develop delirium tremens. Eight patients did not respond to photic stimulation; only one of these had a spontaneous seizure, and none developed delirium tremens. In all 18 patients the serum magnesium levels were significantly lower than in normal control subjects, and the patients with photomyoclonus had lower levels than those who did not respond to photic stimulation (Fig. 2). Furthermore, there was a correlation between the magnesium levels and the photomyoclonus threshold — patients who responded at low frequencies had lower magnesium levels than those who responded at higher frequencies (Fig. 3). Eight of the 10 patients who showed photomyoclonus in the withdrawal period were given magnesium sulfate intravenously in doses of 2 to 6 g (16.7 to 50 mEq). In three patients, administration of 3 g of $MgSO_4$ abolished the response at all fre-

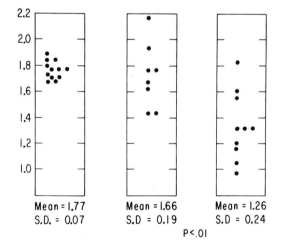

FIG. 2. Serum magnesium (mEq/L) levels in (a) controls (medical students), (b) alcoholics in withdrawal not responding to photic stimulation, and (c) alcoholics responding to photic stimulation. S.D., standard deviation. (From Wolfe and Victor, ref. 25.)

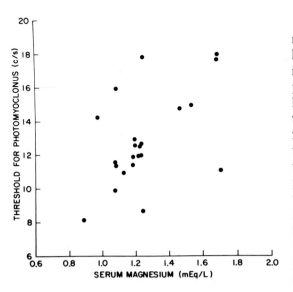

FIG. 3. Relationship between photomyoclonus threshold and serum magnesium levels in the alcohol withdrawal period. (From Wolfe and Victor, ref. 25.)

The close relationship between the photomyoclonus threshold and serum magnesium levels in one of these patients is depicted in Fig. 4. On admission to the hospital, this patient was still intoxicated, at which time he showed no response to photic stimulation. Subsequently, his magnesium level fell and concomitantly a positive response to photic stimulation was elicited. Although the administration of chlordiazepoxide hydrochloride (Librium®) seemed to lessen his tremulousness, it had no significant effect on the photomyoclonus threshold. The intravenous administration of 3 g of $MgSO_4$, however, was accompanied by an elevation of the threshold, and after the second dose of $MgSO_4$ no response to photic stimulation could be obtained.

quencies within minutes after it was given; in the other five patients, all of whom had much lower magnesium levels, there was a significant elevation of the photomyoclonus threshold following the administration of $MgSO_4$.

Thus, the extent to which these patients became hypomagnesemic during alcohol withdrawal correlated closely with a vulnerability to spontaneous seizures and photomyoclonus. The significance of this relationship was supported by the finding that intravenous administration of magnesium sulfate decreased the susceptibility

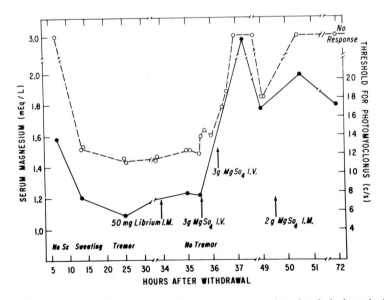

FIG. 4. Relationship of photomyoclonus threshold to serum magnesium level during alcohol withdrawal. ●——●, serum magnesium level; ○— —○, photomyoclonus threshold. (From Wolfe and Victor, ref. 25.)

to photomyoclonus. No such correlation could be made between hypomagnesemia and delirium tremens, however. The three patients in this study who developed delirium tremens had very low levels of serum magnesium at the time of admission to the hospital, and in each case the serum magnesium had returned to normal or near-normal levels at the time of onset of the delirium. Others also have noted that delirium tremens may have its onset after the serum magnesium levels have returned to normal (11,22). Thus, whatever the relationship may be of hypomagnesemia to the early symptoms of withdrawal, it probably is not a significant factor in the genesis of delirium tremens.

ROLE OF RESPIRATORY ALKALOSIS

The study cited above (25) disclosed another consistent abnormality in the withdrawal period, namely, the rapid evolution of an alkalotic state. This was in accord with the observations of Sereny et al. (15), who noted a transient rise in the arterial pH of eight alcoholic subjects during the initial 48-hr period of hospitalization. The alkalemia that characterizes the withdrawal state and its relation to hypomag-

nesemia and photomyoclonus was investigated initially in four volunteer subjects who had been drinking for 60 days before they were withdrawn abruptly (25). The rise in arterial pH values, which could be discerned as early as 8 hr after withdrawal of alcohol, was concomitant with a fall in the serum magnesium level and an increased sensitivity to photic stimulation. These features are illustrated in Figs. 5 and 6. Tremor and hyperreflexia were prominent during the period of hypomagnesemia and alkalosis, and both of these clinical abnormalities abated as the serum magnesium and arterial pH values returned to normal. It is noteworthy that the serum calcium values in these four patients were normal (4.5 to 5.5 mEq/l) throughout the period of intoxication and withdrawal.

The preceding observations prompted a more detailed investigation of the alkalosis that characterizes the alcohol withdrawal state. Nine alcoholics, studied under controlled conditions of drinking and abstinence, were the subjects of this study (24). Following a control period, these patients consumed one to two pints of 100-proof bourbon daily *ad lib*, in addition to an adequate diet, and supplemental vitamins. Four of the patients drank in this way for

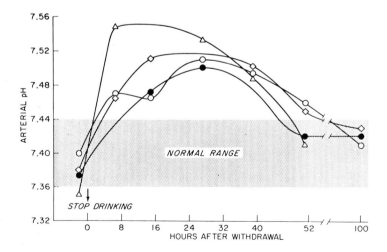

FIG. 5. Arterial pH changes during alcohol withdrawal in four chronic alcoholics, M(●), H(◇), ST(○), and SM(△). (From Wolfe and Victor, ref. 25.)

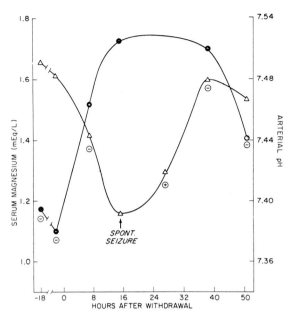

FIG. 6. Relationship between arterial pH, serum magnesium, and photic sensitivity during alcohol withdrawal. ●——●, arterial pH; △——△, serum magnesium; ⊕, photomyoclonus or photoconvulsion response to strobe; ⊖, negative response to strobe. (From Wolfe and Victor, ref. 25.)

60 days; in five patients the drinking period lasted 14 days. Within 8 to 9 hr after the abrupt withdrawal of alcohol there was a significant rise in arterial pH and a concomitant fall in pCO_2, the result of tachypnea and increased depth of respiration (Fig. 7). Furthermore, a correlation could be demonstrated between the severity of the withdrawal symptoms and the magnitude of change of the arterial pH and pCO_2. Only the patients with relatively large changes in pH and pCO_2 (with one exception these were the patients who drank for 60 days) showed spontaneous seizures, photomyoclonus, and severe tremulousness. The fall in serum magnesium levels during the withdrawal period was much greater in the patients who drank for 60 days than in those who drank for 14 days (an average fall of 0.41 mEq/l in the former and 0.10 mEq/l in the latter). Again, serum calcium levels remained in the normal range in all nine patients throughout the study; only two of the nine patients developed acute hypokalemia during the withdrawal period.

The relationships between the clinical and biochemical manifestations of alcohol

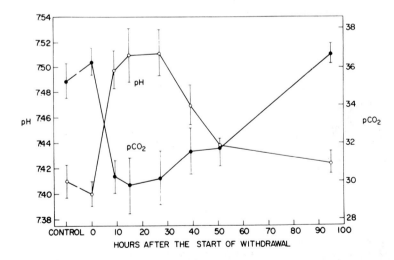

FIG. 7. Arterial pH and pCO_2 during alcohol withdrawal in nine patients. Control values were obtained prior to the drinking period. Values at 0 hr were obtained while the patients were still intoxicated, just prior to cessation of drinking. ○——○——○, pH; ●——●——●, pCO_2; ◯̣, mean ±SEM (9 cases). (From Wolfe et al., ref. 24.)

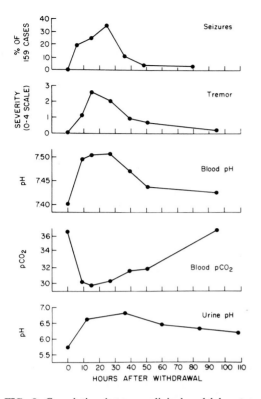

FIG. 8. Correlation between clinical and laboratory findings during withdrawal. (Upper panel represents data from Victor and Brausch, ref. 21); other panels are the mean values of the nine patients in the study of Wolfe et al., ref. 24.)

emergency ward of the Cleveland Metropolitan General Hospital (26). The withdrawal symptoms in this group were much more severe than those of previously-studied patients, allowing us to make observations in nine cases of delirium tremens as well as in 22 patients with the earlier signs of withdrawal (13 patients with tremor and hallucinations and nine patients with seizures).

This study provided confirmatory evidence that the early phase of alcohol withdrawal is consistently associated with respiratory alkalosis and that the severity of the clinical manifestations correlates closely with the magnitude of these biochemical

withdrawal are illustrated in Fig. 8. The upper panel indicates the time of occurrence of spontaneous seizures in relation to the withdrawal of alcohol, based on observations of 159 patients (21). The other data represent the means of values in the nine patients studied by Wolfe et al. (24). The period from 10 to 30 hr following cessation of drinking, during which tremulousness is most severe and most spontaneous seizures occur, coincides with the period of greatest abnormality in arterial pH and pCO_2 and the development of a more alkaline urine.

The foregoing observations, which were made in patients on a metabolic ward during control, drinking, and withdrawal periods, were extended in another study of 31 alcoholics who were admitted from the

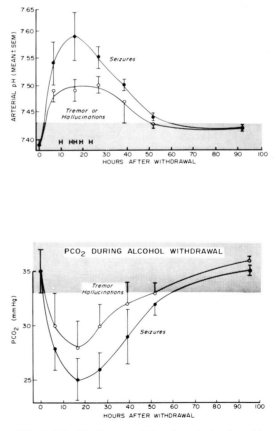

FIG. 9. Arterial pH and pCO_2 values during the withdrawal period in 13 patients with tremor and hallucinations and in nine patients with seizures. (From Wolfe and Victor, ref. 26.)

changes. These features are illustrated in Fig. 9, which shows a maximal degree of respiratory alkalosis between 12 and 21 hr after withdrawal and a concurrence of seizures and hallucinations with the maximal degree of respiratory alkalosis. The reduction in pCO_2 and rise in arterial pH was greater in patients with seizures than in those with tremor and hallucinations alone. The respiratory alkalosis had largely corrected itself by 50 hr after withdrawal, at which time the symptoms were minimal. In patients who went on to develop delirium tremens the pH values did not change significantly, but the pCO_2 values, which had returned to near normal, again decreased coincident with the onset of delirium tremens (Fig. 10), findings that were interpreted to represent a partially compensated respiratory alkalosis.

Finally, it should be emphasized that apart from the changes in serum magne-

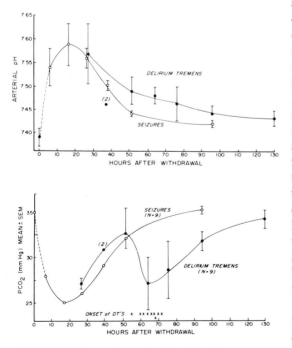

FIG. 10. Comparison of pH and pCO_2 values in patients with alcohol withdrawal seizures and those with delirium tremens. (From Wolfe and Victor, ref. 26.)

sium, arterial pH, and pCO_2, no consistent biochemical abnormalities were found associated with symptoms of withdrawal. Measurements of serum glutamic oxaloacetic transaminase, serum glutamic pyruvic transaminase, serum proteins, etc., were normal and values of serum sodium, chloride, calcium, potassium, and glucose, estimated repeatedly during the withdrawal period, disclosed only a few instances of hypoglycemia and slight depression of the serum potassium in eight of the 31 patients. In these respects, the findings were much the same as in our previous studies, which disclosed no consistent biochemical abnormalities during the period of chronic intoxication as well as during the withdrawal period.

COMMENT

It may be concluded from the foregoing observations that the initial phase of the alcohol withdrawal period (approximately 48 hr after the cessation of drinking) is consistently associated with two abnormalities: (a) acute transient hypomagnesemia and (b) respiratory alkalosis, which is most likely the result of hyperventilation. Furthermore, the severity of the withdrawal symptoms bears a close relationship to the magnitude of change of these biochemical abnormalities. It has been our observation that the administration of magnesium raises the seizure threshold in the initial phase of the withdrawal period and that it may allay other abstinence symptoms as well. Preliminary observations suggest that correction of respiratory alkalosis also may have a salutory effect on withdrawal symptoms, but more data are required to be certain of this effect.

In addition to the experimental evidence presented above, there is considerable indirect evidence to suggest that hypomagnesemia and respiratory alkalosis are important in the causation of withdrawal symptoms. Manifestations of both central and peripheral nervous system irritability have been described repeatedly in states of magnesium deficiency. In several animal species, a deficiency of magnesium has been associated with the occurrence of convulsive seizures, and a lowering of serum magnesium in cattle appears to be responsible for muscular tremor and twitching, apprehensive behavior, and violent convulsions (9,10). In man, magnesium deficiency states may be associated with tremor, twitching, convulsions, carpalpedal spasms, and occasionally with visual and auditory hallucinations, and some of these phenomena can be reversed by the administration of magnesium (5,17). It should be emphasized that this therapeutic effect cannot be attributed simply to the sedative or anesthetic actions of magnesium (16).

It is well known that hyperventilation frequently precipitates seizures in patients with epilepsy and causes a decrease in the frequency of brain waves in normal individuals. It is also well known that respiratory alkalosis caused by hyperventilation may be accompanied by tremors and carpalpedal spasms. A striking example of the effects of hyperventilation is seen in patients with chronic lung disease who have high arterial pCO_2 and normal or slightly decreased pH. When these patients are mechanically hyperventilated, the pCO_2 decreases and arterial pH increases, and if such treatment is prolonged or excessive, the patients may develop disorientation, hallucinations, tremor, hyperreflexia, generalized muscular irritability, seizures, and hyperpyrexia (1,3,8,14). These symptoms have been quickly relieved by simply allowing pCO_2 to increase (14). In some circumstances, alkalosis *per se* appears to be responsible for a state of heightened neuromuscular irritability; for example, an increased incidence of audiogenic seizures occurs in rats pretreated with sodium bicarbonate (12).

The symptoms associated with alkalosis are thought to be due to the direct effect of increased pH on nerve and muscle, or possibly the result of decreased CO_2 tension. They are probably not due to the effects of lowered ionizable calcium, which is invoked frequently as a cause of the so-called tetany that accompanies alkalosis; Walser (23) has pointed out that the changes in ionizable calcium that accompany alterations in blood pH are probably too small to cause these effects.

Studies by Wollman et al. (27) have shown that hyperventilation in normal men, sufficient to lower pCO_2 and produce alkalosis, causes a decrease in cerebral blood flow of as much as 40%. When alkalosis is induced by sodium bicarbonate, however, an increase rather than a decrease in cerebral blood flow occurs, so that cerebral vasoconstriction appears to be caused by lowered CO_2 tension rather than by alkalosis *per se*. Thus, a low pCO_2 may cause cerebral hypoxia, thereby potentiating the direct effect of alkalosis on neural excitability and accounting for many of the symptoms seen during alcohol withdrawal.

It is therefore postulated that the compounded effects of hypomagnesemia and alkalosis, each of which is known to be associated with hyperexcitability of the nervous system, are sufficient to produce photomyoclonus and spontaneous seizures and perhaps other symptoms that characterize the early phase of alcohol withdrawal. The precise relationship between hypomagnesemia and alkalosis is not understood. Possibly, the latter may be responsible for the former by causing a shift of magnesium into bone and other intracellular sites, just as alkalemia causes a shift of potassium from extracellular to intracellular compartments. What it is that induces the respiratory alkalosis in the first place is a matter of speculation. The effect of chronic alcohol intoxication on the neuronal elements in the brainstem that control respirations is to cause a decrease in ventilatory response to carbon dioxide (6). Possibly, removal of the depressant effect of alcohol is followed by a "rebound" phenomenon, resulting in an increased sensitivity of the "respiratory center" to carbon dioxide, and, in turn, hyperventilation.

CONCLUDING REMARKS

The studies reported here have led us to recognize two phases of the withdrawal syndrome—an early or minor phase and a late or major one (delirium tremens). This concept is both of theoretical and practical importance, and the failure to distinguish between these two aspects of the withdrawal syndrome is largely responsible for the confusion in the literature pertaining to the diagnosis and treatment of alcohol withdrawal.

By far the largest number of patients who experience alcohol withdrawal symptoms show only *the minor syndrome,* i.e., varying degrees of tremor, general muscular weakness, insomnia, and anorexia, and less often, of hallucinations and seizures ("rum fits"), having their onset as early as 6 to 8 hr after withdrawal, reaching a peak of severity between 10 and 30 hr, and abating largely by 40 to 50 hr. As has been pointed out, these symptoms correlate closely with vulnerability to photic stimulation, a fall in serum magnesium, and a rise in arterial pH and a drop in pco_2, the result of respiratory alkalosis. These symptoms are almost invariably benign and respond readily to a variety of sedative-hypnotic drugs.

A *small* proportion of patients experience *the major syndrome* or *delirium tremens,* which has its onset between 60 and 80 hr after withdrawal and is characterized by profound confusion, increased psychomotor activity (restlessness, tremor, jactitations, vivid hallucinations), and overactivity of the autonomic nervous system (fever, tachycardia, severe diaphoresis). Spontaneous seizures, if they occur, always precede the onset of delirium tremens, and once delirium tremens becomes estab-

lished the patient is no longer vulnerable either to spontaneous seizures or to photic stimulation. Hypomagnesemia does not seem to be significant in the pathogenesis of delirium tremens, and the relationship to respiratory alkalosis is variable. Delirium tremens is potentially a lethal disease, and its duration and outcome are influenced very little by the administration of sedative-hypnotic drugs; the crucial elements of treatment are the control of dehydration and electrolyte imbalance and the management of hyperthermia and shock, should these complications become manifest.

ACKNOWLEDGMENT

Some of the work reported here was supported by a grant from NINCDS, National Institutes of Health.

REFERENCES

1. Addington, W. W., Kettel, L. J., and Cugell, D. W. (1966): Alkalosis due to mechanical hyperventilation in patients with chronic hypercapnea. *Ann. Rev. Resp. Dis.,* 93:736–741.
2. Flink, E. B., Stutzman, F. L., Anderson, A. R., Lontig, T., and Frasier, R. (1954): Magnesium deficiency after prolonged parenteral fluid administration and after chronic alcoholism complicated by delirium tremens. *J. Lab. Clin. Med.,* 43:169–183.
3. Hamilton, J. D., and Gross, N. J. (1963): Unusual neurological and cardiovascular complications of respiratory failure. *Br. Med. J.,* 2:1092–1096.
4. Heaton, F. W. Pyrah, L. N., Beresford, C. C., Bryson, R. W., and Martin, D. F. (1962): Hypomagnesemia in chronic alcoholism. *Lancet,* 2:802–805.
5. Hirschfelder, A. D., and Haury, V. G. (1934): Clinical manifestations of high and low plasma magnesium. *JAMA,* 102:1138–1141.
6. Hitchcock, F. A. (1941): Some effects of CO_2, anoxia and alcohol on respiration. *Am. J. Physiol.,* 133:328–329.
7. Hughes, J. R., Curtin, M. J., and Brown, V. P. (1960): Usefulness of photic stimulation in routine clinical electroencephalography. *Neurology,* 10:777–782.
8. Kilburn, K. H. (1966): Shock, seizures and coma with alkalosis during mechanical ventilation. *Ann. Intern. Med.,* 65:977–984.
9. Klingman, W. O., Suter, C., Green, R., and Robinson, I. (1955): Role of alcoholism and magnesium

deficiency in convulsions. *Trans. Am. Neurol. Assoc.,* 80:162–165.

10. MacIntyre, I. (1967): Magnesium metabolism. *Adv. Intern. Med.,* 13:143–154.

11. Mendelson, J. H., Wexler, D., Kubzansky, P., Leiderman, H., and Solomon, P. (1959): Serum magnesium in delirium tremens and alcoholic hallucinosis. *J. Nerv. Ment. Dis.,* 128:352–357.

12. Mitchell, W. G., and Ogden, E. (1954): Influence of blood pH on the susceptibility of rats to audiogenic seizures. *Am. J. Physiol.,* 179:225–228.

13. Randall, R. E., Rossmeisl, E. C., and Bleifer, K. H. (1959): Magnesium depletion in man. *Ann. Intern. Med.,* 50:257–287.

14. Rotheram, E. B., Safar, P., and Robin, E. D. (1964): CNS disorder during mechanical ventilation in chronic pulmonary disease. *JAMA,* 189: 993–996.

15. Sereny, G., Rapoport, A., and Hudson, H. (1966): The effect of alcoholic withdrawal on electrolyte and acid-base balance. *Metabolism,* 15:896–904.

16. Somjen, G., Hilmy, M., and Stephen, C. R. (1966): Failure to anesthetize human subjects by intravenous administration of magnesium sulfate. *J. Pharmacol. Exp. Ther.,* 154:652–659.

17. Vallee, B. L., Wacker, W. E. C., and Ulmer, D. D. (1960): The magnesium deficiency tetany syndrome in man. *N. Engl. J. Med.,* 262:155–161.

18. Victor, M. (1968): The pathophysiology of alcoholic epilepsy. *Proc. A. Res. Nerv. Ment. Dis.,* 46:431–454.

19. Victor, M. (1973): The role of hypomagnesemia and respiratory alkalosis in the genesis of alcohol-withdrawal symptoms. *Ann. NY Acad. Sci.,* 215:235–248.

20. Victor, M. (1973): Introductory remarks. *Ann. NY Acad. Sci.,* 215:210–213.

21. Victor, M., and Brausch, C. C. (1967): The role of abstinence in the genesis of alcoholic epilepsy. *Epilepsia,* 8:1–20.

22. Wacker, W. E. C., and Vallee, B. L. (1958): Magnesium metabolism. *N. Engl. J. Med.,* 259: 431–438, 475–482.

23. Walser, M. (1962): Separate effects of hyperparathyroidism, hypercalcemia of malignancy, renal failure and acidosis on the state of calcium, phosphate, and other ions in the plasma. *J. Clin. Invest.,* 41:1454–1471.

24. Wolfe, S. M., Mendelson, J. H., Ogata, M., Victor, M., Marshall, W., and Mello, N. K. (1969): Respiratory alkalosis and alcohol withdrawal. *Trans. Assoc. Am. Physicians,* 82:344–352.

25. Wolfe, S. M., and Victor, M. (1969): The relationship of hypomagnesemia and alkalosis to alcohol withdrawal symptoms. *Ann. NY Acad. Sci.,* 162, Art. 2:973–984.

26. Wolfe, S. M., and Victor, M. (1971): The physiological basis of the alcohol withdrawal syndrome. In: *Recent Advances in Studies of Alcoholism,* edited by N. K. Mello and J. H. Mendelson, pp. 188–199. Publication No. (HSM)71-9045, U.S. Govt. Printing Office, Washington, D.C.

27. Wollman, H., Smith, T. C., Stephen, G. W., Colton, E. T., III, Gleaton, H. E., and Alexander, S. C. (1968): Effects of extremes of respiratory and metabolic alkalosis on cerebral blood flow in man. *J. Appl. Physiol.,* 24:60–65.

Neurotoxicology, edited by L. Roizin, H. Shiraki, and N. Grčević. Raven Press, New York © 1977.

Malnutrition-Alcoholism: Histopathology of Peripheral Nerves and B Vitamins in Nerves, Blood, and CSF

Darab K. Dastur, Anita Dewan, N. Santhadevi, †Daya K. Manghani, and *Zohra A. Razzak

The Neuropathology Unit, Postgraduate Research Laboratories, Grant Medical College and J. J. Group of Hospitals, Bombay–400 008, India

The objective of this investigation was *not* to study alcoholic peripheral neuropathy *per se,* but rather to detect the types of neurologic disorders developing against a background of malnutrition as encountered at two large teaching hospitals in Bombay. During the first half year of this investigation (which lasted about 5 years), it became apparent that the majority of our patients had a history of prolonged intake of alcohol in varying quantities and also, accompanying or often preceding this habit, a history of inadequate intake of food, these patients being drawn from the poorer economic classes.

In the absence of the availability of brain tissue for estimation of vitamin levels, cerebrospinal fluid (CSF) levels probably reflect the status of nutrients such as vitamins better than blood levels of these compounds. This idea is strongly supported by Linus Pauling (24) especially with respect to thiamine. He conceived of improving the mental health of people by providing an "optimum molecular environment for the mind" through maintenance of an adequate concentration of vital substances normally present in the brain. This concept was kept in mind in our investigations, where B vitamins were estimated in the CSF also, whenever it was available. Similarly, whenever possible, thiamine and total vitamin B_6 were estimated in sural nerve biopsy specimens from our patients with malnutrition-alcoholism, no such data being available in published literature. These two aspects, together with the sequential estimation of the blood levels of five or six of the B vitamins under the effect of treatment, constitute some of the new features of our study. New features on the histologic side were quantitation of data on a large number of nerve and muscle biopsies, estimation of density of myelinated nerve fibers, histographic analysis of fiber size spectra, and determination of type of nerve degeneration.

In this chapter, the quantitative histopathology of the sural nerve is given in some depth, an account of B vitamins more briefly, as it has been published elsewhere recently (10), but nerve vitamins are to be stressed. The details of clinical and related features including electromyography and muscle pathology will be reported later.

PATIENTS AND CLINICAL FEATURES

Investigations were carried out on 59 patients ranging in age from 19 to 69 years, with a mean age of 39. All patients

---

* Deceased.

† Present address, Nerve Muscle Research Cell, Bombay Hospital, Bombay–20, India.

were drawn from the poorer socioeconomic groups of greater Bombay; all gave a history of inadequate diet either throughout their life-span or during greater parts of it. Against this background of malnutrition they gave a history of alcohol intake, generally of a local ethanolic brew, for a period varying from 2 to 28 years before admission. Often the alcoholism started during a period of even greater economic stress, and then this habit was accompanied by still greater malnutrition.

All patients presented with sensory neuropathy, parasthesia of tingling and numbness, pins and needles, or burning, more the lower limbs than the upper and more distally. Cutaneous sensory loss of glove and stocking distribution was present in 51 patients, loss of vibration or postural sense, or both, in about three-fourths, and depression or loss of ankle jerks in about two-thirds. The predominant nonneurologic clinical sign in 39 patients was pellagroid pigmentation of the skin. There was a slightly enlarged liver in half the patients, and evidence of glossitis or stomatitis in about a fourth. Mental changes of confusion and disorientation in time and space were present in six of the patients (seven "studies"), who also gave a history of more severe alcoholism, but clinically could not be considered cases of Wernicke-Korsakoff's syndrome (34,35).

LABORATORY AND RELATED METHODS

Blood was collected on the day of admission (or the second day) for the vitamin assays. In about half the patients the CSF was also collected. The electrodiagnostic investigations, followed by the nerve and muscle biopsies, were concluded during the first week of hospitalization during which no specific treatment or vitamin supplements were administered. The treatment schedule is given later under Observations and Comments.

Seven B vitamins were estimated in the blood, six by using microbiologic assays. *Ochromonas danica* was used for thiamine, and *Tetrahymena pyriformis* for riboflavin, nicotinic acid, pantothenic acid, and total vitamin B_6, by the method of Baker and Frank (3). The pyridoxal fraction and serum folates were estimated using *Lactobacillus casei*, by the methods of Anderson et al. (1) and Baker and Frank, respectively (3). Vitamin B_{12} was assayed by the isotopic dilution method of Matthews et al. (19) using [57]Co-cyanocobalamin. Vitamins in the CSF were assayed by the same method. Erythrocyte transketolase activity and the effect of addition of thiamine pyrophosphate (TPP) were estimated by the method of Dreyfus (11), the enzyme activity being expressed as the sedoheptulose-7-PO_4 formed.

Identical vitamin assays were carried out in various categories of asymptomatic control subjects (69 in all in the age range of 20 to 45 years) including vegetarians and nonvegetarians and belonging to medium and low economic groups. None of these was addicted to alcohol. The t-test was used for statistical comparison of data on patients and controls.

The other investigations carried out on the patients were D-xylose absorption by the method of Sammons et al. (28), [57]Co-cyanocobalamin absorption by the method of Armstrong and Woodliffe (2), serum proteins by the Biuret method (39), serum transaminases by the method of Reitman and Frankel (26), total blood counts, examination of bone marrow in all patients, and estimation of gastroacidity in about half.

Thirty-six sural nerve biopsies were available from 35 patients. All of them were processed for paraffin sections, 23 for teased fiber examination, and 12 for araldite sections. The paraffin sections were stained with hematoxylin and eosin; the Picro-Mallory method was used for connective tissue and myelin, and the Holmes' silver method was used for axons. The teased fiber preparations were stained with Sudan black for myelin. One- to two-micron araldite sections were prepared from glutaraldehyde-fixed osmicated portions of nerve cut in cross-section and stained with toluidine blue. These sections were used for counts of myelinated nerve fibers (expressed in mm^2) and for plotting histograms of fiber diameters. Ultrathin sections were cut and electron microscopy (EMscopy) was carried out on three of the nerves, after staining the grids with uranyl acetate and lead citrate.

OBSERVATIONS AND COMMENT

B Vitamins in Blood and CSF

Table 1 summarizes the findings on the blood levels of the seven B vitamins and on the CSF levels of five of these vitamins, with statistical comparisons between control subjects and patients with neuropathy alone (category 1) and between the latter and patients with mental changes as well (category 2). On the one hand, it is seen that in patients of category 1 compared to controls blood levels of all the vitamins except B_{12} were significantly lowered, serum folate and pantothenate being relatively the least affected. On the other hand, in patients of category 2 compared to those of category 1 further significant lowerings of blood level were found only with respect to thiamine and pyridoxal fraction of vitamin B_6. The CSF levels in patients of category 1 compared to controls were also highly significantly lowered for four of the five vitamins estimated. CSF levels revealed more clearly the difference between patients of category 2 and category 1 as shown by thiamine, nicotinate, total vitamin B_6, and its pyridoxal fraction.

The blood and CSF levels in all patients and control subjects were plotted as a scattergram for each of the seven vitamins. Such a scattergram for thiamine (vitamin B_1) is illustrated in Fig. 1. The lesser scatter

of values in the CSF than in the blood of patients is noticeable and is responsible for the more significant difference of CSF levels between patients of categories 1 and 2 (Table 1).

On the one hand, a comparison of the blood thiamine level and the erythrocyte transketolase activity in control subjects and patients of both categories showed that the enzyme concentration failed to reveal a significant difference between controls (158 ± 10 μg sedoheptulose-7-PO_4/ml every hour) and patients with neuropathy only (143 ± 18). On the other hand, the TPP effect showed a significant elevation in patients ($26.0 \pm 8.5\%$) compared to controls ($11.8 \pm 2.9\%$), and in this respect matched the fall in blood thiamine level. In patients with mental change as well, there was a marked fall in the transketolase level (60 μg/ml every hour) and a further rise in the TPP effect (to 67%) compared to patients with neuropathy only, although statistical evaluation could not be carried out because of the very small number of patients. According to Brin (5) a TPP effect greater than 25% indicates vitamin B_1 deficiency, and Dreyfus (12) feels that mental changes become evident when the transketolase activity is reduced to 50% and thiamine level to 20% of the normal concentration in the brain. Applying both these criteria our patients with mental changes showed a poorer status of vitamin B_1 than those with neuropathy alone.

As Table 1 shows, the only vitamin that showed no fall in blood level and, in fact, showed an elevated mean value, although still within normal limits (130 to 730 pg/ml) compared to that in control subjects, was vitamin B_{12}. The only explanation that can be offered for this is an impairment of the normally very rich storage capacity of the liver for vitamin B_{12} due to the moderate hepatic insufficiency that prevailed in these patients as evidenced by the routine liver function tests (10). At this juncture it may also be clarified that none of these patients

TABLE 1. *Mean values and statistical evaluation of seven B vitamins in blood and five in CSF in controls and patients with malnutrition-alcoholic neuropathy*

Controls & categories of patients		Thiamine (ng/ml) Blood	Thiamine (ng/ml) CSF	Riboflavin (ng/ml) Blood	Riboflavin (ng/ml) CSF	Nicotinic acid (μg/ml) Blood	Nicotinic acid (μg/ml) CSF	Pantothenic acid (ng/ml) Blood	Pantothenic acid (ng/ml) CSF	Vitamin B_6 (ng/ml) Total Serum	Vitamin B_6 (ng/ml) Total CSF	Vitamin B_6 (ng/ml) Pyridoxal Serum	Folates (ng/ml) Blood	Vitamin B_{12} Total cyanide extracted (pg/ml) Serum
Normal control subjects	N	69	9	67	5	69	8	64	5	65	7	35	52	69
	Mean	39.0	12.90	272	130	3.63	2.08	277	228	37.20	6.40	4.02	5.45	292
	SD	±6.30	±2.22	±42	±26	±0.47	±0.28	±39	±33	±5.80	±1.20	±1.40	±2.74	±169
1. Patients with peripheral neuropathy only	N	38	21	34	12	38	16	31	10	40	15	20	45	46
	Mean	20.2	6.05	123	69	2.18	1.45	185	176	18.60	3.40	2.90	3.87	540
	SD	±6.6	±2.0	±33	±24	±0.70	±0.17	±51	±54	±3.60	±0.66	±0.42	±3.44	±297
2. Patients with peripheral neuropathy & mental changes	N	7	6	6	3	7	6	6	3	7	5	7	6	6
	Mean	9.40	2.01	108	32 75	1.56	0.84	216	330 150	15.02	1.65	1.71	5.58	514
	SD	±3.1	±0.42	±29	50	±0.50	±0.25	±82	130	±4.4	±0.30	±0.49	±2.30	±292

Statistical comparison symbols between groups (as shown in the table): Thiamine Blood **/**, Thiamine CSF **/**; Riboflavin Blood **/O, Riboflavin CSF **; Nicotinic acid Blood **/*, CSF **/**; Pantothenic acid Blood **/O, CSF O; Vitamin B_6 Serum **/*, Total CSF **/**, Pyridoxal Serum **/**; Folates Blood *; Vitamin B_{12} Serum **.

N, number of subjects; SD, standard deviation; O, not significant; *, p > 0.05; **, p > 0.001.

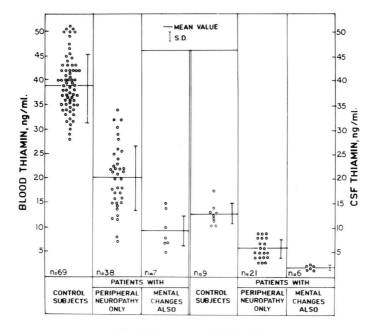

FIG. 1. Scattergram for thiamine.

with malnutrition-alcoholism evidenced any intestinal malabsorption as assessed by the tests mentioned under Laboratory and Related Methods. This was in clear contrast to the intestinal malabsorption noticed in all patients with B_{12}-deficiency neuromyelopathy, who had also shown an elevation of serum folate and a lowering of the vitamin B_6 level but not of the other B vitamins and a megaloblastic bone marrow (9), which was not detected in the present study.

The *treatment schedule* included withdrawal of alcohol and hospital diet only for the first 10 days, 50 mg nicotinic acid i.m. in patients with pellagroid skin changes and 50 mg thiamine i.m. in other patients for the next 10 days, hospital diet only for the following 10 days, another course of 10 injections of nicotinic acid or of thiamine depending on the response to the first course, 50 mg pyridoxine i.m. for 10 days to those who showed persistently low levels of this, 50 mg i.m. of pantothenic acid to those who had burning parasthesia predominantly, and a combination of two or

more of the above vitamins or of vitamin B complex for 10 days.

The result of this schedule was as follows: 18 patients improved on nicotinic acid; 13 on thiamine; six on hospital diet alone; four on a combination of two or three of the above vitamins; two on vitamin B complex; and one each on pantothenate or pyridoxine. On the whole it was apparent that administration of thiamine alone led to its own increase and that of riboflavin, nicotinic acid, and pantothenic acid; of nicotinic acid to its own increase and that of thiamine and riboflavin; and of pyridoxine to its own increase and that of riboflavin. This applied to patients with mental changes as well, four of the six of whom improved considerably, just as did 41 of 43 patients with peripheral neuropathy alone, only 49 in all having taken adequate treatment. Details of the vitaminologic and clinical response of one patient from each of the two categories have been given in our earlier report (10).

In the only other published investigation of estimations of multiple B vitamins in alcoholic subjects with malnutrition, Fennelly et al. (15) observed, like us, a simultaneous decrease in the circulating levels of all the five B vitamins they assayed. Thiamine was the most severely reduced vitamin, and replacement therapy with it alone was associated with maximal clinical benefit. Although they have not done sequential estimation of all the vitamins during treatment with one of them, Fennelly et al. also conclude that the nutriture of the patients before and during the alcoholic habit is the important factor determining the clinical outcome. Moreover, there is increased vitamin requirement in alcoholism, probably to compensate for decreased hepatic storage as well as to repair damaged cells (18). Baker and Frank (4) reported a higher incidence of hypovitaminemia in malnourished alcoholics with cirrhosis or fatty liver than in those without. In decreasing order, folic acid, vitamin B_6, thiamine, nicotinic acid, and riboflavin were found to be the more commonly deficient vitamins in the blood.

The finding of initially very low blood vitamin levels in our patients, the small but significant elevation in these levels on hospital diet alone, and the further rise in level of two, three, or four vitamins after administration of only one of them (as outlined above), strongly suggested an *interrelationship between the B vitamins*. This has been presented elsewhere (10) in the form of a scheme, but the salient features are as follows.

1. Generalized dietetic insufficiency produces deficiency of thiamine, riboflavin, nicotinic acid, pantothenic acid, total vitamin B_6, folates, and proteins.

2. The latter leads to further secondary thiamine deficiency (3).

3. Thiamine deficiency precipitates secondary deficiency of riboflavin by augmenting its urinary excretion (31).

4. In the presence of nicotinate deficiency, body stores of riboflavin tend to be depleted (33).

5. Lack of proteins, especially of milk products, also leads to ariboflavinosis (25).

6. The latter condition causes further pantothenate deficiency (30).

7. With vitamin B_6 deficiency in the presence of insufficient flavine adenine nucleotide there is inadequate formation of the active principle pyridoxal (36).

8. Similarly there is decreased production of active tetrahydrofolate from a primary short supply of folates (33).

Summary and Conclusions

The above observations bring out some interesting features of the problem of malnutrition-alcoholism as we observed it in Bombay.

1. Our patients had a less severe degree of alcoholism and a more chronic background of malnutrition than similar patients from Western countries, such as those reported by Victor and Adams (34) or Leevy and Baker (17) and often had a fairly good response to hospital diet alone, although this diet provided less than the daily minimum requirement of B vitamins (29).

2. A truly complex and multiple B vitamin deficiency prevails in this condition, involving all the B vitamins tested except B_{12}.

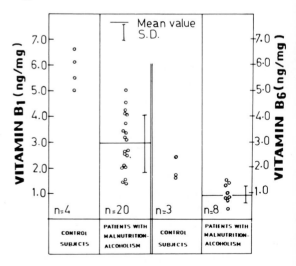

FIG. 2. Scattergram for thiamine levels.

3. Our material has provided an interesting model for the study of metabolic inter-relationships between many of these B vitamins, especially as revealed by the rise in blood levels of two or more vitamins after the therapeutic administration of only one, such as thiamine or nicotinic acid.

4. The effect of alcohol on the nervous system, and at least the peripheral neuropathy, is mediated through malnutrition and particularly a deficiency of the B vitamins that are needed as co-factors in the complete oxidation of ethanol to acetaldehyde and acetic acid (17).

5. The CSF appeared to reflect better than the blood levels the B vitamin status affecting the central nervous system, especially as revealed in the patients with mental changes, who were more severe alcoholics than those with peripheral neuropathy only.

B Vitamins in the Peripheral Nerves

Our observations on nerve vitamins, limited though they are, constitute a legitimate link between the vitamin assays and the nerve histology. Only two of the B vitamins could be assayed in the nerve – thiamine and total vitamin B_6 – and, because of paucity of control material, statistical comparison could not be made between the levels in normal subjects and patients. The scattergram (Fig. 2) shows that in patients the level of thiamine in 19 of 20 nerves and the level of vitamin B_6 in seven of eight

TABLE 2. *Nerve fiber counts and diameters and type of degeneration, and nerve thiamine in patients with malnutrition-alcoholic/peripheral neuropathy*

Serial no.	N-P[b] no.	Age (yr)	Myelinated fibers			Type of nerve degeneration	Nerve thiamine (ng/ml)
			per mm^2	2 μm <(%)	8 μm >(%)		
1.	F/941	45	3,007	31	3	Myelin clefts ++ Normal +	—
2.	G/397	40	9,280 7,882	29 21	26 4	Axonal + Normal +	—
3.	G/398	23	3,240 4,643 10,070	2 3 4	52 55 0	Myelin clefts ++ Axonal + Normal +	4.50
4.	G/447	38	1,430	2	43	Axonal + Normal +	3.70
5.	G/471	26	4,510 3,182 1,900	5 7 6	17 40 63	Axonal + Segmental + Normal +	2.45
6.	G/536	31	4,292	0	46	Axonal + Segmental + Normal +	2.07
7.	G/558	42	3,438	0	57	Axonal ++ Normal +	4.20
8.	G/712	30	1,786	0	38	Axonal ++ Segmental + Normal +	1.35
9.	G/925	50	3,180	—	—	Axonal ++ Segmental + Normal +	—
10.	H/289	45	7,273	36	13	---	3.40
11.	H/608	61	2,898	20	26	Axonal ++ Normal +	4.10
12.	H/655	42	945	13	7	---	—
	Means:	39.4	4,292[a]	11.0	30.6		

[a] Seventeen bundles in 12 nerves
[b] N-P, neuropathology reference number

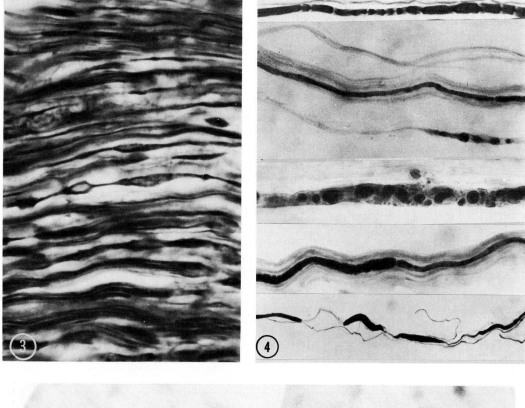

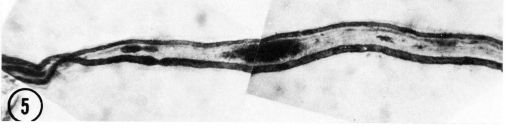

FIG. 3. (NP/F-472). Degenerating axons in the center with irregular thickenings or varicosities; thin fibers in small groups along the sides. Holmes' silver. ×880.

FIG. 4. Composite picture of five nerve fiber groups from four different nerves. The upper three pictures show three different stages of axonal degeneration, the earliest (*upper fiber*) showing cutting of myelin into unequal segments at points of increase of Schmidt-Lantermann incisures. The second and third group show advanced axonal degeneration with formation of myelin droplets filling the Schwann tube (*third picture*) and empty sheaths representing degenerated fibers (*second picture*). The lower two fiber groups show two stages of segmental demyelination, the fourth showing contrast between normal internode and thinner partially (?) demyelinated or regenerated (?) internode. The fifth picture shows clear demyelinated segments along two fibers. Teased fibers, Sudan black. From above downwards. ×180, ×260, ×480, ×140, ×70, respectively.

FIG. 5. (NP/F-455). Montage of a group of three myelinated fibers, the central one showing segmental demyelination in the left half, a large mass of degenerated myelin in the center, and total axonal degeneration in the right half of the picture. The upper and lower fibers are well myelinated. Sudan black. ×150.

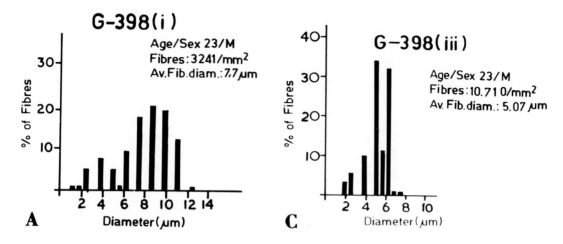

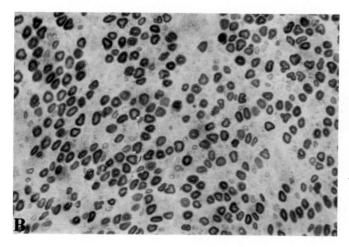

FIG. 6. (NP/G/398). **A:** Myelinated fiber-size spectrum of one nerve bundle showing over 50% of fibers above 8 μm in size, despite the very low fiber count. **B:** Another funiculus of same nerve showing good preservation of fibers of an almost uniform size. Semithin araldite section, toluidine blue. ×625. **C:** Histogram of this showing majority of fibers in the narrow range of 5 to 7 μm.

nerves was clearly lower than the lowest level in the nerves from normal subjects. As there seems to be no published data whatsoever on vitamin levels in nerves, one cannot compare the mean values we obtained for thiamine (2.95 ng/mg) and for total vitamin B_6 (0.92 ng/mg) in patients with malnutrition-alcoholism with the vitamin levels in the nerve in any other disease. Table 2 gives the nerve thiamine level in eight of the 12 patients listed. On the whole there appeared to be fair correlation between the level of B vitamins in the nerves

and the histologic changes observed in them. Thus in cases 3, 5, and 8 there was fair correlation, low fiber counts and severe axonal degeneration accompanying low thiamine levels. Occasionally there was no clear correlation as in cases 7 and 11 (Table 2).

It is interesting to recall here the elegant work of Yonezawa, Murray, and their associates (41) on ganglion and Schwann cell cultures, showing that transketolase is essential for myelin-supporting cells. Thiamine deficiency was brought about by using

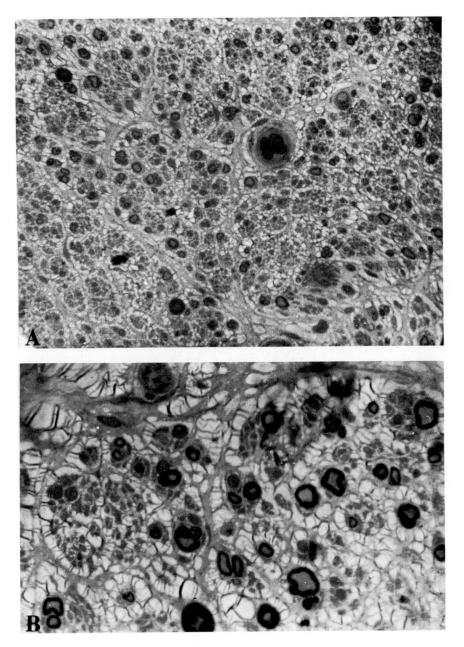

FIG. 7. Legend on facing page.

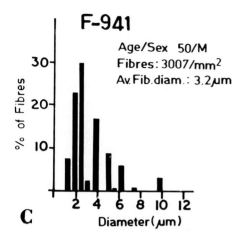

C

FIG. 7. (NP/F-941). **A:** Generalized depletion of large and medium-sized myelinated fibers. Semithin araldite section, toluidine blue. ×250. **B:** Closer view of another part of same bundle, showing that many of the very small myelinated fibers are in groups of two or three and occupy the Schwann cells of unmyelinated fibers which are clearly revealed here. Semithin araldite section, toluidine blue. ×880. **C:** Histogram of the same fiber bundle showing a descending stepladder pattern, with the majority of fibers in the 2 to 4 μm range.

the chemical analog oxythiamine (42), which probably produced inactivation of transketolase, a requirement in the development and maintenance of myelin (12). Yonezawa et al. (43) also produced vitamin B_6 deficiency by using the antivitamin analog desoxypyridoxine, whereby there was primary degeneration of spinal ganglion cells in culture with axonal degeneration and secondary myelin loss. Baker and Frank (4) describe chronic alcoholic subjects with anemia and neuropathy who have an almost selective deficiency of vitamin B_6 and who respond to pyridoxine therapy.

Summary and Conclusions

The peripheral neuropathy of malnutrition and alcoholism appears related to a deficiency of the B vitamins in the nerve, at least of thiamine. Estimations of this and other B vitamins in nerves are called for in other metabolic neuropathies, such as diabetes, and in normal nerves.

Histopathology of Peripheral Nerves

Of the 36 sural nerve biopsies examined through *paraffin sections,* four showed severe degenerative changes, seven moderate, 21 mild, one no appreciable change,

and on three no comment was possible. Moderate diffuse proliferation of Schwann cells, depletion of myelin, patchy loss of axons (especially the thicker ones), and mild diffuse endoneurial fibrosis constituted the principal changes. At sites of loss of large axons there was usually a relative prominence of very fine smooth axons, suggesting attempts at regeneration. Figure 3 shows how degenerating beaded axons were seen alongside groups of very fine fibers, in a silver-impregnated section. That some of the thin axons could belong to remaining unmyelinated fiber groups became apparent when the corresponding myelin preparations (Picro-Mallory stain) showed clearly fewer nerve fibers.

Summarizing the earlier histopathologic findings of alcoholic peripheral neuropathy, Victor (35) stressed the greater involvement of distal segments of nerves, the presence of both myelin and axon degeneration, and the accumulation of myelin breakdown products in the more active stages. These changes have now been shown in the autonomic nerves also (20). Among the first to carry out experimental studies in B vitamin deficiency, especially of thiamine, to study its effect on the nervous system and to compare the changes to those in human alcoholism and beriberi was Zimmerman

(44). Then came the investigations of Swank and Prados (32), Follis (16), and others.

Teased fiber preparations were possible in 23 cases. In 18 nerves a combination of axonal degeneration and of normally myelinated fibers was evident. Only four nerves showed segmental demyelination, and this accompanied fibers undergoing axonal degeneration. The findings in 12 of the nerves are summarized in Table 2. Predominant axonal degeneration has been reported in alcoholic neuropathy in one case each by O'Sullivan and Swallow (23) and Dyck et al. (13), and in a few more cases by Walsh and McCleod (37).

It was interesting to note the stages of axonal degeneration that this material provided. The upper three fibers or fiber groups (from three different cases) in Fig. 4 show this. The uppermost strand demonstrates the earliest stage of an irregular increase in the number of Schmidt–Lantermann clefts in the myelin sheath. This has been shown to be the beginning of axonal degeneration in experimental neurectomy (38) and in at least one other neuropathy in man, that being leprosy (7,8). The second group of fibers in Fig. 4 shows one normal myelinated fiber, another with a few droplets of degenerated myelin remaining, and a number of empty sheaths probably representing remnants of totally degenerate fibers. The third picture from the top (G-536) shows more active degeneration of myelin with droplets of varying size. The fourth and fifth pictures show two stages of segmental demyelination, the upper one (G-925) showing thinning of the fiber with depletion of myelin in the internode on the right. The lowest picture in Fig. 4 shows clear segmental demyelination affecting two fibers.

In two of the 23 nerves examined by the teased fiber technique, the interesting phenomenon of one fiber with both axonal degeneration and segmental demyelination was observed. Thus, in Fig. 5, whereas the upper and lower fibers are normally myelinated, the central fiber shows segmental demyelination (*on left*) and then axonal degeneration, perhaps more distally. Dyck et al. (14) have reported similar axonal degeneration in cases of uremic neuropathy in the distal part of a sural nerve showing segmental demyelination more proximally and have suggested that the demyelination was a consequence of the more severe axonal degenerative change.

Quantitative Histology on Araldite Sections

Myelinated fiber counts were possible in 17 funiculi in 12 of the sural nerves biopsied. These data are summarized in Table 2. The mean fiber density for 17 funiculi was only 4,292 fibers/mm². This is considerably below the average myelinated fiber density in the sural nerve of normal adults of about 7,000 to 10,000/mm² as reported by Ochoa and Mair (21) and Dyck et al. (13). We observed the same in a few control specimens. The nerves from patients with malnutrition-alcoholism showed a marked variation in fiber count from nerve to nerve, the lowest count being 945 and the highest 10,070 fibers/mm² (Table 2). Of equal interest was the fact that there was often a marked difference in counts between two or more bundles of the same nerve, as illustrated by cases 3 and 5 in Table 2.

The histograms of myelinated fiber diameters further brought out the fact that the absence or suppression of the normal bimodal pattern of distribution bore no relationship to the fiber count, relatively normal fiber counts being associated with a loss of large myelinated fibers and vice versa. This is illustrated in Fig. 6 where one bundle with a clearly low fiber count evidences a fair preservation of the larger fibers (Fig. 6A), and another bundle with a

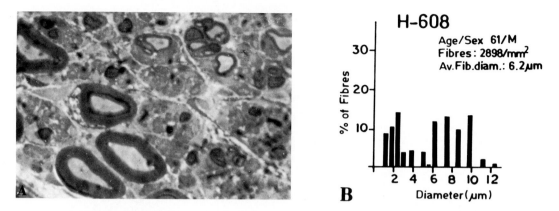

FIG. 8. (NP/H-608). **A:** Semithin section of another nerve with a low fiber count showing well-preserved large myelinated fibers, one with prominent Schmidt-Lantermann cleft and vacuolation of Schwann cytoplasm. Note the probably regenerating small myelinated fibers occupying Schwann cells of unmyelinated fibers and their prominent nuclei. Semithin araldite section, toluidine blue. ×1,400. **B:** Histogram of fibers of the same bundle showing a bimodal pattern of distribution.

normal fiber count, obviously replete with myelinated fibers (Fig. 6B), shows most of them in the narrow range of 5 to 7 μm (Fig. 6C). It is interesting to compare the percentage of fibers below 2 and above 8 μm, respectively, in this and other nerves as given in Table 2. Ochoa and Mair (21) had found that in the normal sural nerve 40 to 50% of the myelinated fibers were more than 8 μm in size. A diffuse depletion of large and prominence of small myelinated fibers are illustrated in Fig. 7A and B and reflected in the histogram (Fig. 7C). Small thin myelinated fibers occupying the Schwann cells of unmyelinated fiber groups, as in Figs. 7B and 8A, suggested regenerat-

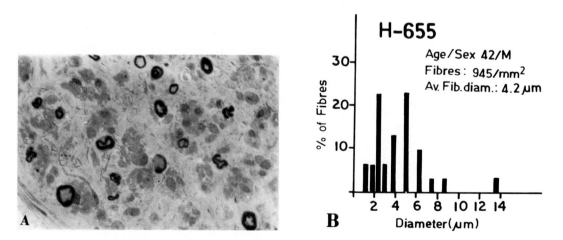

FIG. 9. (NP/H/655). **A:** A part of the bundle shows severe depletion of myelinated fibers, most of the remainder being of small size; prominence of nuclei of Schwann cells of unmyelinated fibers. **B:** Histogram of fibers of the same bundle (with the lowest count in this series) showing peaks at 3 and 5 μm, respectively.

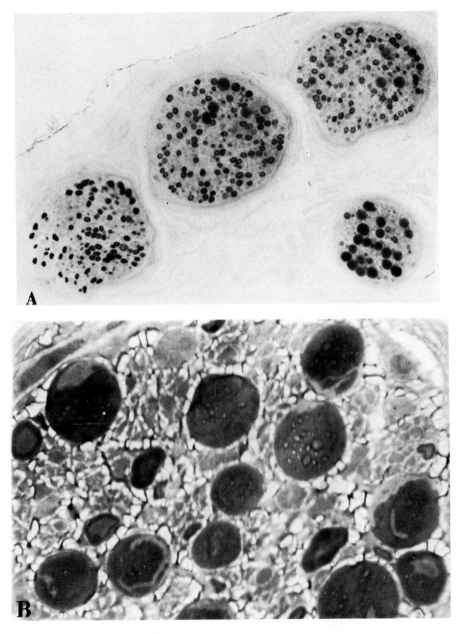

FIG. 10. Legend on facing page.

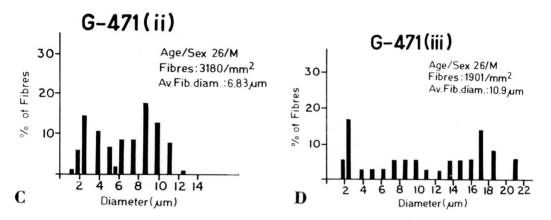

FIG. 10. (NP/G-471). **A:** Four complete funiculi in one semithin section, showing both loss of myelinated fibers and variation in their size. Note the small bundle with swollen osmiophilic fibers. Semithin araldite section, toluidine blue. ×120. **B:** Closer view of the large osmiophilic fibers in the small funiculus presenting a homogenous vacuolated appearance suggesting degeneration. Semithin araldite section, toluidine blue. ×880. **C:** Histogram of large bundle in the center of **A** showing a bimodal pattern of distribution. **D:** Histogram of the fibers in the small bundle showing excessive variation of fiber size and 50% of fibers above 12 μm in size (including most of the degenerating fibers).

ing fibers. The striking preservation of large myelinated fibers in the nerve in Fig. 8A finds correspondence in the typical bimodal histogram in Fig. 8B, despite the reduced fiber density (case 11, Table 2). The nerve most severely depleted of myelinated fibers (case 12 in Table 2 and Fig. 9A) had most of the remaining fibers in the 2 to 7 μm range (Fig. 9B).

Possible degeneration in the remaining large or medium-sized myelinated fibers was encountered in seven of the 17 funiculi. This generally took the form of swelling, osmiophilia, and homogenization of the fiber as seen in the small nerve bundle in Fig. 10A and B. The very large-sized fibers above 12 μm in size in Fig. 10D were possibly degenerating, and should really be discounted in computing the fiber count and diameters. Corrected this way, the myelinated fiber count in the small funiculus in Fig. 10A falls to a fourth of the already low count of 1,900 fibers/mm² (Table 2). This nerve (Fig. 10A) also exemplifies the variation in fiber populations in the funiculi of one nerve; the other three funiculi showed obviously greater densities and

fewer degenerating fibers than the small bundle.

The *fine structural changes* observed in three of these nerves, confirmed, on the one hand, the loss or degeneration of the large myelinated fibers, and revealed, on the other hand, changes in the unmyelinated fibers. Figure 11A shows the formation of myelin ovoids in one of the fibers and the commencement of myelin degeneration and accumulation of debris in the split in the myelin sheath, which possibly represented a distended Schmidt-Lantermann cleft. Fig. 11B shows a few remaining unmyelinated fibers floating in a sea of collagen. There are also proliferated Schwann cell membranes arranged in stacks and devoid of axons, suggesting formation of bands of Büngner at sites of degeneration of unmyelinated fibers. Both these patients were aged 45 years, but similar changes in myelinated and unmyelinated fibers have been reported in normal aging (22).

Two experimental studies worth recalling here are those of Collins et al. (6) and Roy et al. (27). The former found that rats manifested comparable neuropathy after

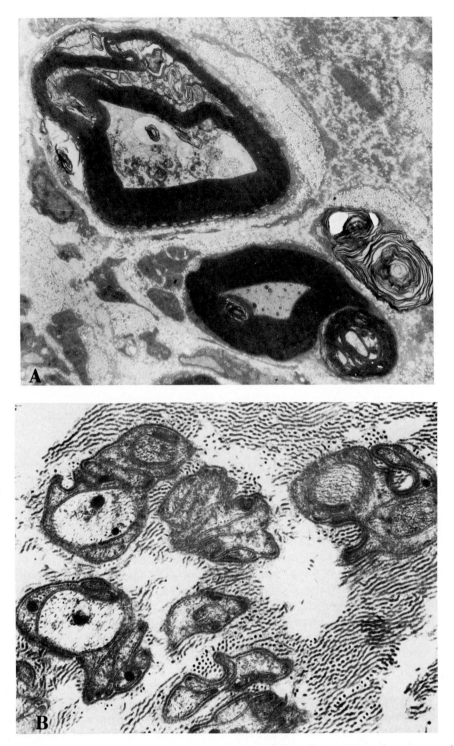

FIG. 11. A: (NP/H-289). One large and one medium-sized myelinated fiber, with prominent axon and myelin degeneration in the large fiber where myelin figures have accumulated in a widened Schmidt-Lantermann cleft. The smaller fiber with a large myelin ovoid in the Schwann cytoplasm measured 8.8 μm in diameter with an axon of 2.8 μm. Note increased collagen, fibroblasts, and Schwann cell processes in the endoneurium. B: (NP/F-941). Remaining unmyelinated fibers and Schwann cells with basement membrane in another nerve (same as in Fig. 7). Note the fan-like stack of Schwann processes in the center forming a band of Büngner. Osmicated araldite sections, stained with uranyl acetate and lead citrate. A: ×3,880. B: ×21,000.

prolonged restriction of food or after with-drawal of thiamine from the diet. EMscopy of the nerves suggested primary changes in the axons, with secondary myelin break-down. Roy et al., studying the effects of protein deficiency in rhesus monkeys, re-ported changes in peripheral nerves in 9 weeks, with the formation of irregular myelin nodules compressing the axons.

SUMMARY AND CONCLUSIONS

Our histologic studies on sural nerve biopsies from patients with peripheral neuropathy caused by malnutrition-alcohol-ism emphasize the value of quantitative data. The myelinated fiber count has been found to vary from the very low to the normal, with overall reduction in a group of 12 patients, the count also varying be-tween different funiculi of the same nerve. Fiber-diameter spectra showed more fre-quent depletion of the larger fibers, with a roughly unimodal distribution or a shift of the normal bimodality to the left. Both enlarged degenerating or small regenerating fibers (utilizing Schwann cells of unmyeli-nated fibers), or both, were encountered in about half the specimens and indicated an active neuropathy. EMscopy in three cases confirmed the myelin degeneration and also showed degeneration of unmyelinated fibers and proliferation of their Schwann cells.

Teased fiber preparations revealed ax-onal degeneration in various stages in 22 of 23 nerves stained for myelin. Four of these showed segmental demyelination as well, the two processes being at times en-countered on the same fiber. Silver im-pregnation showed degenerating and possi-bly regenerating axons, and connective tissue stain varying endoneurial fibrosis.

ACKNOWLEDGMENTS

These studies were made possible by Research Grant No. 01.011-1 from the National Institutes of Health, Bethesda, Maryland during 1970-1973, through donations collected by the Neuropathology Unit from the Public of Bombay during 1974-1975, and by being operated by The Research Society—Grant Medical College and J. J. Group of Hospitals. Grateful acknowledgment is due Dr. N. H. Wadia, Honorary Professor of Neurology, Dr. M. M. Desai of the J. J. Hospitals, Dr. E. P. Bharucha, Emeritus Professor of Neurol-ogy, Dr. P. G. Varaiya of the K. E. M. Hospital, Bombay, for the clinical col-laboration, the late Dr. F. C. R. Avari for the liver function tests, the Council of Scientific and Industrial Research for the support of one of us (Dr. Manghani), Dr. E. V. Quadros for the vitamin B_{12} assays, V. P. Kate for the routine histology, and N. Solanki for photographic printing at the Neuropathology Unit.

REFERENCES

1. Anderson, B. B., Peart, M. B., and Fullford Jones, C. E. (1970): The measurement of serum pyridoxal by a microbiological assay using Lactobacillus casei. *J. Clin. Pathol.,* 23:232–242.
2. Armstrong, B. K., and Woodliffe, H. J. (1970): Studies on the ^{57}Co vitamin B_{12} plasma level absorption test. *J. Clin. Pathol.,* 23:569–571.
3. Baker, H., and Frank, O. (1968): Chapters 1, 2, 4, 5, 6, and 7. In: *Clinical Vitaminology: Methods and Interpretations,* pp. 1–238. Wiley (Inter-science), New York.
4. Baker, H., and Frank, O. (1968): Vitamin status in metabolic upsets. In: *World Review of Nutri-tion and Dietetics,* Vol. 9, pp. 124–160. Karger, Basel.
5. Brin, M. (1962): Erythrocyte transketolase in early thiamine deficiency. *Ann. NY Acad. Sci.,* 98:528–541.
6. Collins, G. H., Webster, H. de F., and Victor, M. (1964): The ultrastructure of myelin and axonal alterations in sciatic nerves of thiamine deficient and chronically starved rats. *Acta Neuropathol.* (*Berl.*), 3:511–521.
7. Dastur, D. K., and Razzak, Z. A. (1971): De-generation and regeneration in teased nerve fibers. I: Leprous neuritis. *Acta Neuropathol. (Berl.),* 18:286–298.
8. Dastur, D. K., Ramamohan, Y., and Shah, J. S. (1973): Ultrastructure of lepromatous nerves. Neural pathogenesis in leprosy. *Int. J. Lepr.,* 41:47–80.
9. Dastur, D. K., Santhadevi, N., Quadros, E. V.,

Gagrat, B. M., Wadia, N. H., Desai, M. M., Singhal, B. S., and Bharucha, E. P. (1975): Inter-relationships between the B-vitamins in B_{12} deficiency-neuromyelopathy. A possible mal-absorption-malnutrition syndrome. *Am. J. Clin. Nutr.*, 28:1255–1270.

10. Dastur, D. K., Santhadevi, N., Quadros, E. V., Avari, F. C. R., Wadia, N. H., Desai, M. M., and Bharucha, E. P. (1976): The B-vitamins in malnutrition with alcoholism. A model of inter-vitamin relationships. *Br. J. Nutr.*, 36:143–159.

11. Dreyfus, P. M. (1962): Clinical application of blood transketolase determinations. *N. Engl. J. Med.*, 267:596–598.

12. Dreyfus, P. M. (1967): Transketolase activity in the nervous system. In: *Thiamine Deficiency: Biochemical Lesions and Their Clinical Signifi-cance*, Ciba Found. Study Group No. 28, edited by G. E. W. Wolsten Holme, p. 103. Churchill, London.

13. Dyck, P. J., Gutrecht, J. A., Bastron, J. A., Karnes, W. E., and Dale, A. J. D. (1968): Histo-logic and teased-fiber measurements of sural nerve in disorders of lower motor and primary sensory neurons. *Proc. Mayo Clin.*, 43:81–123.

14. Dyck, P. J., Johnson, W. J., Lambert, E. H., and O'Brien, P. C. (1971): Segmental demyelination secondary to axonal degeneration in uremic neuropathy. *Proc. Mayo Clin.*, 46:400–431.

15. Fennelly, J., Frank, O., Baker, H., and Leevy, C. M. (1964): Peripheral neuropathy of the alcoholic. I: Aetiological role of aneurin and other B-complex vitamins. *Br. Med. J.*, 2:1290–1292.

16. Follis, R. H. (1948): The pathologic anatomy of specific tissues. A recapitulation and comparison. In: *The Pathology of Nutritional Disease*, edited by R. H. Follis, p. 234. Charles C Thomas, Springfield, Ill.

17. Leevy, C. M., and Baker, H. (1963): Metabolic and nutritional effects of alcoholism. *Arch. Environ. Health*, 7:453–

18. Leevy, C. M., Thompson, A., and Baker, H. (1970): Vitamins and liver injury. *Am. J. Clin. Nutr.*, 23:493–498.

19. Matthews, D. M., Gunasegaram, R., and Linnell, J. C. (1967): Results with radioisotopic assay of serum B_{12} using serum binding agent. *J. Clin. Pathol.*, 20:683–686.

20. Novak, D. J., and Victor, M. (1974): The vagus and sympathetic nerves in alcoholic polyneurop-athy. *Arch. Neurol.*, 30:273–284.

21. Ochoa, J., and Mair, W. G. P. (1969): The normal sural nerve in man. I: Ultrastructure and numbers of fibres and cells. *Acta Neuropathol. (Berl.)*, 13:197–216.

22. Ochoa, J., and Mair, W. G. P. (1969): The normal sural nerve in man. II: Changes in the axons and Schwann cells due to aging. *Acta Neuropathol. (Berl.)*, 13:217–239.

23. O'Sullivan, D. J., and Swallow, M. (1968): The fibre size and content of the radial and sural nerves. *J. Neurol. Neurosurg. Psychiatry*, 31:464–470.

24. Pauling, L. (1968): Orthomolecular psychiatry. *Science*, 160:265–271.

25. Rasmussen, F. (1958): The riboflavin requirement of animals and man and associated metabolic relations. Part II: Relation of requirement to the metabolism of protein and energy. *Nutr. Abstr. Rev.*, 28:369–386.

26. Reitman, S., and Frankel, S. (1957): A calori-metric method for the determination of serum glutamic oxalacetic acid and glutamin pyruvic transaminases. *Am. J. Clin. Pathol.*, 28:56–63.

27. Roy, S., Singh, N., Deo, M. G., and Rama-lingaswami, V. (1972): Ultrastructure of skeletal muscle and peripheral nerve in experimental protein deficiency and its correlation with nerve conduction studies. *J. Neurol. Sci.*, 17:399–409.

28. Sammons, H. G., Morgan, D. B., Frazer, A. C., Montgomery, R. D., Philip, W. M., and Philips, M. J. (1967): Modification in the xylose absorp-tion test as an index of intestinal function. *Gut*, 8:348–353.

29. Santhadevi, N. (1974): Nutritional disorders of the nervous system. The B-vitamins. Thesis, pp. 1–147. Univ. Bombay, India.

30. Spies, T. D., Hightower, D. P., and Hubbard, L. H. (1940): Some recent advances in vitamin therapy. *JAMA*, 115:292–297.

31. Sure, B. (1944): Vitamin interrelationships. III: Influence of suboptimum doses of thiamine on urinary excretions of riboflavin. *J. Nutr.*, 27:447–452.

32. Swank, R. L., and Prados, M. (1942): Avian thiamine deficiency. II. Pathologic changes in the brain and cranial nerves (especially the vestibular) and their relation to the clinical be-haviour. *Arch. Neurol. Psychiatr. (Chic.)*, 47:97–131.

33. Tamburro, C., Frank, O., Thompson, A. D., Sorrell, M. F., and Baker, H. (1971): Quoted by Santhadevi, N., ref. 29 above.

34. Victor, M., and Adams, R. D. (1953): The effect of alcohol upon the nervous system. *Assoc. Res. Nerv. Ment. Dis. Proc.*, 32:526–573.

35. Victor, M. (1965): The effects of nutritional deficiency on the nervous system. A comparison with the effects of carcinoma. In: *The Remote Effects of Cancer on the Nervous System*, edited by L. Brain, and F. H. Norris, Jr., p. 134. Grune & Stratton, New York.

36. Wada, H., and Snell, E. E. (1961): The enzymatic oxidation of pyridoxine and pyridoxamine phos-phates. *J. Biol. Chem.*, 236:2089–2095.

37. Walsh, J. C., and McLeod, J. G. (1970): Alco-holic neuropathy: An electrophysiological and histological study. *J. Neurol. Sci.*, 10:457–469.

38. Webster, H. de F. (1965): Research in demyeli-nating diseases. *Ann. NY Acad. Sci.*, 122:29–38.

39. Wooton, I. D. P. (1964): Plasma proteins. In: *Microanalysis in Medical Biochemistry*, p. 146. Churchill, London.

40. Wortis, H., Stein, M. H., and Joliffe, N. (1942): Fibre dissociation in peripheral neuropathy. *Arch. Intern. Med.*, 69:222–237.

41. Yonezawa, T., Bornstein, M. B., Peterson, E. R.,

and Murray, M. R. (1962): A histochemical study of oxidative enzymes in myelinating cultures of central and peripheral nervous tissue. *J. Neuropathol. Exp. Neurol.,* 21:479–487.

42. Yonezawa, T., and Iwanami, H. (1966): An experimental study of thiamine deficiency in nervous tissue, using tissue culture techniques. *J. Neuropathol. Exp. Neurol.,* 25:362–372.

43. Yonezawa, T., Mari, T., and Nakatani, Y. (1969): Effects of pyridoxine deficiency in nervous tissue maintained in vitro. *Ann. NY Acad. Sci.,* 166: 146–157.

44. Zimmerman, H. M. (1943): Pathology of vitamin B group deficiencies. *Res. Publ. Assoc. Nerv. Ment. Dis.,* 22:51–79.

Neurotoxicology, edited by L. Roizin, H. Shiraki, and N. Grčević. Raven Press, New York © 1977.

Hepatotropic Effects of Phenothiazines and Narcotics: Histopathologic and Electron Microscope Observations

*Albert Goldfield, **Leon Roizin, **Shigeo Hashimoto, and **Jevons C. Liu

*Buffalo Psychiatric Center, Buffalo, New York 14213; and **New York State Psychiatric Institute, New York, New York 10032

It is not our aim to review, in this neurotoxicologic volume, the complete spectrum of liver dysfunctions or pathology associated with the use of neuropsychotropic agents. This would require another volume. Here we would like merely to draw attention to the fact that among the viscerotropic effects of neuropsychotropic agents the hepatobiliary system may also present adverse and toxic reactions following the administration of phenothiazines and narcotics.

PHENOTHIAZINES

Human Studies

A sample of the clinicopathologic aspects of the liver biopsies and postmortem material is summarized in Table 1.[1]

Material and Methods

Selected liver specimens from biopsies and postmortem material were processed for histopathologic methods including the use of frozen and paraffin sections stained with hematoxylin and eosin, Masson's trichrome, phosphotungstic-acid-Schiff (PAS) for mucopolysaccharides, Best for glycogen, and Sudan III for lipids (44). Unstained sections were examined with polarized and ultraviolet microscopes.

Results

The study of a total of 322 postmortem cases and nine biopsies revealed that liver dysfunctions were more frequently observed in females than in males, that it occurred predominantly with chlorpromazine treatment, that its duration varied between 4 to 130 days, and that it developed at variable dosages, i.e., 25 to 1,600 mg per day. Thus, it would seem that liver dysfunction is not directly related to dosage or duration of treatment.

In the vast majority of cases, the jaundice and liver dysfunction were confirmed by laboratory tests and/or liver biopsies. In both instances, it appeared that they were related predominantly to a biliary stasis, and in those cases in which biopsy of the liver was done, the architecture of the liver was well preserved, except in a few instances in which moderate lipid degeneration was noted. In the large majority of the

---

[1] This material was obtained through the kind cooperation of psychiatric and developmental centers of the Mental Hygiene Department of the State of New York.

TABLE 1. *Clinical-pathological aspects of liver biopsies and autopsy material of patients treated with phenothiazines*

Diagnosis	Age, sex	Drug dosage daily	Duration of Rx	Clinical findings	Outcome	Pathological findings
D.P. paranoid type. Epileptic seizures?	43, M	Chlpr. 100–1200, Equanil 100 mg, ECT 6.	158 days	Epileptic seizures?	Death due to pulmonary edema.	Gross: Chronic interstitial pneumonia, bilateral, severe. Acute congestion of viscera. Arteriosclerosis, coronary arteries.
D.P. catatonic type.	55, F	Chlpr. 300 mg	14 days	Liver dysfunction. Laparotomy, external drainage of common bile duct.	Death due to postcholedochostomy with secondary infection, pulmonary congestion and edema.	Gross: Icterus of tissue and viscera, abscess of drainage tract, serofibrinous peritonitis, acute enlargement of spleen, fibrosis of ovaries, obesity, Laennec's cirrhosis.
D.P. hebephrenic type.	53, F	Chlpr. 150–250 mg., Dilantin 1½ gr., Phenobarbital 1 g, Phenergan unknown, Cogentin 2 mg	142 days	Post-lobotomy epileptiform seizures.	Death due to bronchopneumonia, bilateral, severe.	Gross: Bronchopneumonia, coronary artery disease, chronic congestion of abdominal viscera.
Mental deficiency.	14, M	Serpasil 1–2.5 mg. Chlpr. 200–150 mg with electrostim. (10)	102 days	Epileptic seizures.	Death due to cardiac arrest with acute dilatation of heart.	Gross: Acute dilatation of heart, right ventricle; apneumatosis of lungs, acute congestion of kidneys, liver, and spleen. Microscopic: Periportal and mild peribiliary fibrosis with slight lymphocytic infiltration.
Manic-depressive psychosis, manic state, alcoholism.	52, F	Serpasil 12 mg, Chlpr. 100 mg plus Serpasil 4 mg.	97 days	Discoloration of body, unsteady gait, sialorrhea, difficulty in swallowing.	Death due to pulmonary edema and congestion from aspiration of feeding tube, 32 days after first symptom.	Gross: Acute pulmonary edema and congestion, hydrothorax, pachymeningitis hemorrhagica with contusion of skull, chronic cholelithiasis and cholecystitis. Microscopic: Peribiliary and periportal fibrosis, biliary pigments in renal tubules.

Diagnosis	Age, Sex	Drug/Dosage	Duration	Clinical findings	Outcome	Pathology
D.P. paranoid type.	49, F	Chlpr. 68 mg Cogentin 3 mg.	21 days	Agranulocytosis.	Death due to bronchopneumonia and agranulocytosis.	Gross: Bronchopneumonia, petechial hemorrhages lungs, liver, myocardium, kidneys, spleen. Generalized adenitis. Microscopic: Petechial hemorrhages on surface and around hepatic lobules (fig. XVIII.8).
Huntington's chorea with psychosis.	58, M	Chlpr. 150–300 plus Serpasil 1–3 mg.	112 days	PEG cortical atrophy. Internal hydrocephalus. Temperature 103.	Death due to bronchopneumonia? aspiration pneumonia? 14 days after first fever.	Gross: Congestion of liver and kidneys, edema of brain. See neuropathologic table XVIII.2.
D.P. paranoid type.	51, F	Chlpr. 75 mg.	127 days	Temperature 101. Loose stools. Vomiting. Acutely ill.	Death due to acute hemorrhagic pancreatitis due to stenosis of papilla of Vater.	Gross: Pulmonary congestion and edema, hemorrhagic pancreatitis, fatty infiltration of liver. Microscopic: Fatty infiltration of liver.
Psychosis with cerebral arteriosclerosis.	58, M	Chlpr. 50 mg i.m.	120 days	Jaundice, obstructive type.	Death 13 months after the onset, due to hepatorenal disease.	Gross: Generalized jaundice of tissues. Microscopic: Biliary stasis, central portion of lobules, with biliary thrombi; mild fatty degeneration of hepatic cells, central zone.
D.P. paranoid type.	38, M	Chlpr. dosage unknown.	Unknown	Jaundice.	Recovery 180+ days later.	Biliary stasis with biliary thrombi, central portions of lobules. Biliary pigments in hepatic cells of central zone. Periportal mononuclear infiltrations.
D.P. paranoid type.	26, F	Chlpr. 300 mg.	31 days	Bile in urine, bilirubinogen in serum 14.5. Laparotomy: bile tract negative.	Recovery in 180 days.	Biliary stasis with biliary thrombi and biliary pigments, central portions of lobules.
D.P. catatonic type.	27, F	Chlpr. 1. 150–300 mg 2. 300 mg.	1. 129 days 2. 47 days	Fever 106–104. Combiotic Rx. Jaundice. BUN 96 mg.%; WBC 20,000.	Death due to bronchopneumonia, 15 days after 1st symptom.	Jaundice of viscera. Bronchopneumonia, pulmonary congestion and edema, fatty infiltration of liver (fig. XVIII.6). Fibrosis around central veins with biliary stasis. Biliary casts in renal tubules (fig. XVIII.7).

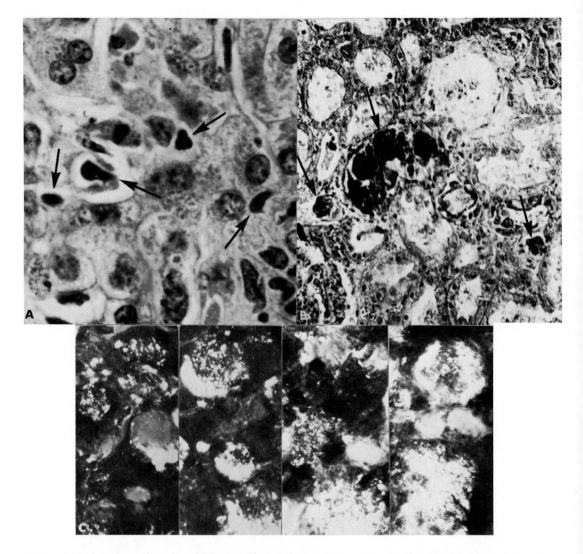

FIG. 1.A: Liver biopsy. Patient treated with chlorpromazine (300 mg/day; 31 days), with jaundice, bile in the urine, bilirubinogen in the serum. Biliary plugs (*arrows*) and biliary pigments in the hepatic cells of the central zone (poorly visualized in black and white illustrations). H.&E. stain. **B:** Kidney (postmortem) showing biliary casts in the renal tubules and bile pigment in the epithelial cells of the renal tubules. Masson's trichrome stain. **C:** Lipid products visualized in polarized light. Sudan III stain. Medium-power magnification. **A, B,** and **C:** ×250.

cases, the liver dysfunction appeared to be transitory and reversible (4 to 240 days). However, there were a few cases in which it lasted for a longer period of time, was associated with preexisting liver pathology, or terminated fatally. In some of these instances biochemical examination of fresh (unfixed) liver tissue and bile revealed the presence of a high concentration of the drug. (Bile contained 21.4 and liver 13.5 μ/g wet tissue; for more details, see ref. 20.)

The most common histopathologic changes appear to be caused by an obstructive type of biliary stasis (1,81,87). In our cases, as well as in those reported in the lit-

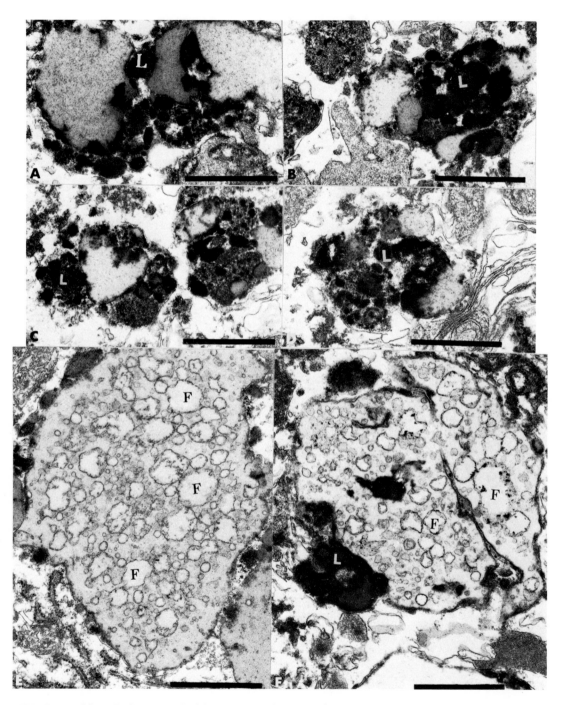

FIG. 2.A–D: Liver. Patient treated with chlorpromazine (50 mg/day i.m.; 120 days, jaundice, hepatorenal syndrome) demonstrating in particular composite lipid products of degeneration (L). **E** and **F**: Lipid material in advanced stages of digestion with numerous vacuoles and translucid fenestrations (F). Uranyl acetate and lead citrate. RCA-EMU-3G. **A–F**: ×27,400. Electron microscope scale = 1 μm.

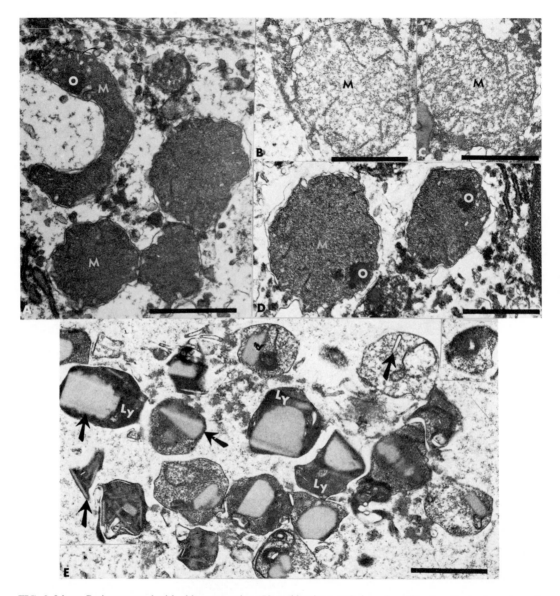

FIG. 3. Liver. Patient treated with chlorpromazine (50 mg/day i.m.; 120 days, jaundice, hepatorenal syndrome). Note in particular mitochondria with dense matrix (**A** and **B**) and few cristae, and (**D**) some containing dense osmiophilic material (0). **B** and **C**: Mitochondria with light osmiophilic matrix. **E**: Shows a congregation of organelles, principally pleomorphic lysosome (Ly) with incorporated material, some of which present crystalloid-like features (*arrows*). Uranyl acetate and lead citrate. RCA-EMU-3G. M, mitochondria. **A**: ×30,500. **B–E**: ×27,400.

erature, the biliary stasis was sometimes associated with biliary thrombi in the central canaliculi and with deposits of biliary pigment in the hepatic parenchymal cells and Kupffer cells (Fig. 1A). In a few instances, this pigment was noted in the epithelium of the kidney tubules, and bile casts were observed in the lumina of the renal tubules (Fig. 1B). Various amounts of fat-stainable material were often evident in the hepatocytes, particularly in the central region of the hepatic lobules (additional data are reviewed in the section on pathogenesis). Although some fine structures appeared altered (disorganized, disrupted, or fragmented, etc.) by various postmortem artifacts, some degenerative changes, in the light also of observations in experimental fresh material, were considered of an *in vivo* occurrence. For instance, lipid deposits of various amounts, osmiophilia, and morphology were observed particularly in the cytoplasm of hepatocytes and in various stages of degeneration or metabolization. It was frequently incorporated in lysosomes and, in some instances, assumed the appearance of large irregular, multivacuolar or multivesicular structures with translucid fenestrations of various shapes and sizes (Fig. 2).

Among the cytoplasmic organelles the mitochondria or pleomorphometabolosomes (PMS) showed marked quantitative and qualitative variations. At times they appeared concentrated around or in the perinuclear region; at others, in random groups. In these instances, they displayed pleomorphism with light matrix and average cristae or dense matrix and fewer cristae (Fig. 3). Here and there, intra-PMS osmiophilic deposits or inclusions were also encountered.

Lysosomes were noticed undergoing different stages of metamorphosis, particularly during the process of degradation of necrobiotic material. Among the latter, "crystaloid-like" products were detected (Fig. 3). Cytosomes and occasionally intracytoplasmic membrane-bound composite polymorphic bodies were found in areas of more pronounced degenerative changes. It contained a variety of necrotic residuals, amorphous and homogeneous, osmiophilic material intertwined with degenerating and disintegrating organelles (of questionable identification), and smudgy membranes. Figure 4 is an example of these "composite polymorphic bodies" that seems to resemble "Mallory's body." No information was available about the drinking habits of the patient. These bodies were frequently in the vicinity of or surrounded by polymorphic lysosomes.

Membranes, lamellar and filamentous or fibrous bodies were also detected. The arrays varied in pattern. They assumed frequently a concentric or parallel arrangement, but "zebra-like" types were also apparent. Although these membranous bodies were generally isolated or in groups of two or three, in some instances they appeared confluent forming more extensive formations (Fig. 5).

Experimental Investigations

Clinical, biochemical, and neuropathologic studies in rats and monkeys already have been described (66,67,88).

Material and Methodology

Acute experiments were carried out in a total of 230 rats (Sherman-Dawley strain). The dosage of chlorpromazine varied between 10 and 50 mg/100 g body weight. The duration of the experiment lasted from 1 to 72 hr. *Short-term experiments* consisted of a total of 88 rats (same species as above). The dosage of chlorpromazine varied between 0.6 and 2.5 mg/100 g body weight, and the duration of the experiments lasted for 2 to 9 weeks. *Chronic experiments* included a total of 107 rats and 10 *Macacus* rhesus monkeys. The dosage of the drug varied between 0.1 and 1.5 mg/100 g body weight. Duration of experiments in rats lasted from 3 to 8 months and in the monkeys was prolonged for up to 20 to 34 months.

Results

Since these studies have been previously reported (63,66,67), we extrapolate

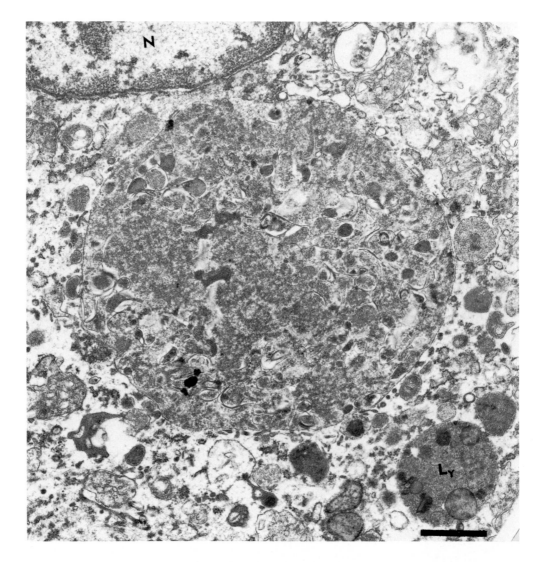

FIG. 4. Postmortem liver of a patient treated with chlorpromazine (50 mg/day i.m.; 120 days, jaundice, hepato-renal syndrome). It illustrates in particular a partially membrane-bound intracytoplasmic body containing a variety of residuals of necrotic products, fine densely osmiophilic material intertwined with degenerating (un-recognizable) organelles and smudgy membranes. It resembles, to a certain degree, Mallory's "hyalin" body. Uranyl acetate and lead citrate. RCA-EMU-3G. ×17,600. N, nucleus; Ly, lysosome.

only some demonstrative examples pertinent to our topic of discussion.

Biochemical Studies

Biochemical studies in acute and chronic chlorpromazine experiments in rats and monkeys, previously reported (88), disclosed high concentrations of the drug in the liver as compared with other body tissues and central nervous system (CNS).

Histopathologic Studies

Histopathologic studies revealed, in some chronic experiments, various degrees of sudanophilia and some degenerative changes of the hepatic cells (66,67).

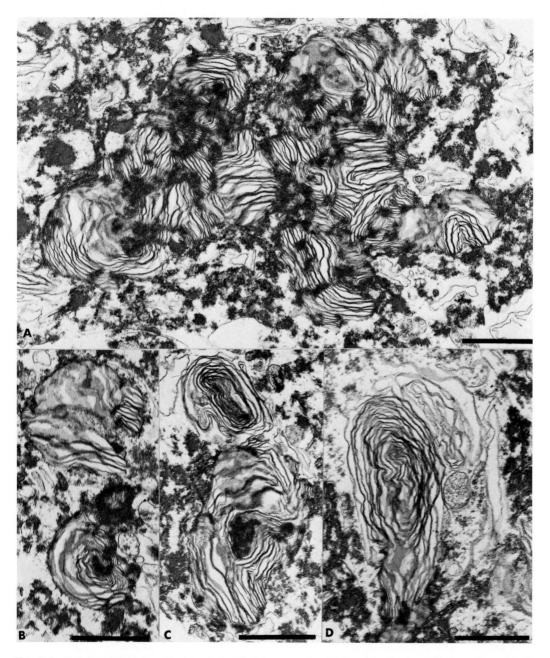

FIG. 5. Postmortem liver of a patient treated with chlorpromazine (200 mg/day for 2 weeks, thereafter gradually increased to 1,500 mg/day for 4 days; sudden death). Cytoplasm of a hepatocyte undergoing degenerative changes with arrays of membranes assuming predominantly "zebra-like" (**A–C**) and concentric patterns (**C** and **D**). Uranyl acetate and lead citrate. RCA-EMU-3G. **A–D:** ×27,400.

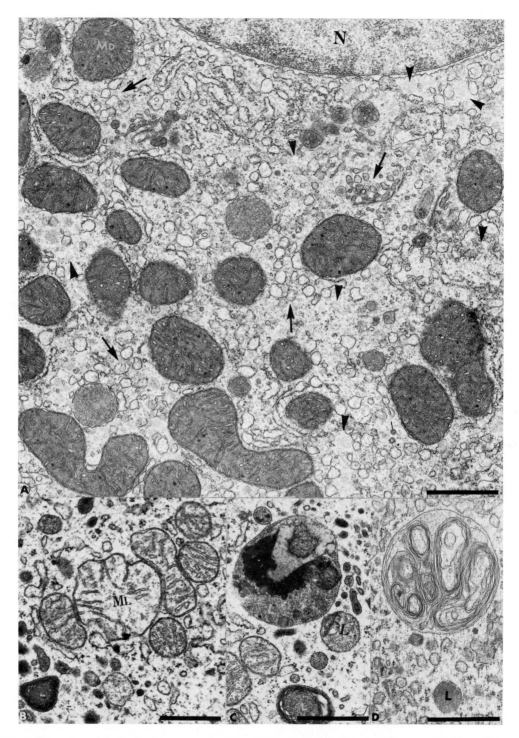

FIG. 6. Liver of rat treated with chlorpromazine (5 mg/100 g, for 11 months). **A:** Hepatocyte showing especially marked proliferation of the endoplasmic reticulum (*long arrows*) with irregular distribution and decrease of ribosomes (*short arrows*); there is also increased number of mitochondria with dense matrix (Md), as compared with a congregation of mitochondria with light matrix (**B:**ML). **C:** Concentration of various organelles in the vicinity of a large lysosome (L) containing digestive material. **D:** Arrays of several concentric fibrillary structures within a cytosome. Uranyl acetate and lead citrate. RCA-EMU-3G. **A, C,** and **D:** ×27,400; **B:** ×23,400.

Ultrastructural Changes

Among the *ultrastructural changes* of note were qualitative variations in distribution and concentration of mitochondria or PMS (Fig. 6). The qualitative changes were manifested by marked PMS pleomorphism associated with alterations of the limiting membranes, cristae, and matrix. At times, the disorganization of the matirix was associated with the presence of variously shaped electron-dense osmiophilic particles or material. Concentrically laminated osmiophilic material or structures, as well as osmiophilic microbodies or osmiophilic amorphous material, were also observed randomly distributed in the liver parenchyma or macrophages. In this regard it is also of interest to note that biochemical studies have shown inhibition of oxidative phosphorylation of PMS (21), whereas chemical analyses revealed that phenothiazines were strongly bound to PMS and microsomes of the liver and different organs (8).

Various degrees of fine ultrastructural changes of the Golgi complex were noted during various phases of the acute and short-term experiments. These were frequently associated with the presence of various pleomorphic organelles. The most remarkable changes, however, were noted in the chronic phases. These were characterized by extensive proliferation and vesiculation of the smooth endoplasmic reticulum (Fig. 7).

Pleomorphic lysosomes were particularly prominent in some liver specimens of monkeys subjected to prolonged (up to 28 months) treatment with chlorpromazine (Fig. 8). In these conditions membranous and filamentous bodies with arrays arranged predominantly in concentric patterns were also noticed. In addition some organelles and isolated PMS appeared to be walled off or surrounded by multiconcentric arrays of fine filaments (Fig. 8).

In Vitro Studies

In vitro studies of liver fractions were carried out in order to ascertain whether the mitochondrial (PMS) reactions were or were not directly affected by chlorpromazine. In comparing the control with the *in vitro* chlorpromazine-treated PMS, the latter showed distinct ultrastructural and osmiophilic alterations of the cristae, matrix, and overall configuration, similar to some of those observed *in vivo* (68).

Experimental Potentiation of Phenothiazine Toxicity

We have previously indicated that some histopathologic features of human hepatic lesions seem to suggest that they possibly existed prior to the initiation of drug therapy and that they, probably under the pharmacodynamic stress of the drug, became aggravated or reactivated. In order to test this impression we carried out the following three experimental investigations:

1. One group of rats was maintained on an ethionine diet for 8 to 14 months until they developed liver dysfunctions, which were estimated by the increased transaminase level in the blood taken periodically prior to the administration of the phenothiazines. In addition, clinicopathological, biochemical, histochemical, and electron microscope investigations were carried out at various intervals of time.

2. When hepatic disorders were determined by the above procedures, then these animals were placed on a control (average) rat diet for 2 weeks. Thereafter, they were treated with intramuscular injections of chlorpromazine (Thorazine®, SKF, 1 mg/100 g (body weight).

3. Control rats of the same sex and age as group 2 were maintained on normal average rat diet and injected with the same

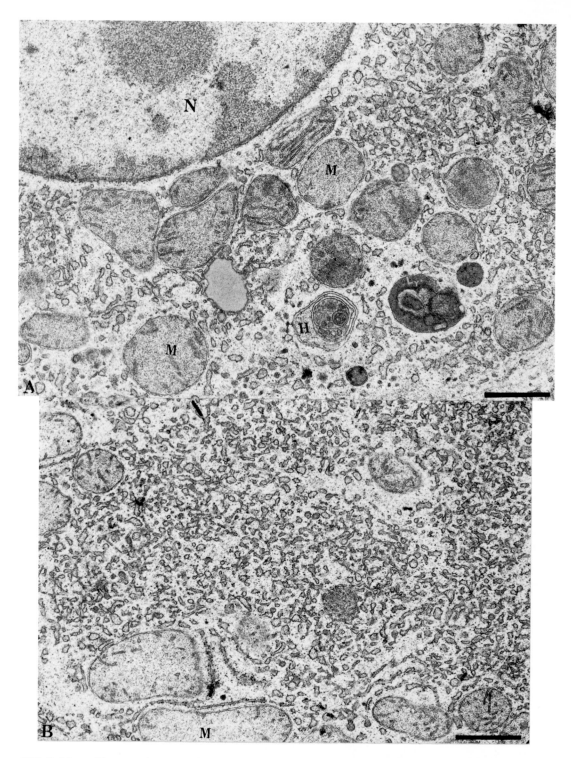

FIG. 7. Liver. *Macacus* rhesus monkey treated with chlorpromazine (1.0 mg/kg gradually increased to 15.0 mg/kg, during a period of 28 months). **A:** Perinuclear region of a hepatocyte showing accumulation of pleomorphic mitochondria, lysosomes (Ly), and a heteromorphic body within an area with marked proliferation of the endoplasmic reticulum, and **B:** demonstrating especially an exuberant hyperplasia of the smooth component of the endoplasmic reticulum. Uranyl acetate and lead citrate. RCA-EMU-3G. ×24,700.

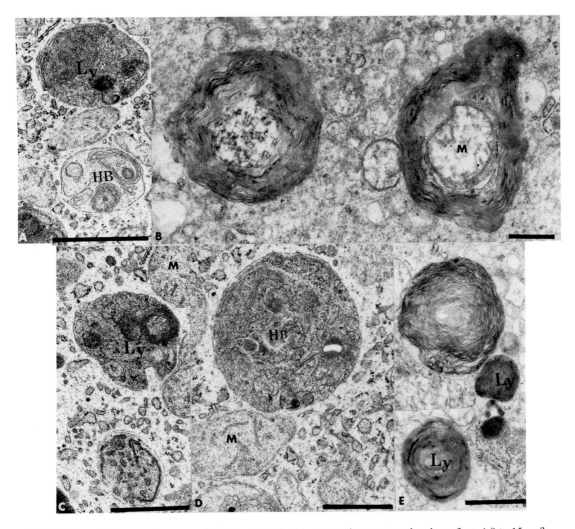

FIG. 8. Liver of *Macacus* rhesus monkey (treated with chlorpromazine, progressive doses from 1.0 to 15 mg/kg for 28 months). Pleomorphic lysosomes (Ly) and heteromorphic bodies (HB). Note also marked variations in the arrangement patterns and proliferation of fine filaments. Uranyl acetate and lead citrate. RCA-EMU-3G. **A:** ×36,600; **B:** ×17,800; **C:** ×30,500; **D:** ×26,900; **E:** 23,400.

phenothiazines and in the same manner as group 2.

These three groups of animals were also compared with another general control group of rats maintained on a regular rat diet and injected with sterile saline in equivalent amounts and in the same manner as the phenothiazine-treated animals. Group 2 rats showed: (a) a decreased tolerance to phenothiazines and an in-creased mortality rate, (b) higher concentration of the chemical agents in the liver (9.5 μg/g as compared with 4.4 μg of group 3) (4), (c) abundant deposits of lipid material associated with vacuolization of the hepatic cells as shown by histopathologic studies of the liver, and (d) various degrees of involvement, disclosed by electron microscopic examinations, of the Golgi complex, rough endoplasmic reticulum, lysosomal pleomorphism (with dense osmiophilic granular and particulate material), and cytosomes, containing necrobiotic material, multiconcentric lamellar structures, and swollen PMS. In addition, at times, PMS appeared surrounded by concentrically laminated structures. In other instances, similar and variable concentric lamellar and dense osmiophilic formations were dispersed within the cytoplasm of the hepatic cells (61) (Figs. 5, 8, 12, and 14).

The possible *pathogenic mechanisms* of the hepatic dysfunctions and injuries associated with phenothiazine therapy have been discussed in detail by several authors. Only some of the main issues are reviewed here. For more detail the reader should consult the following important publications: see refs. 6,7,9,13,15–19,23,24,26,29, 32,34,35,37,38,40–42,48,51–53,55,58,59, 62,73,77,79,85,86,89–93. In summary the morphologic changes in some patients treated with phenothiazines resemble biliary cirrhosis and intrahepatic cholestasis associated, at times, with accumulation of copper pigment at the periphery of hepatocytes and minimal to moderate portal inflammation of mononuclear character with the predominance of lymphocytes and plasma cells.

A significant number of authors consider the hepatic injury a manifestation of a hypersensitivity reaction (30,36,60,78,80, 91,93).

As to the pathogenesis of the intrahepatic cholestasis, Popper and Schaffner (54), on the basis of ultrastructural studies, have postulated that an alteration of the smooth endoplasmic reticulum of the hepatocytes is the primary process. Secondary events include additional damage by cholestasis on a mechanical basis.

All of these findings indicate that: (a) the observed liver dysfunctions are of a low percentage of incidence, are mild, transitory and reversible in character, and thus might indicate some possible idiosyncracy similar to that described by Hanger and Gutman (25), and (b) the

severity of the dysfunctions and pathologic findings appear, at times, related to pre-existing abnormalities of the hepatobiliary tract or to the coexistence of other disease processes that might have an effect on the liver (such as chronic alcoholism, gastroenteric disorders, history of recovered hepatitis, etc.).

Electron Microscope Studies

Since some of these studies have been reported (20,62,67), only the salient findings are briefly summarized.

It is also of interest to note that prenatal administration of drugs may affect not only the CNS but also some functions of the liver, since almost all drug metabolizing pathways[2] in the liver of fetal or newborn subjects may be incomplete, and therefore may become affected structurally as well as biochemically by extended prenatal drug treatment.

NARCOTICS

Human Studies

Histochemical, histopathologic, and electron microscope observations of the CNS have already been reviewed (65,69a and b).

Material and Methods

The essential clinico-pathologic data of a sample of patients are summarized in Table 2 (65).

Selective specimens from the liver were processed for chemical analysis, histologic (H&E and trichrome stains), histochemic (lipids, PAS, Best for glycogen, acid phosphatase, thiamine pyrophosphatase, and glucose-6-phosphatase), and electron microscope methodologies.

---

[2] Essential biochemical activities required for the conjugation, detoxification, and excretion of drugs may be altered, to some extent, by the placental transfer of chlorpromazine (24,46,74).

TABLE 2. *Clinical-pathological aspects of heroin addicts consuming methadone and other multiple chemical agents or alcohol*

Case number	Age and sex	Drug and dosage	Duration of treatment	Clinical findings (drug habits)	Toxicologic findings and general comments
4821 (B.R.)	52; M	Methadone: (180 mg. before death)	Meth. progr.	Alcohol; codeine; barbiturates (addiction to all; cardiac disorders)	Urine: Morphine: + − Methadone: + Quinine: + Codeine: − Barbiturates: −
4825 (D.H.)	19; M	Methadone	Unknown	Heroin addict Methadone	No Urine
4830 (W.D.)	24; M	Methadone: 140 mg. per day	2 mos.	Heroin addict for 4 years; Heroin and Methadone	Urine: Methadone: very strongly + Morphine: − Quinine: −
4831 (P.P.)	19; F	Methadone: 90 mg. per day	Meth. progr.	Heroin addict; asthma Methadone	Urine: Methadone: + very faint reaction; traces
4838 (P.C.)	22; M	Methadone: (20 mg. bid) thorazine: (75 mg tid) Methadone overdosage	Meth. progr.	Heroin addict; Methadone, Thorazine Clorox	Urine: Morphine: − Quinine: − Methadone: + Barbiturates: − Unknown Others: +
4856 (J.J.)	30; M	Methadone: overdosage	Meth. progr.	Heroin and methadone	Urine: Morphine: + − Quinine: − Methadone: − found in street
4882 (R.J.)	32; M	Methadone: overdosage	Unknown	Heroin addict and methadone	No urine
4928 (J.J.)	65; M	Methadone: 80 mg.; Heroin	1 mo. Meth. progr.; narcotics 40 yrs.	Heroin and meth.; Quinine; Naline; Digitalis; Daryan; cardiac disorders	Urine and serum: +
4939 (B.M.)	18; F	Methadone: 100 mg before death	Unknown		Collapsed at a party; flat ECG. pneumothorax. Insufficient amount of urine.
4957	20; M	Heroin overdosage	Methadone program	Heroin and methadone	Urine: Morphine: + Quinine: − Methadone: − Barbiturates: −
4972	58; M	Methadone: overdosage	Methadone program	Narcotics: 10 yrs. +	Urine: Methadone: +
4986	18; M	Methadone: overdosage	Not on methadone program	Heroin addict	Urine: Morphine: + Quinine: + Methadone: + Unknown Others: +
4989 (J.F.)	31; M	Methadone: (80 mg.)	Unknown	Alcohol (severe)	Urine: Morphine: − Quinine: − Methadone: +
4997	23; M	Methadone: overdosage	Unknown		Urine: Morphine: − Quinine: − Methadone: +

Results

The hepatic cells, in particular, were affected by various degrees of degenerative changes, associated with deposits of variable amounts of lipid-stainable material (Fig. 9A and B). Some liver specimens presented mild to pronounced hepatitis (Fig. 1C and D). In these instances, the inflammatory exudate consisted predominantly of mononuclear cells.

The electron microscope studies of human material present the well-known difficulties caused by postmortem changes. However, certain findings in the light of the experimental observations that follow are considered of significance, for instance: (a) abnormal distribution and concentration of composite lipids and glycogen (Fig. 10), and necrobiotic material, and (b) distribution and disorganization of the endoplasmic reticulum (particularly the Golgi complex component), qualitative and quantitative changes of the PMS and lysosomes with frequent inclusions of necrobiotic products undergoing various stages of metabolization or digestion (Fig. 11). Polymorphic membranous bodies with irregularly or concentrically arranged membranes (at times, filaments or lamellae) were detected intermixed with the above-described organelles, isolated (Fig. 12), or in small groups (64).

Experimental Investigations

Material and Methods

These were carried out on 45 young adult rats (Sherman-Dawley strain) injected with methadone in the amounts of 1.1 mg/100 g body weight (for 12 to 24 hr) and 0.11 mg/100 g body weight (6 to 24 months). Selected specimens from the surface and the central regions of the liver were processed for regular electron microscope as well as for combined histochemic procedures for acid phosphatase, thiamine

pyrophosphatase, and glucose-6-phosphatase.

Results

The salient ultrastructural findings consisted of:

1. Numerical variations in the distribution of PMS (Fig. 13). PMS with dense matrix and few cristae appeared predominant in some specimens, PMS with light matrix and variable number of cristae were also encountered, and marked PMS pleomorphism associated, at times, with large or giant PMS were randomly observed as in human cases, some of them measuring 2μm in diameter and 4μm in length.

2. Various degrees of disorganization of the rough endoplasmic reticulum.

3. Irregular distribution or depletion of ribosomes.

4. Moderate to exuberant proliferation of the Golgi complex as demonstrated in Fig. 14.

5. Pleomorphic membranous bodies, like those described in humans, intermixed with other organelles or independently (Fig. 14). This remarkable proliferation of membranes or filaments appeared also surrounding in a concentric fashion certain altered organelles and mitochondria.

6. Lysosomal pleomorphism and metamorphosis in areas undergoing degenerative or necrobiotic degradation similar in character to some of those observed in human material.

7. Some lipid deposits of variable osmiophilia undergoing various stages of digestion.

8. Irregular distribution and concentration of glycogen products, at times, associated with the above-mentioned fine structural changes of the organelles and endoplasmic reticulum. In addition, the combined histochemic and electron microscope preparations disclosed irregular or abnormal concentration of thiamine pyro-

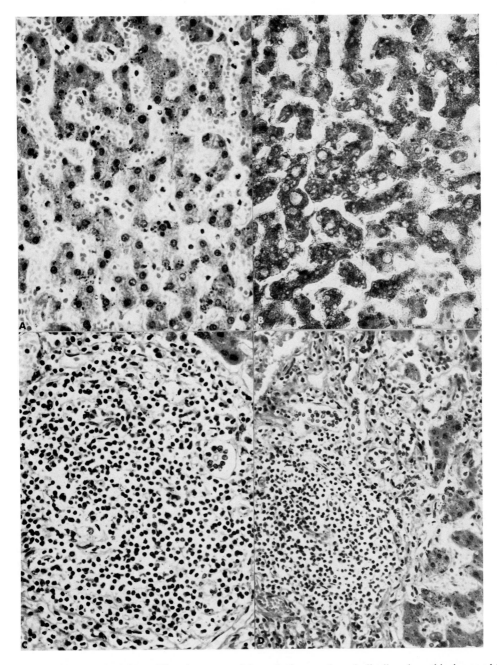

FIG. 9. Liver of chronic heroin addict also consuming methadone and, periodically, phenothiazines and barbiturates. **A:** Deposits of biliary pigments (poorly visualized in black and white illustrations) and **B:** variable amounts of lipid-stainable material and vacuolization of hepatic cords. **C** and **D:** Hepatitis, inflammatory exudate consisting predominantly of mononuclear cells. **A, C,** and **D:** H. & E. Stain, and **B:** Sudan III. Medium-power magnification. **A** and **B:** ×460; **C:** ×370; **D:** ×575.

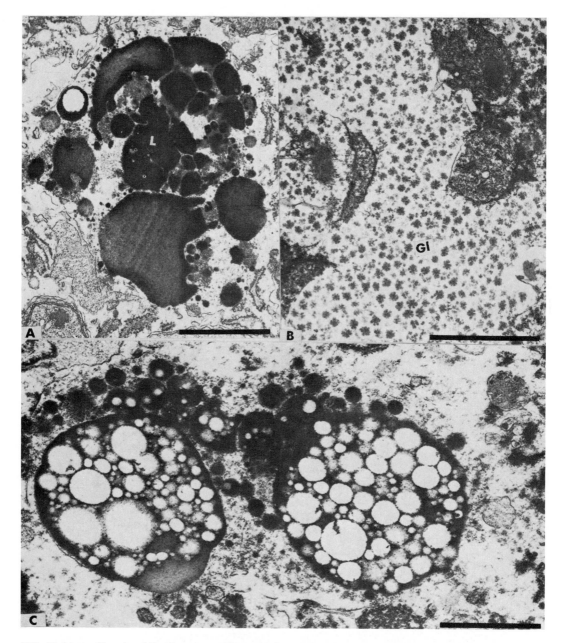

FIG. 10. Liver of heroin addict also consuming methadone and, periodically, other drugs of abuse but more often phenothiazines. The most salient changes are manifested by irregular distribution of various amounts of composite lipid products (A:L) and glycogen (B:GL) associated with disorganization of the fine structural architecture of the cellular cytoplasm. **C:** Two large multivesicular and vacuolar structures in advanced stages of lipid metabolization with participation of lysosomal reaction. Uranyl acetate and lead citrate. RCA-EMU-3G. **A:** ×30,300; **B:** ×36,600; **C:** ×33,200.

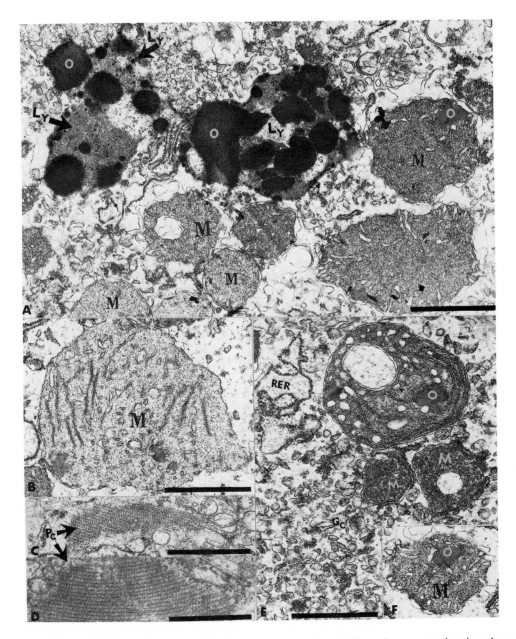

FIG. 11. Liver of a chronic heroin addict (dead after an overdose of methadone; also consumed various drugs of abuse, Table 2B; #4882) illustrating in particular quantitative and qualitative changes of intracytoplasmic organelles of hepatic cells. **A:** Lysosomes (Ly) with incorporated osmiophilic products (O) and pleomorphic mitochondria (M) with dense matrix and few cristae. **B:** Giant mitochondrion (at times of 2 μm in diameter and up to 4 μm in length) with irregular distribution and alterations of the cristae. **C:** Paracrystalline structures (Pc) found in various locations as well as in mitochondria. **D:** Mitochondria (M) of various shapes and sizes with irregular distribution of cristae and osmiophilic deposits (O) in the matrix. Of note also are irregular enlargements of the rough endoplasmic reticulum (RER) and marked proliferation of its smooth component (Gc). Uranyl acetate and lead citrate. RCA-EMU-3G. **A, B,** and **E:** ×28,600. **C** and **D:** ×27,400.

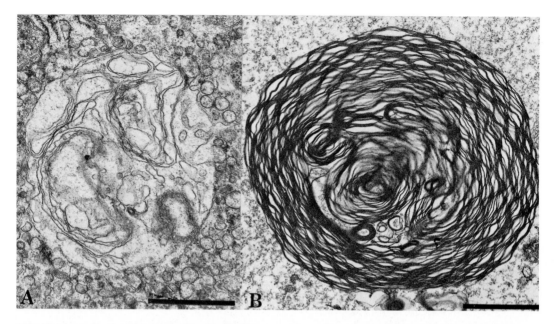

FIG. 12. Liver of a chronic heroin addict (dead after an overdose of heroin) illustrating polymorphic membranous bodies with erratically (**A**) or concentrically (**B**) arranged structures that, at times, appear as fine filaments or lamellae or ribbons. RCA-EMU-3G. Uranyl acetate and lead citrate. **A:** ×29,800; **B:** ×28,600.

phosphatase reaction products in the cytoplasm along the distribution of the smooth endoplasmic reticulum.

The pathogenesis of the liver dysfunctions observed in some heroin addicts is much debated. Earlier studies (especially from 1929 up to the 1950s) assumed that a direct hepatotoxic effect of opiates was the etiologic basis for the high incidence of abnormal liver function tests in narcotic addicts (45). It was even emphasized that a certain pattern of abnormal liver function, including elevated transaminase level, might be a valuable adjunct in recognizing and diagnosing heroin and cocaine use (45) and that a sudden rise in transaminase may be one of the earliest signs of relapse. However, some authors (41) emphasized that a certain percentage (7/21) of addicts showed no abnormalities of transaminase, although they continued to take heroin. In addition in a detailed study, Gorodetsky et al. (22), with uncontaminated morphine solutions administered subcutaneously with sterile technique, demonstrated that six of 20

carefully selected subjects did not show any abnormality in transaminase levels during the course of addiction and that of the 14 who did show transaminase elevation, there was no pattern indicating a rise on initiation of morphine administration or during any given period of the addiction cycle. On this basis, these authors concluded that the incidence of abnormal liver function observed in morphine and heroin addicts is not due to a direct hepatotoxic effect of the opiate. Examinations of Federal prisoners at the Addiction Research Center (Lexington, National Institute of Mental Health) by Sapira et al. (75) have revealed a high incidence of hepatomegaly sometimes accompanied by abnormal liver function tests. In addition, some patients without hepatomegaly had intermittently abnormal liver function tests. In addition to the routine battery of liver function tests, including serum glutamic oxalacetic transminase (SGOT), serum glutamic pyruvic transminase, (SGPT), cephaline floculation, and thymol turbidity. All patients examined

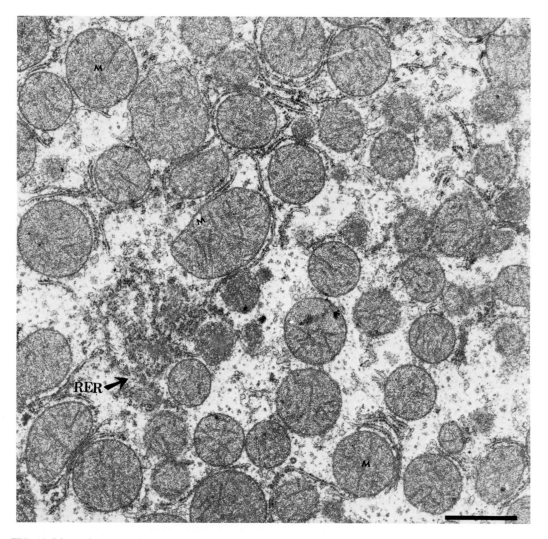

FIG. 13. Liver of rat treated with methadone (0.22 mg/100 g. body weight for 5 months) revealing the accumulation of a large number of mitochondria in a portion of the cytoplasm of a hepatocyte with concomitant disorganization of the underlying fine cytoarchitecture. Uranyl acetate and lead citrate. RCA-EMU-3G. ×27,400. RER, rough endoplasmic reticulum.

or reexamined at the Addiction Research Center were evaluated with regard to: (a) history of the actual duration of needle exposure after correcting for periods of voluntary or enforced abstinence, (b) the details of needle care and frequency of crossexposure to the blood products of other addicts, (c) any history of hepatitis or episode of jaundice following needle use that was compatible with hepatitis (such patients were not included in this study), (d) the position of the right diaphragm as estimated by percussion in those patients with a palpable liver (the majority of the palpable livers were estimated to be greater than 15 cm from the percussed upper border in the midclavicular line), and (e) "addict's lymphadenopathy," a reactive hyperplasia of the epitrochlear and axillary lymph nodes presumably due to long-term intravenous injection of drugs contaminated with particulate matter.

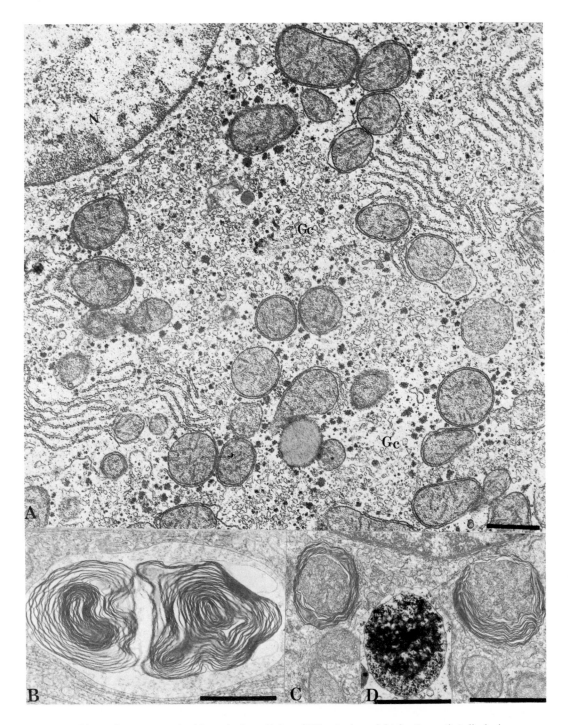

FIG. 14. A: Liver of a rat treated with methadone (2.2 mg/100 g body weight for 6 months) disclosing a very pronounced proliferation of the smooth endoplasmic reticulum (Gc) that imparts to the cytoplasm a "vesicular-like" appearance. **B:** Liver of rat treated with methadone (0.22 mg/100 g body weight for 2 hr) illustrating two adjacent polymorphic membranous bodies with concentric arrays. **C:** Methadone (0.22 mg/100 g body weight for 8 hr) degenerating organelles (more likely mitochondria) surrounded by concentrically arranged membranes. **D:** Methadone (2.2 mg/100 g body weight for 16 hr) lysosome containing amorphous and fine granular material. Uranyl acetate and lead citrate. RCA-EMU-3G. **A:** ×19,900; **B, C,** and **D:** ×29,000.

A total of 32 patients was accepted for final analysis. Of these, five patients had a history of serum hepatitis. Of the 26 patients without history of icterus or hepatitis, nine had hepatomegaly (of whom seven had abnormal liver function tests). Of the remaining 17 patients, 11 had at least one abnormal liver function test, leaving only six residual patients without historic, physical, or laboratory evidence of liver disease. Of these, one had always used drugs by nasal insufflation and, hence, had never been parenterally exposed to serum hepatitis. Thus, approximately five out of six drug addicts who used hypodermic equipment had some evidence of liver disease.

The impression was also given that "if an addict is tested frequently enough over a reasonable period of time, regardless of the clinical status, the likelihood of having an abnormal liver function test will continue to increase" (75). Another methodologic problem was the reliability of the addicts' answers to questions used in this study—"age at onset of drug use entered in the computation of the total months of drug exposure after correcting for periods of no hyperdermic use;" less than 50% gave the same age for starting drug use to both the admission clerk and the interviewer from the Addiction Research Center (75). In reviewing also the pertinent literature related in particular to viral hepatitis (2,3,5, 11,12,27,36,50,56,71,82) and the possibility of multiple reinfections (41,71), Sapira et al. (75) suggested that many narcotic addicts have a long-term intermittent serum hepatitis, "chronic addiction serum hepatitis (CASH)," due to exposure to hypodermic-contaminated equipment. It is also of interest to note that these findings are supported by:

1. Experimental hepatitis in Marmosets inoculated with materials from patients with human hepatitis. This disease showed changes in the length of the incubation period during the course of serial passages through Marmosets (31).

2. Chronic hepatic injury following experimental viral hepatitis in the dog (57). On the other hand, an abnormality of sulfobromophthalein retention was noted in the dog following a short-term administration of high doses of morphine (70). However, Sapira et al. (75) suggested that it could have been caused also by hypoxia and circulatory disorders since the dogs were "noted to become cyanotic."

3. Occurrence of serum hepatitis in LSD users who administered their drugs intravenously with shared syringes (47); and

4. Carriers of hepatitis virus in the blood and transfusion recipients with viral hepatitis in blood (14).

The variability in histopathologic reports of biopsies and autopsy specimens of human cases should not be surprising in light of the above-mentioned clinicopathologic observations. Sapira et al. (75) have also reviewed the pertinent literature up to 1968. Therefore, we limit our comments here to some fundamental features only. In essence, various authors have noted in biopsies and postmortem material various degrees of hepatitis such as "thinny collections of lymphocytes" (27), fulminant (28), acute hepatitis (49), acute yellow atrophy (11), round-cell infiltrations (41,56), various inflammatory abnormalities (33), chronic hepatitis (41), cirrhosis or chronic hepatitis and perilymphangiitis (5), postnecrotic cirrhosis transitional to Laennec's (76), and various transitional or combination features of the above (36,39,43,45).

As to the possible pathogenic mechanisms, on the basis of review of the pertinent literature and our own studies, the following factors should be taken into consideration: (a) differences in sampling specimens in relation to the duration course or evolution of the pathologic processes, i.e., in some cases several episodes of icterus with normal bilirubin and SGOT levels between the attacks were noted (71) (in this instance the liver biopsy was repeated after the third attack; in the latter the histopathology was different than that of the biopsy taken during the original attack), (b) discrepancies related to the intermittent character of the disease probably related to episodes of recovery and relapses of the clinicopathologic process and the importance of performing repeated liver function tests as well as differences in the time of sampling; (c) possible potentiation, aggravation, compounding, and interaction of narcotic pharmacodynamic properties with alcohol (39,65,83), phenothiazines (12,52,53,65,94), sedatives (65, 84); or (d) sympathomimetics (10); and (e) miscellaneous biologic cofactors (inborn or acquired, ref. 72).

CONCLUDING REMARKS

The neural and visceral reactions induced by neuropsychotropic agents are principally related to the interaction between the "target" or the "bioreceptors" of the affected tissue constituents and the direct or indirect effects of the drug's pharmacodynamic properties. Histopathologic lesions (cellular or architectural) may be minimal, nonspecific, or absent in rapid-acting toxicity and/or deaths occurring within a short period of time after drug intake. The survival period must be long enough to permit development of lesions.

When liver dysfunctions occur following the use of phenothiazines, they are generally mild, transitory, and reversible in character (except in some more severe cases with prolonged course and a few fatalities). In these instances, the morphologic changes resemble biliary cirrhosis and include pseudoxanthomatous changes, peripheral necrosis, cholestasis with biliary plugs and destruction of interlobular bile ducts, minimal to moderate portal inflammation of a mononuclear character with predominance of lymphocytes and plasma cells, and, at times, accumulation of copper pigment at the periphery of hepatocytes (32).

The most common pathogenic mecha-nisms of the hepatobiliary disorders or injuries are attributed to toxic intrahepatic-cholestasis (cholangiolitic hepatitis, refs. 26,40, or "Cholestatischen Hepatose," ref. 73) and/or hypersensitivity (allergic colangiolitis, refs.80,91). Some authors (54) have hypothesized, on the basis of ultra-structural studies, that the intrahepatic cholestasis is due to a primary involvement of the Golgi apparatus of the hepatocytes.

The pathogenesis of the hepatic dysfunctions and hepatitis (predominantly of a mononuclear character) in narcotic addicts is considered an expression of compounded effects of the impurity of the drug, the contamination of the syringes, and the recurrence or reactivation of preexisting (predrug) liver pathology caused by the pharmacodynamic stress of the drug with frequent interaction with multiple drugs of abuse, with alcohol, and with malabsorption syndrome.

The development, severity, and evolution of the liver dysfunctions or injuries in humans related to phenothiazine administration and/or narcotics may be modified by the participation of several inborn or acquired pathobiologic cofactors.

In experimental animals some of the structural, and particularly ultracellular, and histochemic reactions seem to be related to direct or indirect (intermediary metabolites) effects of the pharmacodynamic properties of the drug. In some experimental models the hepatotoxic effects of chlorperazine and prochloperazine were potentiated by predrug induced biochemical and structural injuries of the liver.

Individual variations (inborn and acquired) in compatibility, susceptibility, and vulnerability of the liver to chemogenic stress occur in humans as well as in some animal species.

In prenatal condition, through placental transfer, not only the CNS, but also the functions and structures of the liver may be affected by extended maternal drug administration.

ACKNOWLEDGMENTS

The author gratefully acknowledges the assistance and cooperation of J. C. Liu, K. M. Wu, and S. Avrin for electron microscopy procedures, V. Bystron for illustrations, W. Rivers for bibliography, and P. VanCleef for secretarial work.

REFERENCES

1. Albot, G., Lunel, J., and Pagniez, V. (1966): Physiopathologie des icteres a la chlorpromazine. *Actual. Hepatogastroent.*, 2:467–487.
2. Alter, A. A., and Michael, M. (1958): Serum hepatitis in a group of drug addicts. *N. Engl. J. Med.*, 259:387–389.
3. Altschul, A., Foster, P. D., Paley, S. S., and Turner, L. (1952): Incidence of hepatitis among narcotic addicts in the Harlem Hospital, New York. *Arch. Intern. Med.*, 89:24–31.
4. Alexander, G. J., Machiz, S., Gray, R., Liu, J. C., and Roizin, L. (1971): Elevated phenothiazine levels in chronic liver poisoning in guinea pigs. *Fed. Proc.*, 30:562.
5. Appelbaum, E., and Kalkstein, M. (1951): Artificial transmission of viral hepatitis among intravenous diacetylmorphine addicts. *JAMA*, 147:222–224.
6. Baggenstoss, A. H., Foulk, W. T., Butt, H. R., and Bahn, R. C. (1964): The pathology of primary biliary cirrhosis with emphasis on histogenesis. *Am. J. Clin. Pathol.*, 42:259–276.
7. Bailey, B. H., and Kay, R. E. (1960): Prolonged phenothiazine hepatitis: Report of a case. *Am. J. Psychiatry*, 117:557–558.
8. Bickel, M. H. (1974): Binding of phenothiazines to related compounds to tissues and cell constituents. In: *The Phenothiazines and Structurally Related Drugs*, edited by I. S. Forrest, C. J. Carr, and E. Usdin. Raven Press, New York.
9. Bjorneboe, M., Iversen, O., and Olsen, S. (1967): Infective hepatitis and toxic jaundice in a municipal hospital during a five year period. *Acta Med. Scand.*, 182:491–501.
10. Brunson, J. G., Eckman, P. L., and Campbell, J. B. (1957): Increasing prevalence of unexplained liver necrosis. *N. Engl. J. Med.*, 257:52–56.
11. Cardon, P. V., and Beck, E. M. (1952): Recent occurrence of hepatitis among drug addicts of New York City. *NY State J. Med.*, 52:1037–1038.
12. Castleman, B., and McNeely, B. U. (editors): Case records of the Massachusetts General Hospital No. 6–1965, *N. Engl. J. Med.*, 272:254–259.
13. Cohen, I. M., and Archer, J. D. (1955): Liver function and hepatic complications in patients receiving chlorpromazine. *JAMA*, 159:99–101.
14. Cohen, S. N., and Dougherty, W. J. (1968): Transfusion hepatitis arising from addict blood donors. *JAMA*, 203:427.
15. Craddock, W. L. (1956): Toxic effects of chlorpromazine: Hepatitis and agranulocytosis. *US Armed Forces Med. J.*, 7:1726–1740.
16. Crandell, A., and Ma, J. Y. (1959): Jaundice precipitated prochlorperazine (Compazine) in the treatment of alcoholic psychiatric disturbance. *J. Med. Soc. NJ*, 56:553–554.
17. Danhof, I. E. (1958): Factors in the etiology of chlorpromazine jaundice: An experimental study. *Texas Biol. Med.*, 16:443–457.
18. Devore, J. K., Dougherty, C., and Schneider, E. M. (1956): The effect of chlorpromazine on hepatic function and morphology. *Gastroenterology*, 31:391–398.
19. Dundee, J. W. (1957): Chlorpromazine and liver function: The effects of prolonged oral administration. *Anaesthesia*, 12:215–222.
20. Forrest, F. M., Forrest, I. S., and Roizin, L. (1963): Clinical, biochemical and postmortem studies on a patient treated with chlorpromazine. *Agressologie*, 4:259–263.
21. Gallagher, C. H., Koch, J. H., and Mann, D. M. (1965): The effect of phenothiazine on the metabolism of liver mitochondria. *Biochem. Pharmacol.*, 14:789–797, 799–811.
22. Gorodetsky, C. W., Sapira, J. D., Jasimski, D. R., and Martin, W. R. (1968): The role of the drug. Liver disease in narcotic addicts. *Clin. Pharmacol. Ther.*, 9:720–739.
23. Gupta, N. N., Pant, S. S., and Mehrotra, R. M. L. (1962): Toxic effects of chlorpromazine with special reference to jaundice. *Indian J. Med. Sci.*, 16:315–323.
24. Hammond, J. E., and Toseland, P. A. (1970): Placental transfer of chlorpromazine. *Arch. Dis. Child.*, 45:139–140.
25. Hanger, F. M., Jr., and Gutman, A. B. (1940): Postarsphenamine jaundice apparently due to obstruction of intrahepatic biliary tract. *JAMA*, 115:263.
26. Harrower, H. W., and Cooper, P. (1955): Obstructive jaundice due to chlorpromazine. *RI Med. J.*, 38:391.
27. Havens, W. P., Jr. (1956): Viral hepatitis: Multiple attacks in a narcotic addict. *Ann. Intern. Med.*, 44:199–203.
28. Helpern, M., and Rho, Y. M. (1966): Deaths from narcotism in New York City. *NY State J. Med.*, 66:2391–2408.
29. Hodges, H. H., and La Zerte, G. D. (1955): Jaundice and granulocytosis with fatality following chlorpromazine therapy. *JAMA*, 158:114–116.
30. Hollister, L. E. (1957): Allergy to chlorpromazine manifested by jaundice. *Am. J. Med.*, 23:870–879.
31. Holmes, A. W., Capps, R. B., and Deinhardt, F. (1967): Experimental hepatitis in marmosets. *Presented at American Society of Clinical Investigations, May, Atlantic City.*
32. Ishak, K. G., and Irey, N. S. (1972): Hepatic injury associated with the phenothiazines. Clinicopathologic and follow-up study of 36 patients. *Arch. Pathol.*, 93:283–304.

33. Kaplan, K. (1963): Chronic liver disease in narcotic addicts. *Am. J. Dig. Dis.*, 8:402–410.

34. Keup, W. (1959): Effect of phenothiazine derivative on liver function. *Dis. Nerv. Syst.*, 20 (Suppl. 5):161–175.

35. Klatskin, G. (1969): Toxic and drug-induced hepatitis. In: *Diseases of the Liver*, 3rd ed., edited by L. Schiff, pp. 498–601. Lippincott, Philadelphia.

36. Koff, R. S., Grady, G. F., Chalmers, T. C., Mosley, J. W., Swartz, B. L., and the Boston Inter-Hospital Liver Group (1967): Viral hepatitis in a group of Boston hospitals. III. Importance of exposure to shellfish in a non-epidemic period. *N. Engl. J. Med.*, 264:549–550.

37. Kohn, N., and Myerson, R. M. (1961): Cholestatic hepatitis associated with trifluoperazine. *N. Engl. J. Med.*, 264:549–550.

38. Kohn, N. N., and Myerson, R. M. (1961): Zanthomatous biliary cirrhosis following chlorpromazine. *Am. J. Med.*, 31:665–670.

39. Kushner, D. S., and Szanto, P. B. (1958): Heart failure, fever, and splenomegaly in a morphine addict. *JAMA*, 166:2162–2167.

40. Levine, R. A., Briggs, G. W., and Lowell, D. M. (1966): Chronic chlorpromazine cholangiolitic hepatitis. *Gastroenterology*, 50:665–670.

41. Levine, R. A., and Payne, M. A. (1960): Homologous serum hepatitis in youthful heroin users. *Ann. Intern. Med.*, 53:164–178.

42. Lindsay, S., and Skahen, R. (1956): Jaundice during chlorpromazine (Thorazine) therapy. *Arch. Pathol.*, 61:84–90.

43. Louria, D. B., Hensle, T., and Rose, J. (1967): The major medical complications of heroin addiction. *Ann. Intern. Med.*, 67:1–22.

44. Luna, L. G. (editor) (1968): *Manual of Histologic Staining Methods of the Armed Forces Institute of Pathology*, 3rd ed. McGraw-Hill, New York.

45. Marks, V., and Chapple, P. A. L. (1967): Hepatic dysfunction in heroin and cocaine users. *Br. J. Addict.*, 62:189–195.

46. Marx, G. F. (1961): Placental transfer and drugs used in anesthesia. *Anesthesiology*, 22:294–313.

47. Materson, B. J., and Barrett-Connor, E. (1967): LSD "main lining." A new hazard to health. *JAMA*, 200:1126–1127.

48. Nasser, W., and Caroli, J. (1957): Ictere et chlorpromazine: Etude critique. *Rev. Int. Hepat.*, 7:335–385.

49. Norris, R. F., and Potter, H. P. (1965): Hepatic inflammation of narcotic addicts. *Arch. Environ. Health*, II:662–668.

50. Oura, E. (1967): Influence of some alcohols and narcotics on the adenosine phosphates in the liver of the mouse. *Ann. Med. Esp. Biol. Fenn.*, 45:57–62.

51. Popov, C. S. (1974): Effect of phenothiazine drugs on the stability of rat liver subcellular particles. *Adv. Biochem. Psychopharmacol.*, 9:229–243.

52. Popper, H., Rubin, E., Gardiol, D., Schaffner, F., and Paronetto, F. (1965): Drug-induced liver disease. *Arch. Intern. Med.*, 115:128–136.

53. Popper, H., and Schaffner, F. (1959): Drug-induced hepatic injury. *Ann. Intern. Med.*, 51:1230–1252.

54. Popper, H., and Schaffner, F. (1970): Pathophysiology of cholestasis. *Hum. Pathol.*, 1:1–24.

55. Popper, H., Schaffner, F., Rubin, E., Barka, T., and Paronetto, F. (1963): Mechanisms of intrahepatic cholestasis in drug-induced hepatic injury. *Ann. NY Acad. Sci.*, 104:988–1013.

56. Potter, H. P., Cohen, N. N., and Norris, R. F. (1960): Chronic hepatic dysfunction in heroin addicts. *JAMA*, 174:2049–2051.

57. Preisig, R., Gocke, D., Morris, T., and Bradley, S. E. (1966): Chronic hepatic injury following experimental viral hepatitis in the dog. *Experientia*, 22:701–702.

58. Read, A. E., Harrison, C. V., and Sherlock, S. (1961): Chronic chlorpromazine jaundice. *Am. J. Med.*, 31:249–258.

59. Rodin, A. E., and Robertson, D. M. (1958): Fatal toxic hepatitis following chlorpromazine therapy: Report of a case with autopsy findings. *Arch. Pathol.*, 66:170–175.

60. Rodriguez, M., Paronetto, F., Schaffner, F., and Popper, H. (1969): Antimitochondrial antibodies in jaundice following drug administration. *JAMA*, 208:148–150.

61. Roizin, L., Akai, K., Alexander, G. J., Machiz, S., and Liu, J. C. (1971): Phenothiazine pathogenic mechanisms in rats with liver dysfunctions. *Fed. Proc.*, 30:574.

62. Roizin, L., Eros, G., Gold, G., Weinberg, F., English, W. H., and Wodraska, T. (1959): Histopathologic findings in the liver and C.N.S. following administration of tranquilizing drugs. *Dis. Nerv. Syst.*, 20:1–4.

63. Roizin, L., Gold, G., Kaufman, M. A., Fieve, R., Alexander, G. J., Ueno, Y., Liu, J. C., Keoseian, S., and Gray, R. (1968): Experimental potentiation of phenothiazine toxicology. 1. Effect of liver disorders. *Agressologie*, 9:379–381.

64. Roizin, L., Baden, M., Hashimoto, S., and Liu, J. C. (1973): Ultrastructural changes of the liver in the Drug Narcotism Syndrome. *Fed. Proc.*, 32:837 (Abstr.)

65. Roizin, L., Helpern, M., Baden, M., Kaufman, M. A., Hashimoto, S., Liu, J. C., and Eisenberg-Gelber, B. (1972): Methadone fatalities in heroin addicts. *Psychiatr. Q.*, 46:393–410.

66. Roizin, L., Kaufman, M. A., and Casselman, B. (1961): Structural changes induced by neuroleptics. *Rev. Can. Biol.*, 20:221–229.

67. Roizin, L., True, C., and Knight, M. (1959): Structural effects of tranquilizers. *Proc. Assoc. Res. Nerv. Ment. Dis.*, 37:285–323.

68. Roizin, L., Wechsler-Berger, M., and Brock, D. (1964): Ultracellular, functional, and pathological mechanisms. V. In vivo and in vitro CNS and liver mitochondria following administration of phenothiazines. *Trans. Am. Neurol. Assn.*, 89:247–248.

69a. Roizin, L., Hashimoto, S., Liu, J. C., Tom, K. J., and Eisenberg, G. (1971): Methadone effects upon the central nervous system, TPP, AcP and G-6-P. *J. Histochem. Cytochem.*, 19:720–721.

69b. Roizin, L., Hashimoto, S., Tom, K. J., and Liu, J. C. (1974): Methadone effects upon hypothalamic neuronal organelles. *J. Neuropathol. Exp. Neurol.*, 33:176–177.

70. Rosenthal, S. M., and Bourne, W. (1928): The effect of anesthetics on hepatic function. *JAMA*, 90:377.

71. Rosenstein, B. J. (1967): Viral hepatitis in narcotics users. *JAMA*, 199:698–700.

72. Rubin, E., and Lieber, C. S. (1968): Malnutrition tion and liver disease: An overemphasized relationship. *Am. J. Med.*, 45:1–6.

73. Ruttner, J. R., von Rondez, R., and Maier, C. (1962): Chlorpromazine-Ikterus, eire Form der cholostalischen Hepatose. *Dtsch. Med. Wochenschr.*, 87:1107–1110.

74. Salmorajski, T., Ordy, J. M., and Rolsten, C. (1965): Prenatal chlorpromazine effects of liver enzymes, glycogen and ultrastructure in mice offspring. *Am. J. Pathol.*, 47:803–831.

75. Sapira, J. D., Jasinski, D. R., and Gorodetzky, C. D. (1968): Liver disease in narcotic addicts. II. The role of the needle. *Clin. Pharmacol. Ther.*, 9:725–737.

76. Schaefer, J. W., Schiff, L., Call, E. A., and Oikawa, Y. (1967): Progression of acute hepatitis to postnecrotic cirrhosis. *Am. J. Med.*, 42:348–358.

77. Schoenfeld, M. R., Shacknow, N., Farian, K., and Messeloff, C. R. (1964): On the severity of hepatitis among heroin addicts. *J. New Drugs*, 4:79–81.

78. Shay, H., and Siplet, H. (1958): Relationship of chemical structure of chlorpromazine to its liver-sensitizing action. *Gastroenterology*, 35:16–24.

79. Sherlock, S. (1968): *Diseases of the Liver*, 4th ed. Davis, Philadelphia.

80. Sherlock, S. (1969): Factors determining the hepatic reactions to drugs. *Ann. NY Acad. Sci.*, 160:775–782.

81. Sims, J. L., Bremer, E. M., and Huston, E. S. (1955): Chlorpromazine changes in hepatic histology in the absence of jaundice. *J. Lab. Clin. Med.*, 46:952(Abstr.)

82. Steigmann, F., Hyman, S., and Goldbloom, R. (1950): Infectious hepatitis (homologous serum type) in drug addicts. *Gastroenterology*, 15:642–646.

83. Stimmel, B. (1972): Hepatic dysfunction in heroin addicts. The role of alcohol. *JAMA*, 222:811–812.

84. Sun, S. C., Chuong, S. M., and Fresh, J. W. (1965): A viral hepatitis study on Taiwan. *Arch. Intern. Med.*, 115:261-265.

85. Sutherland, J. M., and Light, I. J. (1965): The effects of drugs on the developing fetus. *Pediatr. Clin. North Am.*, 12:781–806.

86. Tanikawa, K., and Tanaka, M. (1966): Electron microscope observations of thioridazine-induced hepatitis. *Kurume Med. J.*, 13:15–21.

87. Walker, C. O., and Combes, B. (1966): Biliary cirrhosis induced by chlorpromazine. *Gastroenterology*, 51:631–640.

88. Wechsler-Berger, M., and Roizin, L. (1960): Tissue levels of chlorpromazine in experimental animals. *Br. J. Psychiatry*, 106:1501–1505.

89. Werther, J. L., and Korelitz, B. I. (1957): Chlorpromazine jaundice: Analysis of 22 cases. *Am. J. Med.*, 22:351–366.

90. Zaki, F. G. (1966): Ultrastructure of hepatic cholestasis. *Medicine (Baltimore)*, 45:537–545.

91. Zelman, S. (1959): Liver cell necrosis in chlorpromazine jaundice (allergic cholangiolitis). *Am. J. Med.*, 27:708–729.

92. Zimmerman, H. J. (1963): Clinical and laboratory manifestations of hepatoxicity. *Ann. NY Acad. Sci.*, 104:954–987.

93. Zimmerman, H. J. (1968): The spectrum of hepatoxicity. *Perspect. Biol. Med.*, 12:135–161.

94. Zweifler, A. J. (1960): Agranulocytosis and jaundice during therapy with meprobamate and promazine. *N. Engl. J. Med.*, 262:1229–1231.

Neurotoxicology, edited by L. Roizin, H. Shiraki, and N. Grčević. Raven Press, New York © 1977.

Pathologic Aspects of the Blood-Brain Barrier

Igor Klatzo

Laboratory of Neuropathology and Neuroanatomical Sciences, National Institute of Neurological and Communicative Disorders and Stroke, Bethesda, Maryland 20014

The neurotoxicity of a substance is determined by its direct effect on the cellular components of neuronal tissue as well as by its ability to penetrate and reach the nervous system. The fact that certain substances may not penetrate from the blood into the brain was first demonstrated by Ehrlich (11) and led to the development of the blood-brain barrier (BBB) concept.

Historically, there has been a considerable evolution in the interpretation of the BBB phenomenon starting from a notion of some simple "barrier" protecting the brain from the entry of noxious blood-borne substances to the current recognition of very complex "barrier systems" responsible for a homeostatically regulated biochemical environment, optimal for the normal function of the brain.

NORMAL ASPECTS

It can be now assumed that the barrier systems involve mechanisms on various structural and biochemic levels. It also becomes increasingly evident that these mechanisms reside primarily in the *cerebral endothelial cell,* which is clearly endowed with some unique features different from endothelial cells of other organs. Structurally, the most characteristic feature of cerebral endothelium is the presence of *tight junctions,* formed by close membrane apposition at certain points of adjacent cells. Using electron microscopically de-

monstrable tracers, e.g., horseradish peroxidase, it has been shown that these tight junctions effectively restrict the diffusion between endothelial cells of macromolecular substances, such as proteins (7). A further support for the assumption that the tight junctions provide an effective barrier for proteins is also provided by the fact that certain "special" BBB regions, such as neurophypophysis, pineal body, median eminence, area postrema, and choroid plexus, that are permeable to proteins are devoid of tight junctions between the endothelial cells (6). The only exception among vertebrates to the existence of a barrier created by tight junctions is the shark brain, where intravenously injected peroxidase passes between endothelial cells separated by electron-lucent spaces of 40 Å and readily accumulates in the subendothelial spaces (8). On the other hand, the perivascular glia in the shark brain is endowed with tight junctions, and this may account for an observation that even drastic traumatic injuries of the shark brain are not followed by perivascular exudates and development of the vasogenic type of brain edema (21).

Developmentally, establishment of the BBB to proteins and formation of the tight junction system takes place quite early. Observations of Olsson et al. (34) indicate that in rat embryos the cerebral blood vessels are impermeable to albumin as early as the 15th day after fertilization.

At this moment, the main function that can be ascribed to tight junctions is the mechanical obstruction to free diffusion of macromolecular substances, such as proteins, through the endothelial layer. The mechanisms involved in the breakdown of this layer to the passage of proteins remain a somewhat controversial matter and are discussed later.

Since the tight junctions seem to form an effective barrier, at least for macromolecular substances, the remaining routes for penetration across the endothelium must be related either to transcellular passage or to vesicular transport. With regard to transcellular passage, cell membrane permeability features as well as transport phenomena unique for cerebral endothelium are now considered.

Concerning features of *general cell membrane permeability,* since the membranes are composed of a bimolecular layer of lipoprotein, the penetration of nonelectrolytes is obviously related to their lipid solubility, whereas an ionic transfer is provided by globular proteins or ionophores interspersed in the lipid layer. Lipid-soluble, apolar substances penetrate into brain with least hindrance, e.g., faster penetration of heroin in comparison with morphine can be explained by their relative lipid solubility. In the case of organic acids or bases, their penetration can be predicted by their fractional concentration of un-ionized species multiplied by their lipid solubility (the partition parameter), the un-ionized part of compound being, as a rule, much more lipid soluble and more permeable than the ionized part (39). Otherwise, *protein binding* of a substance will reduce its penetration by decreasing the concentration of its free form available for diffusion into the brain (4). Thus protein binding of bilirubin reduces markedly its neurotoxicity (10), and even severely icteric adult patients may show very little yellow staining of the brain tissue.

Superimposed on general features of cell membrane permeability, cerebral endothelial cells have unique physiologic properties enabling a facilitated or active transport of various compounds essential to proper functioning of the brain.

The *carrier-mediated facilitated transport* serves primarily for the rapid, nonenergetic transfer of nutrients, such as glucose and certain amino acids. Being carrier-mediated, the systems are saturable as can be demonstrated by kinetic assays using both labeled and unlabeled compounds. The transport carriers are stereospecific, with the L form of amino acids, for example, being mostly favored (33). In addition to monosaccharides and amino acids, a facilitated mechanism has been demonstrated for the transport of short-chain monocarboxylic acids, such as lactic and pyruvic acids (31). Since the facilitated transport is generally bidirectional and the transport capacity of the system for organic acids is rather low, this factor may adversely affect elimination from the brain of lactate in hypoxic and, especially, ischemic conditions, as is discussed later.

The *energy-dependent active transport* mechanism has been extensively investigated as regards the Na–K exchange pump with adenosine triphosphate as the energy source. In addition to this general cellular mechanism that pumps Na out and K into the cell, cerebral endothelium presumably has some special mechanism of active transport that is expressed through the remarkable performance of maintaining considerable ionic gradients between plasma and brain (e.g., K being about 40% lower in the extracellular fluid of the brain than in plasma) and presumably of regulating the movement of water between these compartments. Involvement of cerebral endothelium in energy-dependent transport systems is supported by the observation of Oldendorf (32) describing in brain endothelial cells five times as many mitochondria as in similar cells in skeletal muscle.

Both the active and facilitated transport

systems require some special proteins and enzymes to act as carriers. The development of a special enzymatic composition of cerebral endothelial cells can be surmised from histochemic observations on growing endothelium *in vitro* (41). A comparison between cultured endothelial cells derived from various tissues indicated that cerebellar capillaries show selectively a high activity of butyryl cholinesterase, which is absent in pia-arachnoidal microvessels or in those derived from skin or rib cultures. High activity of two other enzymes believed to be involved in the BBB *in situ,* alkaline phosphatase and γ-glutamyl transpeptidase, is present in capillaries of both brain and meninges but not in those of skin or rib cultures. Otherwise, *in vivo* the cerebral endothelium shows strong histochemic reactions with a variety of oxidative and hydrolytic enzymes. The role of these enzymes in transport mechanisms, however, remains unclear, although coincidentally they are equally prominent also in renal tubules and intestinal epithelium, i.e., cellular structures with well-recognized transport systems (22).

In addition to special proteins involved in active and facilitated transports, the cerebral endothelium possesses specific enzymatic systems regulating passage of certain amines. Best known in this respect are monoamine oxidase and DOPA-decarboxylase, which are involved in restricting movement of biogenic amines in and out of brain (3).

Perhaps, the most fascinating and, so far, the least evaluated is the *vesicular transport* occurring across the cerebral endothelium. Vesicular transport is related to pinocytotic activity of cell membranes represented by their movement creating invaginations and engulfing an extracellular fluid that thus becomes trapped in membrane-bound pinocytotic vesicles. The pinocytotic vesicles can be "digested" intracellularly by lysosomes, or they can migrate to an opposite side of a cell and discharge their contents outside. The pinocytotic activity or "drinking" (in Greek *pinein* means to drink) by the cells is nonselective, and even large molecules can be engulfed in vesicles; at the same time, it provides in the case of cerebral endothelium a mechanism for movement of serum proteins across its layer. In the normal brain, pinocytotic vesicles in cerebral capillaries are rather rare, and this may account for the relative impermeability of brain capillaries to proteins. On the other hand, Westergaard and Brightman (48) recently described an endothelial uptake of blood-injected peroxidase at certain segments of brain arterioles, suggesting that these sites may provide a *locus* for some limited entry of proteins into the brain parenchyma (in addition to the penetration of proteins into "special" BBB areas). Vesicular transport is thought to be bidirectional and generally moves substances from higher to lower concentrations. Its main role and significance appear to occur in pathologic conditions, as is discussed below.

PATHOLOGIC DISTURBANCES OF THE BBB

The normally functioning mechanisms of the BBB can be disturbed singly or in any multiple combination.

With regard to the system of *tight junctions,* it has been recently shown that they remain remarkably intact even in areas where brain parenchyma may reveal severe ischemic injury (50). Otherwise, the cerebral endothelium, being devoid of contractile proteins, does not react to systemically injected histamine, serotonin, or norepinephrine with an increasing permeability to proteins (9,47), as occurs in nonneural tissue due to contraction and separation of the endothelial cells (26). According to electron microscopic observations with peroxidase tracer, hypertonic salt solutions like urea, applied to the arachnoidal surface or perfused via the internal carotid artery, seem to produce an opening of tight junctions (5,40). However, absolute proof is lacking here, since a demonstration of continuous opening of tight junctions traced from luminal to abluminal surface has not yet been provided. Unquestionably, tight junctions can be disrupted in more drastic injuries of brain tissue, but this is usually associated with destruction of the endothelium itself. Otherwise, a reversible opening of BBB, such as can be achieved by application of hyperosmotic compounds, offers a possibility for introducing into the brain various therapeutic agents, the entry of which is otherwise restricted by the BBB; and experimental studies concerning this subject have been carried out by Rapoport (39).

The *malfunction of facilitated transport* for monosaccharides or amino acids is reflected in a variety of pathologic conditions. A reduction in transport of glucose analogs was shown (45,46) to occur following intracarotid perfusions with $HgCl_2$ in low concentrations, whereas perfusions with higher $HgCl_2$ concentrations resulted in increased brain uptake of glucose analogs. Such increased uptake was associated with breakdown of the BBB for proteins and could not be inhibited by saturating the carrier system with unlabeled glucose. Spatz et al. (42,44) showed a decrease in brain uptake of glucose analogs and amino acids (with few exceptions) in severe hypoxia and hypercapnia, whereas an inhibitable increase or no change in uptake was observed in hypocapnia. The marked increase in uptake of glucose occurring in ischemia is discussed later with other BBB disturbances observed in this condition.

Recognized clinical entities associated with malfunctioning facilitated transport are those in which an excessive accumulation of some sugar or amino acid in blood due to an inborn metabolic error results in competitive inhibition in the transport into the brain of vital nutrients, such as glucose or essential amino acids. Thus, in *galactosemia,* characterized by enzymatic deficiency, an excessive accumulation of galactose and its metabolic derivatives is associated with a competitive inhibition of glucose transport that exerts adverse effects on brain function (19,30). A similar mechanism of competitive inhibition is operative in *phenylketonuria* in which due to deficiency of phenylalanine hydroxylase (15,51) there is an excessive accumulation in blood of phenylalanine and its derivatives. A high level of phenylalanine by drastically changing its concentration ratio to other essential amino acids inhibits their transport into the brain, and this leads to reduction of protein synthesis (1) as well as of brain serotonin by lowering transport of tryptophan (35). In *maple syrup disease,* another neurologic disorder associated with inborn aminoaciduria, a deficient metabolism of leucine, isoleucine, and valine results in interference of these excessively accumulated compounds with the transport of other important amino acids (27).

The disturbance of *vesicular transport* can be recognized by an increased number of pinocytotic vesicles in the cerebral endothelium, and this is usually associated with evidence of abnormal passage of proteins when tested with horseradish peroxidase tracer. Pinocytotic activity in cerebral endothelium was shown to be stimulated by divalent ions (18), serotonin, norepinephrine, and cyclic AMP (47). A previously observed increase in the permeability of the BBB to Evans Blue tracer in acute hypertension (6,16) has been reported by Westergaard and Bronsted (49) to depend on a greatly increased vesicular transport of peroxidase in cerebral endothelium, in their study of animals subjected to an acute hypertension with metaraminol (Aramine®). The assumption that the changes of the BBB are due to elevation of the blood pressure *per se,* and not to pharmacologic action of vaso-pressant drugs used is supported by the fact that BBB changes characteristic of hypertension can be produced also by a simple clamping of the thoracic aorta (17). Whether an increased vascular permeability to protein tracers that is observed following *epileptic seizures* (2,23,25) can be specifically ascribed to convulsions or whether the BBB changes merely represent effects of an acute elevation of blood pressure occurring in convulsive experiments remains unclarified. Otherwise, the BBB changes in acute hypertension and in convulsive states (24) were shown to be similarly of a patchy character and associated with intense pinocytotic uptake of peroxidase tracer, which is especially conspicuous in the endothelium of some arterioles.

Mostly, the disturbances of the BBB involve *several mechanisms*. To present a complexity of BBB changes especially in the relationship of their effect upon the brain parenchyma, a neurologically important condition, i.e., *ischemic brain edema,* is now discussed in detail.

It has been increasingly evident that cerebral edema and ischemia are closely interrelated, as an abnormal accumulation of fluid in the brain tissue is characteristic for both conditions. Recent studies (12) indicate that ischemia of even 5-min duration is sufficient to produce an abnormal fluid uptake in various elements of the brain parenchyma (especially in perivascular astrocytic structures). This may be considered an expression of disturbance in energy-dependent cellular osmoregulation, developing acutely in ischemia. However, a change confined to a swelling of cellular elements of brain parenchyma would result merely in water shifting from extracellular into intracellular compartments. Therefore, the fact that there is a net increase of water in brain tissue at these early stages of cerebral ischemia indicates also a change in the movement of water at the BBB level. The

concept that there is a *barrier system* for *water* at the cerebral capillary level has been implied in several investigations (36, 37), which also suggested some central noradrenergic system as responsible for regulation of water permeability. In this connection, it could be demonstrated that a stimulation of the locus coeruleus (38) produced a prompt increase in brain water permeability and a reduction of the cerebral blood flow (CBF).

A dissociation that may exist concerning disturbances in water movement between blood and brain tissue, facilitated transport of nutrients, and increased cerebrovascular permeability to proteins is clearly shown in our recent studies on ischemic brain edema (12). After carotid artery occlusion in the gerbil, the uptake of water, without other demonstrable changes in the BBB permeability, is followed by an increased facilitated transport of glucose analogs (43). The breakdown of the BBB for proteins occurs at a relatively later stage (12) and is associated with increased pinocytotic transport of peroxidase across the cerebral endothelium (50). Such an opening of the BBB to proteins is of a transitory nature and is seemingly independent of CBF levels or development or necrotic changes in brain parenchyma. The uptake of glucose analogs during this stage, however, must be related to other mechanisms of passage than to facilitated transport, since it cannot be inhibited by saturation with unlabeled glucose analogs (43).

Our studies on cerebral ischemia revealed also the existence of a "maturation" phenomenon with regard to the behavior of the BBB (20). According to the principle of this phenomenon, the maturation or the progression of injury, expressed in various parameters, is related to the intensity of an ischemic insult, a lesser intensity resulting in slower development of the lesions. The maturation phenomenon in cerebral ischemia was described with regard to histopathologic development of the ischemic lesions (14) and the behavior of energy metabolites and biogenic amines in postischemic periods (28,29). Concerning the BBB, insults of relatively low intensity may delay development of an increased cerebrovascular permeability to proteins (13), and the well-known delay in clinical appearance of positive scanning using radioactive protein tracers may be related to a gradual maturation of BBB injury in these patients.

The variety of pathologic conditions associated with BBB changes is too great to be considered adequately within the scope of this chapter. Just briefly can be mentioned the importance of the BBB behavior in *brain tumors,* which may determine the accessibility of neoplastic tissue to chemotherapeutic agents. Similarly BBB changes in various *inflammations* and *auto-immune reactions* are of paramount relevance to the efficacy of therapeutic measures. Most of all, it should be evident from the above considerations that the multiplicity of factors that constitute the present concept of the BBB are of major influence in determining the neurotoxicity of substances, and thus the BBB becomes an essential and integral part of modern neurotoxicology.

REFERENCES

1. Appel, S. H. (1966): Inhibition of brain protein synthesis: An approach to the biochemical basis of neurological dysfunction in the amino acidurias. *Trans. NY Acad. Sci.,* 29:63–70.
2. Bauer, K. F., and Leonhardt, H. (1956): A contribution to the pathological physiology of the blood-brain barrier. *J. Comp. Neurol.,* 106:363–370.
3. Bertler, A., Falck, B., Owman, C. H., and Rosengren, E. (1966): The localization of monoaminergic blood-brain barrier mechanisms. *Pharmacol. Rev.,* 18:369–385.
4. Bird, A. E., and Marshall, A. C. (1967): Correlation of serum binding of penicillin with partition coefficients. *Biochem. Pharmacol.,* 16:2275–2290.
5. Brightman, M. W., Hori, M., Rapoport, S. I., Reese, T. S., and Westergaard, E. (1973): Osmotic opening of the tight junctions in cerebral endothelium. *J. Comp. Neurol.,* 152:317–326.
6. Brightman, M. W., Klatzo, I., Olsson, Y., and Reese, T. S. (1970): The blood-brain barrier to proteins under normal and pathological conditions. *J. Neurol. Sci.,* 10:215–239.
7. Brightman, M. W., Reese, T. S., and Feder, N. (1970): Assessment with the electron microscope of the permeability to peroxidase of cerebral endothelium and epithelium in mice and sharks. In: *Capillary Permeability,* edited by C. Crone and N. A. Lassen, pp. 463–478. Munksgaard, Copenhagen.
8. Brightman, M. W., Reese, T. S., Olsson, Y., and Klatzo, I. (1971): Morphologic aspects of the blood-brain barrier to peroxidase in elasmobranchs. In: *Progress in Neuropathology,* edited by H. M. Zimmerman, pp. 146–151. Grune & Stratton, New York.
9. Broman, T., and Lindberg-Broman, A. M. (1945): An experimental study of disorders in the permeability of the cerebral vessels ("the blood-brain barrier") produced by chemical and physico-chemical agents. *Acta Physiol. Scand.,* 10:102–125.
10. Diamond, I. (1969): Bilirubin binding and kernicterus. *Adv. Pediatr.,* 16:99–119.
11. Ehrlich, P. (1885): *Das Sauerstoff-Bedürfniss des Organismus: eine farbenanalytische Studie.* Hirschwald, Berlin.
12. Fujimoto, T., Walker, J. T., Jr., Spatz, M., and Klatzo, I. (1976): Pathophysiologic aspects of ischemic edema. In: *Dynamics of Brain Edema,* edited by H. Pappius and W. Feindel, pp. 171–180. Springer-Verlag, Heidelberg and New York.
13. Ito, U., Go, K. G., Walker, J. T., Jr., Spatz, M., and Klatzo, I. (1976): Experimental cerebral ischemia in Mongolian gerbils. III. Behaviour of the blood-brain barrier. *Acta Neuropathol. (Berl.),* 34:1–6.
14. Ito, U., Spatz, M., Walker, J. T., Jr., and Klatzo, I. (1975): Experimental cerebral ischemia in Mongolian gerbils. I. Light microscopic observations. *Acta Neuropathol. (Berl.),* 32:209–223.
15. Jervis, G. A. (1947): Studies on phenylpyruvic oligophrenia: The position of the metabolic error. *J. Biol. Chem.,* 169:651–656.
16. Johansson, B., Li, C.-L., Olsson, Y., and Klatzo, I. (1970): The effect of acute arterial hypertension on the blood-brain barrier to protein tracers. *Acta Neuropathol. (Berl.),* 16:117–124.
17. Johansson, B., and Linder, L. E. (1974): Blood-brain barrier dysfunction in acute arterial hypertension induced by clamping of the thoracic aorta. *Acta Neurol. Scand.,* 50:360–365.
18. Joó, F. (1971): Increased production of coated vesicles in the brain capillaries during enhanced permeability of the blood-brain barrier. *Br. J. Exp. Pathol.,* 52:646–649.
19. Kalcklar, H. M., Kinoshita, J. H., and Donnell, G. N. (1973): Galactosemia: Biochemistry, genetics, pathophysiology, and developmental aspects. In: *Biology of Brain Dysfunction,* edited by G. E. Gaull, pp. 31–88. Plenum Press, New York.
20. Klatzo, I. (1975): Pathophysiologic aspects of

cerebral ischemia. In: *The Nervous System. The Basic Neurosciences*, Vol. 1, edited by D. B. Tower, pp. 313–322. Raven Press, New York.

21. Klatzo, I., and Steinwall, O. (1965): Observation on cerebrospinal fluid pathways and behaviour of the blood-brain barrier in sharks. *Acta Neuropathol. (Berl.)*, 5:161–175.

22. Landers, J. W., Chason, J. L., Gonzales, J. E., and Palutke, W. (1962): Morphology and enzymatic activity of rat cerebral capillaries. *Lab. Invest.*, 11:1253–1259.

23. Lee, J. C., and Olszewski, J. (1961): Increased cerebrovascular permeability after repeated electroshocks. *Neurology (Minneap.)*, 11:515–519.

24. Lorenzo, A. V., Hedley-Whyte, E. T., Eisenberg, H. M., and Hsu, D. W. (1975): Increased penetration of horseradish peroxidase across the blood-brain barrier induced by Metrasol seizures. *Brain Res.*, 88:136–140.

25. Lorenzo, A. V., Shirahige, I., Liang, M., and Barlow, C. F. (1972): Temporary alteration of cerebrovascular permeability to plasma protein during drug-induced seizures. *Am. J. Physiol.*, 223:268–277.

26. Majno, G., Shea, S. M., and Leventhal, M. (1969): Endothelial contraction induced by histamine-type mediators: An electromicroscopic study. *J. Cell Biol.*, 42:647–672.

27. Morris, M. D., Lewis, B. D., Doolan, P. D., and Harper, H. A. (1961): Clinical and biochemical observations on an apparently nonfatal variant of branched-chain ketoaciduria (maple syrup urine disease). *Pediatrics*, 28:918–923.

28. Mrsulja, B. B., Mrsulja, B. J., Ito, U., Walker, J. T., Jr., Spatz, M., and Klatzo, I. (1975): Experimental cerebral ischemia in Mongolian gerbils. II. Changes in carbohydrates. *Acta Neuropathol. (Berl.)*, 33:91–103.

29. Mrsulja, B. B., Mrsulja, B. J., Spatz, M., Ito, U., Walker, J. T., Jr., and Klatzo, I. (1976): Experimental cerebral ischemia in Mongolian gerbils. IV. Behaviour of biogenic amines. *Acta Neuropathol. (Berl.)*, 36:1–8.

30. Nadler, H. L., Inouye, T., and Hsia, D. Y. Y. (1969): Classical galactosemia: A study of fifty-five cases. In: *Galactosemia*, edited by D. Y. Y. Hsia, pp. 127–139. Charles C Thomas, Springfield, Illinois.

31. Oldendorf, W. H. (1973): Carrier-mediated blood-brain barrier transport of short-chain monocarboxylic organic acids. *Am. J. Physiol.*, 224:1450–1453.

32. Oldendorf, W. H. (1975): Permeability of the blood-brain barrier. In: *The Nervous System. The Basic Neurosciences*, Vol. 1, edited by D. B. Tower, pp. 279–289. Raven Press, New York.

33. Oldendorf, W. H. (1973): Stereospecificity of blood-brain barrier permeability to amino acids. *Am. J. Physiol.*, 224:967–969.

34. Olsson, Y., Klatzo, I., Sourander, P., and Stein wall, D. (1968): Blood-brain barrier to albumin in embryonic, new-born and adult rats. *Acta Neuropathol. (Berl.)*, 10:117–122.

35. Pare, C. M. B., Sandler, M., and Stacey, R. S. (1957): 5-Hydroxytryptamine deficiency in phenyl-ketonuria. *Lancet*, 272:551–553.

36. Raichle, M. E., Eichling, J. O., and Grubb, R. L. (1974): Brain permeability of water. *Arch. Neurol.*, 30:319–321.

37. Raichle, M. E., Eichling, J. O., Straatmann, M. G., Welch, M. J., Larson, K. B., and Ter-Pogossian, M. M. (1976): Blood-brain barrier permeability of C^{11} labeled alcohols and O^{15} labeled water. *Am. J. Physiol.*, 230:543–552.

38. Raichle, M., Eichling, J., Grubb, R. L., Jr., and Hartman, B. K. (1976): Central noradrenergic regulation of brain microcirculation. In: *Dynamics of Brain Edema*, edited by H. Pappius and W. Feindel, pp. 11–17. Springer-Verlag, Heidelberg and New York.

39. Rapoport, S. I. (1976): *Blood-Brain Barrier in Physiology and Medicine*. Raven Press, New York.

40. Rapoport, S. I., Brightman, M. W., and Reese, T. S. (1973): Reversible osmotic opening of the blood-brain barrier (BBB) by opening tight junctions of cerebrovascular endothelium. *Biophysics J.*, 13:230a.

41. Renkawek, K., Murray, M. R., Spatz, M., and Klatzo, I. (1976): Distinctive histochemical characteristics of brain capillaries in organotypic culture. *Exp. Neurol.*, 50:194–206.

42. Spatz, M., Fujimoto, T., and Go, K. G. (1976): Transport studies of schemic cerebral edema. In: *Dynamics of Brain Edema*, edited by H. Pappius and W. Feindel, pp. 181–186. Springer-Verlag, Heidelberg and New York.

43. Spatz, M., Fujimoto, T., and Go, K. G. (1976): Transport studies in ischemic cerebral edema. In: *Brain and Edema: Resolution and Formation*, edited by H. Pappius. Springer-Verlag, West Germany. *(In press.)*

44. Spatz, M., and Klatzo, I. (1976): Pathological aspects of brain transport phenomena. In: *Transport Phenomena in the Nervous System*, Vol. 69, edited by G. Levi, L. Battistin, and A. Lajtha, pp. 479–495. Plenum Press, New York.

45. Steinwall, O. (1968): Transport inhibition phenomena in unilateral chemical injury of the blood-brain barrier. In: *Brain Barrier Systems. Progress in Brain Research*, Vol. 29, edited by A. Lajtha and D. H. Ford, pp. 357–364. Elsevier, Amsterdam.

46. Steinwall, O., and Klatzo, I. (1966): Selective vulnerability of the blood-brain barrier in chemically induced lesions. *J. Neuropathol. Exp. Neurol.*, 25:524–549.

47. Westergaard, E. (1975): The effect of serotonin, norepinephrine and cyclic AMP on the blood-brain barrier. *J. Ultrastruct. Res.*, 50:383.

48. Westergaard, E., and Brightman, M. W. (1973): Transport of proteins across normal cerebral arterioles. *J. Comp. Neurol.*, 152:17–29.

49. Westergaard, E., and Bronsted, H. E. (1975): The effect of acute hypertension on the vesicular transport of proteins in cerebral vessels. In:

VIIth Int. Congr. Neuropathology, Budapest,
Hungary, September 1–7, 1974, edited by St.
Kornyey, St. Tariska, and G. Gosztonyi, pp.
619–622. Excerpta Medica, Amsterdam, Akademiai Kiado, Budapest.

50. Westergaard, E., Go, G., Klatzo, I., and Spatz, M.
(1976): Increased permeability of cerebral vessels to horseradish peroxidase induced by
ischemia in Mongolian gerbils. *Acta Neuropathol.,*
35:307–325.

51. Wiltse, H. E., and Menkes, J. H. (1972): Brain
damage in the aminoacidurias. In: *Handbook of*
Neurochemistry, Vol. 7, edited by A. Lajtha, pp.
143-167. Plenum Press, New York.

Neurotoxicology, edited by L. Roizin, H. Shiraki, and N. Grčević. Raven Press, New York © 1977.

Effects of Central Nervous System Active and Nonactive Drugs on the Fetal Central Nervous System

W. F. Geber

Department of Pharmacology, Medical College of Georgia, Augusta, Georgia 30902

One of the major points of contention in accepting the relevance or application of teratogenic studies in animals to humans lies in the fact that many animal investigations employ concentrations or dosages of drugs or other compounds that far exceed those to which the pregnant human may be expected to be exposed, except under unusual and extreme conditions. One of the primary objectives of the science of teratology is eventually to explain the mechanisms of induction of abnormal fetal development in the majority of human situations in order to develop preventive measures. Therefore, it is imperative that the teratologist attempt to develop an animal model (including doses) that more closely approximates the usual or probable human situation.

Related to the problem of teratogenic dose levels is an evolving concept having far-reaching ramifications: the possibility that *extremely* low levels of a wide range of compounds that produce "no" measurable embryotoxic effect when introduced as single entities into a pregnant female may be potent contributory or co-factors in the etiology of a number of types of pathological states in humans and animals (1,10). The quantitative definition of what constitutes a "very low level" of a toxic substance presents some difficulty both from the standpoint of the animal model and from the standpoint of relating the data to the situation as it may exist in the human environment. Some investigators consider the "low level—no response" concept to have no practical or theoretical basis and, indeed, to be a "nonconcept" at best (5). I believe the major difficulty in establishing the existence of a positive, pathological input into a biological system by a single, potentially toxic substance at very low concentrations has been the lack of an adequate model to demonstrate the presence of an effect when "no effect" is evident. Utilizing two well-established biological concepts, i.e., potentiation and summation, an animal model system was developed for the induction of fetal anomalies as an endpoint indicator of the presence or absence of teratogenic activity of low concentrations of a wide range of compounds. These substances, with several exceptions, were chosen for possessing both dissimilar molecular structures and different physiological and pharmacological activities. Morphine and hydromorphone are structurally similar, as are methadone and propoxyphene, whereas all four compounds are analgesics. The one characteristic all compounds share in common is their teratogenic activity, particularly in the developing central nervous system. Included in the study were morphine, hydromorphone, methadone, vitamin

A, isoproterenol, trypan blue, dimethyl-tryptamine, cocaine, propoxyphene, caffeine, nicotine, salicylate, harmine, and hexachlorophene.

METHODS

All drugs and other chemicals were obtained from the following commercial sources: hydromorphone hydrochloride, Knoll; morphine sulfate, Merck; methadone hydrochloride, cocaine hydrochloride, Mallinckrodt; propoxyphene hydrochloride, Lilly; N,N-dimethyltryptamine, isoproterenol hydrochloride, harmine hydrochloride, nicotine, Aldrich; vitamin A palmitate, Nutritional Biochemical; caffeine, California Foundation for Biochemical Research; trypan blue lot no. 2–977, J. T. Baker; hexachlorophene, Sindar; and sodium salicylate, Pfaltz and Bauer.

The various drug and chemical components of the solutions were dissolved in sterile saline immediately before injection. The more complex nine- and 12-component mixtures required constant agitation to retard precipitation of some of the compounds from the solution. It was necessary to add 0.05 ml of absolute ethanol per 20 ml hexachlorophene solution to obtain dissolution of the compound when it was studied alone in the initial maternal-dose, minimal-fetal-teratogenic-response phase of the present investigation. However, when hexachlorophene was utilized as a component of the 12-compound solution, the caffeine was found to aid in the water solubilization process, and no ethanol was required.

Timed pregnant Lakeview outbred (Lak: LVC) golden hamsters were utilized throughout the study. Day one of pregnancy was calculated as the day following introduction of the receptive female into the cage of the male. Age range of the animals was 105 to 120 days, and weight range, 110 to 125 g at the time of breeding. All pregnant animals were individually caged

in a quiet, temperature- and humidity-controlled room, i.e., $23 \pm 1°C$, a light/dark cycle of 12 hr on, 12 hr off, and 45 to 50% humidity. Food and water were available *ad libitum.*

All drug solutions were administered as single, subcutaneous injections on day 8 of gestation. Following drug injection, the females were returned to their cages, observed for drug-induced behavioral activity, and left undisturbed until day 12 of gestation when they were sacrificed with an excess of ether. The uterus was removed, total implantation sites counted, resorptions noted, and fetuses removed and evaluated. Examination of each fetus included determination of viability and inspection for gross anatomical malformations. Following initial evaluation, all fetuses were placed in 10% buffered formaldehyde to allow for tissue hardening and further gross anatomical study.

In the development of the total data of this study, four steps were taken as follows: (a) a three-component solution of hydromorphone, isoproterenol, and trypan blue (HIT) was utilized to demonstrate, in a limited-component mixture, the marked potentiation of the teratogenic effects of the individual substances; (b) a six-component solution of hydromorphone, morphine, methadone, vitamin A, isoproterenol, and trypan blue was utilized to build on the original three-compound mixture; (c) a nine-component solution was used to reduce the number of narcotic type compounds to one, and to add additional, structurally unrelated teratogens; and (d) a 12-component solution was used adding the remainder of the teratogens previously studied as single entities. An additional breakdown of the components of the six-component solution was studied combining hydromorphone, morphine, and methadone as one solution, and vitamin A, isoproterenol, and trypan blue as the second solution.

Some interpolation is necessary when

comparing data from single and composite dose levels of individual compounds throughout the study since it was not possible to duplicate exact dose levels throughout all experiments because of inherent weight differences within and between groups of animals treated with the varying dose levels and combinations of compounds.

RESULTS

As previously mentioned the number of compounds administered in the composite teratogenic mixture was increased from three to 12 as experience was gained in finding and evaluating compounds possessing significant teratogenic effects on the developing embryonic central nervous system. Maternal-dose, minimal-or-no-teratogenic-response curves were established initially for each of the substances. Table 1 lists the concentrations (maternal dose in mg/kg) and the fetal teratogenic response (percent congenital malformations) to the various compounds. The complete dose-response data are not included in the table since the objective of the present study was the teratogenic response of the lower end of the concentration curve. It was considered more important to demonstrate summation and potentiation of the lowest effective concentrations rather than the higher dose levels. Complete dose-response curves for a number of the compounds have been published elsewhere (9).

The concentrations of the individual components in the composite solutions were set by several considerations. It was believed necessary to have the concentration of at least one or two of the components of the mixture at a maternal-dose level that would be within the effective teratogenic dose range for that component so as to be able to follow a "positive marker" of teratogenic activity. Therefore, either trypan blue or isoproterenol was chosen to be utilized for this objective. In the studies on the three-component mixtures of either HIT or vitamin A, isoproterenol, and trypan blue (VIT), maternal-dose levels of the two marker compounds were well within the positive low-teratogenic-response range. In the other studies on the more complex mixtures, trypan blue and isoproterenol maternal-dose levels were, in general, decreased to the minimal

TABLE 1. *Determination of minimal effective teratogenic dose level*

Compound	Dose (mg/kg)[a]			Mean no. fetuses/litter			Percent CM		
Morphine	25	35	88	11.9	10.8	11.0	0.0	2.3	10.0
Methadone	26	31	67	12.3	12.1	12.2	0.0	2.9	6.2
Hydromorphone	14	19	39	11.7	11.5	11.9	0.0	3.5	14.3
Trypan blue	0.9	1.5	5.6	9.1	8.4	7.8	1.1	4.2	8.3
Isoproterenol	15	25	50				0.0	2.5	7.0
Vitamin A	34*	74**	150	11.8	11.4	11.6	0.0	0.0	2.2
DMT (Dimethyltryptamine)	90*	300**	430	11.0	11.0	10.7	0.0	0.0	5.2
Cocaine	80	125	740	11.2	11.9	10.8	0.0	5.1	12.0
Harmine	90*	120	170	11.9	11.6	11.8	0.0	2.6	5.1
Propoxyphene	85	203	415	12.0	11.0	12.0	0.0	1.0	16.6
Caffeine	49	74	170	11.3	10.8	10.1	0.0	1.0	11.0
Salicylate	37*	45	89	11.4	10.9	10.6	0.0	0.0	2.8
Nicotine	2.7	5.6	8.0	10.5	9.8	9.4	0.0	1.0	5.8
Hexachlorophene	40**	53	113	10.9	10.9	9.6	0.0	1.4	2.6

Twenty litters analyzed for each concentration of each compound, except * = 19 litters and ** = 18 litters.
[a] Dose expressed as the base compound.

TABLE 2. *Component concentrations in composite mixtures of teratogens*

	12 D (mg/kg)	9 D (mg/kg)	6 D (mg/kg)	HIT (mg/kg)	HMM (mg/kg)	VIT (mg/kg)	Saline
Hydromorphone	2.1/4.3/8.7	1.4/2.8	2.9/8.7	14.4	8.0	—	—
Trypan blue	0.6/1.3/2.7	0.5/0.9	1.1/3.9	4.9	—	2.9	—
Vitamin A	3.0/5.9/12	2.0/4.1	4.6/14.3	—	—	13.0	—
Isoproterenol	4.9/9.5/19.5	3.2/6.5	7.4/23	41	—	21.4	—
Morphine	—	—	2.9/8.7	—	8.0	—	—
Methadone	—	—	2.9/8.7	—	8.0	—	—
DMT	12/24/49.2	8/16	—	—	—	—	—
Cocaine	10.7/21.4/43.6	7.1/14.2	—	—	—	—	—
Harmine	9.1/18.2/39.4	6.5/13	—	—	—	—	—
Propoxyphene	10.6/21.6/44.2	7.2/14.4	—	—	—	—	—
Caffeine	12/24/49.2	8/16	—	—	—	—	—
Salicylate	9.1/18.3/38.6	—	—	—	—	—	—
Nicotine	0.4/0.8/1.7	—	—	—	—	—	—
Hexachlorophene	4/8/16	—	—	—	—	—	—
Percent CM	5.9 13.4 25.4	10.8 19.4	8.0 39.8	48.0	0.0	10.8	0.0
	(21) (47) (90)	(36) (68)	(35) (172)	(155)	(0)	(20)	(0)
No. litters	30/30/30	30 30	40 40	40	20	20	44
Mean no. fetuses	11.8 11.7 11.8	11.2 11.6	11.0 10.8	8.1	11.4	9.3[a]	11.9
per litter ±SEM	±0.2 ±0.4 ±0.4	±0.3 ±0.2	±0.3 ±0.4[b]	±0.4[a]	±0.4	±0.3	±0.3

[a] Difference from control $p = <0.01$.
[b] Difference from control $p = <0.5, > 0.2$.

or below minimal teratogenic-response-dose level.

Three Component Solutions (HIT, VIT)

The fetal teratogenic response to the mixture HIT indicated that a marked degree of potentiation of teratogenic effect had occurred between the components. Forty eight percent of the fetuses from females receiving this solution were malformed compared to an estimated 19% that would have been malformed if the three components had acted by summation alone. By way of contrast, the mixture VIT appeared to act by summation of the teratogenic effects of its components. Approximately 11% of the fetuses from females exposed to the mixture were malformed compared to an estimated 8% that would have been malformed if the individual components had acted alone.

Six-Component Solution (6D)

The lower dose level of the 6D solution appeared to produce a percentage of malformed fetuses that was definitely higher than that estimated for the concentration of the trypan blue component alone. The concentrations of the remainder of the components were well below that expected to produce a positive teratogenic response if they were acting alone. The higher dose level of the 6D mixture produced additional evidence of potentiation of the components of the mixture. However, it was impossible to determine which component(s) were interacting with each other and to what extent.

Nine- (9D) and Twelve- (12D) Component Mixture

As the number of additional components in the composite mixtures was enlarged, it became increasingly less clear which components were potentiating and which were summating their individual teratogenic effects. However, one can still distinguish the fact that the individual components, now at relatively low concentrations compared to the three-component mixture, continued to contribute a definitive influence on the overall teratogenic effect of the mixture. Therefore, the actual percentage of malformed fetuses remained much above an estimated percentage that could be calculated or predicted from the summation of the individual maternal-dose, fetal-teratogenic-response data for each component.

Maternal and Fetal Mortality

No maternal mortality occurred in any of the experimental or control groups. Significant fetal mortality was limited to the VIT and HIT groups in which the toxicities of trypan blue and isoproterenol were clearly evident since neither the vitamin A nor hydromorphone data indicated any tendency to produce fetal death at the maternal concentrations studied. Some residual effect on fetal viability was still evident in the 6D high-maternal-dose-level groups although the results are on the border line of statistical significance.

The data from the 9D and 12D groups, at all maternal-dose levels, exhibited little or no evidence of summation of the fetal lethality effects of trypan blue and isoproterenol even though the compounds did manifest the previously mentioned summation and potentiation activities of their teratogenic properties. In addition, the other components in the 9D and 12D mixtures apparently do not contribute to a summation or potentiation effect of the fetal lethality of the solution.

Single Versus Multiple Doses

An interesting additional factor was added to the complex interplay of the

TABLE 3. *Single versus multiple dose effects of two low-concentration multiple-teratogen solutions*

Compound	Dose (mg/kg)[a] Soln. A	Soln. B	Mean no. fetuses/litter[b] Soln. A	Soln. B	Percent CM[c] Soln. A	Soln. B
Hydromorphone	0.37	3.0				
Morphine	0.31	2.6				
Methadone	0.38	3.1				
Vitamin A	0.45	5.5				
Isoproterenol	0.71	8.9				
Trypan blue	0.09	1.2				
Single dose			11.6 ± 0.2	10.2 ± 0.3	0.0 (0)[e]	12.3 (25)[e]
Multiple dose			6.7 ± 0.3^d	5.0 ± 0.1^d	28.3 (38)[e]	54.0 (54)[e]
Saline						
Single dose			11.9 ± 0.2	$11.4 \pm 0.3**$	0.0 (0)[e]	0.0 (0)[e]
Multiple dose			$11.7 \pm 0.2*$	11.2 ± 0.2	0.0 (0)[e]	0.0 (0)[e]

[a] Dose expressed as the base compound.
[b] Twenty litters analyzed in each group, except * = 19 litters, ** = 17 litters.
[c] CM, congenital malformations; figures in parenthesis represent the number of CM fetuses.
[d] Significant difference form saline control $p = <0.01$.
[e] Total number of fetus/dose level.

various teratogens by administering to the pregnant females the composite 6D mixture at much lower concentrations than previously studied, and on three successive days, i.e., days 7, 8, and 9 of gestation. Table 3 compares the results of a single injection of maternal dose levels of the 6D composite mixture with those obtained following three maternal injections. Note that the dose levels of the individual components of the lowest dose level mixture (Soln. A) are well below the levels utilized to determine the noneffective, i.e., nonteratogenic, dose levels in Table 1. A single maternal injection of the lowest dose level mixture (Soln. A) produced no detectable fetal external malformations, whereas following three successive daily injections, 40% of the fetuses exhibited external congenital lesions. The other 6D composite mixture (Soln. B) contained approximately 10 times the maternal-dose level of each compound in the mixture as the low dose level mixture. The single injection of this higher dose mixture (Soln. B) gave a positive, detectable teratogenic response of 12% compared to 54% response following the three injections.

DISCUSSION

On balance, the vast majority of published data in teratology concentrates on identifying a specific pathway believed to be responsible for the teratogenic activity of a particular factor or compound studied in the various laboratories (18). I propose that a different approach may yield interesting and valuable clues to the mechanism of teratogenesis in general. This alternate method of teratogenic factorial analysis would tend to ignore or relegate to secondary importance the differences in physical characteristics and physiological/pharmacological functions or activities of the wide spectrum of effective teratogens. Those compounds not initially teratogenic and requiring metabolic alteration by either the maternal or fetal organism, or both, would enter the common pathway following the necessary structural changes. Admittedly, one must work with "blinders" on and with some degree of prejudice since the range of factors or chemical substances capable of disrupting the normal sequence of fetal development is becoming increasingly wide and complex.

Can some single or relatively simple scheme account for the fact that the same fetal anomaly can be produced by many apparently unrelated teratogenic factors or chemical substances? First of all, it must be recalled that this fact about teratogens is a major tenet of the science of teratology and has been recognized as such for some time (15). However, it is seldom the focal point of experimental investigations of a comparative nature.

Another problem arises in choosing the maternal concentration or intensity of the individual teratogenic compound or factor. Acting alone in most experimental systems utilized for teratogenic studies, the teratogen is present generally in what many outside the field of teratology consider unphysiological amounts. Hence, the commonly expressed thought, "If you put enough of anything in, you'll get an effect." Certainly to some extent this criticism is justified. However, if again we refer to basic teratogenic tenets, we find that teratogens are capable of summation and potentiation (16). Therefore, if two or three teratogenic substances or factors are present simultaneously during the critical period of organogenesis, only one-half, one-third, or less of the amount of each teratogen acting alone may be required to effectively produce abnormal fetal development of any selected organ or tissue. Tentatively, it may be assumed that as the number of teratogens simultaneously present increases, the amount of each required is decreased by a factor related to the total number of teratogens. Whether the factor represents and relates to simple additive teratogenic effects or the more important potentiation aspect is, as of now, not fully studied and elucidated. If each additional teratogen that is added to a complex mix-

ture of teratogens causes the composite group to exert an increase in teratogenicity by a geometric or logarithmetic amount, then each component may need to be present in only a very small fractional percentage of the concentration or intensity required when it is operating as the sole effective teratogen.

With these background relationships as a frame of reference, it may be possible to begin to postulate what constitutes a common pathway or series of converging mechanisms that account for the fact that extremely diverse types of teratogenic agents can produce a common abnormality of fetal development. Since established teratogens have been shown to possess extremely varied physical and physiochemical characteristics, it may be that the only way to explain teratogenesis from any single teratogen may be its action on a specifically selected and limited organelle, i.e., lysosome, cell membrane, microtubules or microfilaments, or DNA synthetic pathway, working in combination with some other basic biological system, i.e., vascular system, hypophysis, hypothalamus, or adrenal gland.

Probably the extremely active DNA and RNA synthetic pathways that characterize the entire range of differentiating and growing fetal organ systems during the critical period of organogenesis would be the logical site for the ultimate influence by whatever type of disruptive forces or substances present in the fetal tissues following passage through the uteroplacental tissues. Many investigators have demonstrated in a number of experimental systems the wide variety of factors capable of influencing the DNA/RNA synthetic pathways. Included among these are narcotics, anoxia, noise, X-rays, catecholamines, etc. (2–4,7,11,13,17).

Another factor, decreased uterine blood flow, has been implicated in various fetal responses, including abnormal development (6–8,14). The mechanism(s) involved

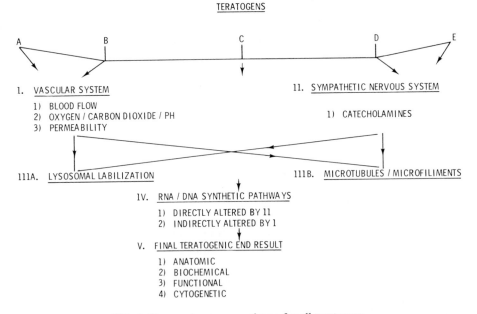

FIG. 1. Proposed common scheme for all teratogens.

probably include the induction of a state of anoxia or hypoxemia in the fetus. The decreased blood flow most certainly induces a concomitant increase in carbon dioxide concentrations in the blood and an alteration in tissue pH in all fetal cells.

Possible causative factors involved in the decreased uteroplacental blood flow should be considered now since some may play a dual role in producing fetal responses. This point can be illustrated by the activation of the sympathetic nervous system or by exogenous catecholamine injection. Both of these situations could decrease uterine blood flow, and the passage of excess endogenously released or exogenously injected neurohormones could pass into the developing fetus and alter differentiating cellular pathways. Apparently these latter phenomena do occur although, again, the exact final locus and mechanism of the series of related actions is not completely known at this time.

Exogenous drugs or chemicals (either teratogenic in their original structural configuration or after metabolic change)

probably bring about their effects by at least two different mechanisms. First, their inherent pharmacological actions may include the ability to produce vasoconstriction, and second, they may cause a release of catecholamines from various storage sites. The combination of vasoconstriction originating from either autonomic nervous system activation, drug injection, or indirect release of catecholamines by a substance and the concomitant hypoxemia and catecholamine effect on DNA/RNA synthetic pathways may also be involved in the final step in the induction of teratogenesis by many other factors in our environment. Heat and cold are known to produce abnormal fetal development, and both are capable of intense activation of the sympathetic nervous system.

Lysosomal labilization is postulated to play some part in the overall action of at least some if not all teratogenic agents. Since the lysosomes contain a wide variety of enzymes, some of which are capable of actions on proteins, it may be reasonable to suggest that the release of these enzymes by the teratogen would lead to a disruption of normal fetal synthetic pathways. A recent review has shown that membranes can be labilized by some compounds known to be teratogenic (12).

Figure 1 summarizes the proposed interrelationships involved in the induction of abnormal fetal development by either single or multiple teratogenic agents A through E, all varying in their physical or biochemical structure or function.

It is obvious to anyone familiar with the literature that all reported teratogens do not produce the same spectrum of congenital anomalies. However, this conclusion may be somewhat misleading for the following reasons: (a) very few investigations are comparative studies carried out on a large number of compounds that are not structually or functionally related, and (b) dose-response curves are usually not run for each day of the critical period of organogenesis. It is well established that each developing fetal organ system and tissue has its own most sensitive period during which time it may be most easily and markedly deviated from the normal developmental pathways, and it may be that each teratogen is most effective at a particular dose level at various times within the defined most critical period of a particular fetal tissue. This may explain in part why some teratogens appear to be associated more with one type of specific congenital anomaly and another teratogen with another specific type of anomaly.

REFERENCES

1. National Primary and Secondary Air Quality Standards (1971): *Code of Federal Regulations 42*, Chapter 4, Part 410. U.S. Government Printing Office, Washington, D.C. Also *Federal Register 36*, No. 84, 8186.
2. Barka, T. (1965): Induced cell proliferation: Effect of isoproterenol. *Exp. Cell Res.*, 37:662–679.
3. Barka, T. (1968): Stimulation of protein and ribonucleic acid synthesis in the rat submaxillary gland by isoproterenol. *Lab. Invest.*, 18:38–41.
4. Clouet, D. H. (1971): Protein and nucleic acid metabolism. In: *Narcotic Drugs: Biochemical Pharmacology*, edited by D. H. Clouet, pp. 216–228. Plenum Press, New York.
5. Dinman, B. D. (1972): Non-concept of no-threshold:Chemicals in the environment. *Science*, 175:495–497.
6. Franklin, J. B., and Brent, R. L. (1964): The effect of uterine vascular clamping on the development of rat embryos three to fourteen days old. *J. Morphol.*, 115:273–290.
7. Geber, W. F. (1966): Developmental effects of chronic maternal audiovisual stress on the rat fetus. *J. Embryol. Exp. Morphol.*, 16:1–16.
8. Geber, W. F. (1970): Cardiovascular and teratogenic effects of chronic intermittent noise stress. In: *Physiological Effects of Noise*, edited by B. L. Welch and A.S. Welch, pp. 85–90. Plenum Press, New York.
9. Geber, W. F., and Schramm, L. C. (1975): Congenital malformations of the central nervous system produced by narcotic analgesics in the hamster. *Am. J. Obstet. Gynecol.*, 123:705–713.
10. Runner, M. N. (1967): Comparative pharmacology in relation to teratogenesis. *Fed. Proc.*, 26:1131–1136.
11. Russell, L. B., and Montgomery, C. S. (1966): Radiation sensitivity differences within cell division cycles during mouse cleavage. *Int. J. Radiat. Biol.*, 10:151–164.
12. Seeman, P. (1972): The membrane actions of anesthetics and tranquilizers. *Pharmacol. Rev.*, 24:583–655.
13. Way, E. L., and Shen, F. H. (1971): Catecholamines and 5-hydroxytryptamine. In: *Narcotic Drugs: Biochemical Pharmacology*, edited by D. H. Clouet, pp. 229–253. Plenum Press, New York.
14. Wigglesworth, J. S. (1966): Fetal growth retardation. *Br. Med. Bull.*, 22:13–15.
15. Wilson, J. G. (1971): General principles in experimental teratology. In: *Int. Conf. Congenital Malformations*, edited by J. G. Wilson, pp. 187–194. Lippincott, Philadelphia.
16. Wilson, J. G. (1964): Teratogenic interaction of chemical agents in the rat. *J. Pharmacol. Exp. Ther.*, 144:429–436.
17. Wilson, J. G. (1953): Effects of irradiation on embryonic development. II. X-ray on the ninth day of gestation in the rat. *Am. J. Anat.*, 92:153–177.
18. Woollam, D. H. M., and Millen, J. M. (1960): The modification of the activity of certain agents exerting a deleterious effect on the development of the mammalian embryo. In: *Ciba Found. Symp. Congenital Malformations*, edited by G. E. W. Wolstenholm and C. M. O'Conner, pp. 158–177. Little, Brown, Boston.

Neurotoxicology, edited by L. Roizin, H. Shiraki, and N. Grčević. Raven Press, New York © 1977.

Effects of Prolonged Administration of "Street Heroin" On the Chromosomes of *Macaca mulatta* (Rhesus) Monkeys

*Harlow K. Fischman, **Leon Roizin, *Emilia Moralishvili, *Catherine Joy, and *John D. Rainer

*Department of Medical Genetics, and **Department of Neuropathology and Neurotoxicology, New York State Psychiatric Institute, New York, New York 10032

This investigation was undertaken in order to examine the possible effects of narcotic addiction on heredity. It formed part of a collaborative project of the Department of Medical Genetics and the Department of Neuropathology and Neurotoxicology for studying the effects of heroin on the chromosomes and central nervous system (CNS) under controlled conditions.

Macaca mulatta monkeys were chosen for the study because their relatively close evolutionary relationship to man makes it more likely that the results would be applicable to human beings. "Street heroin" is a variable mixture of several substances. Despite the obvious problems inherent in its experimental use, it was felt that since addicts are exposed to similar material and substances contained may have additive or synergistic effects its use would be appropriate. Definitive identification of the individual chromosomes of *Macaca mulatta* greatly aids in making a critical evaluation of the possible damage caused by heroin to them. A Giemsa banding technique for monkey chromosomes was devised that, through its elucidation of the longitudinal differentiation of the chromosomes, permits, in addition to chromosome identification, the analysis of structural rearrangements, both within an individual chromosome and between homologous and nonhomologous chromosomes.

METHODS AND MATERIALS

From 5 to 7 ml of venous blood was drawn into a syringe containing 100 U of heparin. The needle was removed and the blood transferred into a Difco separation vial. After the red blood cells settled, the lymphocyte-rich supernatant was removed and 1 ml of it inoculated into each culture vessel, containing growth medium. (MEM, 6.5 ml; fetal calf serum, 2.0 ml; antibiotics, 0.1 ml; phytohemagglutinin in 0.2 ml.) After 72 hr of culture, vinblastine (Velban®) was added to the culture. One hour later, the contents of the culture were transferred to a centrifuge tube and spun down at 800 rpm for 10 min. The supernatant was discarded, and the cells resuspended in KCl at 37°C for 10 min. They were centrifuged again, the supernatant removed, and fixed in 3:1 methanol-acetic acid at 4°C for 1 hr. The fixative was changed twice, and the cells were finally suspended in 0.5 ml of fresh fixative. Drops of cell suspension were placed on a chilled, wet slide and air dried. Slides that were less than 1 week old were used for banding. Trypsin-Giemsa banding was carried out by a modification of the method of Moorthy and Mitra (3). The slides were treated with Grand Island Biological Co. trypsin (2 ml of trypsin plus 48 ml of Hanks BSS without Mg^{++}). They were then washed twice in saline and stained with Giemsa in 6.8 pH phosphate buffer (1.5 ml of 0.1 citric acid + 50 ml of distilled water, which was adjusted to pH 6.8 with 0.2 M sodium phosphate). The slides were then washed in buffer, air dried, and mounted in Permount. Photographs of well-banded metaphases were taken through a Zeiss Photomicroscope, equipped with a 100 X planapochromat objective, using Kodak 35 mm High Contrast Copy film.

Fifteen karyotypes were used for measurements. Initially the average total length (A) of each chromosome was determined $\left(\frac{\Sigma L}{n} = A, \; n = 15\right)$. Although the 15 karyotypes chosen were of sufficiently good quality for length measurements, it was not always possible to measure band locations on all karyotypes for all chromosomes. Therefore, the 10 best chromosomes were chosen individually for each chromosome 1 through 20, plus X and Y from among the 15 karyotypes. Band measurements were done by assigning a value of zero to the centromere and measuring out toward the telomere of each arm. A measurement was taken at each boundary of a positively and negatively stained region, with the final measurement being the end of the arm, which is equivalent to the total length of the arm. Since the degree of condensation of the chromosomes varied, it was necessary to convert all the band measurements to percentages of total chromosome length (Z) along the respective arms $\left(Z = \frac{Y}{X}\right) \times 100$ where X = total absolute length of the chromosome in question and Y = band measurement in absolute units in order to arrive at an average value. For the purpose of constructing a karyo-

type, these average values were converted to unit values $\left(W = A \times \frac{Z}{100}\right)$, using the average total chromosome length computed from all 15 karyotypes as the A value. If the arm ratio is then computed from the final average long and short arm unit lengths (see Table 1), it will be found to be the same as the average arm ratio computed from the 10 samples.

Ten monkeys were used in the experiment. Six were adults (five females and one male) who were exposed to street heroin. Another was the female baby of a heroin-exposed mother. Three adults (two females and one male) were used as controls. Heroin monkeys were placed on a regular regime of intravenous injections of increasing concentrations of heroin for up to 2 years. Appropriate methods for examining chromosomes from these monkeys' blood, bone marrow, and meiotic cells were perfected, and a technique for culturing monkey leukocytes was established (details to be published elsewhere). Both regular and Giemsa-banded karyotypes were completed for each animal.

Data on chromosome aberrations found in lymphocyte cultures were obtained from detailed analyses of 100 metaphases per monkey. A statistical comparison between the heroin-exposed monkeys and their controls, for chromosome and chromatid breaks as well as for total aberrations, was accomplished by means of a comparison of proportions, based on a binomial distribution.

RESULTS

Figure 1 shows the proposed G-band karyotype, which consists of five rows of chromosomes, arranged in such a way that they are most readily identified. The top row consists of six large- to medium-sized submetacentric chromosomes. The second row contains five medium-sized submetacentrics. The third row has two large, one

TABLE 1. *Measurements of* Macaca mulatta *chromosomes*

	1	2	3	4	5	6	7	8	9	10	11	12	13	14	15	16	17	18	19	20	X	Y
											Absolute units											
Short arm	21.3	16.8	14.8	13.6	13.6	11.6	11.3	10.9	8.9	8.1	6.5	16.8	15.2	12.1	11.0	8.8	8.5	11.7	9.1	12.9	14.9	2.5
Long arm	36.5	31.5	29.5	29.6	28.5	23.0	22.7	21.1	23.2	22.2	20.7	26.5	23.8	16.7	13.0	14.0	12.3	12.3	11.0	17.9	26.0	10.8
Total length	57.8	48.3	44.3	43.2	42.1	34.6	34.0	32.0	32.1	30.3	27.2	43.3	39.0	28.8	24.0	22.8	20.8	24.0	20.1	30.8	40.9	13.3
											% of Total haploid genome length											
Short arm	3.14	2.47	2.18	2.00	2.00	1.71	1.66	1.60	1.31	1.19	0.96	2.47	2.24	1.78	1.62	1.30	1.25	1.72	1.34	1.90	2.19	0.37
Long arm	5.37	4.64	4.34	4.36	4.19	3.38	3.34	3.11	3.41	3.27	3.04	3.90	3.50	2.46	1.91	2.06	1.81	1.81	1.62	2.63	3.83	1.59
Total length	8.51	7.11	6.52	6.36	6.19	5.09	5.00	4.71	4.72	4.46	4.00	6.37	5.74	4.24	3.53	3.36	3.06	3.53	2.96	4.53	6.02	1.96
Arm ratios	1.71	1.88	1.99	2.18	2.10	1.98	2.01	1.94	2.61	2.74	3.18	1.58	1.57	1.38	1.18	1.59	1.45	1.05	1.21	1.39	1.74	4.32

The lengths of the short and long arm and total length of each chromosome are expressed both in absolute units, and as percentages of the total haploid autosomal complement, together with the arm ratio.

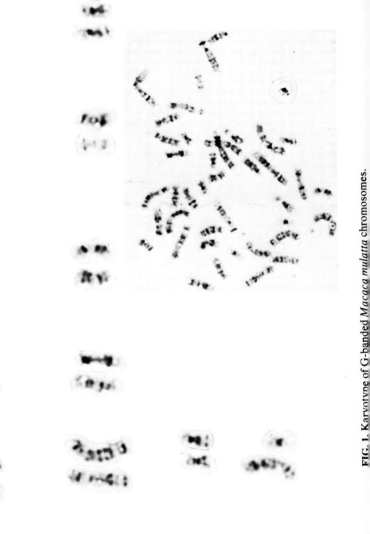

FIG. 1. Karyotype of G-banded *Macaca mulatta* chromosomes.

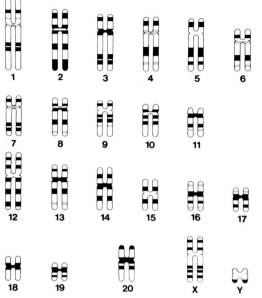

FIG. 2. Idiogram of G-banded *Macaca mulatta* chromosomes ("Type A").

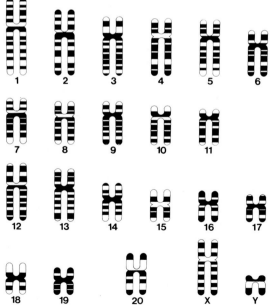

FIG. 3. Idiogram of G-banded *Macaca mulatta* chromosomes ("Type B").

medium, and three small metacentrics. The fourth row contains two small metacentrics. The fifth row contains one medium-sized metacentric, which is distinguished by a prominent secondary constriction in the short arm and the two sex chromosomes. The X is a large metacentric and the Y an acrocentric or subterminal, the smallest chromosome in the complement. Figure 2 is an idiogram showing the most consistently staining bands (Type A). In particularly well-stained preparations, other fainter bands do appear. These are demonstrated in Fig. 3 (Type B). A more detailed analysis of the banding, including measurements of the band locations will be published elsewhere.

The data on chromosome damage (Table 2) demonstrate that there is a significant difference between those animals exposed to heroin and those which were not, both with respect to chromosome breaks and the total number of aberrations. This difference is within the 95% confidence range. Data on chromosome damage have also been collected on the heroin-exposed monkeys' bone marrow chromosomes. The frequencies of chromosome and chromatid gaps and breaks and total aberrations are high (28.1, 8.65, and 36.9%, respectively).

DISCUSSION

Nonbanded karyotypes of *Macaca mulatta* have been published (1,2,4). Recently, Stock and Hsu (5) and DeVries and his group (6,7) published G-banded karyotypes, however, chromosome measurements were not included in these reports.

The unequivocal identification of individual *Macaca mulatta* chromosomes, by means of G banding has enabled us to obtain accurate measurements of chromosome lengths and arm ratios. These data, together with our experience in examining monkey chromosomes in our laboratory, have made clear that it is advantageous to

TABLE 2. *Effects of prolonged administration of street heroin on lymphocyte chromosomes of* Macaca mulatta *(rhesus) monkeys*

| Monkey (No.) | Cells evaluated | Aneuploid cells | Experimentals | | | |
			Gaps	Breaks	Frags.	Total aberrs.
2	100	12	4	7	2	11
3	100	6	1	3	1	5
5	100	6	7	5	0	12
6	100	8	8	2	1	10
7	100	7	2	3	1	5
[a]7'	100	3	8	7	2	15
Total	700	44	32	29	8	62
Mean	100	6.29	4.57	4.14	1.14	8.86
			Controls			
19D	100	11	3	2	1	5
16A	100	3	6	0	0	6
17B	100	2	0	1	0	1
Total	300	16	9	3	1	12
Mean	100	5.33	3.00	1.00	0.33	4.00

[a] Baby of #7.

arrange the karyotypes as shown in Fig. 1. Here the chromosomes are organized principally in terms of arm ratios and secondarily by means of lengths. This most closely fits the manner in which they are identified under the microscope. An exception is made for chromosome number 20, which by virtue of its singular secondary constriction, has a quite different appearance from the other medium-sized metacentrics.

This is to our knowledge the first report on the effects of heroin on primate chromosomes. This is not surprising, considering the difficulties imposed by making such a study conform as much as possible to conditions under which drug addicts are exposed to heroin. The high percentage of chromosome aberrations found in heroin monkeys suggests that heroin addicts are being genetically damaged. It has been clearly demonstrated in many organisms that most agents causing damage to chromosomes in somatic cells also damage those of reproductive cells and produce gene mutations.

Another group of monkeys has recently been placed on a regime of chemically pure heroin. Examination of their chromosomes will establish whether or not it is the heroin itself that causes the damage. Chromosome aberration analyses were done on these monkeys before their first exposure to heroin, and they will serve as their own controls for an analysis of the possible effects of heroin on the chromosomes and CNS. Chromosome aberration analyses will be made both during and at the termination of heroin exposure.

In addition, the chromosomes of pregnant female monkeys on a heroin regime will be analyzed, as will those of their offspring, as part of an effort to determine whether or not there is an interaction between heroin addiction and pregnancy, with regard to genetic and CNS damage.

ACKNOWLEDGMENTS

The authors are grateful to Dr. Amini Moorthy of New York University for her important contributions toward the development of adequate G band and bone marrow techniques.

This investigation was supported by General Research Support Grant No. RR05650 from the National Institutes of Health.

Diacetyl morphine HCl (heroin) was obtained through the courtesy of Dr. Monique C. Braude and Jacqueline R. Bryant from FDA/NIDA Drug Abuse Research Advisory Committee and Biomedical Research Branch Division of Research, National Institute on Drug Abuse, Rockville, Maryland.

REFERENCES

1. Dzhemilev, Z. A. (1973): Marked chromosome associations in monkeys. I. The association frequency of nucleolus-organizing chromosomes in cultured lymphocytes at different X-ray doses and the quantitative analysis of nucleoli. *Tsitologiia,* 15(8):1043–1048.

2. Fernandez-Donoso, R., Lindsten, J., and Norrby, E. (1970): The chromosomes of the cynomolgus macaque (*Macaca fasicularis*). *Hereditas,* 65:269–276.

3. Moorthy, A. S., and Mitra, J. (1972): Banding patterns in chromosomes of Chinese hamster (*Cricetulus griseus*). *Mam. Chrom. Newsl.,* 13(4):154–155.

4. Schmager, J. (1972): Cytotaxonomy and geographical distribution of the Papinae. *J. Hum. Evol.,* 1:477–485.

5. Stock, A. D., and Hsu, T. C. (1973): Evolutionary conservatism in arrangement of genetic material: A comparative analysis of chromosome banding between the rhesus macaque ($2n = 42$, 84 arms) and the African green monkey ($2n = 60$, 120 arms). *Chromosoma,* 43:211–224.

6. Vries, G. F., De, France, H. F., De, and Schevers, J. A. M. (1975): Identical Giemsa banding patterns of two *Macaca* species: *Macaca mulatta* and *Macaca fascicularis. Cytogenet. Cell Genet.,* 14:26–33.

7. Vries, G. F., De, Geleijnse, M. E. M., France, H. F., De, and Hogendoorn, A. M. (1975): Lymphocyte cultures of *Macaca mulatta* and *Macaca fasicularis. Lab. Anim. Sci.,* 25(1):33–38.

Neurotoxicology, edited by L. Roizin, H. Shiraki, and N. Grcević. Raven Press, New York © 1977.

Primary and Secondary Alterations in Cerebellar Morphology in Carnivore (Ferret) and Rodent (Rat) After Exposure to Methylazoxymethanol Acetate

R. Haddad, Ausma Rabe, Judy Shek, Sheila Donahue, and Ruth Dumas

Institute for Basic Research in Mental Retardation, Staten Island, New York 10314

Methylazoxymethanol is a naturally occurring neurotoxin. It is an alkylating agent that methylates DNA, RNA, and proteins. Dividing nerve cells are especially vulnerable to its neurotoxic action. Consequently, various brain structures can be selectively altered depending on the time of exposure. Jones et al. (3) have reviewed methylazoxymethanol neurotoxicity, and Langman et al. (4) have provided an interesting survey of closely related research.

STUDIES IN THE FERRET

Injection of the pregnant jill with 15 mg/kg of methylazoxymethanol acetate

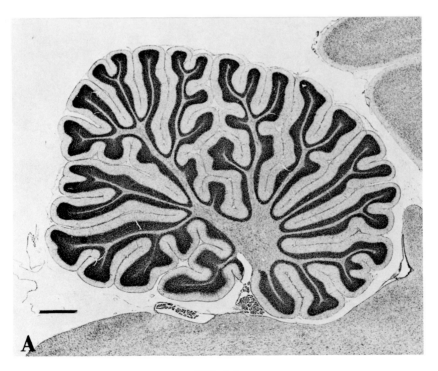

FIG. 1.A.

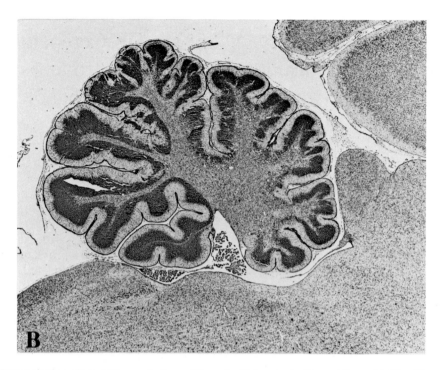

FIG. 1. Parasagittal sections of the cerebellum of 6-week-old ferrets. **A:** Normal ferret. **B:** Kit of ferret given 15 mg/kg of MAM Ac, i.p., on gestation day 40. Note that in the normal cerebellum the external granular layer has almost disappeared by this age. Line is 1 mm long. Nissl stain.

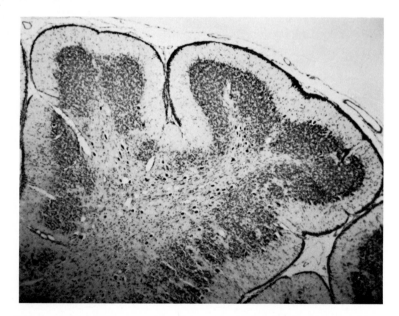

FIG. 2. Detail of lobule V from the treated brain of Fig. 1 showing scattered Purkinje cells and abnormal thickness of the external granular layer. ×40.

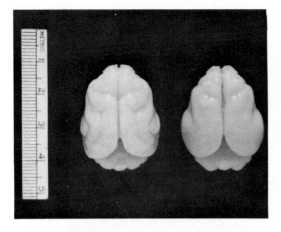

FIG. 3. Brains of 6-week-old ferrets. Normal on left. The lissencephalic brain on the right is from a kit of an animal that was injected with 15 mg/kg, i.p., of MAM Ac on gestation day 32.

(MAM Ac) on gestation day 40 (full term is 42 days), when the cerebellar external granular layer is rapidly proliferating, results in a considerable cerebellar dysplasia in the kits. Not only is the cerebellum substantially reduced in size, but it is not fully differentiated, the anterior vermis being especially hypoplastic. Histological examination at weaning (6 weeks of age) shows an abnormal persistence of the external granular layer and a massive loss of

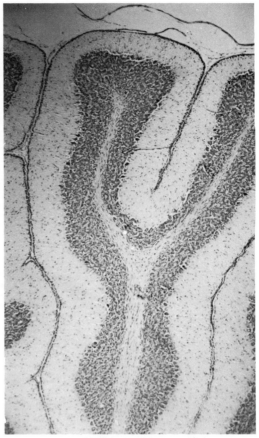

FIG. 5. Detail of lobule V from a Nissl-stained parasagittal section of the cerebellum of a 6-week-old lissencephalic ferret similar to one shown in Fig. 3. Note the thickness of the external granular layer. ×40.

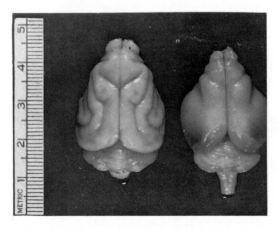

FIG. 4. Same treatment as in Fig. 3, 12 months of age. Normal on the left. Note hydrocephaly as well as lissencephaly in brain of treated animal on right.

granule cells which gives a moth-eaten appearance to the cerebellar lobules (Fig. 1). Many Purkinje cells are scattered through the internal granular and medullary layers (Fig. 2).

Treatment given earlier in gestation has less effect on the cerebellum and more on the cerebrum. Injection of the pregnant jill on gestation day 32 with 15 mg/kg of MAM Ac interferes with the development of the cerebral convolutions, resulting in lissencephaly in the kits. The normal ferret brain has well-defined convolutions, whereas the kits of the MAM Ac-injected jills show a rather smooth cerebral cortex

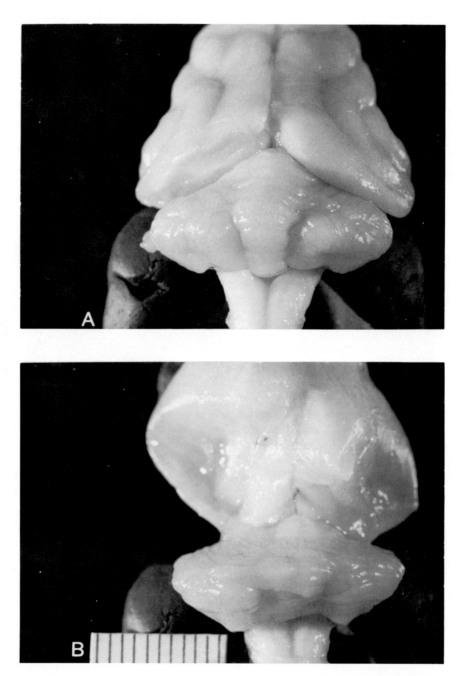

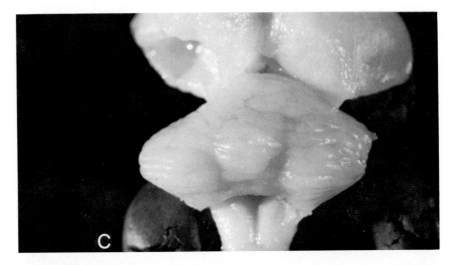

FIG. 6. Ferret brains at 12 months of age showing secondary cerebellar alterations. **A:** Normal ferret. The posterior end of the left hemisphere has been amputated to more fully expose the cerebellum. **B:** Kit of a ferret given 15 mg/kg of MAM Ac, i.p., on gestation day 32. Note the flattened anterior aspect and distorted posterior outline of the cerebellum. Hydrocephalic cerebral hemispheres collapsed after removal of the brain. **C:** Another ferret also exposed to the same dose of MAM Ac on gestation day 32. Note the asymmetric flattening of the anterior aspect as well as the changed posterior outline of the cerebellum. Scale is in millimeters.

with little convolutional development. At weaning, a mild degree of hydrocephaly is also present (Fig. 3), whereas at maturity the hydrocephaly is usually more severe, with bilateral thinning of the cerebral cortex in the lateral occipital region (Fig. 4).

The cerebellum of the lissencephalic ferrets is not only likely to be smaller than that of the normal ferret but usually shows irregularities in the internal granular and Purkinje cell layers. These changes are a consequence of a primary cerebellar lesion. Examination of the fetal brain 48 hr after injection of the jill with 15 mg/kg of MAM Ac permits observation of the distribution of necrotic cells. When treated on gestation day 32, by far the greater damage is done to the developing cerebral cortex, throughout which a heavy scattering of necrotic cells can be seen. However, necrotic cells can also readily be found in the cerebellar rudiment, particularly in its anterior region. Histological sections of the cerebellum show consequent alterations in cerebellar development—a heavier than normal external granular layer still present

at weaning (Fig. 5), anomalies in the development of the internal granular layer, and occasional scattering of Purkinje cells deep in the internal granular layer, some being found at the edge of the medullary layer.

Fourteen such lissencephalic ferrets were maintained for about 1 year. In 10 of them, the neopallium over the occipital pole of the lateral ventricles was thinned to the point of translucency. In four of the 10, a flattening of the anterior aspect of the cerebellum was found (Fig. 6B). This anomaly in cerebellar morphology is presumably secondary to the cerebral pathology. It was found only in mature animals in which extreme hydrocephalic alterations were present. When the hydrocephaly was markedly asymmetric, so too was the cerebellar flattening (Fig. 6C).

The posterior aspect of the cerebellum also shows a distorted outline (Fig. 6B and 6C). This change may be secondary to dilatation of the fourth ventricle (Fig. 7B). So far no obstructions have been found that might account for the hydrocephaly.

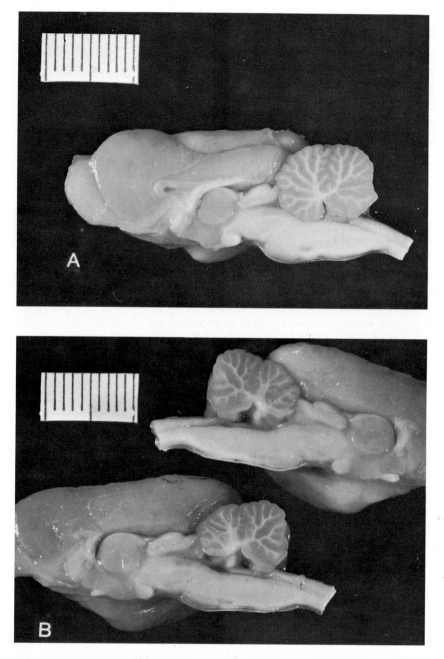

FIG. 7. Sagittal view of the brains shown in Fig. 6A and B. Note the enlarged fourth ventricle in the treated ferret (**B**). **A** is normal. Scale is in millimeters.

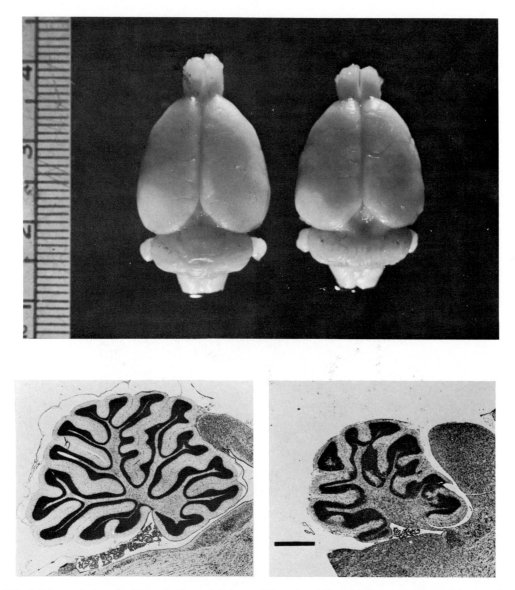

FIG. 8. Primary lesions in the cerebellum of adult rats. Normal on left. On right, rats injected with 50 mg/kg of MAM Ac, s.c., on the day of birth. Line is 1 mm.

STUDIES IN THE RAT

Both direct and indirect effects of exposure to MAM Ac on cerebellar development also occur in the rat. Perinatal treatment, at the time the cerebellar cortex is developing, results in a primary alteration of cerebellar morphology, whereas treatment on gestation day 15, when the cerebrum is beginning to develop, results in an indirect alteration.

Treatment at birth, when the cells of the external granular layer of the rat cerebellum are the most rapidly proliferating cells of the body, results in substantial lesions of the cerebellar cortex. The size and shape of the cerebellum is permanently altered by a single injection of 50 mg/kg, s.c., of

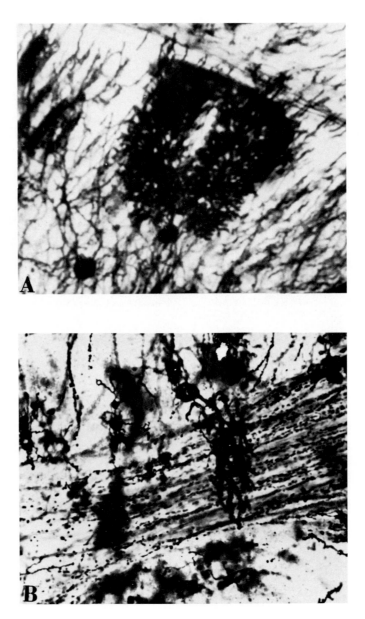

FIG. 9. Golgi-stained sections of cerebellum of 4-month-old rats showing a normal (**A**) and an abnormal (**B**) Purkinje cell. The abnormal cell has a dendritic arborization that not only is reduced but also is abnormally oriented, extending into the medullary layer. ×225.

MAM Ac on the day of birth. Parasagittal sections of such a cerebellum show not only a reduction of cerebellar size but also a poorer differentiation of the cerebellar lobules and an irregular internal granular layer (Fig. 8). Many Purkinje cells are embedded in the internal granular layer. Golgi-stained sections have shown them to have a reduced dendritic arborization and a massive deficit of dendritic spines. Moreover, they are frequently abnormally oriented (Fig. 9).

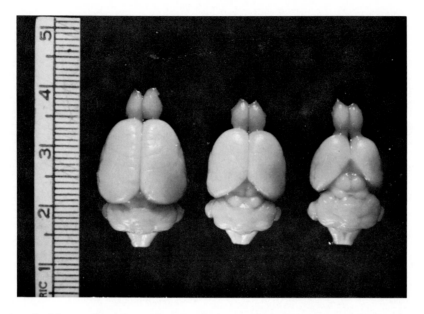

FIG. 10. Brains of adult rats showing two degrees of micrencephaly and concomitant alteration of cerebellar shape. Such graded effects in the offspring can be obtained by injecting pregnant rats with 20 to 30 mg/kg of MAM Ac, i.p., on either gestation day 14 or 15.

Treatment of the pregnant rat with 20 to 30 mg/kg of MAM Ac on gestation day 15 results in micrencephaly in all of the young (Fig. 10). Note that the shape of the cerebellum of the treated animals is also affected. Regional dissection, however, has shown that even though the cerebellar shape is altered in the micrencephalic rat, the mass is changed little or not at all. [We have found no change in the cerebellar mass of severely micrencephalic Long-Evans rats of the Blue Spruce substrain. However, Fischer et al. (2) have reported a slight loss of cerebellar mass in another substrain of Long-Evans rats.] Although microscopic examination of Nissl-stained sections shows irregularities in the lobular pattern exceeding the normal range of variation (Fig. 11B), Bodian- and Golgi-stained sections have not shown cytological anomalies in the cerebellum of our micrencephalic rats. A reduction in the number of Purkinje cells would be expected in the cerebellum of the micrencephalic rat since it has recently been shown that the Purkinje cells of the rat are proliferating on gestation day 15 (1). Such a loss has been reported by Pfaffenroth (5) in rats treated with ethylnitrosourea, another teratogenic alkylating agent, on gestation day 15. However, we have not yet determined the Purkinje cell density in our micrencephalic rats.

Examination of parasagittal sections of the cerebellum of normal, micrencephalic, and cerebellar-lesioned rats (Fig. 11) suggests an explanation of the altered appearance of the cerebellum in the micrencephalic rat. The cerebellum of the micrencephalic rat can be seen to be flattened. This, we believe, is a secondary consequence of the reduced height of the skull over the developing cerebellum. We propose that the severely reduced size of the developing cerebral hemispheres of the micrencephalic brain results in the formation of a skull with a lessened height of the cerebral vault and that this in turn deter-

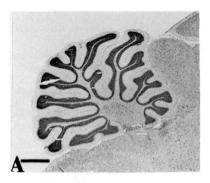

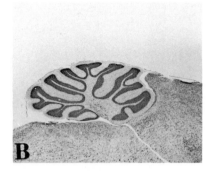

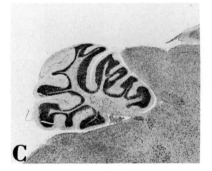

FIG. 11. Nissl-stained parasagittal sections of 28-day-old rat cerebelli. **A:** Normal. **B:** Micrencephalic rat (offspring of a rat injected with 25 mg/kg of MAM Ac, i.p., on gestation day 15). **C:** Rat with cerebellar hypoplasia resulting from injection with 50 mg/kg of MAM Ac, s.c., at birth. Line is 1 mm.

mines the shape of the space into which the cerebellum can develop. Consequently, we view the altered shape of the cerebellum in the micrencephalic rat as a secondary, rather than a primary, effect of exposure to MAM Ac.

ACKNOWLEDGMENTS

This work was supported in part by grants # 1 RO 1 NS 10409–01A1 and # HD-08346–01–02 awarded by the National Institutes of Health, Department of Health, Education and Welfare.

We thank Dr. George A. Jervis for making it possible for us to conduct this research at the Institute for Basic Research in Mental Retardation.

REFERENCES

1. Das, G. D., and Nornes, H. O. (1972): Neurogenesis in the cerebellum of the rat: An autoradiographic study. *Z. Anat. Entwicklungsgesch.,* 138:155–165.
2. Fischer, M. H., Welker, C., and Waisman, H. A. (1972): Generalized growth retardation in rats induced by prenatal exposure to methylazoxymethyl acetate. *Teratology,* 5:223–232.
3. Jones, M., Mickelsen, O., and Yang, M. (1973): Methylazoxymethanol neurotoxicity. In: *Progress in Neuropathology,* Vol. 2., edited by H. M. Zimmerman, pp. 91–114. Grune & Stratton, New York.
4. Langman, J., Webster, W., and Rodier, P. (1975): Morphological and behavioral abnormalities caused by insults to the CNS in the perinatal period. In: *Teratology,* edited by C. L. Berry and D. E. Poswillo, pp. 182–200. Springer Publ., New York.
5. Pfaffenroth, M. J. (1976): Teratogenic effects of ethylnitrosourea on the development of the rat cerebellar cortex. *Anat. Rec.,* 184:501 (Abstr.).

Neurotoxicology, edited by L. Roizin, H. Shiraki,
and N. Grčević. Raven Press, New York © 1977.

Chemogenic Lesion:
A Multifactor Pathogenic Concept

Leon Roizin

Department of Neuropathology, New York State Psychiatric Institute, New York, New York 10032

The molecule is the common denominator of all biological organizations; while its morphochemistry
mediates the functional versatility and selective vulnerability.

In recent years, there has been a rapid growth in the use of chemicals to control numerous undesirable biological, environmental, and ecological conditions as well as a rapid proliferation of industrial chemicals. In addition, we have also seen an increased use of chemical agents for therapeutic purposes. These biological factors, coupled with the current overwhelming growth of drug abuse and/or drug addiction, have contributed to the occurrence of frequent adverse clinical, biochemical, toxicological, and pathological unwarranted reactions (including fatalities) in patients of various ages (23,45,57,58,76,86,94,100, 101,112,115a,120,121,131,137,144,150, 178,179, etc.).

These observations led us to explore with a multidisciplinary methodology the mode of action and, in particular, some histochemical, histopathological, and electron microscopic reactions in the central nervous system (CNS) and liver to adverse or toxic effects of a variety of neuropsychotropic agents in human and experimental models (142b,148,151,153–155,157,161–163,166–168).

MATERIAL AND METHODOLOGY

Over the last 20 years we have examined the following material:

1. Human central nervous system and viscera from patients who had consumed: (a) tranquilizers and who had developed adverse or toxic reactions, organic brain syndrome, and/or coma caused by accidental or intentional overdosage; (b) opiates and narcotics (including methadone); (c) monoamine oxidase inhibitor (MAO) antidepressants; (d) hallucinogens; and (e) lithium. These drugs were used individually as well as in various combinations and, at times, included also alcohol. The investigative and control material was obtained with the cooperation of the directors of the clinicopathological laboratories of the various hospitals and institutions of the New York State Department of Mental Hygiene, through the Neuropathologic Registry at the NYS Psychiatric Institute, and from the Chief Medical Examiner's Office of the Forensic Institute, New York City. This material, combined with the review cases from the literature, amounted to a total of 1,725 cases.

2. Experimental material from: (a) a total of 4,033 animals that had been used for acute and chronic neurotoxicological studies, including mice, rats, and monkeys of both sexes and of variable ages (from embryos to adults); (b) spinal cord ganglia tissue cultures; (c) subcellular fractions of the CNS; and (d) chromosomes of the

TABLE 1. *Materials and methodologies in multidisciplinary studies with neuropsychotropic agents*

Clinical correlates:	1) Medical examinations 2) Neurological examinations 3) Psychiatric examinations 4) Ancillary examinations 5) Therapy

Drug correlates:
(neurotoxicology)
	1) Body fluids } a. drug identification }
	    and } b. drug profile } qualitative
	2) Tissues } c. drug metabolites } and
	3) Catecholamines, neurotransmitters & } quantitative
	    neuromodular substances }
	4) Liver profile
	5) Kidney profile
	6) Sequential Multiple Analyzer-12/60 (SMA)
	7) Special chemoanalyses (when indicated)

Structural correlates:
  Histology:
	1) Gross anatomopathological findings
	2) Standard histologic stains
	3) Differential neurohistologic methods
	4) Histochemical methods for identification of
	    degenerative products (when indicated)

Histochemistry:	1) Enzymes: a) oxidoreduc. sys. & b) hydrolases
	2) RNA & DNA: a) stains & b) microspectrophotometry
	3) Catecholamines: fluorescence } qualitative
	    autoradiography } and
	    } quantitative
	4) Neurosecretory products (hypothalamus)

Electron microscopy:	1) Standard + stains 2) Enzymes 3) Autoradiography 4) Neurosecretory products (hypothalamus)
In vitro Tissue culture:	1) Neuronal differentiation 2) Enzymes: hydrolases 3) Electron microscopy 4) Electron microscopy + enzymes 5) Neurosecretory prod. (hypothalamus)
Subcellular fractions:	1) Organelles [a) morphology and { and 2) Subunits [b) enzymes
Chromosomes:	1) Mitosis [a) qualitative morphology { b) quantitative characteristics 2) Meiosis [c) binding properties

white blood cell (WBC) and bone marrow. Tables 1 and 2 summarize our multidisciplinary methodologies.

RESULTS

Since this volume was planned on a multidisciplinary basis and some of our studies have been included here (refs. 3,71,163, and 204, *this volume*), to avoid redundancy, I extrapolate only some demonstrative examples from the phenothiazine and narcotic studies presented in this volume and supplement my discussion with some additional findings as they relate in particular to the topic under discussion.

TABLE 2. *Experimental model in multidisciplinary investigations of neuropsychotropic agents*

Clinical correlates:	1) Type of animals: pedigree and anamnesis
	2) Environment and nutrition: diet[a]
	3) Treatment: dosage:
	      route of administration
	      frequency and duration
	4) Behavior: records and special exams[b]
	5) Collection of investigatory material:
	   a) body fluids: 4 types
	   b) body tissues: fresh
	            fixed: perfusion ⎱
	                   immersion ⎰

Drug correlates: ⎫ Structural correlates: ⎬ (same as in Table 1) *In vitro* ⎭	

[a] According to animal species requirements.

[b] Skinner and motility activity cages, and when feasible electroencephalography.

Phenothiazines

Human Investigations

Clinical observations disclosed a large variety of neuropsychotropic and viscerotropic adverse or toxic reactions, which are summarized in Table 3.

Biochemical and toxicological studies of postmortem specimens of a patient treated for 5 years with phenothiazines and for the last 10 months with chlorpromazine (900 mg/day) revealed the presence of various amounts of this drug, in descending order, in lungs, liver, gall bladder (and bile), intestines, testis, hypophysis, adrenals, pancreas and, in the CNS, thalamus and hypothalamus, temporal lobe and hippocampus, cerebellum, medulla, spinal cord (upper cervical), pons, lenticular nucleus, and corpus callosum (67).

Tissue concentration of chlorpromazine in laboratory animals showed, with some individual variations, the following tissue distributions, in order of decreasing concentrations: lungs, liver, spleen, kidneys, intestine, and, in the CNS, cerebral cortex, basal ganglia, hypothalamus, mesencephalon, spinal cord, and cerebellum. In addition, chlorpromazine tagged with S^{35} (19,32) was studied in 32 rats and 10 *Macacus* rhesus monkeys. One-half of the animals was given S^{35}-labeled preparation (ethane disulfonate, 2.5 mg/100 g body weight) and the other half the plain drug. These animals were sacrificed 1, $6^{1}/_{2}$, and 24 hr after intravenous administration of prochlorperazine (Smith, Klein & French Lab., Philadelphia). Time exposure was 1,2,4,6, 8,12, and 24 weeks. Plotted curves indicated the basal ganglia-diencephalon as the site emitting the highest level of radioactivity. Pharmacodynamically the greatest drug activity was at the 24-hr period.

Histopathological findings in biopsies of the liver of patients with hepatic dysfunctions (144,167) consisted of various degrees of cholestasis associated at times with biliary thrombi in the central canaliculi and deposits of biliary pigment in the hepatic parenchymal and Kupffer cells and, at times, increased sudanophilia of hepatic parenchyma and occasional necrosis. In human postmortem examinations, the most outstanding visceral pathology consisted of cholestasis and/or liver degeneration (at times with hepatitis), nephrosis (at times with biliary plugs),

TABLE 3. *Adverse and toxic reactions in humans to phenothiazines*

Cardiovascular
Variations in blood pressure, tachycardia vasomotor disorders.
Endocrinological and neurohumoral
Galactorrhea, hypertrophy of breasts, amenorrhea, diabetes mellitus, obesity, changes in sexual desire; variable effects on the storage, receptor and transfer of biogenic amines and neuromediators or neurotransmitters and related mechanisms (principally in experimental animals).
Secretory
Dysfunction of secretion of lacrimal, salivary and sebaceous glands, altered secretion of nasal mucosa, effects on neurosecretory mechanisms (rat and humans) hypothalamus-hypophysial-adrenal axis.
Dermatological
Dermatitis and/or erythema, photosensitization, edema.
Liver
Dysfunctions with or without jaundice.
Renal
Oliguria, polyuria.
Articular
Rheumatoid symptoms, activation or aggravation of pre-existing rheumatoid state.
Gastrointestinal
Diarrhea or constipation, anorexia or bulimia, vomiting and pyrosis.
Ophthalmological
Acute myopia corneal opacities, retinal pigments.
Hematological
Blood dyscreasias (3 cases of leukemia), altered coagulation, agranulocytosis, bone-marrow aplasia.
Immunological
Antinuclear antibodies.
CNS
  a. Neurological disorders: CNS depressant, extrapyramidal, dystonic, motor, epileptogenic, thermoregulatory, cerebellar, sphincter control disorders, diabetes insipidus, tardive dyskenisias.
  b. Psychiatric and behavioral: restlessness, emotional oversensitiveness, mental impairment, overestimation of capabilities, tendency to withdraw from social contacts, paranoid states with delusions of persecution, visual, auditory and tactile hallucinations, delirium, violent behavior, confusional states, catatonic-like features, akathisia, acute psychosis withdrawal symptoms; changes in catecholamine content.

This table was compiled on the basis of the information obtained from the following bibliographical references: refs. 2,7,8–10,14,16–18,21,23b,24,26,29,31,34–39,41,43,46,47,54,56,58, 59,62–64,69,70,76–79,81–84,87,88,93,94,100,105–108,111,115a,117,118,124,129,131,134, 137,141b,144,167,174,179,180–182,192,198,200,202,203,206,209.

bronchopneumonia, and petechial hemorrhages in the lungs, liver, myocardium, kidneys, and spleen.

The most significant *neuropathological findings* in human postmortem CNS were expressed by nonspecific variable chromatolysis or anoxic-like changes and various degrees of lipid degeneration, glial satellitosis, and pseudo- or neuronophagia in various areas of the brain cortex, basal ganglia (Fig. 1), cerebellum, and hypothalamus; many neurons of the hypothalamic nuclei (particularly the ventromedial) displayed marked variations in the distribution of the Nissl substance. Some cytoplasmic and extraneuronal material showed also metachromatic reaction (Fig. 2). In some instances, a paucity of neurons and depigmentation of substantia nigra in the mesencephalon were prominent (Fig. 3) (167). Some similar changes were presented in this volume by Jellinger (94), Kaufman (97), and Shiraki (178). Dystrophic alterations of the glia and, at times, increased vascular permeability were encountered.

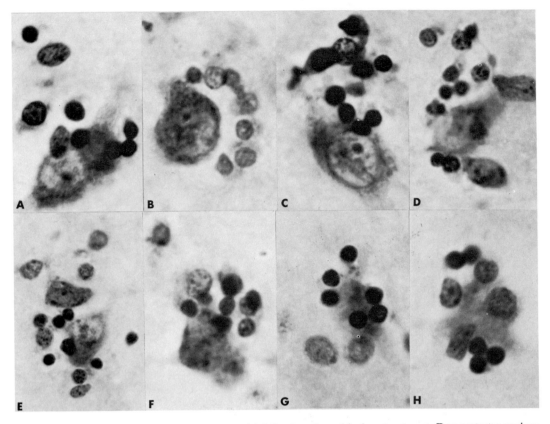

FIG. 1. Basal ganglia. Human postmortem material following phenothiazines treatment. Demonstrates various stages of increased satellitosis (A–E), pseudoneuronophagia (F and G), and neuronophagia (H). Nissl stain. A,F,G, and H: × 1,560; B: × 1,620; C and D: × 1,500 and E: × 1,140.

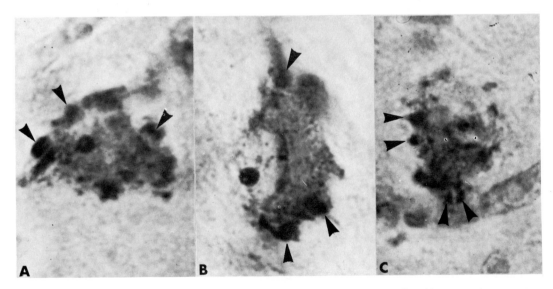

FIG. 2. Hypothalamus, ventromedial nucleus. Human postmortem material following chlorpromazine treatment. Note in particular, irregular distribution of the Nissl substance and metachromatic material (arrows). Nissl stain. A–C: × 1,250.

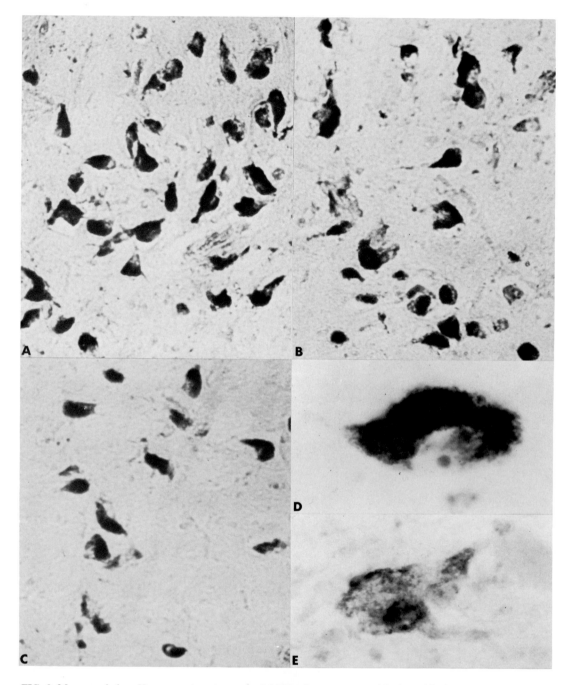

FIG. 3. Mesencephalon. Human postmortem material following treatment with phenothiazines shows **A:** average distribution of neurons in substantia nigra (medial segment), **B** and **C:** irregular distribution and reduction in number of neurons in substantia nigra (similar region to **A**), **D:** high power of a neuron with average pigmentation, and **E:** neuron with marked depigmentation. Nissl stain. **A–C:** × 250; **D** and **E:** × 1,400.

Experimental Investigations

Laboratory animals, in acute phases and mainly after high and toxic dosages, presented also a variety of *histopathological changes* of the liver and CNS. These have already been reported by us (157,159,167). However, here we would like to reiterate that: (a) in *Macacus* rhesus monkeys hypertrophy and hyperplasia of microglia (Figs. 4 and 5) were prominent in the cerebral cortex; (b) various degrees of microglial dystrophy with degenerative changes and tendency to metamorphosis in rod cells were evident in certain areas of the cerebral cortex

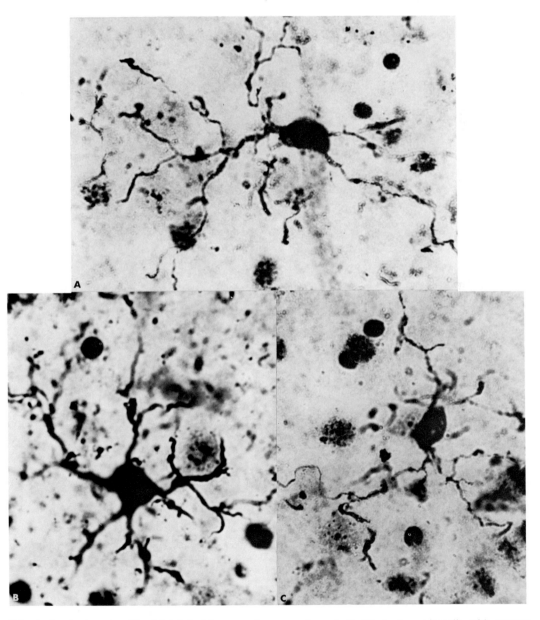

FIG. 4. Cerebral cortex (frontal lobe). *Macacus* rhesus monkey. **A–C:** Illustrating microglia with average morphological features. Hortega silver impregnation method. **A–C:** × 2,130.

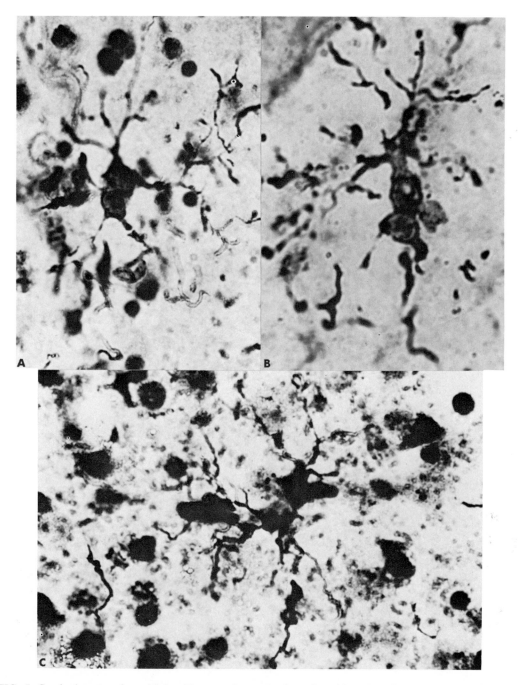

FIG. 5. Cerebral cortex, frontal lobe. *Macacus* rhesus monkey after chlorpromazine (1.0 to 1.5 mg/kg body weight) administration. Various stages of microglial division in the process of hyperplasia. Hortega's silver carbonate impregnation method. **A** and **B:** × 2,130; and **C:** × 1,750.

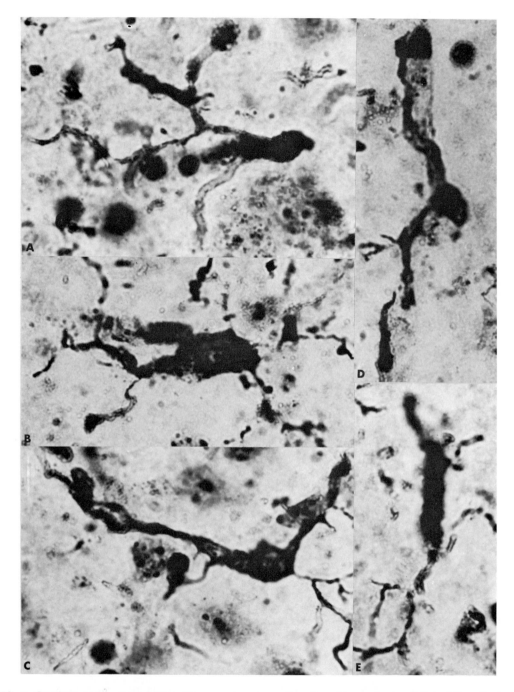

FIG. 6. Cerebral cortex, frontal lobe. *Macacus* rhesus monkey after chlorpromazine (1.0 to 1.5 mg/kg body weight) administration. **A–C:** Dystrophic microglial cells undergoing various degrees of degenerative changes; **D** and **E:** metamorphosis of microglial cells into the "rod cell prototype." Hortega's silver carbonate impregnation method. **A–E:** × 2,200.

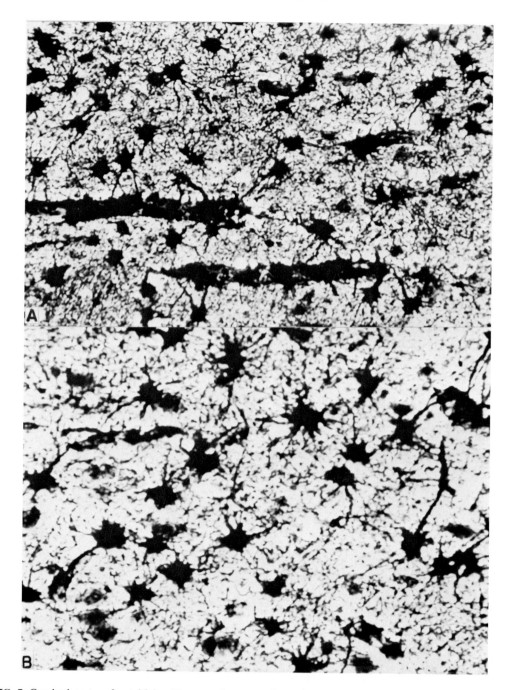

FIG. 7. Cerebral cortex, frontal lobe. *Macacus* rhesus monkey after chlorpromazine administration (0.1 to 1.5 mg/kg body weight). Reveals hypertrophy and hyperplasia of astrocytes in the subcortical white matter (**A**) and gray matter (**B**). Cajal's gold sublimate impregnation method for astrocytes. **A**: × 480; and **B**: × 670.

(Fig. 6); and (c) astrocytes were more prominent around or in the vicinity of blood vessels (Fig. 7). It is also of interest that fast-acting drugs cause no visible structural changes of the nervous system, and if changes do occur they may lack specificity.

Histochemical studies on adenosine triphosphatase (ATP-ase), succinic dehydrogenase and DPNH diaphorase (lactic bound), acid phosphatase (AcP), glucose-6-phosphatase (G-6-P), and thiamine pyrophosphatase (TPP) demonstrated diversified concentrations and distribution of enzyme reaction products in various constituents of the anatomotopographic regions of the CNS (153–155).

Electron microscope examinations of the CNS pointed out, in various experimental conditions, different qualitative and quantitative fine structural alterations of the nucleolar-nuclear system, the endoplasmic reticulum (both smooth and rough components), and related subunits, mitochondria, lysosomes, multivesicular bodies, and cellular processes. In many instances these changes affected the respective unit membranes and/or the matrix of the affected organelles.[1] Regarding the synapses, of particular interest were the marked variations in concentration of the synaptic vesicles (both s^+ and dense core types)[2] in the basal ganglia (164) and hypothalamus (144), which, at times, were also associated with variations of the osmiophilia of the vesicle content, their membranes as well as the synaptic cleft and postsynaptic zone.

Heroin and Methadone[3]

Human Investigations

Clinical observations of adverse reactions are summarized in Table 4.

---

[1] In *in vitro* studies of the CNS (168) and the liver (71,150), similar changes were apparent.

[2] s^+ = spherular.

[3] Heroin addicts under methadone detoxification and maintenance program.

TABLE 4. *Pharmacodynamic properties of methadone*

CNS and vegetative NS:
  Hypnotic, sedative, slowing EEG, respiratory depression, dizziness, blurring of vision, reduced motor activity, transient hallucinations, insomnia, forgetfulness, myoclonic jerks, delirium, reduction in libido to transient impotence. Behavioral disorders: inability to acceptably function in society or antisocial, truancy, or vagrancy, arrests (other than traffic violations and alcoholism); hypothermia, miosis, excessive sweating, pedal edema.
Metabolic functions
  Hyperglycemia, release of antidiuretic hormone (less than 5% daily urine): weight gain
Gastrointestinal and smooth muscle
  Inhibition of spasmogenic effect of ACH. and histamine of strips of isolated intestine: *in vivo* (unanesthetized animal): increased intestinal tone, decreased amplitude of contractions and propulsive constipation, dryness of mouth, biliary tract spasms.
Cardiovascular System
  Peripheral vasodilation, may contribute to orthostatic hypotension: EKG: occasional sinus bradycardia.
Respiratory system
  Diminished pulmonary ventilation, depression, antitussive.
Drug interactions
  Barbiturates, amphetamines, opiates, tranquilizers, alcohol, anesthetics.
Drug dependence
  Physical, long-lasting physiological and psychological.

Biochemical studies revealed the presence of heroin and methadone in various regions of the CNS and body tissues (151).

The most common *anatomopathological findings* in heroin addicts are pulmonary edema (which may also result from hypoxia due to respiratory depression or failure) and pulmonary complications, liver pathology (hepatitis, liver degeneration, and postnecrotic cirrhosis), secondary infections (viral, bacterial, mycotic), trauma (violent deaths, accidents, etc.), cardiovascular and, in some instances, renal insufficiency, chondroosteomyelitis, transverse myelitis, and anaphylactic or allergic mechanisms.

The *neuropathological findings* include a variety of mild to prominent nonspecific neuronal degeneration in various anatomotopographic regions of the CNS, some of

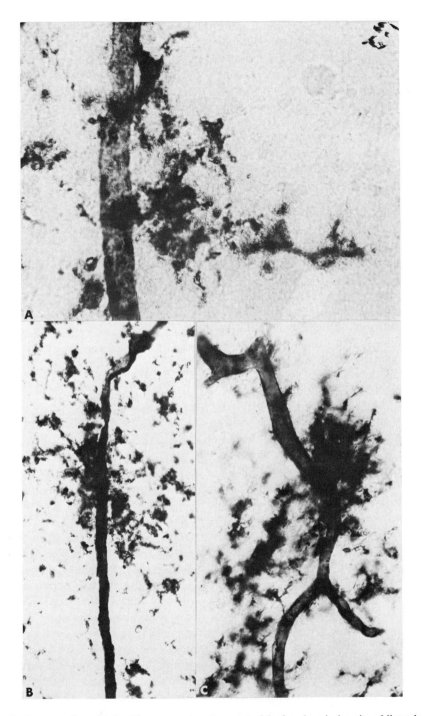

FIG. 8. Cerebral cortex, frontal lobe. Human postmortem material of a chronic heroin addict who has taken methadone prior to demise. Illustrates perivascular glial reactions associated with increased vascular permeability as revealed by TPP method. **A:** × 960; **B:** × 320; and **C:** × 380.

which recall the microscopic features of an anoxic process (150).

Moderate to prominent degrees of alteration in the distribution and concentration of *enzyme reaction* products of TPP, G-6-P, and AcP occurred in various cytoarchitectural and anatomotopographic regions of the CNS. In addition, perivascular glial (principally astrocytic) reactions were more prominent in TPP preparations, which, at times, also showed increased vascular permeability (Fig. 8) (161).

The most pronounced *electron microscope* changes in the CNS were related to the ultrastructure and distribution of the endoplasmic reticulum (particularly Golgi complex), mitochondrial pleomorphism, ribosomes, synaptic complex and their subunits, degenerative products in the cellular cytoplasm, vascular walls, and perivascular regions. Of particular significance was the presence of axonal degeneration and dystrophies as well as some senile plaque-like formations (Fig. 9) (143,150).

The disorganization of the endoplasmic reticulum and related subunits of mitochondria, multivesicular bodies, heterogenous, and membranous structures, and abnormal amounts of lipid products, glycogen granules, as well as necrobiotic material, were prominent in electron microscope preparations of the *liver* (71,148b).

Experimental Investigations

In the acute phases, following administration of heroin and methadone in rats and monkeys: (a) the most salient histochemical observations were represented by marked variations in the intensity of reaction and distribution of the TPP, G-6-P, and AcP reaction products among the neurons of various anatomotopographic areas of the CNS; (b) increased acetylcholinesterase at synaptic and postsynaptic levels (similar to those reported

by Kokko et al., ref. 104) was evident in some areas of the CNS, and (c) variable concentrations and distribution of the dense core vesicles (catecholamines) were detected in the neurons of the ventromedial nucleus of the hypothalamus, as well as in some unmyelinated (and occasionally myelinated) axons and synaptic terminals (Fig. 10). Concomitantly, electron microscope examinations of the same hypothalamic region detected variations in: (a) extension, configuration, and fine structural organization of the endoplasmic reticulum, particularly of the Golgi complex and related subunits, (b) quantitative distribution of ribosomes, (c) numerical distribution and pleomorphisms of mitochondria, lysosomes, and MVB, and (d) organelle content and subunits of the synaptic complex. These ultrastructural changes were predominant during the early phase (1 to 16 hr) of methadone neurotoxicity in rats.

Additional studies, including the use of standard electron microscope combined with TPP preparations revealed: (a) variations in configuration, extension, shape, dimension, and osmiophilia of the canaliculi of the endoplasmic reticulum, particularly the Golgi complex and related subunits (Fig. 11), and (b) alterations of the pattern of distribution of the TPP reaction products (Fig. 11).

In *chronic phases* qualitative and quantitative changes of RNA, smooth and rough endoplasmic reticulum, mitochondria (polymorphometabolosomes or PMS), synapses, and axoplasmic contents were prominent (163).

DISCUSSION

The clinical response and laboratory observations to direct and indirect effects of neuropsychotropic agents, in accordance with the investigative methods, may be expressed in multiple and diversified patterns.

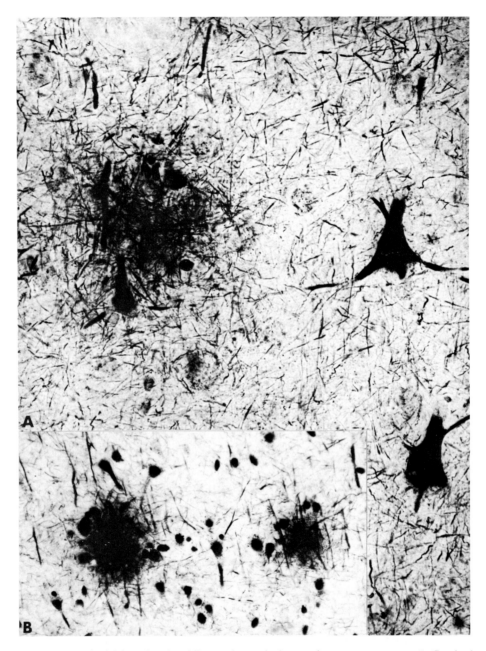

FIG. 9. Postmortem material from heroin addicts under methadone maintenance treatment. **A:** Cerebral cortex (20-year-old female); **B:** cerebellum (23-year-old male) showing senile plaque-like formations as visualized by Gomori acid phosphatase method. **A:** × 1,340; and **B:** × 380.

Clinical Adverse or Toxic Reactions

Table 3 summarizes the most common clinical adverse and toxic reactions of neuroleptics, revealing that the neuropsychotropic agents, in addition to affecting the nervous system, may also have viscerotropic properties. Incidence, fre-

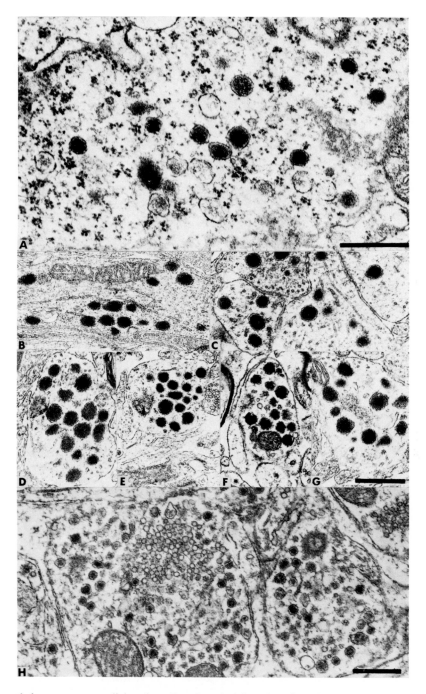

FIG. 10. Hypothalamus, ventromedial nucleus. Rat after administration of methadone (2.2 mg/100 g body weight; duration 4 to 24 hr). Discloses various degrees of qualitative and quantitative changes, particularly of dense core vesicles, in **A:** cytoplasm of neuron; **B–D:** neuropil; and **E:** synaptic terminals. Uranyl acetate and lead citrate. RCA-EMU 3G. **A–C:** × 53,000; **D–H:** × 35,600. Scale = 0.5 μm.

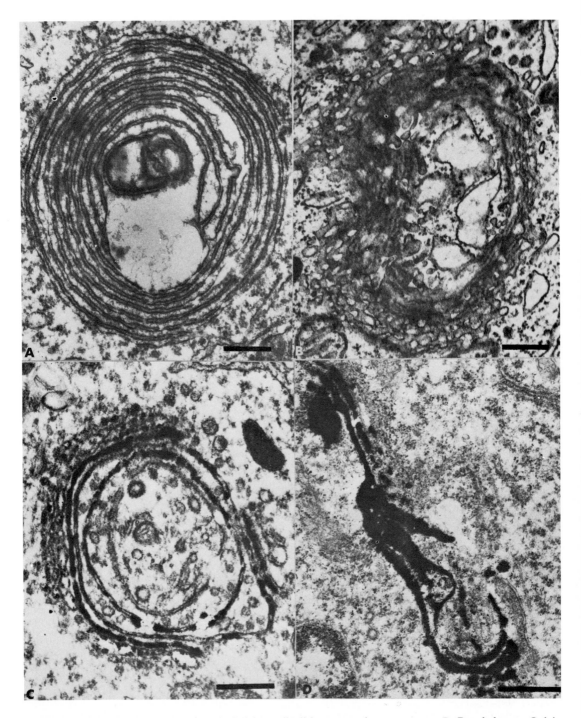

FIG. 11. A: Hypothalamus. Rat control. Golgi canaliculi in concentric arrangement. B: Rat thalamus. Golgi canaliculi undergoing marked disorganization following administration of methadone (1.5 mg/100 g body weight; duration 16 hr). C: Hypothalamus. Rat control. TPP reaction products within the Golgi canaliculi. D: Rat hypothalamus after methadone treatment (4.4 mg/100 g body weight; duration 1 hr). A and C: Regular electron microscope methods. B and D: Combined histochemical procedure (TPP) and regular electron microscope methods. A and B: × 28,600; C: × 36,600; and D: × 40,400. Scale = 0.5 μm.

quency, duration, severity, reversibility, and irreversibility seem to be conditioned by some of the following interacting cofactors.

Drug and Biochemical Cofactors

Pharmacodynamic properties and the mode of action of the neuropsychotropic agents have already been reviewed by Clouet (ref. 28, and Chapter 7, *this volume*), Perel, and Teller (*this volume*). Quite often the safety margin between effective medical dosage and toxicity is very narrow. This may further be handicapped since the chemotherapy is frequently carried out for long periods of time. *Multiple drug* intake resulting in multiphasic drug interactions has been emphasized in a significant number of clinicopathological surveys in the United States (23b,168,193, and Simpson, Chapter 1, *this volume*) and Britain that have shown an average patient in a hospital is frequently treated with several drugs, whereas individual figures up to 20 or 30 have been recorded by Smith et al. (182). Not only may drug interactions affect the absorption, transport, distribution, metabolization, and elimination of the therapeutic agent, but also they could interfere with or change its characteristic pharmacodynamic properties. In order not to deviate from our main topic, for more details concerning a variety of biological confactors, the interested reader is referred to the following bibliographical references: see refs. 23b, 45,76,84,94,120,150. Furthermore, drug interactions may alter the response of the therapeutic agents without modifying their concentration in the plasma. In such instances, the action of a drug is not predictable from knowledge of its pharmacological properties (45).

Pathobiological Cofactors

Virchow (196), in attempting to "place pathology among the biological sciences," remarked that "the contrast between health and disease is not to be sought in a fundamental difference of two kinds of life, nor in alteration of essence, but only alteration of conditions." The conditions are also regulated by metabolic mechanisms constantly undergoing changes related to physiological and environmental adaptive or reactive processes.

This fundamental biological principle served us as a guideline in the evaluation of our research investigations on the pathogenesis of drugs or chemically induced adverse and toxic reactions in human and experimental conditions. However, in comparing the structural findings in human with those obtained in laboratory animals, we must keep in mind that the experimental animals (prior to the administration of the drugs) and their respective controls were selected from healthy groups of the same age, sex, approximate weight, etc., and living in the same average healthy conditions; whereas, human material is obviously much more heterogenous and associated with a variety of diversified biological and pathophysiological factors of neurogenic, psychogenic, and metabolic character (4,54). In addition, the evaluation of the pathological findings related to phenothiazines and particularly narcotics has become more complicated during recent years due to:

1. *Erratic alcohol* consumption (Victor and Smith, *this volume*) and even relatively small amounts of alcohol intake in association with neuropsychotropic agents may cause unwanted adverse reactions (11,151).

2. *Nutritional* factors and their possible role in the pathological processes have already been discussed by Carr and Dastur (*this volume*).

3. In these circumstances, contributing complications may result from additional medical (52,120,179), socioeconomical, and environmental conditions (52,120,179).

In essence, the above-mentioned pharmacodynamic, metabolic, and pathobiolog-

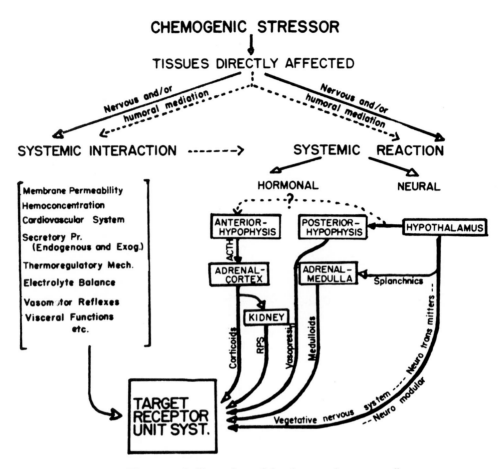

FIG. 12. Diagrammatic illustrations of the chemogenic stressor effects.

ical cofactors mediate their properties through the anatomophysiological correlates of the affected organ or target. Their functional and histochemical potentialities are reviewed below.

Pathogenic mechanisms

In our studies on neuropathogenic mechanisms of drug or chemical adverse reaction, we have adapted and expanded Cannon's (23a) "homeostasis" and Selye's "stress" pathophysiological concepts (173) up to the ultracellular level of the CNS, structural organization. On this basis, we assumed that the pharmacodynamic properties of the drug or chemical

agent induce a chemical stress upon the homeokinesis of the histochemical and functional correlates of the interacting "target" or bioreceptor.[4] This working hypothesis is schematically illustrated in the following figures and tables.

Figure 12 illustrates schematically the mechanisms by which a chemogenic stressor induces a systemic interaction within the homeokinesis of the organisms and the target or receptor unit[4] (*left side of the diagram*) which respond with compensatory reactions (*right side of the diagram*).

---

[4] This may be a component of the cell, organelle, membrane, and their respective molecular organization.

The target or receptor site (in a functioning organism) is not in a static state, but is maintained in normal conditions by a dynamic anatomophysiological synergism (Table 5). This homeokinetic state is regulated in physiological processes in an orderly manner by intrinsic hereditary mechanisms in conjunction with the environmental conditions of the cell. In abnormal conditions correlated structural, metabolic, or functional reversible changes (histometabolic dysergia) take place. However, if such endogenous or exogenous phenomena are repeated or perpetuated without control and exceed the physiological endurance or histochemical compatibility of the target, then, eventually, the disorganization or dissolution of the integrated anatomophysiological synergistic equilibrium follows with consequent irreversible changes of the structural, metabolic, and functional parameters (141a).

When the chemical agents reach the target or receptor site, they react with the available physiological and biochemical adjustments according to: (a) the drug concentration, (b) the interplay with the duration of the chemogenic effects, and (c) the biological conditions of the target. Normally, the chemical agent, like nutrients, coupling at the target or receptor site is gradually metabolized. But, when the drug is given in large amounts or more frequently than the "metabolization rate," then the chemical agent accumulates and may reach toxic concentrations. In addition, individual differences (genetic heterogeneity, biological variables) in receptor response and dose requirements (drug absorption, transport, distribution, and elimination) have also been observed. For instance, a dose that is satisfactory in one patient may be less effective or even ineffective in another or cause adverse reactions or toxicity in a third. Some drugs

TABLE 5. *Diagrammatic illustration of structural, metabolic, and functional (SMF) reaction patterns in normal and abnormal conditions*

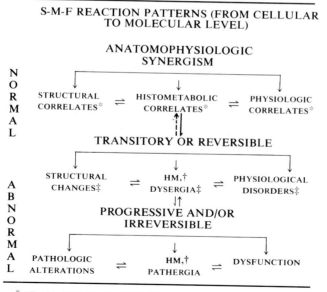

* AT ALL LEVELS OF ORGANIZATION
† HISTOMETABOLIC
‡ ENDOGENOUS AND/OR EXOGENOUS ORIGIN, DISCONTINUED ARROW MEANS PARTIAL REVERSIBILITY.

bind irreversibly to the receptor, and their action may persist long after the concentration in plasma has become unmeasurable (45). Furthermore, some other predisposing, facilitating, or sensitizing cofactors seem to be operating in certain clinicopathological conditions, as for instance:

1. Some schizophrenics treated with neuroleptics showed psychotic exacerbations, such as confusion, disorientation, paranoid ideation, increased agitation and excitement, violent behavior, visual-auditory hallucinations, depersonalization (167), and catatonic behavior (6,7,13, 117,118,203). High plasma levels of chlorpromazine in some patients were associated with aggravation of their schizophrenia. Reduction of dosage resulted in a corresponding reduction of the plasma level and also improvement of the patient's condition (33). All these exacerbations were terminated by anticholinergic therapy, except in some cases who apparently developed irreversible change resulting in "tardive dyskinesias" (Simpson, *this volume*). It is also of interest that depressive conditions are more common with reserpine and tetrabenzaine (20), whereas senile patients are particularly prone to confusion (44). Similar exacerbation of symptoms was observed in some schizophrenics treated with atropine (66), whereas DFP reactivated acute psychotic phenomena in a chronic schizophrenic (169). In addition, psychotic patients or patients who previously displayed only neurotic symptoms usually showed symptom intensification on administration of mescaline and LSD-25. In these instances, it was also stressed that the previous personality often enters and exerts a large influence on the determination of both the form and content of the reaction to drugs (85).

2. Activation of epileptic seizures (15,111) and temporal syndrome (47,65,

194) occurred with therapeutic doses of neuroleptics. Moreover, epileptics appear more prone to convulsions while under treatment with weaker neuroleptics (20, 75), as do patients with history of electroconvulsive therapy, brain injuries, lobotomy, and alcoholism (2,29,74).

3. In support of similar phenomena, although occurring in extraneural structures, I would like to mention the following pathochemical correlates: (a) necrosis of the epithelium of renal tubules, in a manic patient treated with lithium carbonate, showed high concentration of lithium (3.7 mEq/liter) and higher than any analyzed organ (25); (b) interstitial myocarditis in a manic depressive patient treated with lithium carbonate contained extremely high concentration of lithium (2.14 mEq/liter, 191); and (c) livers of rats affected by various degrees of degeneration caused by ethionine diet (8 to 14 months duration) (142a,146) and of rats previously treated for a long time (3 to 9 months) with prochlorperazine (4) showed much higher concentrations of this drug in the liver and brain than controls.

At the ultracellular level, during recent years, "the spotlight" of the gradient morphological measure of the target has been focused upon the "unit membrane." It has been established that in physiological conditions:

1. Energy transformation and most integrated metabolic processes are intrinsic, associated, or membrane-bound (40,72,73,132,133,185,201). In these instances each enzyme serves two capacities: (a) as a group of catalysts in a sequential metabolic process and (b) as an integral part of a membrane system (73,201,etc.).

2. Drugs and chemical agents exercise their pharmacodynamic or biochemical properties by interacting with the target or receptor sites located within unit membranes.

3. In biochemical terms the bioreceptors are "specialized macromolecules" (51) for specific binding or interaction with specific endogenous and exogenous molecules.

4. In the nervous system the receptor sites (chemosensitive, receptive, cognitive) are principally incorporated (embedded) in the postsynaptic membrane, and the molecules of the receptor sites by interacting with drugs are capable of undergoing conformational changes as well as inducing the translocation of ions and producing bioelectrical changes (40). In light of these considerations we used, as a biological model for *in vivo* and *in vitro* (168) studies, the reactions of the mitochondrial organelle or PMS (140b) and their respective subunits, since they are one of the most widely studied organelles in various biological conditions (72, 109). As a matter of fact, it has been established that: (a) chlorpromazine, imipramine, and other basic lipophilic drugs are strongly bound to liver microsomes and PMS (14a), and (b) chlorpromazine inhibits the oxidative phosphorylation of PMS (67a,164,197).

Table 6 summarizes the fundamental structural, chemical, and functional correlates in physiological conditions.

Table 7 summarizes the structural, functional, and histometabolic interdependency of the PMS subunits in pathobiological conditions. It has been established that when the PMS are damaged or disrupted, the enzyme assemblies of the citric-cycle oxidations are apparently detached from the respective units and become water soluble. In these circumstances or when the fragmented organelles are composed principally of paired membranes, the citric-cycle oxidative functions are altered or lost. With subsequent fragmentation of the fine structure (unpaired single membranes), the original functions of the disintegrated organelle are reduced to only the electron transport mechanisms. It is also significant that drugs have no demonstrable effects on membrane-bound enzymes, after the same enzymes have been separated or extracted from the membrane. Thus, the membrane-enzyme associate systems represent the molecular basis of the histometabolism or the biological energy transformation in tissues. Alterations of the fine membrane systems and

TABLE 6. *The structural, chemical, and functional correlates of the mito-chondrion*

Structure	Chemistry	Function
Outer and inner limiting membranes:	DPN, flavoproteins cytochromes, ECE	ETP, K inner membrane
Matrix:	Enzymes, Krebs' and fatty acid oxidation cycles	Oxidation, Krebs', tricarboxylic acid cycle; "respiratory assemblies," conversion of ADP in ATP; trans. H_2O and certain m
Cristae:	Stratified proteins and phospholipid molecules	ETP, fatty acid and some NH-acid oxidation; oxidative phosphorilation

ECE, enzyme coupling energy; m, molecular or atomic proportion constituents; DPN, diphosphophyridine nucleotide; ETP, electron transport particles; ADP, adenosine diphosphate; ATP, adenosine triphosphate; NH-acid, amino acids.

TABLE 7. *Illustrates the ultrastructural and three main functional correlates of the mitochondrion in physiological and pathobiological processes affecting principally the membrane systems of the mitochondrion.*

Structure		Functions		
		Citric cycle oxidation	Oxidative phosphorylation	Electron transp. part.
	Intact PMS	+	+	+
	Paired chains (membranes)	−	+	+
	Unpaired chains (membranes)	−	−	+

subunits of the mitochondria were observed by us in humans and especially in various experimental conditions *in vitro* (166,168) and *in vivo* following the administration of various neuropsychotropic agents. For instance, qualitative and quantitative changes of PMS were seen in the cytoplasm of the neurons in spinal cord ganglia tissue cultures treated with LSD-25 (Fig. 13). In human heroin and methadone fatalities (151), in addition to PMS pleomorphism, we observed also various degrees of disorganization of the cristae and variations in the osmiophilia of the matrix (Fig. 14). Figure 15 illustrates, in particular, variations in pattern of distribution (Fig. 15A–E),

and an increase in number (Fig. 15F and G) of the PMS cristae, as well as abnormal membranous formations (Fig. 15). Marked variations in the osmiophilic character of the matrix of the PMS were prominent in the neurons of the lenticular nucleus of rats treated with prochlorperazine (Fig. 16A–E). Intra-PMS osmiophilic deposits or inclusions were also noted in various human and experimental CNS material following administration of neuropsychotropic agents (Fig. 16F–J).

Besides the mitochondrion or the PMS, other cellular organelles and their unit membrane systems could also act as target or receptor sites.

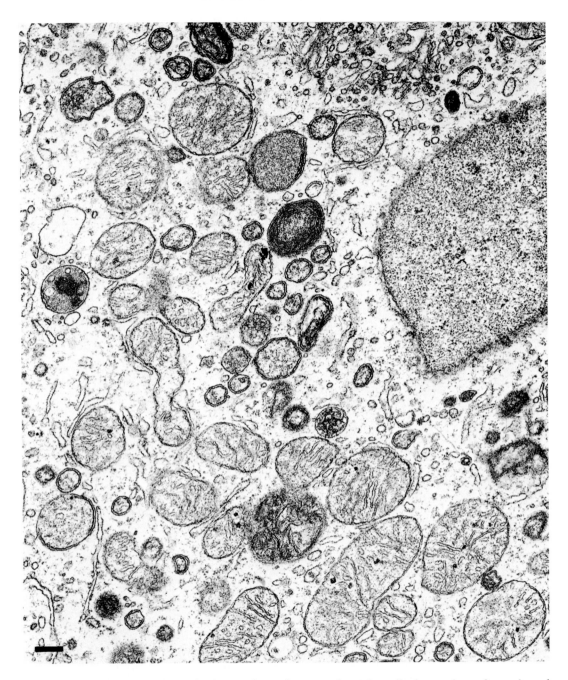

FIG. 13. A: Large number of PMS in the cytoplasm of a neuron in cord ganglia tissue culture after prolonged administration of LSD. Uranyl acetate and lead citrate. RCA-EMU 3G. × 14,700. Scale = 0.5 µm. (From Roizin et al., ref. 166.)

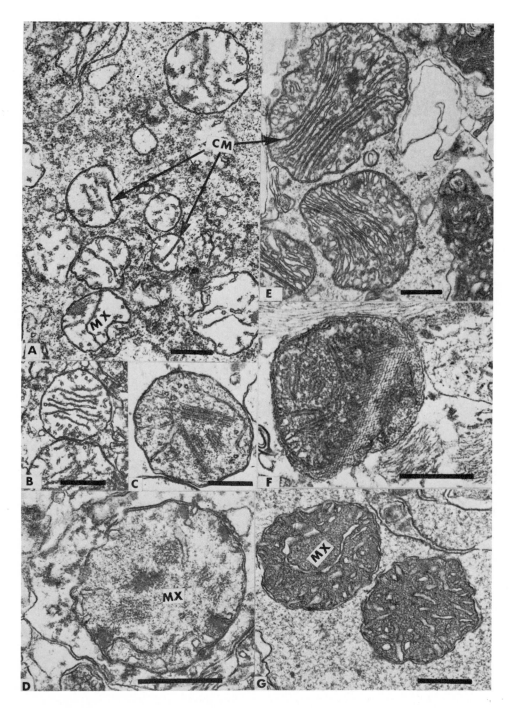

FIG. 14. Cerebral cortex. Human postmortem material. Heroin addict who died following the use of large doses of methadone. **A** and **B**: Average variety of PMS; **C–E**: in particular, variations and changes of the cristae mitochondriales; **F**: alterations of the cristae and matrix; and **G**: PMS with dense matrix. Uranyl acetate and lead citrate. RCA-EMU 3G. **A–C**: × 30,480; **D**: × 57,150; **E**: × 28,580; **F**: × 51,050; and **G**: × 37,150. Scale = 0.5 μm. Cm, cristae mitochondriales; Mx, matrix.

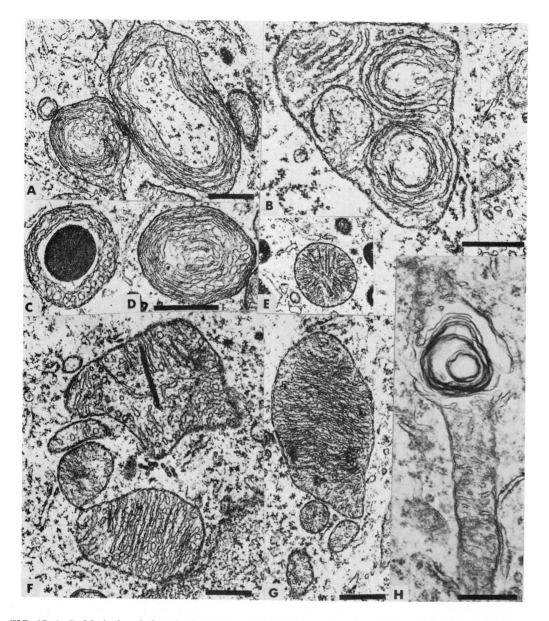

FIG. 15. A–G: Marked variations in the pattern of distribution and number of the cristae in the cells of spinal cord ganglia treated with prolonged LSD-25. **H:** Abnormal membranous whorl-like formation in a PMS of a neuron from the lenticular nucleus of a rat treated for 6 months with prochlorperazine (0.5 mg/100 g body weight). Uranyl acetate and lead citrate. RCA-EMU 3G. **A,E,F,** and **G:** × 29,000; **B,D,** and **H:** × 40,500; and **C:** × 42,000. Scale = 0.5 μm. (A–G, from Roizin et al., ref. 166.)

In the nervous system, the target or receptor sites may be located along the neuronal surfaces, their processes, and, after crossing the cellular and organelle membranes, the ultracellular components of the nucleonucleolar system and cellular cytoplasm. There is common agreement that: (a) the synapses, or rather the synaptic complex (including the axonal or presynaptic terminals, synaptic vesicles, presynaptic

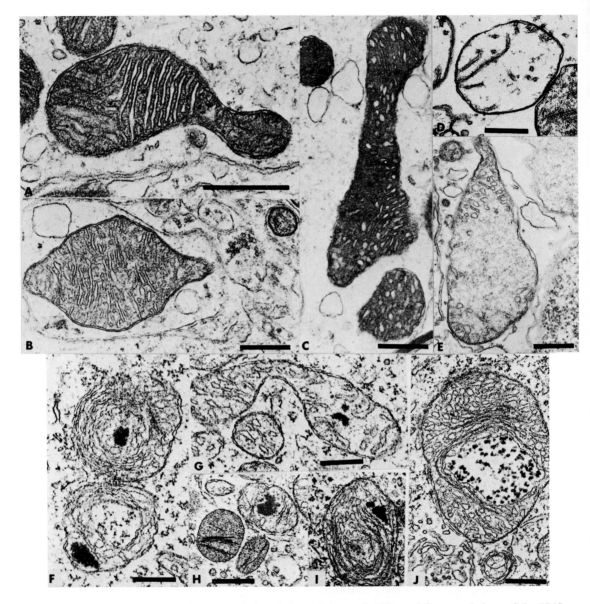

FIG. 16. Demonstrates, in particular, marked variations of the osmiophilia and fine morphology of the PMS matrix. **A,B,** and **C:** Neurons of the rat lenticular nucleus treated with prochlorperazine (0.5 to 1.0 mg/100 g body weight) for 10, 15, and 24 months, respectively. **D:** PMS from postmortem cerebral cortex of a chronic heroin addict who also took methadone. **E:** PMS from the rat lenticular nucleus treated with prochlorperazine (0.5 mg/100 g body weight) for 6 months. **F–I:** PMS from cells of spinal cord ganglia tissue cultures following prolonged LSD-25 treatment. Note also the presence of dense amorphous material within the matrix [**E** (*upper side*), **F,** and **G**] and between the cristae [**E** (*lower side*), and **H**] and glycogen-like granules (**J**). Uranyl acetate, lead citrate. RCA-EMU 3G. **A:** × 59,000; **B** and **C:** × 34,400; **D:** × 30,500; **E–J:** × 29,000. Scale = 0.5 μm. (F–J, from Roizin et al., ref. 166.)

membrane, synaptic cleft, and postsynaptic membrane), are uniquely specific organelles of the nervous system, (b) they are principally related to transmission (communication) of neural activity (action potentials and related integrative functions), and (c) they compartmentalize the metabolic processes concerned with the storage, transport, release, and reuptake of neurochemical transmitters (16,50,92,127,128). It is beyond the scope of this discussion to review the fast growing and extensive literature on the fine morphology, biochemistry, and physiology of synapses except to reiterate that, although the synaptic functions and particularly the postsynaptic membrane have been designated as the opiate receptor interaction (28,51,130) in the nervous system, extraneural target and receptor sites also occur (42). Furthermore, there is evidence suggesting interactions of morphine (42), and probably other neuropsychotropic agents, with one or more neurotransmitters, and that some neurotransmitters (catecholamines) exercise also extraneural effects. The following extraneural effects have been observed: (a) alteration of the permeability of the hepatic cells to inorganic ions (80), (b) acceleration of hepatic glycogenesis, and (c) release of potassium from the liver resulting in increased potassium concentration in plasma (48,49).

In the final evaluation of these pathogenic mechanisms (particularly in humans), in addition to previously mentioned biological cofactors, growth and aging processes as essential morphometabolic constituents of the target must also be taken into consideration. During recent years it has been demonstrated in humans and in experimental conditions that: (a) CNS from its origin through embryonal morphochemical metamorphosis, functional differentiation, and maturation shows selective vulnerabilities (95,165,205), (b) various chemical agents, particularly of low molecular weight, pass through the placental barrier, and (c) they are bound or retained and become more

concentrated in the fetus than in the mother (2,115b,188). As a result of these three factors, or some as yet unknown factors, various chromosomal, teratogenic, and embryopathic processes have occurred (95,162, Fischman et al. and Haddad et al., *this volume*) following the use of various neuropsychotropic drugs and chemical agents. As far as the role of the age factor at the involutional (senile) phase is concerned, very little is known about characteristic effects of neuropsychotropic agents on the body tissues except that some senile patients following the intake of neuroleptics are prone to confusion. It is also of interest to note that we have observed senile plaque-like formations, axonal dystrophies, lipofuscin pigment, and lipid products of degeneration in amounts more than usual in two young (20- and 23-year-old) chronic heroin addicts.

On the basis of the multi- and interdisciplinary methodologies in human and in various experimental conditions, we believe that the histochemical and ultrastructural changes described above are the expression of the interaction of the drug or chemical agents (or their metabolic by-products) with multiple neural and extraneural target or receptor sites. These are represented by specialized bimodel molecules embodied in the framework of the involved organelles, their unit membrane, or their metabolic products (neurotransmitters, biogenic amines, polypeptides, or amino acids, 40,51,132,205). Since this chain of histometabolic and structural reactions was initiated by chemical mechanisms at the molecular level of organization, we propose to designate them "chemogenic" or "chemomolecular lesions." The development (predisposition, facilitation, precipitation) and evolution (aggravation, modification, reversibility or irreversibility) of these chemopathological processes depend also on the "total biological reality" (141b), which consists of the interaction between the compounded inborn and acquired biological

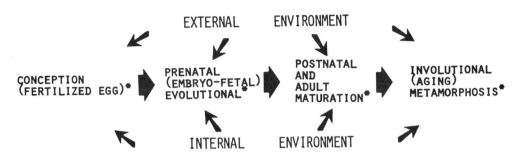

FIG. 17. Schematic illustration of the total biological reality of an organism from conception to senility. The arrows indicate possible environmental effects upon the structural-chemical-functional correlates of the organism through the various biological phases of its life-span.

processes of the organisms, throughout its life-span, with internal and external environmental conditions, as schematically outlined in Fig. 17.

SUMMARY AND CONCLUDING REMARKS

Multidisciplinary studies have revealed clinical adverse or toxic reactions of the CNS and peripheral nervous system, and cardiovascular, gastrointestinal, hepatic, renal, hematological, endocrinological and neural-humoral, secretory, dermatological, articular and immunological functions following the intake of neuropsychotropic agents.

Prenatal effects have also been reported in the literature and in this volume.

Particular attention was focused upon the pathogenic mechanisms of the adverse or toxic reactions affecting the CNS and liver.

Neural and extraneural, reversible and irreversible, fine ultrastructural and histochemical changes affecting some organelles (including their respective ultrastructures and unit membrane systems) were observed in human and experimental (*in vivo* and *in vitro*) conditions.

Thus, the so-called neuropsychotropic agents possess also "visceral" and "histometabolic tropism."

The discussed multidisciplinary findings seem to suggest that the described clinical and pathological adverse and toxic reactions may be considered the expression of

the interaction of multiple targets or bioreceptor sites of the affected organelles and respective ultrastructures with the drug or chemical agent or their biochemical by-products.

According to several investigators, the target or receptor sites consist of bimodal molecules that are integral components of the lipoprotein membranes or are specific molecules incorporated within the framework of the organelles and their respective subunits (including their metabolic by-products). These ultrastructures bear specialized physicochemical sites that bind or interact with specific endogenous and exogenous chemical molecules (40,51,132,205). By interacting with the drug, the molecules of the respective receptor sites in the nervous system may also undergo conformational changes capable of inducing the translocation of ions and producing corresponding bioelectrical changes (40) or converting ionophores to a conductive state (80). Since in physiological conditions the interaction between the target or receptor sites and the chemical agents takes place at their respective molecular levels of organization, it is surmised that the adverse or toxic reactions induced by the drug or chemical agent are also the expression of molecular interactions. On this basis we consider the above-described adverse or toxic reactions the expression of a *chemogenic or chemomolecular lesion* of reversible or irreversible character resulting from *in vivo* or *in vitro* molecular interactions among the chemical agents and morphochemical correlates of the vital units of the organism.[5]

The selective vulnerability, reversibility, or irreversibility of the chemogenic lesion depend upon the degree, extension and the anatomotopographic distribution of the interaction between: (a) targets and bioreceptors (including the inborn and acquired constitutional organization and its biological condition); (b) drug and biochemical cofactors (including biochemical properties and pharmacokinetics, dosage, mode of administration and duration of treatment) and; at times, (c) participation of accessory medical, pathobiological, and pathochemical cofactors (total biological reality).

In the final analysis it is hoped that the identification of the mechanisms involved in the initiation and evolution of the chemogenic lesions will help to develop antidotes, and establish preventive or prophylactic measures to safeguard the patients' health from the occurrence or recurrence of unwarranted chemical effects.

ACKNOWLEDGMENTS

The author gratefully acknowledges the assistance and cooperation of J. C. Liu, K. M. Wu, and S. Avrin for electron microscopy procedures, V. Bystron for illustrations, W. Rivers for bibliography, and I. Tyburczy for secretarial work.

REFERENCES

1. Adelson, L. (1952): Pathologic findings in patients dead of common poisons. Am. J. Clin. Pathol., 22:509–519.

---

[5] Schleiden (171), Schwann (172), and Virchow (195) with the light microscope classified them as "cells." However, on the basis of more recent histochemical, electron microscope, tissue culture, refrigerated gradient ultracentrifugation, etc., investigations, it seems to me justified to include in the same category the organelles, their respective ultrastructural components, and the active unit membrane systems up to their molecular level of organization.

2. Aivazian, G. H., and Reese, H. C., Jr. (1959): Clinical evaluation of prosazine therapy for schizophrenia. Dis. Nerv. Syst., 20:472–477.

3. Akai, K., Roizin, L., and Liu, J. C. (1977): Ultrastructural findings in experimental lithium neurotoxicology. In: Neurotoxicology, edited by L. Roizin, H. Shiraki, and N. Grčević. (This volume.)

4. Alexander, F., and French, T. N. (1948): Studies in Psychosomatic Medicine. Roland Press, New York.

5. Alexander, G., Machiz, S., Gray, R., Liu, J. C., and Roizin, L. (1971): Elevated phenothiazine levels in chronic liver poisoning in guinea pigs. Fed. Proc., 30:562.

6. Angus, J. W. S., Ignal, F., Igbal, J., and Simpson, G. M. (1967): A year's trial of thiothiaxene in chronic schizophrenia. Int. J. Neuropsychiatry, 3:408–412.

7. Angus, J. W. S., and Simpson, G. M. (1970): Hysteria and drug induced dystonia. Acta Psychiatr. Scand. [Suppl.], 212:25–58.

8. Anton-Stephens, D. (1954): Preliminary observations on the psychiatric use of chlorpromazine (Largactil). J. Ment. Sci., 100:543–557.

9. Arnold, O. H. (1959): Klinische Erfahrungen mit dem Neuroleptikum Truxal. Wein. Med. Wochenschr., 109:892–898.

10. Azima, H., and Ogle, W. (1954): Effects of Largactil in mental syndromes. Can. Med. Assoc. J., 71:116–121.

11. Baden, M. M. (1974): Alcoholism as related to drug addiction. A medical examiner's review. In: Drug Abuse, edited by W. Keup, p. 64. Charles C Thomas, Springfield, Ill.

12. Bailey, B. H., and Kay, R. E. (1960): Prolonged phenothiazine hepatitis: Report of a case. Am. J. Psychiatry, 117:557–558.

13. Behrman, S. (1972): Mutism induced by phenothiazines. Br. J. Psychiatry, 121:599–604.

14. Bersohn, I., and Wallace, B. V. (1955): Chlorpromazine (Largactil) jaundice. South African Med. J., 29:677–683.

14a. Bickel, M. H. (1974): Binding of phenothiazines and related compounds to tissues and cell constituents. In: The Phenothiazines and Structurally Related Drugs, edited by I. S. Forrest, C. J. Carr, and E. Usdin, pp. 163–166. Raven Press, New York.

15. Blair, D., and Braday, D. M. (1958): Recent advances in the treatment of schizophrenia. J. Ment. Sci., 104:625–634.

16. Bloom, F. E., and Costa, E. (1974): The effects of drugs on serotonergic nerve terminals. In: Cytopharmacology, Vol. 1: 1st Int. Symp. Cell Biol. & Cytopharmacol., edited by F. Clementi, and B. Ceccarelli, p. 379–396. Raven Press, New York.

17. Boardman, R. H. (1954): Fatal case of toxic hepatitis implicating chlorpromazine. Br. Med. J., 2:579.

18. Bobon, J., Collard, J., and Demaret, A. (1961): Un vouveau neuroleptique a effet hypnogene differe: Le Dipiperone (R 3345), butyrophenone

carbamidee. *Acta Neurol. Psychiatr. Belg.*, 61:611–630.

19. Bollard, B., Roizin, L., Sabbia, R., and Horwitz, W. A. (1963): Distribution of free and S^{35} labelled prochlorperazine (Compazine) in mammalian tissue. *Fed. Proc.*, 22:317 (Abstr.)

20. Brauchitsch, H. V. (1962): Die klinische Wirkung des Benzoquinolizinderivates Nitoman bei der chronischen Schizophrenie. *Nervenarzt*, 33:60–66.

21. Brooks, G. W., and Mac Donald, M. G. (1961): Effects of trifluoperazine in aged depressed female patients. *Am. J. Psychiatry*, 117:932–933.

22. Buchtal, A. B., and Jenkinson, D. H. (1970): Effects of isomers of the α-agonist amidephrine on arterial and tracheal muscle in vitro. *Eur. J. Pharmacol.*, 10:293–296.

23a. Cannon, W. B. (1932): *The Wisdom of the Body*. W. W. Norton, New York.

23b. Cares, R., Asrican, E., Fenishel, M., Sack, P., and Severino, J. (1957): Therapeutic and toxic effects of chlorpromazine among 3,014 hospitalized cases. *Am. J. Psychiatry*, 114:318–327.

24. Carfagno, S. C., and Magee, J. T. (1961): Granulocytopenia due to chlorpromazine: A report of 11 cases. *Am. J. Med. Sci.*, 241:44–54.

25. Chapman, A. J., and Lewis, G. (1972): Iatrogenic lithium poisoning: A case report with necropsy findings. *J. Okla. State Med. Assoc.*, 65:491–494.

26. Chatagnon, P., Chatagnon, C., Wilkin, M. O., Fournier, M., and Lorcy, P. (1961): Syndrome dyskinétique facio-bucco-lingual et chorétique avec hémiballisme d'étiologie chlorpromazinique. *Ann. Med. Psychol.*, 119:310–318.

27. Childers, R. T., Jr. (1961): Hyperpyrexia, coma and death during chlorpromazine therapy. *J. Clin. Exp. Psychopathol. Q. Rev. Psychiatr. Neurol.*, 22:163–164.

28. Clouet, D. H. (1972): Theoretical biochemical mechanisms for drug dependence. In: *Chemical and Biological Aspects of Drug Dependence*, edited by S. J. Mulé and H. Brill, pp. 545–561. CRC Press, Cleveland.

29. Cohen, H., and Freireich, A. Z. (1958): Trilafon in the treatment of chronically psychotic hospitalized patients. *Am. J. Psychiatry*, 115:452–454.

30. Cooper, J. R., Bloom, F. E., and Roth, R. H. (1974): *The Biochemical Basis of Neuropharmacology*, 2nd ed. Oxford Univ. Press, New York.

31. Cornu, F., and Hoffet, H. (1961): Clinical experience with Tarcatan. *Dis. Nerv. Syst.*, 22:40–44.

32. Cuatico, W., Roizin, L., Sabbia, R., Horwitz, W. A., and Wodraskia, G. (1965): S^{35} prochlorperazine autoradiography of the central nervous system. *Int. J. Neuropsychiatry*, 1:364–370.

33. Curry, S. H., Marshall, J. H. L., Davis, J. S., and Jankowsky, D. J. (1970): Chlorpromazine plasma levels and effects. *Arch. Gen. Psychiatry*, 22:289–296.

34. Darling, H. F. (1959): Fluphenazine: A preliminary study. *Dis. Nerv. Syst.*, 20:167–170.

35. Darling, H. F. (1961): Acetophenazine (Tindal) and thiopropazate (Dartal) in ambulatory psychoneurotic patients. *Am. J. Psychiatry*, 118:358–359.

36. David, H. (1957): Experimentelle Leberveränderungen nach kurzfristiger und chronischer Gabe von Chlorpromazin. *Z. Ges. Exp. Med.*, 128:471–481.

37. Deberdt, R. (1961): Experiences avec la thioridazine (TP 21). *Acta Neurol. Psychiatr. Belg.*, 61:652–657.

38. Denber, H. C. B., and Bird, E. G. (1957): Chlorpromazine in the treatment of mental illness. IV. Final results with analysis of data of 1,523 patients. *Am. J. Psychiatry*, 113:972–978.

39. Denber, H. C. B. (1958): Some preliminary results with a new phenothiazine derivate: Prochlorperazine. *Psychiatr. Res. Rep.*, 9:16–22.

40. De Robertis, E. (1973): The isolation and molecular properties of the receptor proteolipids. In: *Drug Receptor: A Symposium*, edited by H. P. Rang, p. 257. Univ. Park Press, Baltimore.

41. Devore, J. K., Daugherty, C., and Schneider, E. M. (1956): The effect of chlorpromazine on hepatic function and morphology. *Gastroenterology*, 31:391–398.

42. Diab, I. M., Dinerstein, R. J., Watanabe, M., and Roth, L. J. (1976): (3H) Morphine localization in myenteric plexus. *Science*, 193:689–691.

43. Dickes, R., Schenker, V., and Deutsch, L. (1957): Serial liver function and blood studies in patients receiving chlorpromazine. *N. Engl. J. Med.*, 256:1–7.

44. Divry, P., Bobon, J., and Collard, J. (1960): Rapport sur l'activite neuropsychopharmacologique du Halopéridol (R 1625). *Acta Neurol. Belg.*, 60:7–19.

45. Dollery, C. T. (1976): Drug interactions. *Rassegna Med.*, 53:76–81.

46. Doughty, R. B. (1955): The incidence of jaundice associated with chlorpromazine therapy. In: *Chlorpromazine and Mental Health*, p. 195. Lea & Febiger, Philadelphia.

47. Doussinet, P., D'Alteroche, R., and Soucachet, P. (1956): Douze observations d'accidents comitiaus avec localisations e'lectriques temporales survenus chez des malades mentaux en traitement á la chlorpromazine. *Sem. Hôp. Paris*, 32:3334.

48. D'Silva, J. L. (1934): The action of adrenaline on serum potassium. *J. Physiol. (Lond.)*, 82:393–398.

49. D'Silva, J. L. (1937): Action of adrenaline on serum potassium. *J. Physiol. (Lond.)*, 90:303–309.

50. Ecles, J. C. (1964): *The Physiology of Synapses*. Academic Press, New York.

51. Ehrenpreis, S., and Teller, D. N. (1972): Interaction of drugs of dependence with receptors. In: *Chemical and Biological Aspects of Drug Dependence*, edited by S. J. Mulé and H. Brill, p. 177. CRC Press, Cleveland.

52. Elliot, R. N., Schrut, A. W., and Marra, J. (1956): Fatal acute aseptic necrosis of the liver associated with chlorpromazine. *Am. J. Psychiatry*, 112:940.

53. Ellis, S. (1967): The effects of sympathomimetic amines and adrenergic blocking agents on metabolism. In: *Physiological Pharmacology*, Vol. 4, edited by W. S. Root, and F. G. Hofman, p. 179. Academic Press, London.

54. Engel, G. L. (1954): Selection of clinical material in psychosomatic medicine: The need for a new physiology. *Psychosom. Med.*, 16:368–373.

55. Enna, S. J., Bennett, J. P., Jr., Bylund, D. B., Cneese, I., Burt, L. R., Charness, M. E., Yamamura, H. T., Simantov, R., and Snyder, S. H. (1977): Neurotransmitter receptor binding: Regional distribution in human brain. *J. Neurochem.*, 28(1):233–236.

56. Enss, H., Hartmann, K., Hippius, H., and Richter, H. E. (1958): Klinische Erfahrungen mit einem neuen Piperazine-Derivat des Phenothiazins in der Neuro-Psychiatrie. *Arch. Psychiatr. Z. Neurol.*, 197:534–550.

57. Farber, I. J. (1957): Drug fatalities. *Am. J. Psychiatry*, 114:371–372.

58. Feldman, P. E., and Statman, J. (1957): Agranulocytosis during treatment with methylpromazine. *Am. J. Psychiatry*, 114:464–465.

59. Finke, H. (1956): Beitrag zur Reserpin-Therapie in der Psychiatrie. *Munch. Med. Wochenschr.*, 98:872–874.

60. Fischer, A., and Gottreich, N. S. (1960): Anemia as a complication of prochlorperazine therapy. *Am. J. Psychiatry*, 116:932–933.

61. Fischman, H. K., Moorthy, A. S., Roizin, L., Rainer, J. D., and Moralishvili, E. (1976): Effects of prolonged administration of "street heroin" on lymphocyte chromosomes of Macaca Mulatta (Rhesus) monkeys. In: *Neurotoxicology.*, edited by L. Roizin, H. Shiraki, and N. Grcevic. (*This volume.*)

62. Flegel, H. (1960): Klinische Erfahrungen mit Nitoman, einem neuartigen Psychopharmakon. *Nervenarzt*, 31:556–557.

63. Flegel, H., Rasper, A., and Lauber, H. (1960): Klinisch therapeutische Studie über Haloperidol (Fluoro-Piperidino-Butyrophenon). *Nervenarzt*, 31:133–136.

64. Flegel, H., Harling, H. O., and Wödl, H. (1961): Truxal in psychiatrischen Krankenhaus und ambulanter Nachbehandlung. *Psychiatr. Neurol. (Basel)*, 142:176–187.

65. Flor-Henry, P. (1969): Schizophrenic-like reactions and affective psychosis associated with temporal lobe epilepsy. *Am. J. Psychiatry*, 1263:148–152.

66. Forrer, G. R. (1951): Atropine toxicity in the treatment of mental disease. *Am. J. Psychiatry*, 108:107–112.

67. Forrest, F. M., Forrest, I. S., and Roizin, L. (1963): Clinical, biochemical and postmortem studies on a patient treated with chlorpromazine. *Agréssologie*, 4:259–265.

67a. Gallagher, C. H., Koch, J. H., and Mann, D. M. (1965): The effect of phenothiazine on the metabolism of liver mitochondria. *Biochem. Pharmacol.*, 14:789–797.

68. Gambescia, J. M., Imbriglia, J., Galamaga, P., and Winkelman, W. (1956): Jaundice associated with the administration of chlorpromazine. *Gastroenterology*, 30:735–751.

69. Garmany, G., May, A. R., and Folkson, A. (1954): The use and action of chlorpromazine in psychoneuroses. *Br. Med. J.*, 2:439–441.

70. Gaulhofer, W. K., and van der Helm, H., Jr. (1961): Icterus veroorzaakt door chlorpromazine. *Ned. Tijdschr. Geneeskd.*, 105:477–481.

71. Goldfield, A., Roizin, L., Hashimoto, S., and Liu, J. C. (1977): Liver pathology: Drugs of abuse and narcotic addiction. In: *Neurotoxicology*, edited by L. Roizin, H. Shiraki, and N. Grčević. (*This volume.*)

72. Green, D. E., and Fleischer, S. (1962): On the molecular organization of biological transducing system. In: *Horizons of Biochemistry*, edited by M. Kasha, and B. Pullman, p. 381. Academic Press, New York.

73. Green, D. E., and Goldberger, R. F. (1967): *Molecular Insights into the Living Process*, p. 222. Academic Press, New York.

74. Gross, H., Kaupeny, F., Plavec, J., and Steininger, E. (1960): Thioridazin (Melleril), ein neues Neuroleptikum für die klinische und die ambulante Psychiatrie. *Wien. Med. Wochenschr.*, 110:844–850.

75. Gross, H., and Kaltenbäck, E. (1961): Tarcatan (Chlorprothixene) as a neuroleptic drug in clinical psychiatry. *Dis. Nerv. Syst.*, 22:502–509.

76. Haase, H. J., and Janssen, P. A. J. (1965): The Action of Neuroleptic Drugs. A psychiatric and and pharmacological investigation. *Chicago, Year Book Med., Publ.*, pp. 5–174.

77. Haeger, K. H. M., and Ryd, H. (1956): Potenzierende Pharmaka vor Allgemeinnarkose in der Brut-und Bauchchirurgie. *Chirurg*, 27:33–37.

78. Hartnett, B. S. (1955): Liver damage and eosinophilia following chlorpromazine therapy. Report of a case. *Br. Med. J.*, 1:1458–1459.

79. Haworth, K., Jones, L. M., and Mandel, W. (1961): Clinical experience with a new phenothiazine (Piperacetazine). *Am. J. Psychiatry*, 117:749–750.

80. Haylett, D. G., and Jenkinson, D. H. (1973): Action of the catecholamines on the membrane properties of the liver cells. In: *Drug Receptors: A Symposium*, edited by H. P. Rang, p. 15. Univ. Park Press, Baltimore.

81. Heinrich, K., and Richert, J. (1960): Chlorperphenazin in der psychiatrischen und neurologischen Therapie. *Nervenarzt*, 31:128–133.

82. Hippius, H. (1966): Psychiatric side effects of psychotropic drugs. In: *Psychosomatic Medicine: Proc. 1st Int. Congr. Acad. Psychosom.*

Med., edited by E. Dunlop, and M. N. Weisman, pp. 133–136. Excerpta Medica Foundation, Amsterdam.

83. Hippius, H., and Kanig, K. (1958): Agranulozytose unter neuropsychiatrischer Phenothiazin-Therapie. *Ärztl. Wochenschr.,* 13:501–507.

84. Hoch, P. H., Cattell, J. P., Malitz, S., and Lesse, S. (1955): Investigations on chlorpromazine in psychiatric practice. *J. Nerv. Ment. Dis.,* 121:184–185.

85. Hoch, P. H., Pennes, H. H., and Cattell, J. P. (1953): Psychosis produced by administration of drugs. In: *Metabolic and Toxic Diseases of the Nervous System,* edited by H. H. Merritt, and C. C. Hare. *Proc. Assoc. Res. Nerv. Ment. Dis.,* 32:287.

86. Hodges, H. H., and LaZerte, G. D. (1955): Jaundice and agranulocytosis with fatality following chlorpromazine therapy. *JAMA,* 158:114–116.

87. Hofmann, G., and Kryspin-Exner, K. (1960): Klinische Erfahrungen mit einem neuen Neuroleptikum (TP 21, Melleril). *Wien. Med. Wochenschr.,* 110:897–901.

88. Holman, W. T. (1958): High dosage Compazine in chronic schizophrenia. *Dis. Nerv. Syst.,* 19:309–310.

89. Hooper, J. H., Jr., Welch, V. C., and Shackelford, R. T. (1961): Abnormal lactation associated with tranquilizing drug therapy. *JAMA,* 178:506–507.

90. Hormia, M., Hormia, A., and Hakola, P. (1957): Effect of chlorpromazine and reserpine on liver parenchyme in the white rat. *Ann. Med. Exp. Biol. Fenn. Helsinki.,* 35:316–323.

91. Isaaks, B., McArthur, J. G., and Taylor, R. M. (1955): Jaundice in relation to chlorpromazine therapy. *Br. Med. J.,* II:1122–1124.

92. Iversen, L. L. (1971): Role of transmitters uptake mechanisms in synaptic neurotransmission. *Br. J. Pharmacol.,* 41:571.

93. Jacoby, M. G. (1958): High dosage chlorpromazine therapy after previous agranulocytosis. *Am. J. Psychiatry,* 114:1040.

94. Jellinger, K. (1977): Morphological effects of neuroleptic long-term therapy on human brain. In: *Neurotoxicology,* edited by L. Roizin, H. Shiraki, and N. Grčević. (*This volume.*)

95. Kalter, H. (1972): Teratogenicity, embryolethality and mutagenicity of drug of dependence. In: *Chemical and Biological Aspects of Drug Dependence,* edited by S. J. Mulé and H. Brill, p. 413. CRC Press, Cleveland.

96. Kato, T. K., Jarvik, L. R., Roizin, L., and Morashivili, E. (1970): Chromosome studies in pregnant Rhesus Macaque given LSD-25. *J. Nerv. Ment. Dis.,* 31:245–250.

97. Kaufman, M. A. (1977): Alternate diagnoses of tardive dyskinesia: Neuropathological findings in three suspected cases. In: *Neurotoxicology,* edited by L. Roizin, H. Shiraki, and N. Grčević. (*This volume.*)

98. Kelsey, J. R., Moyer, J. H., Brown, W. G., and Bennett, H. D. (1955): Chlorpromazine jaundice. *Gastroenterology,* 29:865–876.

99. Kemp, J. A. (1957): Jaundice occurring during administration of promazine. *Gastroenterology,* 32:937–938.

100. Keup, W. (editor) (1972): *Drug Abuse.* Charles C Thomas, Springfield, Ill.

101. Kinross-Wright, V. (1955): Complications of chlorpromazine treatment. *Dis. Nerv. Syst.,* 16:114–119.

102. Kinross-Wright, V., and Moyer, J. H. (1956): Chlorpromazine and hepatic function. *Arch. Neurol. Psychiatry (Chic.),* 76:675–680.

103. Kohn, N., and Myerson, R. M. (1961): Cholestatic hepatitis associated with trifluoperazine. *N. Engl. J. Med.,* 264:549–550.

104. Kokko, A., Mautner, H. G., and Barrnett, R. J. (1969): Fine structural localization of acetylocholinesterase use acetylmethylthiocholine and acetylselenocholine as substrates. *J. Histochem. Cytochem.,* 17:625–640.

105. Kruse, W. (1957): "Paradoxical" effect of chlorpromazine in a case of periodic catatonia. *Am. J. Psychiatry,* 114:463–464.

106. Labhardt, F. (1955): Einige allgemeine und psychiatrische Gesichtspunkte zur Behandlung mit neuroplegischen Medikamenten. *Dermatologica,* III:177.

107. Lang, A. W., and Moore, R. A. (1961): Acute toxic psychosis concurrent with phenothiazine therapy. *Am. J. Psychiatry,* 117:939–940.

108. Lapolla, A. (1961): Fluphenazine in the treatment of hospitalized psychotic females. *West Med.,* 2:110–116.

109. Lehninger, A. L. (1965): *Bioenergetics: The Molecular Basis of Biological Energy Transformations.* Benjamin, New York.

110. Loftus, R., Huizenga, K. A., Stauffer, M. H., Rome, H. P., and Cain, J. C. (1955): Jaundice caused by chlorpromazine (Thorazine). *JAMA,* 157:1286–1288.

111. Logothetis, J. (1967): Epileptic seizures in the course of phenothiazine therapy. *Neurology (Minneap.),* 17:869–875.

112. Lomas, J., Boardman, R. H., and Markowe, M. (1955): Complications of chlorpromazine therapy in 800 mental-hospital patients. *Lancet,* 24:1144–1147.

113. MacDonald, G. E. (1956): Chlorpromazine (Thorazine) hepatitis; report of three cases. *N.Y. State J. Med.,* 56:3004–3006.

114. Mahrer, P. R., Bergman, P. S., and Estren, S. (1958): Atropine-like poisoning due to tranquilizing agents. *Am. J. Psychiatry,* 115:337–339.

115a. Maier, C., and Rüttner, J. R. (1955): Toxische Hepatose unter dem Bild des intrahepatischen Verschluβikterus nach Chlorpromazin, Atophan, Salvarsan und Methyltestosteron-Medikation. *Schweiz. Med. Wochenschr.,* 85:445–448.

115b. Martland, H. S., and Martland, H., Jr. (1950): Placental barrier carbon monoxide, barbiturate, and radium poisoning. *Am. J. Surg.,* 50:270–279.

116. Mathov, E. (1961): Complicaciones indeseables de las psicodrogas. Algunas experiencias personales. *Acta Neuropsiqu. Arg.*, 7:144–145.

117. May, R. H. (1959): Catatonic-like states following phenothiazine therapy. *Am. J. Psychiatry*, 115:1119–1120.

118. May, R. H., Selymes, P., Weekley, R. D., and Potts, A. M. (1960): Thioridazine therapy: Results and complications. *J. Nerv. Ment. Dis.*, 130:230–234.

119. McLean, D. D., Martin, H. R., Ellingson, R. J., and Smith, J. A. (1958): Seizures during therapy with phenothiazine derivates. *Am. J. Psychiatry*, 114:934.

120. Meyer, L. (1968): Drug induced disease. In: *Drug Induced Disease*, edited by L. Meyer and H. M. Peac, p. 7. Excerpta Medica Foundation, Amsterdam.

121. Nijdam, S. J. (1960): Die therapeutische Wirkung der Neuroleptika allein und in Kombination mit anderen Therapien. *Wien. Med. Wochenschr.*, 110:722–725.

122. Nishikawa, K., and Roizin, L. (1966): The fine structures of synapses of the CNS and their content following administration of phenothiazines. In: *Proc. 6th Int. Cong. Electron Microscopists*, edited by R. Uyeda, pp. 441–442. Moruzen Co., Ltd., Kyoto, Japan.

123. Olivier, H. R., and Sugar, M. (1961): Complications in Trilafon therapy. *Dis. Nerv. Syst.*, 22:32–34.

124. Ollendorf, R. H. V. (1960): High dosage chlorpromazine therapy in acute and chronic schizophrenia. *Am. J. Psychiatry*, 116:729–736.

125. Paganini, A. E., and Zlotow, M. (1958): Two year follow-up study of the relationship of chlorpromazine and the incidence of convulsions in fifty post-lobotomy patients. *Am. J. Psychiatry*, 114:839–840.

126. Paganini, A. E., and Zlotow, M. (1959): Hairy tongue in patients receiving phenothiazines: Preliminary report. *Am. J. Psychiatry*, 116:362–363.

127. Pappas, G. D., and Purpura, D. P. (editors) (1972): *Structure and Function of Synapses.* Raven Press, New York.

128. Pappas, G. D., and Waxman, S. G. (1972): Synaptic fine structure-morphological correlates of the chemical and electronic transmission. In: *Structure and Function of Synapses*, edited by G. D. Pappas, and D. P. Purpura, p. 1. Raven Press, New York.

129. Pellerat, J., and Rives, H. (1961): Frequence des accidents cutanes induits par les neuroleptiques chez les malades mentaux. *Revue Lyonnaise de Medicine*, 10:598.

130. Pert, C. B., and Snyder, S. H. (1973): Opiate receptor: Demonstration in nervous tissue. *Science*, 179:1011–1014.

131. Petersen, M. C., Carey, B., and Rhoads, D. V. (1958): Blood discrasias due to phenothiazine derivates: Report of four cases. *Am. J. Psychiatry*, 115:257.

132. Radouco-Thomas, C. (1971): Introduction. In: *Advances in Cytopharmacology: 1st Int. Symp. Cell Biol. & Cytopharmacol.*, edited by F. Clementi, and B. Ceccarelli, pp. XI–XVII. Raven Press, New York.

133. Rang, H. P. (editor) (1973): *Drug Receptors.* Univ. Park Press, Baltimore.

134. Ravn, J. (1960): Truxal, ein neuartiges Psychopharmacon. *Wien. Klin. Wochenschr.*, 72:192–196.

135. Read, A. E., Harrison, C. V., and Sherlock, S. (1961): Chronic chlorpromazine jaundice, with particular reference to its relationship to primary biliary cirrhosis. *Am. J. Med.*, 31:249–258.

136. Reinert, R. E. (1959): EEG changes with promazine. *Am. J. Psychiatry*, 115:742–743.

137. Reinert, R. E., and Hermann, C. G. (1960): Unexplained death during chlorpromazine therapy. *J. Nerv. Ment. Dis.*, 131:435–442.

138. Reinhart, M. J., Silverstein, B. S., and Cross, T. N. (1957): A case of agranulocytosis following "Sparine" administration. *Am. J. Psychiatry*, 114:462–463.

139. Roizin, L. (1948): Histometabolic changes and neuropathologic selectivity in the light of recent investigations (histometabolic dysergia). *J. Neuropathol. Exp. Neurol.*, 7:216–233.

140a. Roizin, L. (1960): Review of ultracellular structures and their functions with special reference to pathogenic mechanisms at a molecular level. *J. Neuropathol. Exp. Neurol.*, 19:591–621.

140b. Roizin, L. (1971): Evolution of fundamental CNS pathogenic concepts. In: *The World Biennial of Psychiatry and Psychotherapy*, edited by S. Arieti, pp. 560–602. Basic Books, New York.

141a. Roizin, L. (1971): Introduction to metabolic disorders. In: *Textbook of Neuropathology*, Vol. 2, edited by J. Minckler et al., pp. 1267–1273. McGraw-Hill, New York.

141b. Roizin, L. (1975): Neuropathologic aspects of adverse and toxic reactions of neuropsychotropic agents. In: *Int. Encyclopedia of Neurology, Psychiatry, Psychoanalysis and Psychology*, edited by B. B. Wolman. Aesculapius Publ., New York. (*In press.*)

142a. Roizin, L., Akai, K., Alexander, G., Machiz, S., and Liu, J. C. (1971): Phenothiazine pathogenic mechanisms in rat with liver dysfunctions. *Fed. Proc.*, 30:574.

142b. Roizin, L., Akai, K., Lawler, C., and Liu, J. C. (1970): Lithium neurotoxicologic effects—acute phase (preliminary observations). *Dis. Nerv. Syst. (GWAN Suppl.)*, 31:38–44.

143. Roizin, L., Baden, M., Kaufman, M. A., Willson, N., Alexander, G., Hashimoto, S., Liu, J. C., and Eisenberg-Gelber, B. (1975): *Neuropathology of Drug-Narcotism Syndrome: Pathogenic Considerations*, pp. 343–348. Excerpta Medica, Amsterdam.

144. Roizin, L., Eros, G., Gold, G., Weinberg, F., English, W. H., and Wodraska, T. (1959): Histopathologic findings in the liver and CNS

following administration of tranquilizing drugs. *Dis. Nerv. Syst.,* 20:176–179.

145. Roizin, L., Gold, G., Alexander, G., Miles, B., Kaufman, M. A., Lawler, C., and Akai, K. (1972): Prenatal effects of hallucinogens. In: *Drug Abuse: Current Concepts and Research,* edited by W. Keup, p. 123. Charles C Thomas, Springfield, Ill.

146. Roizin, L., Gold, G., Kaufman, M. A., Fieve, R., Alexander, G., and Ueno, Y. (1968): Experimental potentiation of phenothiazine toxicology. 1. Effects of liver disorders. 2. Int. Symp. Action Mechanisms and Metabolism of Psychoactive Drugs. *Agréssologie,* 9:379–381.

147. Roizin, L., Hashimoto, S., Liu, J. C., Tom, K. J., and Eisenberg, B. (1971): Methadone effects upon the central nervous system, TPP, AcP, and G-6-P. *J. Histochem. Cytochem.,* 19:720–721.

148a. Roizin, L., Hashimoto, S., Liu, J. C., and Tom, K. J. (1973): Methadone neurotoxicity. III. Electron microscope investigations. *J. Neuropathol. Exp. Neurol.,* 32:180.

148b. Roizin, L., Baden, M., Hashimoto, S., and Liu, J. C. (1973): Ultrastructural changes of the liver in the Narcotism-Drug Syndrome. *Fed. Proc.,* 32:1837A.

149. Roizin, L., Hashimoto, S., Tom, K. J., and Liu, J. C. (1974): Methadone effect upon hypothalamic neuronal organelles. *J. Neuropathol. Exp. Neurol.,* 33:176–177.

150. Roizin, L., Helpern, M., Baden, M., Kaufman, M. A., Hashimoto, S., Liu, J. C., and Eisenberg, B. (1972): Neuropathology of drug dependence. In: *Chemical and Biological Aspects of Drug Dependence,* edited by S. J. Mulé, and H. Brill, p. 389. CRC Press, Cleveland.

151. Roizin, L., Helpern, M., Baden, M., Kaufman, M. A., Hashimoto, S., Liu, J. C., and Eisenberg, B. (1972): Methadone fatalities in heroin addicts. *Psychiatr. Q.,* 46:393–410.

152. Roizin, L., Helpern, M., Baden, M., Kaufman, M. A., and Akai, K. (1972): Toxosynpathes (a multifactor pathogenic concept). In: *Drug Abuse: Current Concepts and Research,* edited by W. Keup, p. 97. Charles C Thomas, Springfield, Ill.

153. Roizin, L., Iyengar, V. K. S., DiVirgilio, G., and Robinson, E. (1965): Cytochemical patterns of ATP-ase (mitochondrial) in the CNS. 2. Diversified neuronal reaction in normal rats and after prochlorperazine administration. *Fed. Proc.,* 24:493.

154. Roizin, L., Iyengar, V. K. S., DiVirgilio, G., Wodraska, G., and Liu, J. C. (1965): Effects of prochlorperazine on the rat CNS succinic dehydrogenase and diphosphopyridine nucleotide diaphorase (lactive linked). *J. Cell Biol.,* 27:88A–89A (Abstr.)

155. Roizin, L., Iyengar, V. K. S., Marquez-Alba, E., and Yahr, M. D. (1965): Correlated neuropathologic and cytoenzymatic studies following atropine administration. *Trans. Am. Neurol. Assoc.,* 90:281–282.

156. Roizin, L., Kaufman, M. A., Bollard, B., Sabbia, R., and Horwitz, W. A. (1962): Clinical and tissue studies of prochlorperazine in rats and monkeys. Int. Cong. Action Mechanisms and Metabolism of Psychoactive Drug Derived from Phenothiazine Structurally Related Compounds. *Psychopharm. Serv. Cont. Bull.,* 2:81–83.

157. Roizin, L., Kaufman, M. A., and Casselman, B. (1961): Structural changes induced by neuroleptics. Extrapyramidal system and neuroleptic. *Rev. Can. Biol.,* 20:221–229.

158. Roizin, L., Kaufman, M. A., Gold, G., Iyengar, V. K. S., Liu, J. C., and Keosian, S. (1966): A multidisciplinary investigation of the phenothiazines. *Mental Hygiene,* 50:574–579.

159. Roizin, L., Kaufman, M. A., and Miles, N. (1960): Short-term experiments with chlorpromazine in rats. 1. Histologic studies. *Fed. Proc.,* 19:391 (Abstr.)

160. Roizin, L., Kaufman, M. A., and Rugh, R. (1966): Irradiation effects upon the fetal central nervous system of Macacus rhesus monkeys. Effects on lysosomes. *Acta Radiol.,* 5:161–176.

161. Roizin, L., Hashimoto, S., Liu, J. C., Tom, K. J., and Eisenberg, B. (1971): Methadone effects upon CNS, AcP, TPP and G-6-P. *J. Histochem. Cytochem.,* 19:720–721.

162. Roizin, L., Lazar, M., and Gold, G. (1966): Prenatal effects of phenothiazines. *Fed. Proc.,* 25:353.

163. Roizin, L., and Liu, J. C. (1976): Ultrastructural investigation of the hypothalamus in heroin chronically addicted monkeys. In: *Neurotoxicology,* edited by L. Roizin, H. Shiraki, and N. Grčević. (*This volume.*)

164. Roizin, L., and Nishikawa, K. (1965): The Golgi complex of the CNS. Anatomo-topographic studies following administration of prochlorperazine (compazine, S.K.F.). *J. Neuropathol. Exp. Neurol.,* 24:165–166.

165. Roizin, L., Rugh, R., and Kaufman, M. A. (1962): Neuropathologic investigations of the x-irradiation embryo rat brain. (I. Effects of 150 r. at 9.5 and 8.5 g.d.) *J. Neuropathol. Exp. Neurol.,* 21:219–243.

166. Roizin, L., Schneider, J., Willson, N., Liu, J. C., and Mullen, C. (1974): Effects of prolonged LSD-25 administration upon neurons of cord ganglia tissue cultures. *J. Neuropathol. Exp. Neurol.,* 33:212–225.

167. Roizin, L., True, C., and Knight, M. (1959): Structural effects of tranquilizers. The effect of pharmacologic agents. *Proc. Assoc. Res. Nerv. Ment. Dis.,* 37:285–324.

168. Roizin, L., Wechsler-Berger, M., and Brock, D. (1964): Ultracellular functional and pathogenic mechanisms. V. In vivo and vitro CNS and liver mitochondria following administration of phenothiazines. *Trans. Am. Neurol. Assoc.,* 89:247–248.

169. Rowntree, D. W., Nevin, S., and Wilson, A. (1950): The effects of DFP in schizophrenia and manic depressive patients. *J. Neurol. Neurosurg. Psychiatry,* 13:47–52.

170. Salomon, M. I., King, E. J., and Gallo, G. (1971): Renal functional damage during the course of lithium therapy: A case report with renal biopsy findings. *Dis. Nerv. Syst.,* 32: 483–485.

171. Schleiden, M. J. (1838): ·Beiträge zür Phytogenesis. *Arch. f. Anat. Physiol. u. Wissensch. Med.,* 4:137–176.

172. Schwann, T. (1847): Microscopical Researches into the Accordance in the Structure and Growth of Animals and Plants. (Translated from the German by H. Smith.) C. and J. Alard, Printers, London, 1947, p. 186.

173. Selye, H., and Fortier, C. (1950): Adaptive reactions to stress. In: *Life Stress and Body Disease,* edited by H. G. Wolff, S. G. Wolff, and C. C. Hare. Williams & Wilkins, Baltimore. *Proc. Ass. Res. Nerv. Ment. Dis.,* 29:3.

174. Serpe, S. J., and Norins, A. L. (1961): Allergic purpura after administration of trifluoperazine. *N.Y. State J. Med.,* 61:3517–3518.

175. Shanon, J. (1959): Neuromuscular symptoms simulating conversion hysteria caused by perphenazine (Trilafon). *Dis. Nerv. Syst.,* 20:24–26.

176. Shawver, J. R., and Tarnowski, S. M. (1960): Thrombocytopenia in prolonged chlorpromazine therapy. *Am. J. Psychiatry,* 116:845–846.

177. Shay, H., and Siplet, H. (1957): Study of chlorpromazine jaundice, its mechanism and prevention. *Gastroenterology,* 32:571–591.

178. Shiraki, H. (1977): Morphological background (grumous degeneration of cerebellar nucleus) for tardive dyskinesia induced by antipsychotic drugs in schizophrenia. In: *Neurotoxicology,* edited by L. Roizin, H. Shiraki, and N. Grčević. (*This volume.*)

179. Simpson, G. M., Varga, E., and Haher, J. (1976): Psychotic exacerbations produced by neuroleptics. *Dis. Nerv. Syst.,* 37:367–369.

180. Sims, J. L., Bremer, E. M., and Huston, E. S. (1955): Chlorpromazine: Changes in hepatic histology in the absence of jaundice. *J. Lab. Clin. Med.,* 46:952.

181. Sloane, R. B., and Haden, P. (1961): Use of thioridazine (Mellaril) in psychological disorders. *Dis. Nerv. Syst.,* 22:330–334.

182. Smith, Ch. E., Harris, J. R., and Garrett, A. L. (1959): Chlorpromazine in the treatment of the chronic mental patient in a prison hospital. *Dis. Nerv. Syst.,* 20:134–137.

183. Snell, G. D., Dausset, J., and Nathenson, G. (1976): *Histocompatibility,* p. 446. Academic Press, New York.

184. Snyder, S. H. (1975): Opiate receptor in normal and drug altered brain function. *Nature,* 257: 185–189.

185. Snyder, S. H., and Simantov, R. (1977): The opiate receptor and opioid peptides. *J. Neurochem.,* 28:13–20.

186. Stanley, W. J. (1959): Prolonged hypotension due to chlorpromazine. *Am. J. Psychiatry,* 115: 1124–1126.

187. Stevanovic, D. V. (1961): Photosensitivity due to certain drugs. *Br. J. Dermatol.,* 73:233–237.

188. Strassmann, G. (1954): Pathologic findings in poisoning. In: *Legal Medicine,* edited by R. B. H. Gradwhol, p. 285. Mosby, St. Louis.

189. Sussman, R. M., and Sumner, P. (1955): Jaundice following the administration of 50 mg of chlorpromazine. *N. Engl. J. Med.,* 253:499–502.

190. Swain, J. M., and Litteral, E. B. (1960): Prolonged effect of chlorpromazine EEG findings in a senile group. *J. Nerv. Ment. Dis.,* 131: 550–553.

191. Tseng, Len, H. (1971): Interstitial myocarditis probably related to lithium carbonate intoxication. *Arch. Pathol.,* 92:444–448.

192. Tuteur, W., Stiller, R., and Glotzer, J. (1959): The discharged mental hospital chlorpromazine patient. *Dis. Nerv. Syst.,* 20:512–517.

193. Vallat, J.-N., and Lepetit (1954): Intoxication par la chlorpromazine (Largactil) au cours d'une tentative de suicide. *Presse Méd.,* 62:752.

194. Varga, E., Haher, E. J., and Simpson, G. M. (1974): Neuroleptic induced Kluver-Bucy syndrome. *Biol. Psychiatry,* 101:65–68.

195. Virchow, R. (1858): *The Cellular Pathology.* Hirschwald, Berlin.

196. Virchow, R. (1962): The place of pathology among biological sciences. In: *Disease, Life and Man,* translated with an introduction by L. J. Rather, pp. 165–183. Collier Book, New York.

197. Waelsch, H. (1964): Biochemical mechanisms of drug action. *Neuropsychopharmacology,* Vol. 3, edited by P. B. Bradley, F. Flügel, and P. Hoch, pp. 189–193. Elsevier, New York.

198. Waldrop, F. N., Robertson, R. H., and Vourlekis, A. (1961): A comparison of the therapeutic and toxic effects of thioridazine and chlorpromazine in chronic schizophrenic patients. *Compr. Psychiatry,* 2:96–105.

199. Wechsler-Berger, M., and Roizin, L. (1960): Tissue levels of chlorpromazine in experimental animals. *J. Ment. Sci.,* 106:1501–1505.

200. Weingärtner, L. (1961): Unerwünschte Arzneimittelwirkungen. *Mschr. Kinderheilk.,* 109: 517–526.

201. Weiss, P. (1961): From cell to molecule. In: *The Molecular Control of Cellular Activity,* edited by J. N. Allen, p. 1. McGraw Hill, New York.

202. Whitfield, A. G. W. (1959): Chlorpromazine jaundice. *Br. Med. J.,* 1:784–785.

203. Williams, P. (1972): An unusual response to chlorpromazine therapy. *Br. J. Psychiatry,* 10: 439–440.

204. Willson, N., Roizin, L., and Schneider, J. (1976): Effects of LSD on membranous organelles in cultured neurons. In: *Neurotoxicology,* edited by L. Roizin, H. Shiraki, and N. Grčević. (*This volume.*)

205. Wilson, J. G. (1965): Teratogenic interaction of chemical agents in the rat. *J. Pharm. Exp. Ther.,* 148:429–436.

206. Witton, K. (1961): Orthostatic hypotension

secondary to psychotropic drugs. Treatment with emphasis on parenteral ritalin. *Dis. Nerv. Syst.*, 22:189–192.

207. Wolff, H. G., Wolf, S. G., and Hare, C. C. (editors) (1950): *Life Stress and Bodily Disease*. Williams & Wilkins, Baltimore.

208. Zarowitz, H., and Friedman, I. S. (1957): Jaundice following small amounts of chlorpromazine. *N.Y. State J. Med.*, 57:1922–1924.

209. Zatuchni, J., and Miller, G. (1954): Jaundice during chlorpromazine therapy. *N. Engl. J. Med.*, 251:1003–1006.

210. Zlotlow, M., and Paganini, A. E. (1958): Fatalities in patients receiving chlorpromazine and reserpine during 1956–1957 at Pilgrim State Hospital. *Am. J. Psychiatry,* 115:154–156.

SUBJECT INDEX

Subject Index

Absorption, gastrointestinal, factors affecting, 512

Acetylcholine
brain levels after 6-hydroxydopamine, 15
release affected by opiates, 64

Acetylcholinesterase, activity affected by parathion, 457–467

Acriflavin, inhibiting RNA synthesis, 399–401

Acrylamide, neuropathies from, 427–430

Actinomycin D
inhibiting RNA synthesis, 391–393
mode of action of, 396–399
nuclear changes from, 394–396

Addiction to heroin, and methadone maintenance, 71–79

Additives in foods, hepatic effects of, 513

Adenyl cyclase
inhibition by lithium, 178–179
prostaglandins affecting, 65

Aging
and effects of drugs, 639
and Minamata disease, 241

Akathisia, from tranquilizers, 2–3, 5

Akinesia, from tranquilizers, 3

Alcohol
abuse with polydrug problems, 75–76
interactions with drugs, 503–508, 629
and malnutrition with peripheral neuropathy, 529–545
sural nerve biopsies in, 539–545
vitamin B assays in, 531–539
withdrawal syndromes, 504, 505, 508, 517–526
and delirium tremens genesis, 517–519
respiratory alkalosis in, 521–524
magnesium levels in, 519–521

Alkalosis, respiratory, in alcohol withdrawal, 521–524

Alkylmercury intoxication, see Minamata disease

Aluminum neurotoxicity, 313–314

Alzheimer's disease
aluminum role in, 313
from lead exposure, 293

Amines, tertiary, and choroid plexus lesions, 419–424

Amino acid uptake by brain, disorders in, 580

γ-Aminobutyric acid, and responses to opiates, 64–65

Amitriptyline, long-term use of, cortical atrophy from, 149–155

Ammon's horn, in subacute myeloopticoneuropathy, 337–341

Amphetamines
detection in urine, 93–101
interaction with alcohol, 503
interaction with brain catecholamines, 19, 20

Amyloid bodies in brain
in heroin-addicted monkeys, 118, 128
in paraquat poisoning, 471, 473, 476, 482

Analgesic drugs, narcotic, see Narcotics

Anesthesia, and chronic exposure to low levels of halothane, 137–144

Anorexic agents, and chlorphentermine neuropathy, 485–500

Anthracycline antibiotics, inhibiting RNA synthesis, 399–401

Anticoagulants, and ethyl biscoumacetate interaction with methylphenidate, 147

Antidepressants
lithium toxicity, 171–200. See also Lithium.
long-term use of, cortical atrophy from, 149–155
methylphenidate interactions with other drugs, 147–148
neuronal inclusions from nortriptyline, 163–170
pharmacokinetics of, 157–160

Antimicrobials
actinomycin neurotoxicity, 391–401
choroid plexus lesions from piperazine derivatives, 419–424
hexachlorophene neurotoxicity, 381–410
myeloopticoneuropathy from iodochlorhydroxyquin, 327–368
neuronal storage dystrophy in chloroquine intoxication, 371–379
nitrofurantoin neuropathy, 413–416

Apomorphine, behavioral effects of, 18

Astrocytes, psychotropic drugs affecting, in vitro, 163–170

Astrocytic lamellar processes, hypothalamic, in heroin-addicted monkeys, 114, 127

Ataxia, from lithium, 174

ATPase inhibition in cell membranes
from hexachlorophene, 384
in lead poisoning, 291–292

Atrophy of brain
from antidepressive and neuroleptic drugs, 149–155
in Minamata disease, 235–236
Autonomic nervous system, tranquilizers affecting, 1–2
Autopsy, and certifications of deaths from drug addiction, 103–110
Autoradiography, whole body
in Minamata disease, 247–259
in subacute myelooptico neuropathy, 327–343, 348–349
Axonal dying-back disease, from industrial agents, 427–430

Barbiturates, detection in urine, 93–101
Behavioral effects
of hallucinogens, 221
of 6-hydroxydopamine, 17–18
of tranquilizers, 6
BHA, hepatic effects of, 513
BHT, hepatic effects of, 513
Bithionol, germicidal effects of, 386
Blindness, in Minamata disease, 236
Blood-brain barrier, 577–582
chemotoxic damage to, 271–274
normal aspects of, 577–579
pathologic disturbances of, 579–582
Blood levels of drugs
chlorpromazine, 9–10
hexachlorophene, 382
lithium, 175, 187
mescaline, 219
Bone, lithium distribution in, 176
Brain
atrophy of
from antidepressive and neuroleptic drugs, 149–155
in Minamata disease, 235–236
blood-brain barrier, 577–582
characteristics of cerebral endothelium, 577–579
chlorpromazine affecting cerebral cortex, 616, 619
lithium distribution in, 175–176
mescaline distribution in, 219–220
Bufotenine, biochemical aspects of, 217
Bungner bands, in alcoholic peripheral neuropathy, 543

Caffeine, teratogenic dose level of, 585–593
Calcarine cortex
in methylmercury intoxication, 263
in Minamata disease, 236

Capillaries in brain, in paraquat poisoning, 480–481, 482
Catecholamines
extraneural effects of, 639
6-hydroxydopamine affecting, 15–17
interaction with morphine, 19–20, 63–64
interaction with psychotropic drugs, 19–21
Caudate nucleus, pathology from long-term neuroleptic therapy, 31–36
Central nervous system
and blood-brain barrier, 577–582
chlorphentermine affecting, 497–500
fetal, drugs affecting, 585–593
in lithium toxicity, 173–175, 185–201
in methylmercury intoxication, 263–268
multidisciplinary studies of chemogenic lesions in, 613–641
Cerebellum
grumose degeneration of dentate nucleus, 43–54, 259
in mercury poisoning, 283
methylazoxymethanol affecting, 603–612
in methylmercury intoxication, 264
in Minamata disease, 240, 255
Cerebrospinal fluid
lithium in, after therapy, 176
mescaline levels in, 219
vitamin B levels in alcoholic peripheral neuropathy, 531–535
Cerebrovascular lesions
phlebitis from long-term neuroleptic therapy, 36–38
sclerosis in Minamata disease, 251–253
Cerebrum, see Brain
Certification, of deaths from drug addiction, 103–110
Chemogenic lesions, multidisciplinary studies of, 613–641
Chinoform intoxication, see Myelooptico-neuropathy
Chlordecone poisoning, 443–455
Chlordiazepoxide, interaction with alcohol, 503
p-Chlorophenylalanine, and responses to opiates, 64
Chloroquine, neuronal storage dystrophy from, 371–379
Chlorothiazide, and renal clearance of lithium, 178
Chlorphentermine neuropathy, 485–500
Chlorpromazine, 1–6
detection in urine, 93–101
hepatic effects of, 549–562
lithium with, toxic effects of, 174
long-term use of, cortical atrophy from, 149–155

Chlorpromazine (*contd.*)
  and LSD behavioral activity, 216
  and mescaline-induced behavior, 219
  multidisciplinary studies of, 615–623
  pharmacokinetics of, 9–12
  in psychotic reactions from psychotomimetic drugs, 206
Chorea, Huntington's, from long-term neuroleptic therapy, 36
Choroid plexus lesions, from tertiary amines, 419–424
Chromatin, nuclear, actinomycin affecting, 391–401
Chromatography, and drug detection in biological specimens, 83–86
Chromatolysis, in paraquat poisoning, 471, 473, 482
Chromomycin A$_3$, inhibiting RNA synthesis, 399–401
Chromosomes
  heroin affecting, in monkeys, 595–601
  psychotomimetic drugs affecting, 208–209
Cinerubin, inhibiting RNA synthesis, 399–401
Clioquinol
  intoxication from, *see* Myeloopticoneuropathy
  organ distribution and metabolism of, 348–349
Clozapine, 6
Cocaine, teratogenic dose level of, 585–593
Confusional state, from tranquilizers, 1, 6
Convulsions, *see* Seizures
Copper in brain tissue, lead poisoning affecting, 290–292
Cyclophosphamide, choroid plexus lesions from, 422
Cysts, hydrocephalic, in lead-treated chicks, 303–306
Cytoplasmic inclusions, chlorphentermine-induced, 486–489, 500

Daunomycin, inhibiting RNA synthesis, 399–401
Death
  from drug addiction, certification of, 103–110
  neuroleptic-related, 1–2
Degeneration
  axonal, in industrial neuropathies, 427–430
  choroid plexus, from tertiary amines, 419–424
Delirium tremens, 517–519
Dementias
  and aluminum neurotoxicity, 313–314
  from lead exposure, 293
Dense bodies, in neurons after drug therapy, 163–170
Dentate nucleus, grumose degeneration of, 43–54, 259

electron microscopic findings in, 50–53
  in ethylmercury intoxication, 49–50
  in parkinsonian disorders, 44–45
  in phenothiazine intoxication, 49
  in Ramsay-Hunt syndrome, 45–49
Depression
  antidepressants in, *see* Antidepressants
  and suicide after psychotomimetic drugs, 207
Detection of drugs in biological specimens
  analytical procedures in, 81
  chromatography in, 83–86
    gas, 85–86
    thin-layer, 84–85, 101
  enzyme multiplied immunoassay in, 86–87
  erroneous results in, 88
  extraction techniques in, 81–83
  hemagglutination inhibition technique in, 87, 94, 97–98
  and preliminary treatment of urines with ion exchange papers, 94
  radioimmunoassay in, 87–88, 94–95, 98–101
Detoxification, in methadone maintenance program, 76
Diabetes insipidus, from lithium, 177–178
Diet. *See also* Nutrition.
  and food interactions with drugs, 511–514
Dimethyltryptamine, teratogenic dose level of, 585–593
Diphenylhydantoin
  cerebellar lesions from, 416
  interaction with methylphenidate, 147
DNA
  lithium affecting, 180–181
  neuronal, chronic drug therapy affecting, 155
  psychotomimetic drugs affecting, 208–209
L-Dopa, food interactions with, 512
Dopamine
  brain levels after 6-hydroxydopamine, 15
  striatal turnover of, 65
Dopaminergic activity
  and effects of LSD, 215–217
  and effects of mescaline, 222
Drug abuse
  alcohol, *see* Alcohol
  and detection in biological specimens, 81–101
  and methadone maintenance program, 71–79
  narcotics, *see* Narcotics
  polydrug and alcohol abuse, 75–76
Drug interactions, 629
  with alcohol, 503–508, 629
  with food, 511–514
  methylphenidate, 147–148
  psychotomimetic drugs, 210
  selenium and mercury, 275–281

Dyskinesia, tardive, from tranquilizers, 4–6, 12
  alternative diagnoses to, 57–61
Dystonic reactions, acute, from tranquilizers, 2,
  12

Edema, cerebral
  from hexachlorophene, 384
  in ischemia, 581–582
  in paraquat poisoning, 471
  in triethyltin encephalopathy, 317
Electrocardiogram, in lithium toxicity, 173
Electroencephalogram
  hallucinogens affecting, 221
  lithium toxicity affecting, 173
  in mercurial blood-brain damage, 273
Elzholz bodies, in kepone poisoning, 454
Encephalopathy
  aluminum, 314
  lead, 293
    in chick embryo, 303–311
    rodent models of, 299–302
  from long-term neuroleptic therapy, 27–31
  triethyltin, 317–324
Endoplasmic reticulum
  in CNS cells
    chlorpromazine affecting, 623
    in cortical neurons, affected by low levels of
      halothane, 140
    hypothalamic, in heroin-addicted monkeys,
      114, 126
    lithium affecting, 187
    narcotics affecting, 625
  hepatic
    narcotics affecting, 564
    phenothiazines affecting, 559
Endorphins, 66–67
Endothelial cells, cerebral, tight junctions of,
    577–578
  disruption of, 580
Enkephalins, 66
EnteroVioform toxicity, *see* Myeloop-
    ticoneuropathy
Enzymes
  activity in cerebral endothelium, 579
  in multiplied immunoassay for detection of
    drugs in biological specimens, 86–87
  reaction products of
    chlorpromazine affecting, 623
    narcotics affecting, 625
Epilepsy, *see* Seizures
Ethanol, *see* Alcohol
Ethidium bromide, inhibiting RNA synthesis, 399
Ethyl biscoumacetate, interaction with methyl-
    phenidate, 147

Ethylmercury intoxication, and grumose degen-
    eration of dentate nucleus, 49–50
Exacerbation of psychosis, after therapy, 632
Extrapyramidal disorders, from tranquilizers,
    2–6

Fetal CNS, drugs affecting, 585–593
Flashback phenomenon, from psychotomimetic
    drugs, 207
Folate levels, in alcoholic peripheral neuropathy,
    532
Food and drug interactions, 511–514. *See also*
    Nutrition.

Galactosemia, brain function in, 580
Ganglion cells
  in mercury poisoning, 283, 287
  in paraquat poisoning, 473
  storage dystrophy in chloroquine intoxication,
    375
Geniculate nucleus, in methylmercury intoxica-
    tion, 261, 262, 268
Glia, psychotropic drugs affecting, *in vitro*, 163–
    170
Glucose uptake in brain
  disorders in, 580
  lithium affecting, 180
Golgi complex
  in CNS cells, lithium affecting, 187
  hepatic
    chlorpromazine affecting, 559
    narcotics affecting, 564
  hypothalamic, in heroin-addicted monkeys,
    114, 126
Granule cells, cerebellar
  in mercury poisoning, 283
  in Minamata disease, 240
Green tongue, in subacute myeloop-
    ticoneuropathy, 328, 341, 356
Grumose degeneration, cerebellar, 43–54, 259
Guam parkinsonism-dimentia complex, and
    grumose degeneration of dentate nucleus,
    45

Hallucinogens
  biochemical aspects of, 215–223
  chromosomal effects of, 208–209
  clinical aspects of, 205–211
  flashback phenomenon from, 207
  and homicidal behavior, 207–208
  indolealkylamines, 217
  LSD, 205–211, 215–217, 227–234

Hallucinogens (*contd.*)
  mescaline, 205, 217–222
  organic brain damage from, 208
  psychotic reactions from, 206–207
  and suicidal behavior, 207
Haloperidol
  lithium with, toxic effects of, 174
  and mescaline activity, 219
Halothane, chronic exposure to low levels of, 137–144
Harmala alkaloids, biochemical aspects of, 217
Harmine, teratogenic dose level of, 585–593
Heart, in lithium toxicity, 173
Hemagglutination inhibition technique, for detection of drugs in biological specimens, 87, 94, 97–98
Heroin, *see* Narcotics
Hexacarbon solvents, neuropathies from, 427–430
Hexachlorophene
  absorption and metabolism of, 382
  chemical properties of, 381
  compared to bithionol, 386
  neurotoxicity of, 382–387
    in developing nervous system tadpoles, 403–410
    experimental studies, 382–386
    in humans, 386–387
  teratogenic dose level of, 585–593
Histamine levels, opiates affecting, 65
Homicide, and psychotomimetic drug use, 207–208
Huntington's chorea, from long-term neuroleptic therapy, 36
Hydantoin compounds, neuropathy from, 416
Hydrocephalic cysts, in lead-treated chicks, 303–306
Hydromorphone, teratogenic dose level of, 585–593
Hydropic degeneration, in choroid plexus, from tertiary amines, 419–424
6-Hydroxydopamine, 15–21
  behavioral effects of, 17–18
  effects on catecholamines, 15–17
    modulation of, 16–17
    specificity of, 15–16
  in study of psychotropic drug interactions with catecholamines, 19–21
5-Hydroxytryptamine, *see* Serotonin
Hypertension, blood-brain barrier in, 580–581
Hypothalamus
  chlorpromazine affecting, 616
  in heroin-addicted monkeys, 111–130
    amyloid bodies in, 118, 128
    astrocytic lamellar processes in, 114, 127

    endoplasmic reticulum and lamellar bodies in, 114, 126
    lipofuscin and pigment bodies in, 114, 126
    membranous bodies in, 114, 127
    mitochondria in, 114, 127–128
    neurodystrophic processes in, 114–118, 128
    nucleonucleolar system in, 112, 119–125
    synapses in, 118–119, 128–129
  lithium distribution in, 175–176

Imipramine
  interaction with methylphenidate, 147
  long-term use of, cortical atrophy from, 149–155
  and norepinephrine reuptake in adrenergic tissue, 199
  pharmacokinetics of, 157–160
Immunoassay, in detection of drugs in biological specimens, 86–88, 93–101
Inclusions
  cytoplasmic, chlorphentermine-induced, 486–489, 500
  neuronal, after drug therapy, 163–170
Indolealkylamines, biochemical aspects of, 217
Industrial neuropathies
  from acrylamide and hexacarbon solvents, 427–430
  from kepone, 443–455
  from tri-ortho-cresyl phosphate, 431–440
Inositol metabolism, cerebral, lithium affecting, 180
Interactions of drugs, *see* Drug interactions
Interference microscopy, differential, of tadpole nervous system, 403–410
Iodochlorhydroxyquin toxicity, *see* Myeloopticoneuropathy
Ion exchange papers, treatment of urine specimens with, 93–101
Iron in brain tissue, lead poisoning affecting, 290, 292
Ischemia, and cerebral edema, 581–582
Isoproterenol, teratogenic dose level of, 585–593

Kepone poisoning, 443–455
Kidney
  affected by low levels of halothane, 139, 141
  in lithium toxicity, 172
  in paraquat poisoning, 472, 473
Kuru, from lead exposure, 293

Laminated bodies, concentric, in neurons after drug therapy, 163–170

Lead toxicity, 289–297
  dementias in, 293
  encephalopathy in, 293
    in chick embryo, 303–311
    rodent models of, 299–302
  hydrocephalic cysts in, 303–306
  and lead uptake by blood and brain, 310
  and trace metals in brain tissues, 290–292
Lipidosis, drug-induced, 165, 169–170
Lipofuscin in neurons
  in hypothalamus, in heroin-addicted monkeys, 114, 126
  after lithium, 187
  in paraquat poisoning, 471, 473
  significance of, 481–482
Lithium
  and adenyl cyclase inhibition, 178–179
  diabetes insipidus from, 177–178
  distribution in body, 175–176
    in bone, 176
    in brain, 175–176
  excretion of, 176–177
  in extraneural structures, 632
  and intermediary metabolism, 179–180
  medical uses of, 171
  toxicity of, 171–181
    clinical features of, 172–174
    in nonpsychiatric patients, 171–172
    permanent damage in, 174–175
    in psychiatric patients, 172
    and ultrastructural changes in CNS, 185–201
Liver affected by low levels of halothane, 142
  microsomal enzyme induction from drugs, 513
  multidisciplinary studies of chemogenic lesions in, 613–641
  narcotics affecting, 562–572
  in paraquat poisoning, 472, 473
  phenothiazines affecting, 549–562
LSD
  biochemical aspects of, 215–217
  clinical aspects of, 205–211
  effects of neurons
    in culture, 227–234
    in vitro, 163, 165
  interaction with alcohol, 506
Lysosomes
  in CNS cells
    lithium affecting, 187
    LSD affecting, 228–229
  hepatic
    chlorpromazine affecting, 555, 559
    narcotics affecting, 564

Macroglossia, from tranquilizers, 2
Magnesium levels, in alcohol withdrawal, 519–521
Malnutrition
  and alcoholic peripheral neuropathy, 529–545
  and drug metabolism, 514
Mania, and lithium toxicity, 171–200
Maple syrup disease, brain function in, 580
Marihuana, interaction with alcohol, 505
Melanocyte-stimulating hormone, and action of morphine, 66
Membrane of cells
  ATPase inhibition in
    from hexachlorophene, 384–385
    in lead poisoning, 291–292
  LSD affecting, 233–234
  mescaline affecting, 220
  permeability of, 578
Mental status, lithium affecting, 175
Mercury poisoning
  and blood-brain barrier damage, 271–274
  and mercury content of brain, 245–246, 249, 253–255, 285–286
  and metabolic mechanisms in neurotoxicity, 283–287
  and Minamata disease, 235–246, 247–259, 261
  neuropathology in Niigata, 261–269
  selenium interaction in, 275–281
Mescaline
  biochemical aspects of, 217–222
  clinical aspects of, 205–211
Mesoridazine, affecting neurons and glia *in vitro*, 163–170
Metals
  aluminum neurotoxicity, 313–314
  lead toxicity, 289–311
  mercury toxicity, *see* Mercury poisoning
  triethyltin encephalopathy, 317–324
Methadone
  detection in urine, 93–101
  hepatic effects of, 562–572
  maintenance program for heroin addicts, 71–79
    and antisocial behavior, 74–75
    and detoxification process, 76
    and mortality changes, 76–79
    and problems of polydrug abuse, 75–76
    and retention rates, 72
    and social productivity, 73–74
  multidisciplinary studies of, 623–625
  teratogenic dose level of, 585–593
Methylazoxymethanol, affecting cerebellar morphology, 603–612
  in ferret, 603–608
  in rat, 609–612

Methylmercury intoxication
  in Minamata disease, 235–246, 247–259
  and neuropathology in Niigata, 261–269
Methylphenidate, interactions with other drugs,
    147–148
Microsomal enzymes, induction by drugs, 513
Minamata disease, 235–246, 261
  autoradiography in, 247–259
  brain atrophy in, 235–236
  cerebellar cortex in, 240, 255
  cerebrovascular sclerosis in, 251–253
  cutaneous sensory receptors in, 259
  hemodynamic circulatory disturbance in,
    249–251
  and mercury distribution in brain, 245–246,
    249, 253–255
  neurohistopathology of, 236–241
  peripheral nerves in, 255–259
  selenium levels in, 275
  sural nerve biopsy findings in, 241–245
Mithramycin, inhibiting RNA synthesis, 399–401
Mitochondria
  in CNS cells
    lithium affecting, 287
    LSD affecting, 229–233
  hepatic
    chlorpromazine affecting, 555, 559
    narcotics affecting, 564
  hypothalamic, in heroin-addicted monkeys,
    114, 127–128
  as target or receptor sites, 633–634
Monoamine oxidase inhibitors, and norepine-
    phrine reuptake in adrenergic tissue, 199
Morphine. *See also* Narcotics.
  interaction with brain catecholamines, 19–20,
    63–64
  teratogenic dose level of, 585–593
Mortality, in methadone maintenance program,
    76–79
Multidisciplinary studies, of chemogenic lesions,
    613–641
Multiple drug intake, effects of, 629
  and alcohol abuse, 75–76
Myelin bodies
  in alcoholic peripheral neuropathy, 543
  from chlorphentermine, 490
  in kepone poisoning, 451, 455
Myelination, in Minamata disease, 241–245, 267
Myelinic vacuoles, in triethyltin encephalopathy,
    318
Myelinopathy from hexachlorphene
  in premature infants, 386–387
  in tadpoles, 409
Myeloopticoneuropathy, subacute, 327–343

  Ammon's horn in, 337–341
  clinical features of, 327–328
  differential diagnosis of, 341–342
  dorsal root ganglia in, 329
  epidemiology of, 328–329
  experimental, 345–350, 356–359
  green tongue in, 328, 341, 356
  in humans, 327–343, 353–356
  and *in vitro,* studies of nervous tissue, 361–368
  modifying factors in, 342
  olivary nucleus in, 335
  optic nerve and retina in, 335
  peripheral nerves in, 331–333
  Purkinje cells in, 337
  spinal cord in, 333–335, 346–347, 353
  spinal nerve rootlets in, 329

Naloxone, interaction with alcohol, 503–504
Narcotics, 63–130
  and acetylcholine release, 64
  γ-aminobutyric acid affecting responses to,
    64–65
  and certifications of deaths from drug addic-
    tion, 103–110
  and detection of drugs in biological specimens,
    81–101
  hepatic effects of, 562–572
  heroin affecting monkey chromosomes, 595–
    601
  and histamine release, 65
  hypothalamus in heroin-addicted monkeys,
    111–130
  and methadone maintenance program, 71–79
  morphine interaction with brain
    catecholamines, 19–20, 63–64
  multidisciplinary studies of heroin and
    methadone, 623–625
    in animals, 625
    in humans, 623–625
  and neurotransmitter activity, 63–65
  and peptide hormone activity, 65–66
  and prostaglandin activity, 65
  receptors for, 66
    binding sites in, 63
  and serotonin turnover, 64
Neurodystrophic processes, hypothalamic, in
    heroin-addicted monkeys, 114–118, 128
Neurofibrillary changes
  in aluminum neurotoxicity, 313–314
  in lead poisoning, 293
Neuroleptics, *see* Tranquilizers
Neuronal storage dystrophy, in chloroquine in-
    toxication, 371–379

Neurotransmitters
    extraneural effects of, 639
    and responses to opiates, 63–65
Nicotine, teratogenic dose level of, 585–593
Nicotinic acid levels, in alcoholic peripheral
        neuropathy, 532
Nissl substance, chlorpromazine affecting, 616
Nitrofurantoin neuropathy, sciatic nerves in,
        413–416
4-Nitroquinolin-N-oxide, inhibiting RNA syn-
        thesis, 399
Nogalomycin, inhibiting RNA synthesis, 399–
        401
Norepinephrine
    brain levels after 6-hydroxydopamine, 15
    uptake at receptor sites, drugs affecting, 199
Nortriptyline, affecting neurons and glia *in vitro*,
        163–170
Nuclear chromatin, actinomycin affecting, 391–
        401
Nutrition
    and alcoholic peripheral neuropathy, 529–545
    and drug metabolism, 514

Occipital cysts, in lead-treated chicks, 303–306
Olivary nucleus, in subacute myeloop-
        ticoneuropathy, 335
Olivomycin, inhibiting RNA synthesis, 399–401
Opiates, *see* Narcotics
Optic nerve
    in methylmercury poisoning, 268
    in subacute myelopticoneuropathy, 335, 353
    tadpole, hexachlorophene affecting, 404
Oral movements, tranquilizers affecting, 2, 5
Organic brain damage, from psychotomimetic
        drugs, 208

Pancreas, in paraquat poisoning, 472, 473
Pantothenic acid levels, in alcoholic peripheral
        neuropathy, 532
Paraquat poisoning, cerebral changes in, 469–483
Parathion
    and AChE in nervous system, 457–467
    metabolized to paraoxon, 466, 513
Parkinsonian disorders, and grumose degenera-
        tion of dentate nucleus, 44–45
Peptides, and responses to opiates, 65–66
Peripheral nerves
    in alcoholism with malnutrition, 529–545
    in chloroquine intoxication, 375
    chlorphentermine affecting, 489–495, 500
    hexachlorophene affecting, 385
    in kepone poisoning, 443–455
    in Minamata disease, 255–259
    in subacute myelopticoneuropathy, 331–333

Permeability, of cell membranes, 578
Pesticides
    cerebral changes in paraquat poisoning, 469–
        483
    parathion affecting nervous system, 457–467
Phenothiazines, 1–6
    chlorpromazine, *see* Chlorpromazine
    hepatic effects of, 549–562
    interaction with mescaline, 219
    intoxication with grumose degeneration of den-
        tate nucleus, 49
    lithium with, toxic effects of, 174
    long-term therapy with, 25–38
    multidisciplinary studies of, 615–623
        in animals, 619–623
        in humans, 615–618
    pharmacokinetics of, 9–12
    and ultrastructure of neurons and glia, 163–170
Phenylethylamines, biochemical aspects of,
        217–222
Phenylketonuria, brain function in, 580
Phlebitis, cerebral, from long-term neuroleptic
        therapy, 36–38
Photic responses, in alcohol withdrawal, 518–519
Pica, in iron deficiency, 292–293
Pigment bodies, hypothalamic, in heroin-
        addicted monkeys, 114, 126
Pinocytotic vesicles, in cerebral endothelium,
        579
    disorders of, 580
Piperazine derivatives, choroid plexus lesions
        from, 419–424
Platelets, serotonin uptake in, after lithium, 199
Pleometabolosomes
    in CNS cells, lithium affecting, 187
    hepatic
        chlorpromazine affecting, 555, 559
        narcotics affecting, 564
    hypothalamic, in heroin-addicted monkeys,
        114, 127
Plumbism, *see* Lead toxicity
Pneumoencephalography, after long-term an-
        tidepressant and neuroleptic drugs, 149–
        155
Pregnancy, and effects of low levels of halothane
        in rats, 142–143
Premature infants, myelinopathy from
        hexachlorophene, 386–387
Propoxyphene, teratogenic dose level of, 585–
        593
Prostaglandins, action affected by opiates, 65
Pseudoparkinsonism, from tranquilizers, 3–4
    dosage affecting, 4
Psilocin, biochemical aspects of, 217
Psilocybin, biochemical aspects of, 217

Psychotic reactions, from psychotomimetic drugs, 106–107
Psychotomimetic drugs, *see* Hallucinogens
Psychotropic agents, *see* Tranquilizers
Purkinje cells
   in methylmercury intoxication, 264
   in Minamata disease, 240
   in paraquat poisoning, 471, 473
   in subacute myeloopticoneuropathy, 337
Pyridoxine levels, in alcoholic peripheral neuropathy, 532

Quinoform compounds, myeloopticoneuropathy from, 327–343, 345, 353

Radioimmunoassay, in detection of drugs in biological specimens, 87–88, 94–95, 98–101
Ramsay-Hunt syndrome, and grumose degeneration of dentate nucleus, 45–49
Receptor sites
   chemical agents affecting, 631–640
   for opiates, 66
Reich bodies, in kepone poisoning, 454
Reserpine, interaction with brain catecholamines, 20
Retina
   in methylmercury intoxication, 268
   in subacute myeloopticoneuropathy, 335, 353
Riboflavin levels, in alcoholic peripheral neuropathy, 532
Ribosomes, cortical, mescaline affecting, 220–221
Ritalin, interaction with other drugs, 147–148
RNA
   neuronal, chronic drug therapy affecting, 154–155
   synthesis affected by actinomycin, 391–401
Rotational behavior, from 6-hydroxydopamine, 18

Salicylate, teratogenic dose level of, 585–593
Schizophrenia exacerbation, after therapy, 632
Schwann cells
   in alcoholic peripheral neuropathy, 541, 543
   chlorphentermine affecting, 490–495, 500
   in kepone poisoning, 447, 454
Sciatic nerves, in nitrofurantoin neuropathy, 413–416
Sedative effects, of tranquilizers, 1–2
Seizures
   in alcohol withdrawal, 518–519
   aluminum-induced, 314

blood-brain barrier in, 581
neuroleptic-related, 2, 632
Selenium, interaction with mercury, 275–281
Serotonin
   brain levels
      after 6-hydroxydopamine, 15
      after lithium, 199
      after LSD, 216, 217
   and responses to opiates, 64
SKF-525A, and mescaline activity, 220
Spinal cord, in subacute myeloopticoneuropathy, 333–335, 346–347, 353
Storage dystrophy, neuronal, in chloroquine intoxication, 371–379
Suicide, after psychotomimetic drugs, 207
Sural nerve biopsy
   in alcoholic peripheral neuropathy, 539–545
   in kepone poisoning, 444–455
   in methylmercury intoxication, 267
   in Minamata disease, 241–245
Synapses
   functions and physiology of, 639
   hypothalamic, in heroin-addicted monkeys, 118–119, 128–129
Synaptic vesicles
   chlorpromazine affecting, 623
   lithium affecting, 188, 193–197

Tadpole nervous system, lesions from hexachlorophene, 403–410
Temperature, tranquilizers affecting, 1
Teratogenic activity of drugs, dosage affecting, 585–593
Thiamine levels, in alcoholic peripheral neuropathy, 532
Thiazide, and renal clearance of lithium, 178
Thiopental, interaction with methylphenidate, 147
Thyrotropin releasing hormone, behavioral effects of, 65–66
Tight junctions, of cerebral endothelium, 577–578
Tilorone, affecting lymphoid tissue, 424
Tongue movements, tranquilizers affecting, 2, 5
Tranquilizers, 1–61
   accumulation in CNS, 12
   acute intoxication from, 25–27
   akathisia from, 2–3
   dystonic reaction from, acute, 2, 12
   and grumose degeneration of dentate nucleus, 43–54
   6-hydroxydopamine, 15–21
   hydroxylations of, 11–12
   long-term therapy with, 5, 12, 25–38
      cerebral phlebitis from, 36–38

Tranquilizers (*contd.*)
  long-term therapy with (*contd.*)
    cortical atrophy from, 149–155
    encephalopathy from, 27–31
    experimental studies of, 27
    Huntington's chorea from, 36
    and pathologic changes in brains, 31–36
  neurological effects of, 2–6
  pharmacokinetics of, 9–12
  phenothiazines, *see* Phenothiazines
  plasma levels of, and therapeutic effects, 9–10
  pseudoparkinsonism from, 3–4
    dosage affecting, 4
  sedative and autonomic effects of, 1–2
  tardive dyskinesia from, 4–6, 12
    alternative diagnoses to, 57–61
Transaminase levels, in heroin addicts, 568
Triethyltin, affecting developing mouse brain, 317–324
Tri-ortho-cresyl phosphate
  biochemistry and metabolism of, 431–432
  neurotoxicity of, 432–440
Trypan blue, teratogenic dose level of, 585–593
Tyramine in foods, interaction with drugs, 513–514

Urine
  immunoassay for drug detection in, 93–101
  lithium excretion in, 176–177

Vacuolization
  of choroid plexus epithelium, from tertiary amines, 419–424

  intramyelinic, in triethyltin encephalopathy, 318
Vagus nerve rootlets, in subacute myeloopticoneuropathy, 333
Vasopressin
  and analgesic response to morphine, 66
  lithium affecting responses to, 179
  release in lithium toxicity, 175
Vesicles, synaptic
  chlorpromazine affecting, 623
  lithium affecting, 188, 193–197
Vesicular structures, membrane-bound, in paraquat poisoning, 475
Vesicular transport, in cerebral endothelium, 579
  disturbance of, 580
Visual acuity
  in methylmercury intoxication, 268
  in Minamata disease, 236
  in myeloopticoneuropathy, subacute, 328
Visual perception, hallucinogens affecting, 221
Vitamin A, teratogenic dose level of, 585–593
Vitamin B assays, in alcoholic peripheral neuropathy, 531–539
Vitamin C deficiency, and neuropathy from hydantoin compounds, 416

Weight gain, lithium-induced, 179–180
Withdrawal from alcohol, syndromes with, 504, 505, 508, 517–526

Zinc in brain tissue, lead poisoning affecting, 290